AO TRAUMA

Miquel Videla Cés, J Miquel Sales Pérez, Joan Girós Torres,
Roberto Rivero Sosa

Learning From Failures in Orthopedic Trauma

Key Points for Success

AO
TRAUMA

Miquel Videla Cés, J Miquel Sales Pérez, Joan Girós Torres, Roberto Rivero Sosa

Learning From Failures in Orthopedic Trauma

Key Points for Success

More than 1,100 high-quality x-rays, clinical photographs, and illustrations

Library of Congress Cataloging-in-Publication Data is available from the publisher.

Hazards

Great care has been taken to maintain the accuracy of the information contained in this publication. However, the publisher, and/or the distributor, and/or the editors, and/or the authors cannot be held responsible for errors or any consequences arising from the use of the information contained in this publication. Contributions published under the name of individual authors are statements and opinions solely of said authors and not of the publisher, and/or the distributor, and/or the AO Group.

The products, procedures, and therapies described in this work are hazardous and are therefore only to be applied by certified and trained medical professionals in environments specially designed for such procedures. No suggested test or procedure should be carried out unless, in the user's professional judgment, its risk is justified. Whoever applies products, procedures, and therapies shown or described in this work will do this at their own risk. Because of rapid advances in the medical sciences, AO recommends that independent verification of diagnosis, therapies, drugs, dosages, and operation methods should be made before any action is taken.

Although all advertising material which may be inserted into the work is expected to conform to ethical (medical) standards, inclusion in this publication does not constitute a guarantee or endorsement by the publisher regarding quality or value of such product or of the claims made of it by its manufacturer.

Legal restrictions

Distribution by Georg Thieme Verlag, Rüdigerstrasse 14, 70469 Stuttgart, Germany, and Thieme New York, 333 Seventh Avenue, New York, NY 10001, USA

ISBN: 978-3-13-243456-1
e-ISBN: 978-3-13-243457-8

1 2 3 4 5 6

Foreword

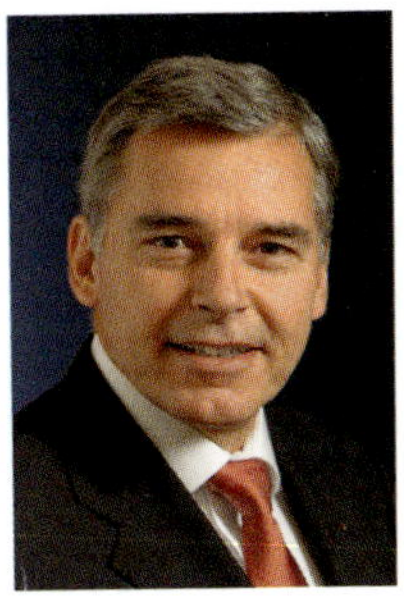

Nikolaus L Renner, Dr med
Head of the Department of Traumatology
Cantonal Hospital Aarau
Tellstrasse 25
5001 Aarau
Switzerland

The success of the AO is attributed, among other things, to the classical four pillars instrumentation (ie, development of new implants and instruments for their application as well as for fracture reduction), research, education, and documentation. Pure documentation, however, is useless if the results are not thoroughly analyzed and discussed and if the ensuing discussion does not lead to recommendations for actual changes in the treatment of future patients.

When the AO was founded by a group of 13 Swiss surgeons, they named their association *Arbeitsgemeinschaft für Osteosynthesefragen*, which was translated as *Association for the Study of Internal Fixation (ASIF)*, that has evolved into a tight-knit community fostering a special AO spirit which was noticed by outsiders right from the beginning. In a quite simplistic way this is also called today the "family spirit" of the AO Foundation, which is much too trivial, though. Surgeons are quite often "alpha individuals" and tend to be loners. To create an environment that allows to admit failures and to discuss them at eye level amongst peers was 60 years ago unthinkable and as disruptive as the revolutionary treatment that was propagated by the group. Yet, it was at least as important for the success of the AO as the classical four pillars. From this perspective, this book is closing a gap since it mirrors a tradition that has been living on in the AO from its beginning but has never before been put down in writing in such a comprehensive way.

Learning from failures appears to be natural and easy. In practice, though, when an operation does not lead to the desired outcome, the main reason for the failure is not always obvious. Quite often there are different factors contributing to the failure and it is thus the editors' merit to provide categories according to which failures can be classified. This is a very helpful starting point for the analysis. If the reader browses only through the table of contents, however, she or he will completely miss the pearls. The real benefit for the reader comes by carefully reading through every illustrative case in each chapter which was diligently selected and analyzed by the authors. Although the failure may be often quite obvious for the more experienced surgeon, he or she will still learn and gain valuable insights from the carefully documented solutions.

Failures can never be completely avoided. First and foremost they have an impact on our patients' lives but are always also a humbling experience for the surgeon. The editors and authors have to be complimented on addressing this sensitive topic and on breaking it up into easily digestible morsels. This book should thus help surgeons to analyze their own failures and prevent them and others from repeating the same mistakes.

Nikolaus L Renner

Preface

This book has been published thanks to the sponsorship of the AO Foundation whose interest in the topic was sparked by Rafael Orozco Delclós' *Errores en la Osteosíntesis*, the first Spanish book on the topic of surgical failures, published in 1993.

Miquel Videla Cés, J Miquel Sales Pérez, Joan Girós Torres, and Roberto Rivero Sosa, the editors of *Learning From Failures*, were Orozco Delclós' colleagues. They shared his interest in surgical failures, be it their own or those of other surgeons, and in learning how to prevent them. The editors have therefore collected cases, documented, and jealously guarded them for this edition.

While reviewing the failures published back in 1993, the editors found that some failures in incorrectly applying the principles of fracture fixation have persisted and are still made today, but the main difference is the evolution in implants to treat fractures. They therefore believe it is essential to insist on teaching the basic principles of fracture fixation and the fundamentals of the AO techniques.

The operative treatment of fractures, for instance, is a highly valuable but difficult therapeutic procedure and carries with it great responsibility.

Failure is human; we all make mistakes because human beings are imperfect or to quote Seneca, "errare humanum est".

Surgeons ought to strive to learn all possible outcomes for each intervention with the resources available to them; however, they have a right to fail on the one condition that they recognize any such failure, make an effort to understand the reasons behind the failure, and then correct it with the means available to them. No surgeon has the right to repeat that failure, though. By investigating the causes of certain unsatisfactory results, surgeons can learn more about the possibilities and limitations of a technique they use. If their documentation is in order, their radiological dossier complete, and their self-criticism objective, they will quickly discover how they can improve their results [1].

We can all make mistakes by misjudging criteria and technique. Patients understand that surgeons and doctors in general are no gods but just human beings. They expect the surgeon to show empathy, understanding, and, above all, honesty.

Failure is always educational as long as it is fully understood and corrected. It is important to recognize failures, whether due to omission, technique, diagnosis, reasoning, or simply ignorance. "If we shut the door to all errors, truth will be shut out," said Rabindranath Tagore.

This book is an update on the 1993 work in Spanish on the failures that can occur owing to a lack of respect for the evolution of the fundamental principles of the AO techniques and compounded by the appearance of new implants.

We apologize for those images that do not meet the highest quality standards, as they were taken at critical moments in the emergency department. We decided to include them, though, as they serve the purpose of teaching and because "a picture is worth a thousand words".

Miquel Videla Cés, MD
J Miquel Sales Pérez, MD, PhD
Joan Girós Torres, MD, PhD
Roberto Rivero Sosa, MD

1 **Müller ME.** Prólogo in: Orozco Delclós R. *Errores en la Osteosíntesis*, Barcelona: Masson; 1993.

Acknowledgments

Learning From Failures in Orthopedic Trauma is the result of many years of reflecting on and documenting how to best treat fractures and their complications. It owes its existence to the invaluable collaboration of the true "protagonists", namely the patients who suffered one or more failures and underwent rescue surgery until a satisfactory outcome was achieved.

When the idea for this project was conceived, it soon developed into a book project to pay homage to the work of R Orozco Delclós and his team from Barcelona in teaching about resolving mistakes and failures in internal fixation. From the very beginning, Jaime Quintero played a key role as a facilitator between the editors, the AOTrauma Education Commission, and AO Education Institute.

This special book would not have been possible without the effort, dedication, and support of an extensive list of contributors. We are very pleased to have been able to work together with such a dedicated group of authors from different backgrounds who are also AO experts.

While there have been many people involved in the project to thank, we would especially like to mention the following group and individuals:

- Members of the AOTrauma Education Commission for recognizing the value of this project as a valid teaching tool and for approving this publication.
- Urs Rüetschi who pushed us to go beyond the impact of just an image of a failure, encouraging us to analyze the failure more in depth and look for the resolution to each problem. This was a task that at first seemed impossible to us.
- The many colleagues from around the world who provided excellent cases and images.
- Nikolaus Renner for writing the foreword to this book.
- Katalin Fekete, Project Manager for this book, for the overall planning and management of this project as well as her guidance, support, and expertise.
- Carl Lau, Manager Publishing, for providing expert advice and support throughout the production process, and Robin Greene for enabling extensive resources to prepare this publication and make it into an invaluable publication.
- Irene Contreras for her fantastic linguistic and cultural support and liaising; Marcel Erismann and Roman Kellenberger for their excellent graphic work, Amber Parkinson and Jecca Reichmuth for their invaluable editorial advice, and the entire Publishing team for their help and professional support.
- Tom Wirth at nougat GmbH for the graphic design and aesthetic aspects of the book which aids the audience in reading and understanding the content.
- Our hospital colleagues (physicians and other staff) for their unconditional daily support, for their understanding and help in facilitating the reflective discussions and enforcing the teaching character of the cases presented in this book.
- And last but not least, our families for their loving support and unwavering faith and encouragement throughout this project. To produce and publish the book *Learning From Failures in Orthopedic Trauma*, we spent much time away from our families and without their understanding this book would not have been possible.

Miquel Videla Cés, MD
J Miquel Sales Pérez, MD PhD
Roberto Rivero Sosa, MD
Joan Girós Torres, MD PhD

Contributors

Editors

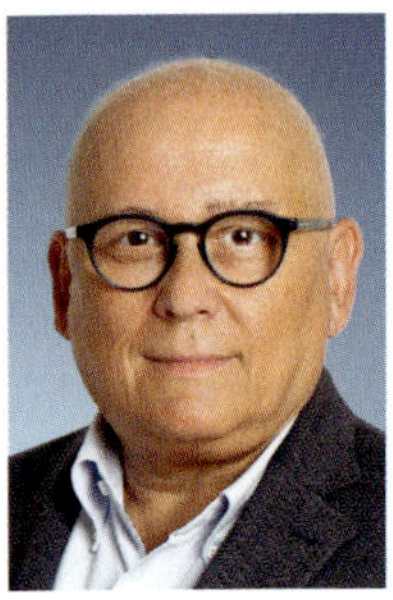

Miquel Videla Cés, MD
Clinical Professor, University of Barcelona
Head of Trauma Unit
Service of Orthopedic Surgery and Traumatology
Consorci Sanitari Integral
Hospital de Sant Joan Despí Moisès Broggi
C. Jacint Verdaguer 90
08970 Sant Joan Despí, Barcelona
Spain

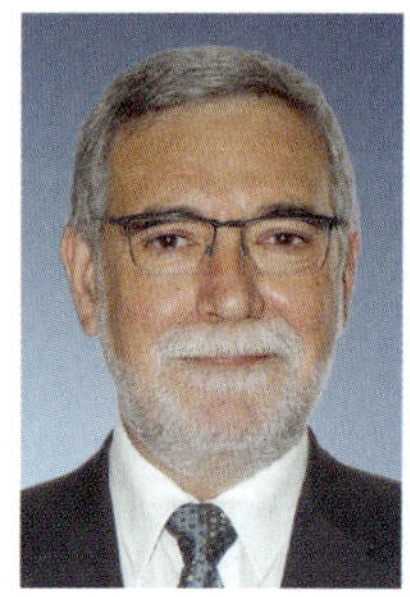

J Miquel Sales Pérez, MD, PhD
Clinical Professor, University of Barcelona
Head of the Orthopedic Surgery and
Traumatology Department
Service of Orthopedic Surgery and Traumatology
Consorci Sanitari Integral
Hospital de Sant Joan Despí Moisès Broggi
C. Jacint Verdaguer 90
08970 Sant Joan Despí, Barcelona
Spain

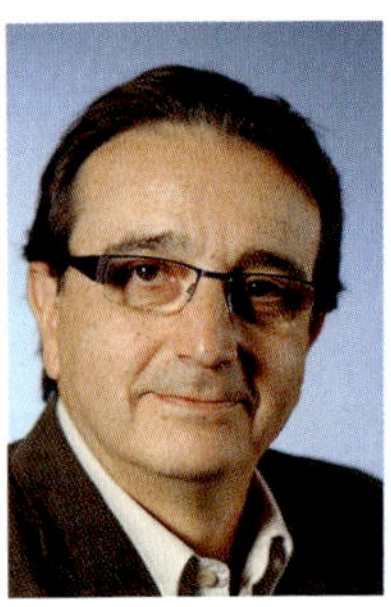

Joan Girós Torres, MD, PhD
Clinical Professor, University of Barcelona
Senior Consultant, Orthopedic Surgery and
Traumatology Department
Service of Orthopedic Surgery and Traumatology
Consorci Sanitari Integral
Hospital de Sant Joan Despí Moisès Broggi
C. Jacint Verdaguer 90
08970 Sant Joan Despí, Barcelona
Spain

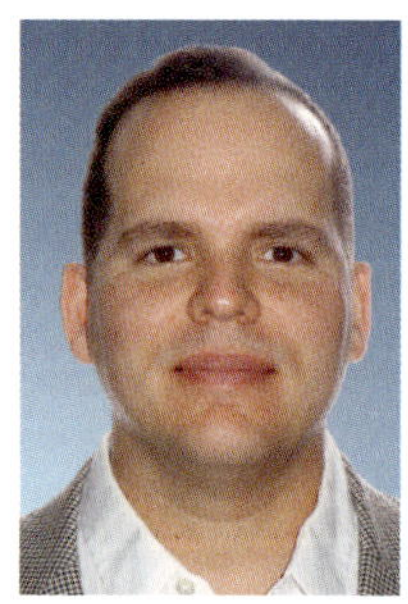

Roberto Rivero Sosa, MD
Consultant, Orthopedic Surgery and
Traumatology Department
Service of Orthopedic Surgery and Traumatology
Consorci Sanitari Integral
Hospital de Sant Joan Despí Moisès Broggi
C. Jacint Verdaguer 90
08970 Sant Joan Despí, Barcelona
Spain

Authors

Terry S Axelrod, MD, MSc, FRCSC
Professor, Division of Orthopaedics
Department of Surgery
Sunnybrook Health Sciences Centre
University of Toronto
Room MG 371
2075 Bayview Ave.
Toronto, ON M4N 3M5
Canada

Reto Babst, Prof Dr med
Vorsteher Department Chirurgie
Chefarzt Unfallchirurgie
Klinik Orthopädie und Unfallchirurgie
Luzerner Kantonsspital
6000 Lucerne 16
Switzerland

Suthorn Bavonratanavech, MD
Chief of Orthopedic and Trauma Network, BDMS.
Senior Director of Bangkok Orthopedic Center
Bangkok Medical Center
2 Soi Soonvijai 7
New Petchaburi Rd.
Bangkok, 10310
Thailand

Christopher A Becker, Dr med
Ludwig Maximilians University Munich
Department for General, Trauma- & Reconstructive
Surgery
Marchioninistrasse 15
81377 Munich
Germany

Frank J P Beeres, Dr med, PhD
Leitender Arzt, Klinik Orthopädie und Unfallchirurgie
Luzerner Kantonsspital Luzern
Spitalstrasse
6000 Luzern 16
Switzerland

Jordi Bertrán Padrós, MD, PhD
Trauma and Orthopaedic Surgeon
Unión de Mutuas
Josep Tarradellas 110
08029 Barcelona
Spain

Jarosław Brudnicki, MD, PhD
Senior Assistant
Department of General Surgery Orthopaedic and Politrauma
University Hospital of Jagiellonian University Cracow
Szpital Uniwersytecki
ul. Mikołaja Kopernika 36
31-501 Kraków
Poland

Arancha Capel Agundez, MD
Trauma Unit
Doce de Octubre
University Hospital
Av. Andalucía s/n
28045 Madrid
Spain

Matej Cimerman, MD
Professor, Director of Traumatology
University Clinical Centre Ljubljana
Zaloška 7
1000 Ljubljana
Slovenia

Peter A Cole, MD
Professor
University of Minnesota
Chairman of Orthopedic SurgeryRegions Hospital
Department of Orthopaedic Surgery
Regions Hospital
640 Jackson Street
Mail Stop 11503L
St. Paul, MN 55101
USA

Anthony J Dugarte, MD
389 E270th St
Euclid, OH 44132
USA

Christian Kammerlander, PD Dr med
Vice Director
Ludwig Maximilians University Munich
Department for General, Trauma- & Reconstructive Surgery
Marchioninistrasse 15
81377 Munich
Germany

Anze Kristan, MD, PhD
University Medical Centre Ljubljana
Zaloška cesta 7
1525 Ljubljana
Slovenia

Björn-Christian Link, Dr med
Leitender Arzt
Klinik für Orthopädie und Unfallchirurgie
Luzerner Kantonsspital Luzern
Spitalstrasse
6000 Lucerne 16
Switzerland

José Juan Mendoza Vera, MD
Servicio de Traumatologíade Fremap Barcelona
Carrer dels Madrazo 8-10
08006 Barcelona
Spain

Josep M Muñoz-Vives, MD
Consultant Orthopaedic Trauma Surgeon
Fundació Althaia
C/ Dr. Joan Soler, 1-3
08243 Manresa, Barcelona
Spain

Rodrigo Pesántez, MD
Professor
Avenida 9# 116-20
Bogotá
Colombia

Jaime Quintero, MD
Assistant Professor
Hospital Universitario Clinica San Rafael
Ortopedia y Traumatologia
Carrera 8 No.17-45 Sur
Bogotá
Colombia

Pol Maria Rommens, Dr med, Dr h.c.
Professor, Director Department of Orthopaedics and Traumatology
University Medical Center
Johannes Gutenberg-University
Langenbeckstrasse 1
55131 Mainz
Germany

Bianka Rubenbauer, Dr med
Ludwig Maximilians University Munich
Department for General, Trauma- & Reconstructive Surgery
Marchioninistrasse 15
81377 Munich
Germany

Eladio Saura-Sánchez, Dr med
Associate Professor Miguel Hernandez University
Chief of Traumatology Unit
University Hospital of Elche
Camino de la Almazara 11
03203 Elche
Spain

Francisco Saura-Sánchez, Dr med
Hip and Foot Unit
Hospital General Universitario Santa Lucia
30202 Santa Lucia, Cartagena
Spain

Mariano Saura-Sánchez, Dr Eng
Associate Professor, Mechanical Engineering
Polytechnic University of Cartagena
30202 Cartagena
Spain

Juan Carlos Serfaty Soler, MD
Head of the Department of Traumatology and Orthopedic Surgery
MC Mutual
Calle Copérnico 58
08006 Barcelona
Spain

Fabian Sommer, Dr med
Ludwig Maximilians University Munich
Department for General, Trauma- & Reconstructive Surgery
Marchioninistrasse 15
81377 Munich
Germany

Matevž Tomaževič, MD
Orthopaedic trauma consultant
University Medical Center Ljubljana
Department of Traumatology
Zaloška cesta 2
1000 Ljubljana
Slovenia

In Memoriam

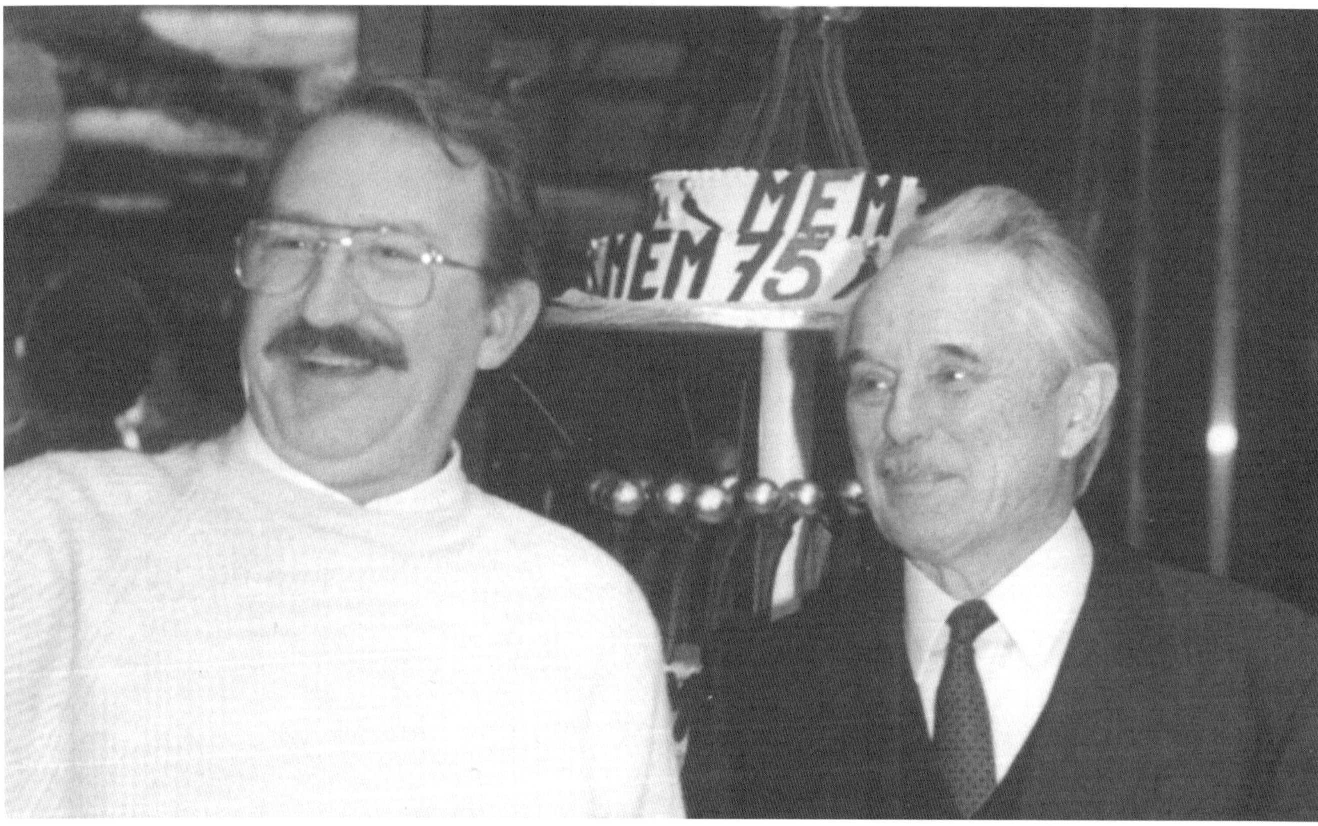

Rafael Orozco Delclós
1938 – 2005

Maurice E Müller
1918 – 2009

Abbreviations

3D	three-dimensional
ABCDE	airway, breathing, circulation, disability, exposure/examination
AP	anteroposterior
ARI	AO Research Institute
ATLS	advanced trauma life support
BMD	bone mineral density
BMI	body mass index
CT	computed tomography
DCP	dynamic compression plate
DCU	dynamic compression unit
DEXA	dual energy x-ray absorptiometry
DHS	dynamic hip screw
ETC	early total care
HLS	head of the locked screw
IM	intramedullary
IS	iliosacra
ISS	Injury Severity Score
K-wire	Kirschner wire
LAP	locking attachment plate
LC-DCP	limited-contact dynamic compression plate
LCP	locking compression plate
LFN	lateral femoral nail
LHS	locking head screw
LISS	less invasive stabilization system
LISS DF	less invasive stabilization system-distal femur
MIPO	minimally invasive plate osteosynthesis
NPWD	negative-pressure wound dressing
NPWT	negative-pressure wound therapy, also called vacuum-assisted wound closure (VAC)
PC-Fix	point contact fixator
PFN	proximal femoral nail
PFNA	proximal femoral nail antirotation
PHILOS	proximal humerus internal locked system
PMMA	polymethylmethacrylate
UTN	unreamed tibial nail
VAC	vacuum-assisted wound closure, see negative-pressure wound therapy (NPWT)
WHO	World Health Organization

Online AO Educational Content

Abundant online educational offerings from across AO are accessible through the QR codes printed on this page. Also included are the journal references linked to PubMed. Using a QR code scanner on a mobile device, readers will be taken to a microsite containing supplemental content curated by the book editors specifically for that chapter topic.

Links to supplemental AO educational content include:
- Webinars and webcasts
- Lectures
- Teaching videos
- AO/OTA Fracture and Dislocation Classification

As the array of online AO educational resources evolves and develops, the offerings in the microsite will be reviewed and updated by the book editors. This will ensure that readers are linked to the latest in AO education.

Table of Contents

Section 1

Introduction to internal fixation

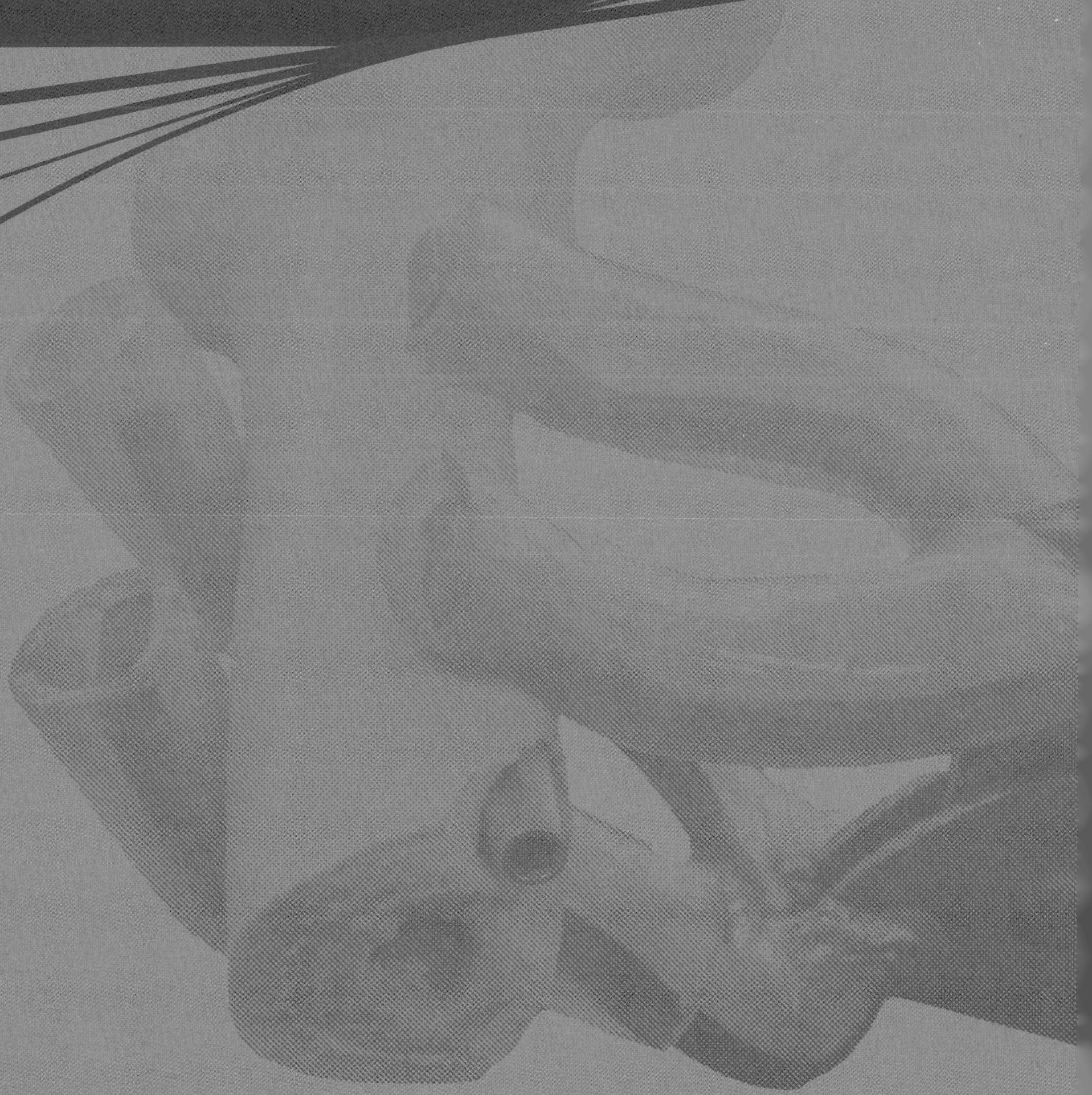

Section 1
Introduction to internal fixation

1.1 The evolution of internal fixation over the last 20 years

Joan Girós Torres
Roberto Rivero Sosa, J Miquel Sales Pérez, Miquel Videla Cés

Every day we know more and we understand less.
Albert Einstein

An elderly professor at medical school who taught the history of medicine used to say that the breakneck speed at which modern medicine was evolving meant that any surgical technique would become obsolete within 30 years. This does not appear to have happened with the techniques proposed by the founding fathers of the AO: Maurice E Müller, Robert Schneider, Hans Willenegger, Martin Allgöwer, Walter Bandi, et al (**Fig 1.1-1**). An exhaustive review of documented and clinically controlled cases has shown that current techniques following their foundational principles have evolved thanks to a better knowledge of the biological response of bone to the materials used for fracture fixation.

Even today, anatomy, stability, biology, and mobilization are still the four fundamental AO principles. They evolved in response to findings from different scientific investigations and clinical observations. The progressive changes in surgical approaches and methods have been based on clinical and laboratory research and resulted in new discoveries that have led to the development of new implants and instruments. The strategy for fracture fixation is dynamic and follows the principles, methods, and techniques of internal fixation.

The progressive evolution of the implants available today is the result of a long-standing collaboration between the AO Research Institute (ARI) and Synthes.

The less invasive stabilization system (LISS) was developed from the point contact fixator (PC-Fix) system while the locking compression plate (LCP) system and anatomically preshaped implants combine the old versions of limited-contact dynamic compression plate (LC-DCP), PC-Fix, and LISS. The "fusion" of the holes of the LC-DCP and LISS plates into a combination hole (combi-hole), developed by Wagner and Frigg [Frigg, 2001; Gautier et al, 2003], allows the use of locking head screws (LHS) (internal fixator) or alternatively, the conventional cortex screws (with dynamic compression).

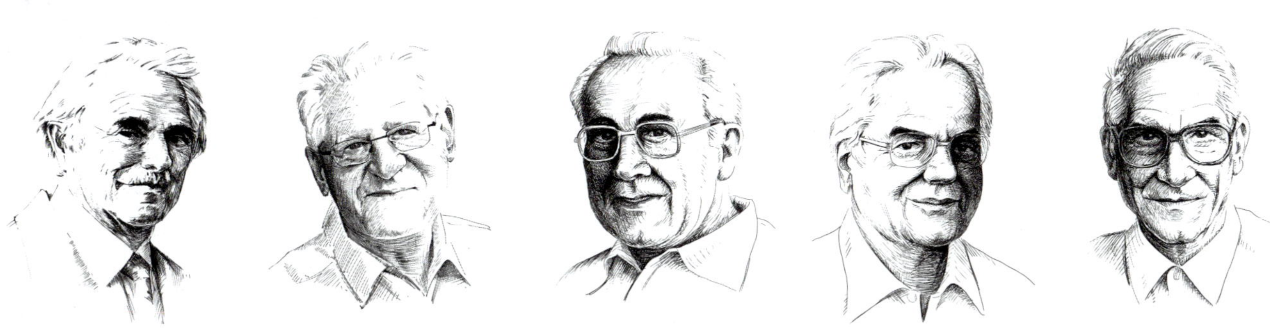

Fig 1.1-1 Founders of the AO (from left to right):
Maurice E Müller, Martin Allgöwer, Walter Bandi, Robert Schneider, Hans Willenegger.
Co-founders of the AO:
Ernst Baumann, Fritz Brussatis, August Guggenbühl, Willy Hunziker, Walter Ott, René Patry, Walter Schär, and Walter Stähli.

From the biomechanical point of view, the LCP is used as an internal fixator that provides angular stability and does not require perfect premolding of the LCP or pressure on the cortical bone. Biologically, since no close contact or pressure on the cortical bone exists, the periosteal circulation will be less compromised.

The LCP system can be used as:

- A conventional plate using only the dynamic compression unit (DCU) in the space for conventional screws.
- A purely internal fixator only using the space for blocked screws, ie, LHS without dynamic compression.
- A combination of the two previous principles in case of limited indications, which requires strict and meticulous planning. Correct indications are segmental fractures with:
  - A simple fracture pattern that would benefit from stabilization by interfragmentary compression techniques and absolute stability criteria.
  - A multifragmentary fracture pattern that should be treated by applying a splint to stabilize the fracture lines, using relative stability criteria and with the implant acting as an internal fixator

  Both situations are treated with the same implant but have a different function and stability criteria.

The basic AO principles (**Fig 1.1-2**) of fracture fixation established by the founders had the main goal of restoring form and function:

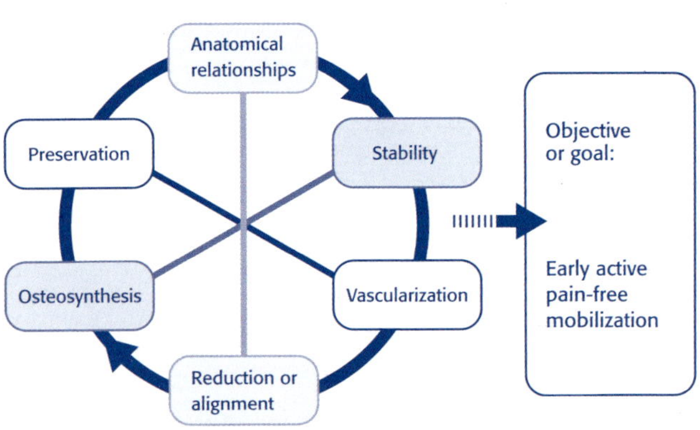

Fig 1.1-2 The AO principles contributing to successful fracture healing are of equal importance without any order of preference.

- **Reduction and fixation** of the fracture to restore its anatomical relationships, ie, restoration of the form.
- **Stabilization by fixation** as required by the characteristics of the fracture and the injury.
- **Preservation of bone and soft-tissue vascularization** through careful manipulation and gentle reduction techniques, ie, respect for the biology requiring a high level of care and technical ability as well as science.
- **Early and safe mobilization** of both the injured part and the patient, ie, restoration of function.

These principles still embody the AO philosophy. However, new implants now allow surgeons to reduce the surgical approaches and damage to surrounding tissues. The reduced surgical approaches and minimally invasive techniques emphasize the biological needs of the different bone segments, the preservation of the fracture hematoma, and the adjacent soft tissues, all important aspects for fracture healing. The new anatomical implants used as internal fixators or conventional implants make it necessary for us to reformulate or be more explicit in the evolution of the AO principles:

Reduction and fixation

Reduction and fixation of the fracture to restore anatomical relationships. Direct or indirect atraumatic reduction and fixation techniques are obligatory. The fracture of a bone results in the loss of its rigidity. This can be temporarily reestablished by osteosynthesis while union definitively restores it. Anatomical reduction is:

- Essential in intraarticular fractures to restore joint congruity, reconstruct the anatomy, expand the compression surface, and obtain a maximum friction coefficient, which are all factors favoring stability.
- Essential in metaphyseal or diaphyseal fractures of a simple transverse or oblique type, if interfragmentary compression techniques are used with absolute stability criteria.
- Not essential in multifragmentary fractures of long bones. Instead axial alignment should be obtained while respecting the length and degree of torsion between diaphysis and metaphysis, ie, functional reduction.

Stabilization by fixation

Fracture fixation providing absolute or relative stability depends on the personality of the fracture, the type of patient, and what the injury requires.

- Compression method principle of absolute stability:
  - Mandatory in joint fractures, achieved through interfragmentary compression.
  - May be indicated in simple transverse or oblique diaphyseal and metaphyseal fractures with little soft-tissue compromise, optimal bone quality, with the aim that the bone contributes to its own stability.
  - Biomechanically, the loading forces during activity pass mainly through the bone and to the least possible degree through the implant. Absolute stability is the absence of micromovement between the bone fragments which has a positive effect on vascularization because the blood vessels can cross the fracture site more easily and promote primary fracture healing.
- Internal fixator method or intramedullary nailing follow the principle of relative stability:
  - Most of diaphyseal fractures with a multifragmentary pattern must be treated with methods with elastic fixation that provide relative stability and secondary fracture healing.
  - Fixation with relative stability aims to maintain the reduction and still keep the mechanical stimulation for fracture repair by callus formation.
  - With relative stability, the bone fragments displace in relation to each other when physiological load is applied across the fracture. Displacement increases with the applied load and decreases with the rigidity of the fixation device.
  - Generally, a fixation method is considered flexible if it allows controlled interfragmentary movement under physiological load.
  - Locked intramedullary nailing is generally accepted as the standard treatment for diaphyseal long-bone fractures. The limitations of nailing are related to the fracture type, location, and pattern.
  - Another method that provides relative stability is the internal fixation with extramedullary bridging plates with a splint protection function.

Preservation of bone and soft-tissue vascularization

Preservation of blood supply to the bone and the surrounding soft tissues. This is achieved through careful manipulation and gentle direct or indirect reduction techniques, using appropriate surgical approaches. Whenever possible, indirect reduction will reduce the surgical trauma. Iatrogenic osteonecrosis, on the other hand, is the result of careless surgical access and rough handling of bone fragments.

With the development and increased use of minimally invasive surgical methods for the fixation of fractures, it is paramount that surgeons are equipped with anatomically preshaped implants and excellent anatomical knowledge.

Early and safe mobilization

Early, safe, and painless active mobilization of the injured part and of the patient is critical. Restoring function is key: "Life is movement and movement is life".

Evolution is an ongoing process. Methods, techniques, and new implants will undergo further development to help facilitate our work as surgeons. However, the general basic principles of the AO technique will remain.

Key points to remember

- "A good osteosynthesis is not the one performed with original implants but the one that follows the AO principles," said Hans Willenegger [Frigg, 2001].
- Anatomy, stability, biology, and mobilization are still the fundamental AO principles. They are all equally important and are not listed in order of preference.
- Surgeons must never forget that a fracture is a soft-tissue injury with a broken bone.
- "Improved surgical techniques may be more important than new implants and prosthesis," said R.K. Marti in his lecture [Gautier et al, 2003; Marti, 2008].

References and suggested reading

Bandi W, Müller ME, Allgöwer M, et al. *Technique of Internal Fixation of Fractures.* Berlin Heidelberg: Springer-Verlag; 1965.
Buckley R, Moran C, Apivatthakakul T. *AO Principles of Fracture Management.* 3rd ed. Stuttgart New York: Thieme; 2017.
Frigg R. Locking Compression Plate (LCP). An osteosynthesis plate based on the Dynamic Compression Plate and the Point Contact Fixator (PC-Fix). *Injury.* 2001 Sep;32 Suppl 2:63–66.
Frigg R. Development of the Locking Compression Plate. *Injury.* 2003 Nov;34 Suppl 2:B6–10.
Gautier E, Sommer C. Guidelines for the clinical application of the LCP. *Injury.* 2003 Nov;34 Suppl 2:B63–76.
Leunig M, Hertel R, Siebenrock KA, et al. The evolution of indirect reduction techniques for the treatment of fractures. *Clin Orthop Relat Res.* 2000 Jun(375):7–14.
Marti RK. Osteotomies for posttraumatic deformities. Lecture presented at: Meeting commemorating AO Spain's 37th anniversary and the AO's 50th; October 2008; Segovia, Spain.
Mast J, Jakob RP, Ganz R. *Planning and reduction technique in fracture surgery.* Berlin: Springer-Verlag; 1989.
Müller M, Allgöwer M, Schneider R, et al. *Manual of Internal Fixation.* 2nd ed. Berlin Heidelberg New York: Springer Verlag; 1979.
Müller ME, Allgöwer M, Schneider R, et al. Manual of Internal Fixation: techniques recommended by the AO-ASIF Group. 3rd ed. Berlin Heidelberg: Springer-Verlag; 1991.
Orozco Delclós R. *Errores en la Osteosíntesis.* Barcelona: Masson; 1993. Spanish.
Perren SM. Evolution of the internal fixation of long bone fractures. The scientific basis of biological internal fixation: choosing a new balance between stability and biology. *J Bone Joint Surg Br.* 2002 Nov;84(8):1093–1110.
Perren SM. Backgrounds of the technology of internal fixators. *Injury.* 2003 Nov;34 Suppl 2:B1–3.
Rozbruch SR, Muller U, Gautier E, et al. The evolution of femoral shaft plating technique. *Clin Orthop Relat Res.* 1998 Sep(354):195–208.
Rüedi TP, Murphy WM. *AO Principles of Fracture Management.* 1st ed. Stuttgart New York: Thieme; 2000.
Schatzker J. Changes in the AO/ASIF principles and methods. *Injury.* 1995;26:B51–B56.
Sommer C. Locking Compression Plate. *Injury.* 2003 Nov;34 Suppl 2:B4–5.
Wagner M. General principles for the clinical use of the LCP. *Injury.* 2003 Nov;34 Suppl 2:B31–42.
Wagner M, Frigg R. *Internal Fixators—Concepts and Cases Using LCP and LISS.* New York: Thieme; 2006.
Willenegger H. Principios y filosofia. AO bases teóricas y principios prácticos des tratamiento quirúrgico de las fracturas. [Principles and philosophy. The AO theoretical basis and practical principles of surgical fracture treatment]. Lecture presented at: AO conference; 1981; Spain. Spanish.

Section 2

Breaches of AO principles

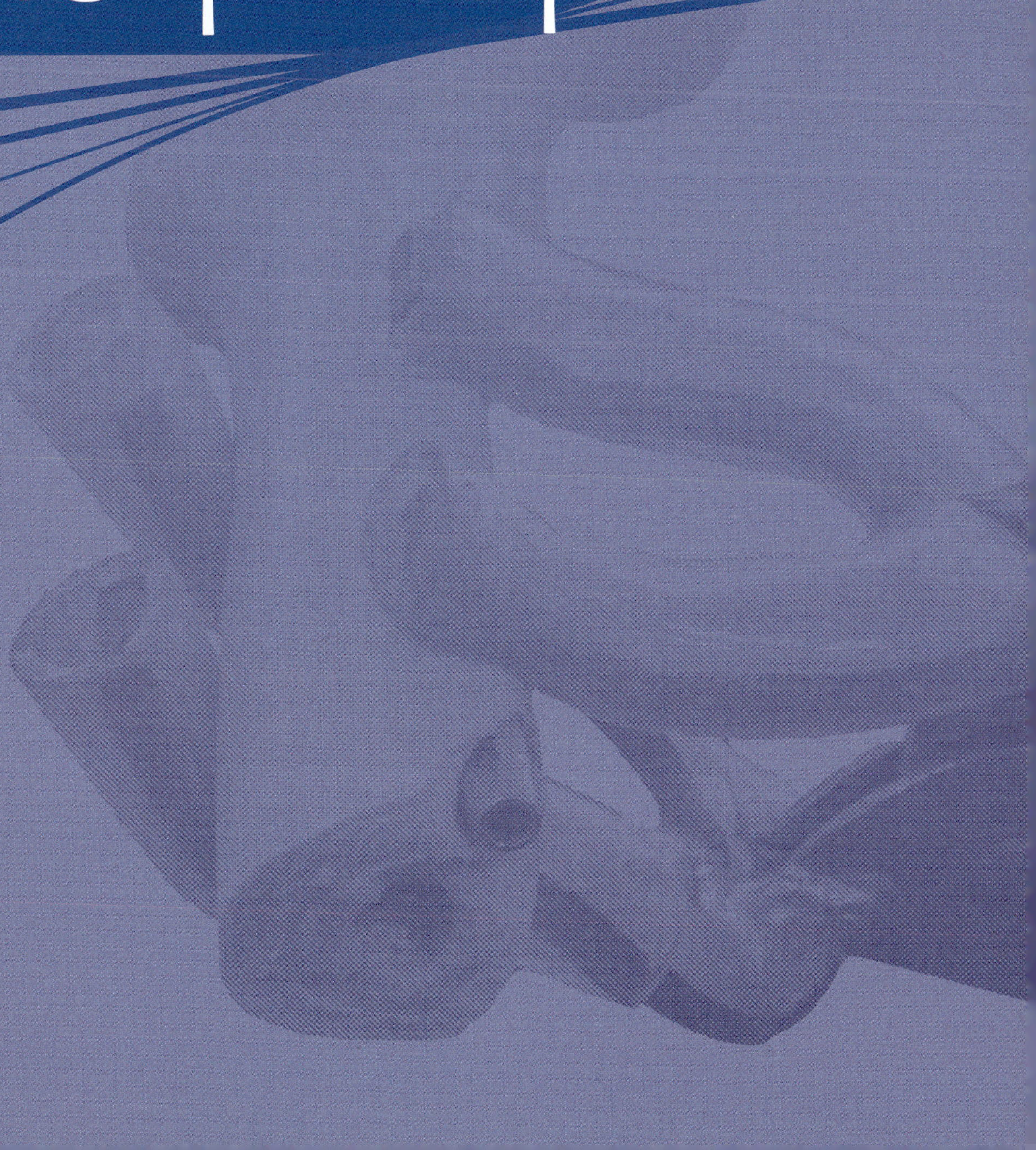

Section 2
Breaches of AO principles

2.1 General considerations on violation of AO principles

J Miquel Sales Pérez
Joan Girós Torres, Roberto Rivero Sosa, Miquel Videla Cés

Why things are as they are and not otherwise?
Evangelista Torricelli

A fracture is usually a combination of bone and soft-tissue injuries, and the fundamental objective of fracture treatment is to completely restore the function of the injured limb.

Before widespread acceptance of surgical fracture treatment, the so-called fracture disease, ie, chronic complex regional pain syndrome, caused by the combination of prolonged immobilization, circulatory disorders, inflammation, and pain could be commonly observed during nonoperative treatment. The absence of weight bearing or physiological stimulus led to joint stiffness, muscle and skin atrophy, and circulatory dysfunction. Nonoperative treatment of fractures also led to a higher number of unions with malpositioned fragments, delayed unions, nonunions, and malunions.

The treatment of fractures has made significant progress through the development of osteosynthesis techniques. Osteosynthesis has fulfilled its objectives when there is no need for external fixation, and early, active, and pain-free mobilization of the muscles and joints is possible. This fundamental principle of the AO and its achievement is possible through a stable, long-lasting osteosynthesis of the bone fragments during the period necessary for the union of the fracture.

The founders of the AO established, from the beginning, the goal of achieving **early pain-free active mobilization** after performing an **anatomical reduction** with **stable fixation** of the bone fragments while **preserving their vascularization**. Thus, the stabilization of the anatomical reduction, especially in joint fractures, achieves biomechanical conditions that lead to direct bone healing without callus formation, via remodeling of the Haversian canals and the blood vessels, while respecting the blood supply of bone and soft tissues to obtain early and pain-free functional restitution.

This goal of osteosynthesis was based on the mechanical principle of stability and on the biological criteria related to vascularization so as to aid uneventful bone healing. The mechanical and biological criteria are closely related, and an acceptable union cannot result if there is imbalance between them. The principles for internal fixation are still valid after decades of research and application, but they have evolved leading to a better understanding of the biological and biomechanical aspects of the injury.

At present these principles and their interrelationship (**Fig 2.1-1**) remain valid and they must be followed but not necessarily in a set order. The importance that was first given

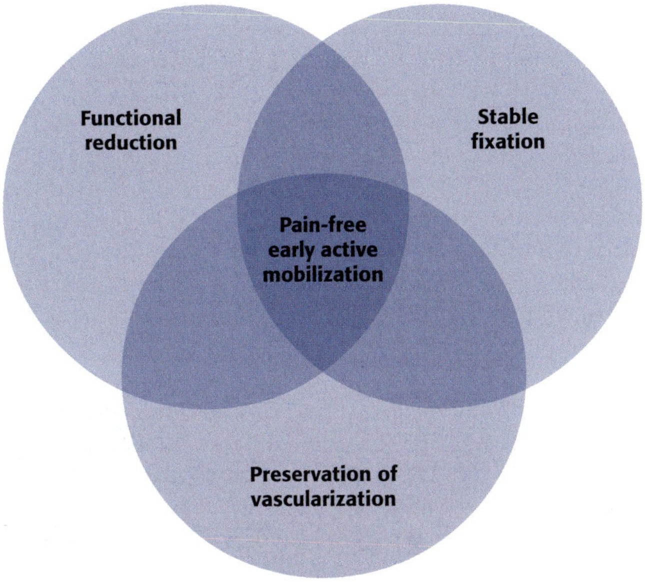

Fig 2.1-1 Graphical representation of how the AO principles interrelate.

to the mechanical concept has been counteracted by the concepts of respect for biology and understanding stability and the way these concepts are applied to the type and site of the fracture.

The interrelationship of the principles has implications for the expected clinical and radiographic results, although other factors, eg, infection or bearing too much weight too quickly, may affect the evolution of the fracture and the functional restoration.

The application of internal fracture fixation was a real revolution in fracture treatment, but it has not resolved all the problems. The presentation of complications such as delayed consolidation and pseudarthrosis did not disappear completely and others such as infection appeared with significant repercussion during the evolution of cases treated with osteosynthesis. For this reason, great efforts have been made to improve the osteosynthesis procedure, minimize complications, and improve the results of the treatment.

The interaction between bone and implant have led to new plate designs to avoid devitalization of soft tissue and bone through contact and pressure of the implant on the periosteum and the bone. If the bone-implant contact is reduced, bone necrosis occurs less often. The anchoring of plates and screws with new designs allows their use in osteoporotic bone. And plates that have been premolded to fit the anatomy of the bone can be applied to fractures in specific sites. A better knowledge of fracture healing has enabled surgeons to better understand the role that soft tissue plays in healing. The use of indirect reduction, without devascularization of the bone fragments, also improves soft-tissue care.

The vascular change in the bone and in the injured soft tissue caused by the fracture has led to surgical changes. Minimally invasive osteosynthesis enables preservation of the fracture hematoma which is essential for the regenerative process of fracture healing. Biology also plays a crucial role in the healing process and respecting it is vital to the healing of the fracture and soft tissues to achieve good function as early as possible.

The principles have been further developed in recent decades due to new issues that surgeons face, like the demographic shift throughout the world and the needs of a rapidly growing older population. There has generally been a large increase in the number of osteoporotic fractures in the elderly, high-energy trauma patients. Lately, surgeons have also seen an increase in the number of periimplant or periprosthetic fractures, ie, fractures that occur proximal or in relation to other osteosynthesis implants or prostheses applied previously due to prior injuries or degenerative diseases.

In osteosynthesis, many factors need to be considered to obtain the expected result. We should remember that despite the indication and availability of implants, the implant is only a means of carrying out principles already described many years ago by the founding AO members. On occasion, in a single traumatic bone injury, various solutions may be offered using different implants, which is acceptable as long as the established principles are fulfilled. Ignorance or violation of the recognized principles of surgical fracture treatment is not only a cause of suboptimal results but in practical terms, a guarantee of failure of treatment. The technical expertise and prior experience of the surgeons must also be considered, which improves with each case treated or studied.

This chapter presents real examples of the violation of three of the principles mentioned: fracture reduction, osteosynthesis stability, and respect for vascularization, which also make the fourth principle of early active and pain-free mobilization impossible. The selection of the cases has sought to provide an array of the most thought-provoking educational examples so that we can discuss the difficulties involved in remedying the injury and each of the AO principles.

Understanding the reason behind a failed osteosynthesis leads to reflection on which of the principle(s) has or have not been respected; on many occasions the errors are multiple or combined. The reasoning behind the causes and understanding the mechanisms behind the unexpected outcome can help avoid repeated similar failures. The solution provided and explained in each case also helps surgeons understand how to correct the problem and can help them with the planning of future cases.

The authors' fundamental aim in presenting these cases is to reflect on and discuss why and how surgeons do what they do. This is the educational value of these cases and the revised solutions.

Key points to remember

- Osteosynthesis is the surgical procedure by which the bone fragments are stabilized using implants. The goal of osteosynthesis is to restore the anatomy of the bone, to achieve sufficient and lasting stability between the bone fragments while the healing callus is formed, allowing immediate function without pain.
- Osteosynthesis is based on the interrelationship of mechanical stability and biological vascularization.
- Violation of the principles of fracture reduction, stability of osteosynthesis, and not respecting vascularization makes pain-free mobilization impossible:
  - Ignorance of or noncompliance with the principles of osteosynthesis lead to failures of the internal fixation.
  - An implant is only a means to fulfill certain functions to treat the fracture and not the end in itself.
  - The main objective in the treatment of fractures is the application of the basic principles of stability while altering the vascularization as little as possible.

References and suggested reading

Buckley R, Moran C, Apivatthakakul T. *AO Principles of Fracture Management.* 3rd ed. Stuttgart New York: Thieme; 2017.
Gautier E, Sommer C. Guidelines for the clinical application of the LCP. *Injury.* 2003 Nov;34 Suppl 2:B63–76.
Gustilo RB, Anderson JT. Prevention of infection in the treatment of one thousand and twenty-five open fractures of long bones: retrospective and prospective analyses. *J Bone Joint Surg Am.* 1976 Jun;58(4):453–458.
Gustilo RB, Mendoza RM, Williams DN. Problems in the management of type III (severe) open fractures: a new classification of type III open fractures. *J Trauma.* 1984 Aug;24(8):742–746.
Gustilo RB, Merkow RL, Templeman D. The management of open fractures. *J Bone Joint Surg Am.* 1990 Feb;72(2):299–304.
Kfuri M, Schatzker J. Revisiting the Schatzker classification of tibial plateau fractures. *Injury.* 2018 Dec;49(12):2252–2263.
Luo CF, Sun H, Zhang B, et al. Three-column fixation for complex tibial plateau fractures. *J Orthop Trauma.* 2010 Nov;24(11):683–692.
Marsh JL, Slongo TF, Agel J, et al. Fracture and dislocation classification compendium — 2007: Orthopaedic Trauma Association classification, database and outcomes committee. *J Orthop Trauma.* 2007 Nov-Dec;21(10 Suppl):S1–133.
Matthews SJ, Nikolaou VS, Giannoudis PV. Innovations in osteosynthesis and fracture care. Injury. 2008 Aug;39(8):827–838.
Meinberg EG, Agel J, Roberts CS, et al. Fracture and Dislocation Classification Compendium-2018. *J Orthop Trauma.* 2018 Jan;32 Suppl 1:S1–s170.
Miclau T, Martin RE. The evolution of modern plate osteosynthesis. *Injury.* 1997;28 Suppl 1:A3–6.
Müller M, Allgöwer M, Schneider R, et al. *Manual of Internal Fixation.* 2nd ed. Berlin Heidelberg New York: Springer Verlag; 1970.
Müller ME, Allgöwer M, Schneider R, et al. *Manual of Internal Fixation: techniques recommended by the AO-ASIF Group.* 3rd ed. Berlin Heidelberg: Springer-Verlag; 1991.
Müller ME, Nazarian S, Koch P, et al. *Classification AO des fractures. 1: Les os longs [AO Fracture Classification. 1 Long bones].* Berlin: Springer-Verlag; 1987.
Müller ME, Nazarian S, Koch P, et al. *The comprehensive classification of fractures of long bones.* Berlin Heidelberg: Springer-Verlag; 1990.
Orozco Delclós R, Sales JM, Videla M. *Atlas of internal fixation: fractures of long bones; classification, statistical analysis, technique, radiology.* Berlin Heidelberg: Springer-Verlag; 2000.
Perren SM. Evolution of the internal fixation of long bone fractures. The scientific basis of biological internal fixation: choosing a new balance between stability and biology. *J Bone Joint Surg Br.* 2002 Nov;84(8):1093–1110.
Rozbruch SR, Muller U, Gautier E, et al. The evolution of femoral shaft plating technique. *Clin Orthop Relat Res.* 1998 Sep(354):195–208.
Sales JM, Videla M, Forcada P, et al. *Atlas de Osteosíntesis. Fracturas de los huesos largos. Vias de acceso quirúrgico.* 2nd ed. Barcelona: Elsevier Masson; 2009. Spanish.
Schatzker J, McBroom R, Bruce D. The tibial plateau fracture. The Toronto experience 1968–1975. *Clin Orthop Relat Res.* 1979 Jan–Feb(138):94–104.
Schatzker J, Tile M. *The rationale of operative fracture care.* 3rd ed. Berlin New York Tokyo: Springer; 1987.
Séquin R, Texhammar R. *AO/ASIF Instrumentation. Manual of Use and Care.* Berlin Heidelberg New York: Springer-Verlag; 1981.
Tscherne H, Oestern HJ. [A new classification of soft-tissue damage in open and closed fractures (author's transl)]. *Unfallheilkunde.* 1982 Mar;85(3):111–115. German.

2.2 Osteosynthesis in unreduced fractures

Joan Girós Torres, Rodrigo Pesantez, Roberto Rivero Sosa, J Miquel Sales Pérez, Miquel Videla Cés

The last thing you know is where to start.

Isaac Newton

The displacement of a fracture can be considered a consequence of the action of deforming forces due to the trauma caused by the bone injury. The reduction of a fracture aims to return the bone to its original anatomical shape and regain its normal functions. Osteosynthesis counteracts the deforming forces on the fracture like the muscular action between agonist and antagonist muscles (eg, biceps and triceps), for instance. The reduction of the fracture creates stability by load transmission on the bone-implant interface until consolidation of the fracture.

The principle of anatomical fracture reduction has evolved in recent years into the concept of functional reduction, as it has become clear that not all fractures require a strictly anatomical reduction to achieve adequate functional outcome for the patient.

There is consensus that fractures occurring at an articular site should be differentiated from those in a diaphyseal site due to their different mechanical needs. This is logical because in articular fractures an exact correction of the articular regions is needed to achieve good functional outcome. Any alteration to the articular surfaces will cause joint incongruity resulting in a decreased range of motion and subsequent sequelae of an arthritic degenerative type, especially in those articulations most subjected to load bearing. The anatomical reduction of the articular surface represents the essential condition for the complete functional restitution of a fractured joint.

Thus, the concept of anatomical reduction and interfragmentary compression and osteosynthesis providing absolute stability to the fracture site can still be found today in the treatment of articular fractures. In this case, joint congruity is achieved and the surfaces of the fracture site have the maximum contact possible so when compressed there exists maximum friction between the fragments, with the bone achieving its own stability. Compression between fragments is the main cause of stability of a reduced fracture. Interfragmentary compression can also be obtained by using traction screws or with anatomically preshaped or molded plates placed to apply compression, for instance. Biomechanically, it is ideal if the load-bearing forces pass mainly through the bone and only to the least possible degree through the implant. The anatomical reduction creates stability and the osteosynthesis reinforces it by compressing the site and neutralizing it or guiding the forces. It permits optimal functioning with early mobilization that favors joint cartilage regeneration and avoids an articular incongruity that would otherwise lead to evolution towards an arthritic process. Interfragmentary compression neither influences the speed of callus formation nor causes resorption or bone necrosis, but it does favor stability and revascularization of the fracture site. Anatomical reduction is essential for normal joint function in articular fractures. The consolidation of a joint fracture, with anatomical reduction and compression, occurs directly by first intention, without formation of bone callus visible radiographically. If a bone callus appears in the control x-rays, this denotes a loss of stability.

Moreover, articular fractures with impaction are not reduced by closed methods and articular depressions are not filled with fibrocartilage; they should be filled with autogenous bone graft.

If the articular fracture is not reduced anatomically, it tends towards instability. The pressures exercised by the load are not distributed physiologically, but concentrate in other areas and the implant must absorb a large part of the load bearing, possibly failing due to fatigue. The formation of the healing callus will be delayed or it will not form and will evolve towards pseudoarthrosis. If the surgeon does not restore the anatomy, the articular function will be compromised and will progress towards definitive sequelae.

In diaphyseal fractures, the function requires a correct alignment of the bone and limb, and a recovery of the bone length and its rotation to achieve correct limb function. Metaphyseal and diaphyseal axial displacements must be reduced to prevent articular overloading. This reduction in diaphyseal fractures, understood as a functional reduction, is not recommended so as to avoid unnecessary surgical access that may devascularize the bone fragments and affect the vascularization of the soft tissues necessary for fracture healing.

In multifragmentary diaphyseal fractures with various intermediate fragments, manipulation of the fragments to achieve better reduction provides no benefits radiologically, if alignment, rotation, and length of the bone are respected. Consolidation of the fragments will benefit from controlled movement at the fracture site through periosteal and endosteal consolidation and will have a radiographically visible callus. It is therefore advisable not to approach the site and to respect the fracture hematoma. In cases of intramedullary nailing with comminution at the fracture site, it will be necessary to stabilize the reduction by locking the nail to avoid collapse and consequent loss of nail length. If plates are used to treat diaphyseal fractures with comminution at the fracture site, they must be applied, wherever possible, through approaches that respect the fracture hematoma and act by bridging the site to also achieve the consolidation favored by the hematoma.

In simple diaphyseal fractures, there is a greater indication for a more closed approach to the site, with osteosynthesis performed using internal fixation such as with the intramedullary nail which acts by bearing the load in a stable way. If contact of the bone fragments exists, greater stability and thus improved transmission of load bearing will result until the fracture's consolidation. In simple factures where plate osteosynthesis through minimal surgical approaches with preservation of vascularization is considered, an osteosynthesis with absolute stability criteria may be indicated. In cases where the fracture occurs in areas that do not permit a stable intramedullary fixation, the osteosynthesis should be extramedullary with plates respecting the site and the soft tissues through anatomical approaches. Fracture site compression is indicated if its vascularization can be respected, but it requires greater technical expertise. Diaphyseal radial and ulnar fractures constitute an exception to the foregoing concept, as they are considered articular fractures and require anatomical reduction to reestablish the combined movement between both bones in pronation and supination maneuvers and in the mobility of the proximal and distal joint regions to recover forearm functionality without sequelae.

Case description

A 28-year-old woman who was hit by a car sustained a contusion in her left knee and presented with an isolated tibial plateau fracture. The fracture was stabilized by external fixation on the day of the accident (AO/OTA 41C3.1) (**Fig 2.2-1**).

A computed tomographic scan was performed along with a three-dimensional reconstruction to obtain additional images and assess the fracture (**Fig 2.2-2**).

Subsequently, surgical intervention was indicated and internal fixation with plate and screws performed to obtain stability. The immediate postoperative x-rays showed a tibial plateau fracture that was not reduced but stabilized with two proximal cannulated screws and a proximal plate over the proximal tibia (**Fig 2.2-3**).

Eight months later, the patient presented with a varus angulated pseudarthrosis of the proximal tibia and a clinical reduction in mobility with a range of -20–80° (**Fig 2.2-4**).

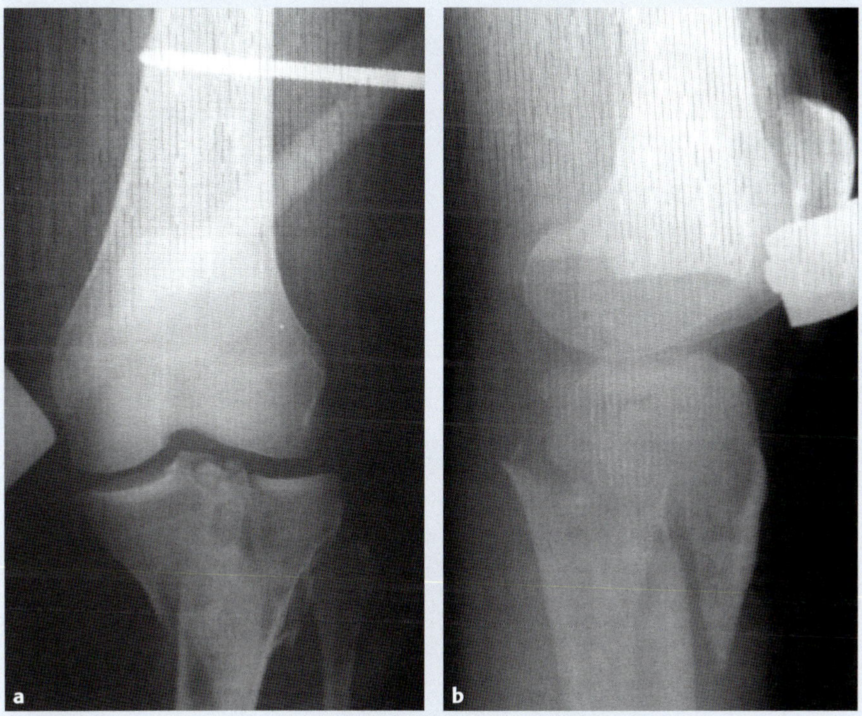

Fig 2.2-1a–b Initial x-rays after external fixation show the tibial plateau fracture.

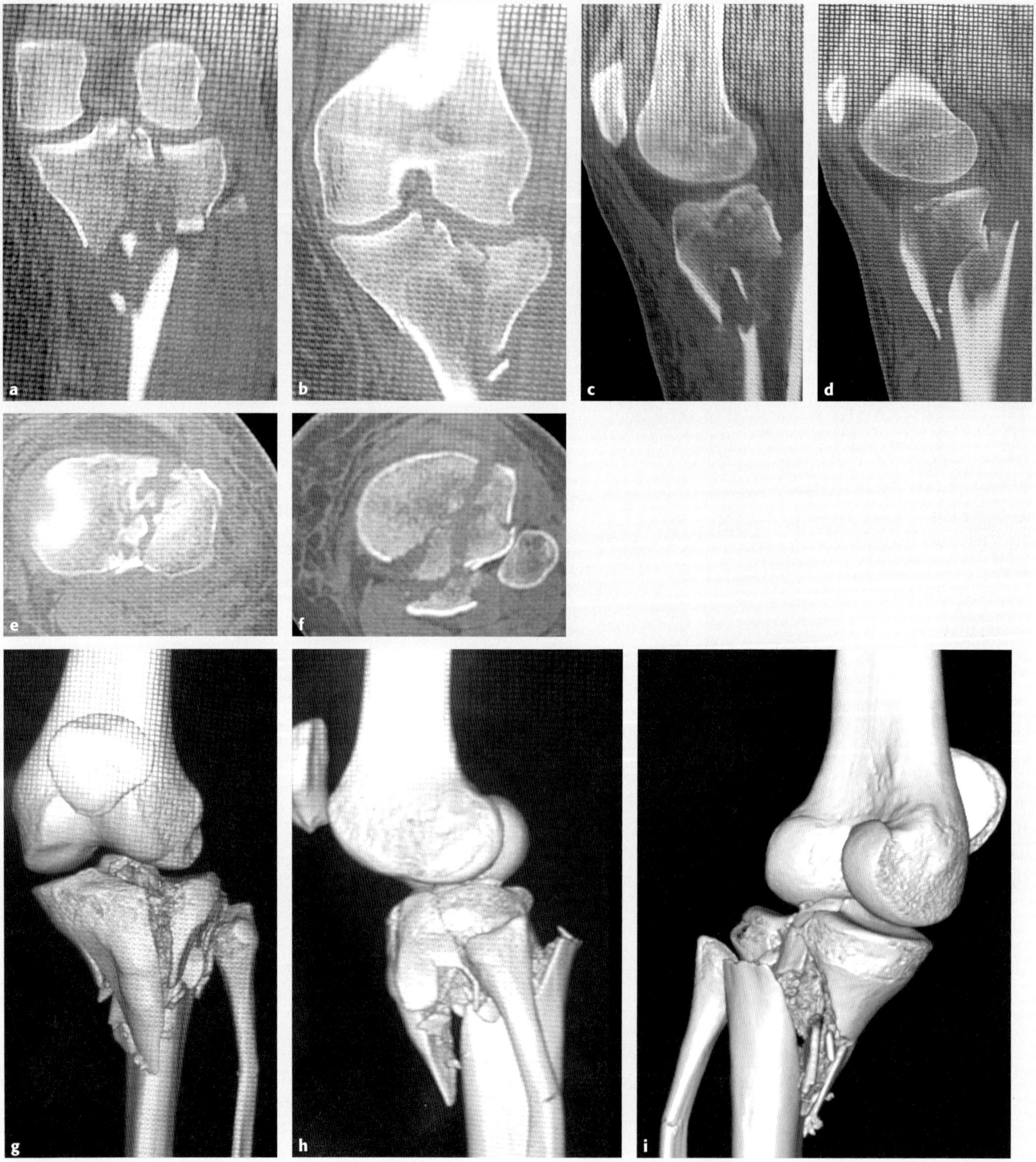

Fig 2.2-2a–i Preoperative computed tomographic (CT) scans of the tibial plateau fracture.
a–b AP views.
c–d Lateral views.
e–f Coronal views.
g–i Three-dimensional reconstruction in AP and lateral views.

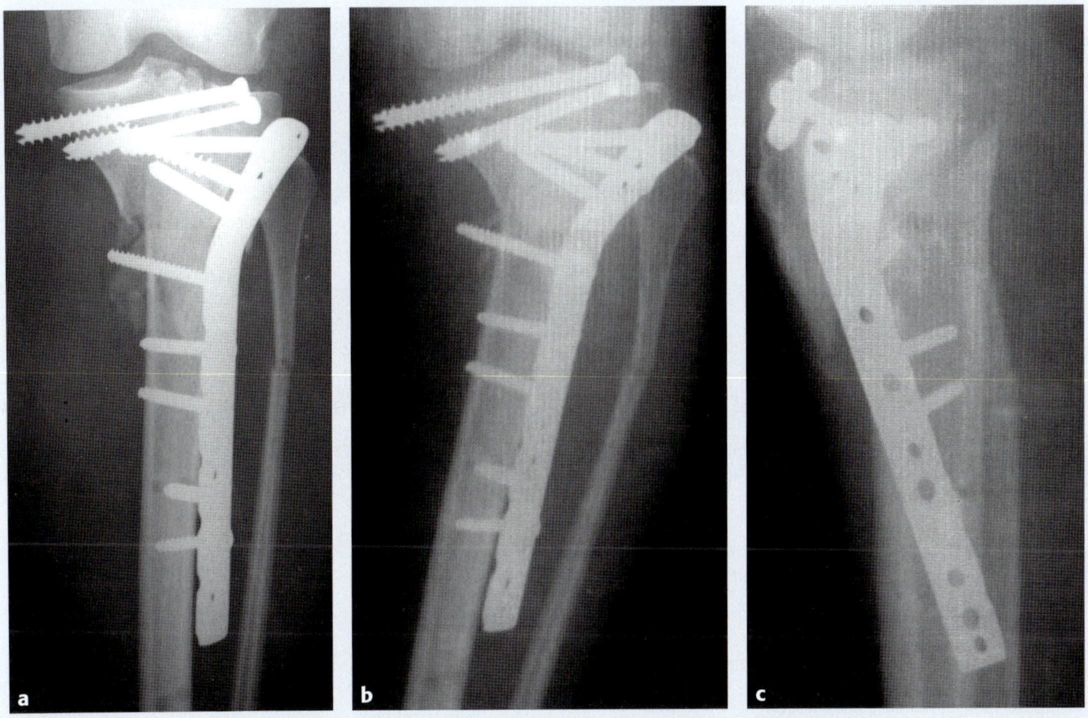

Fig 2.2-3a–c X-rays taken immediately postoperatively following internal fixation. They show the lack of reduction of the fracture and the osteosynthesis performed during the intervention.

Analysis of failure and reflection

Despite studying the fracture preoperatively, the surgeon responsible did not fully understand the fracture to be able to plan how to approach and correct it. Instead she or he performed surgery to treat the fracture. After it was fixed without reduction, patient monitoring was continued; however, the surgeon failed to recognize her or his own inability to understand the principles for treatment of tibial plateau fractures until the fracture showed a lack of consolidation with varus deviation.

The surgeon should have reflected on what should have been done differently: she or he should have tried to understand the anatomy of the fracture, classify it based on the images available, and select the appropriate surgical tactic to approach, reduce, and stabilize this tibial plateau fracture adequately. Continuing without correcting the basic error, which in this case is a lack of anatomical reduction in a joint fracture fixed with osteosynthesis, can never improve the prognosis of an injury, and it will progress towards complications and sequelae.

Final outcome

The patient was subsequently treated with an intraarticular osteotomy of the tibial plateau and bone substitutes to correct the defect (**Fig 2.2-5**). The fracture was fixed with a one-third tubular plate medially and a proximal tibial locking compression plate (**Fig 2.2-6**). The patient was allowed partial weight bearing with crutches according to pain tolerance from the first day and immediate functional rehabilitation was initiated (**Fig 2.2-7**). She managed to achieve a full range of mobility and the alignment of her lower limbs was reestablished (**Fig 2.2-8**).

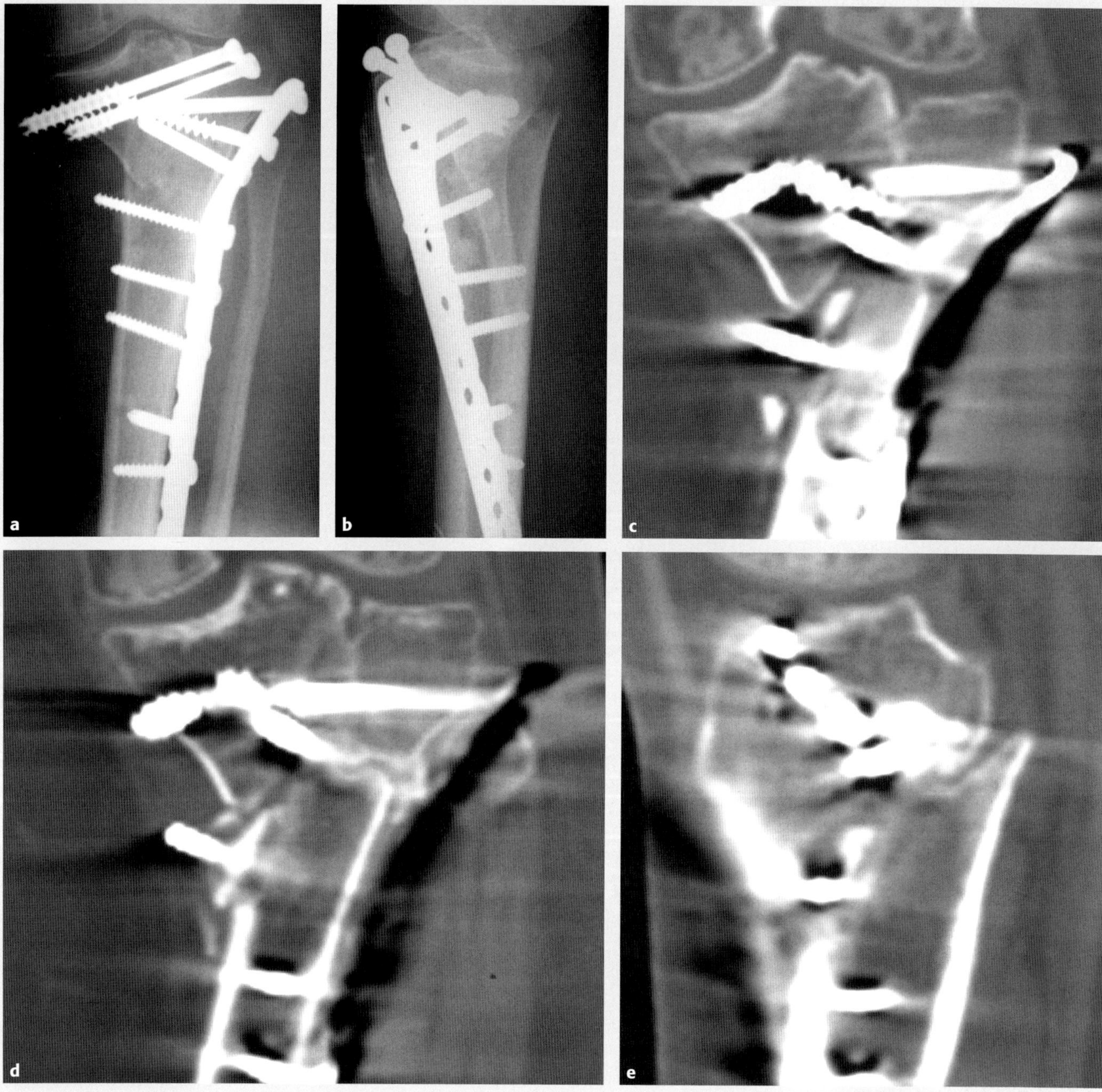

Fig 2.2-4a–e Radiological study of the fracture at 8 months.
a–b X-rays in AP and lateral views showing a varus deviation of the proximal tibia.
c–e Computed tomographic scans presenting a varus pseudarthrosis of the proximal metaphysis of the tibia. The lateral view (**e**) shows the deviation of the fracture in antecurvatum.

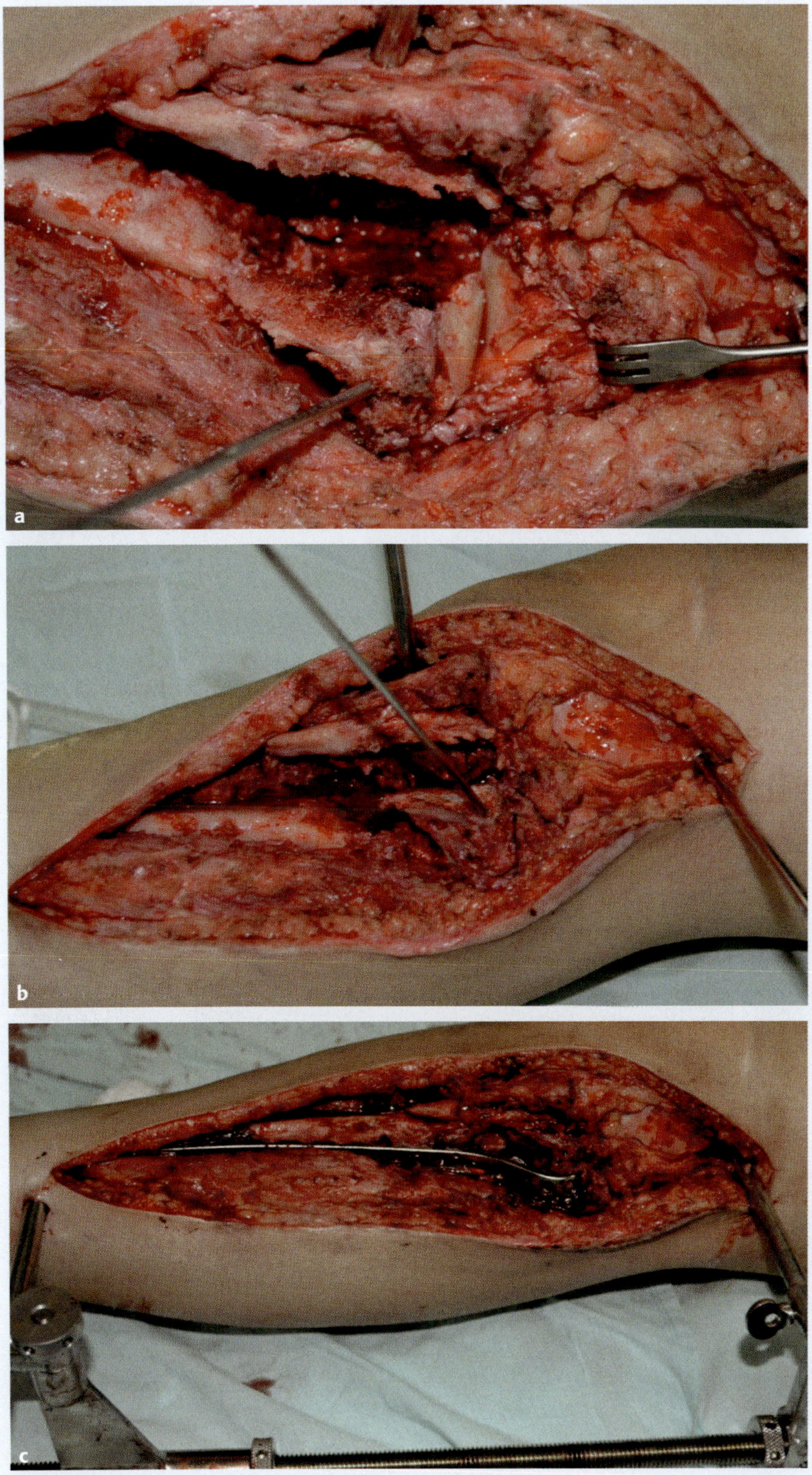

Fig 2.2-5a–c Intraoperative photographs of the surgical correction. With the aid of the distractor, alignment of the limb is achieved, followed by reduction of the fracture, filling of the bone defect with bone substitute, and then stabilization of the fracture site with a new osteosynthesis.

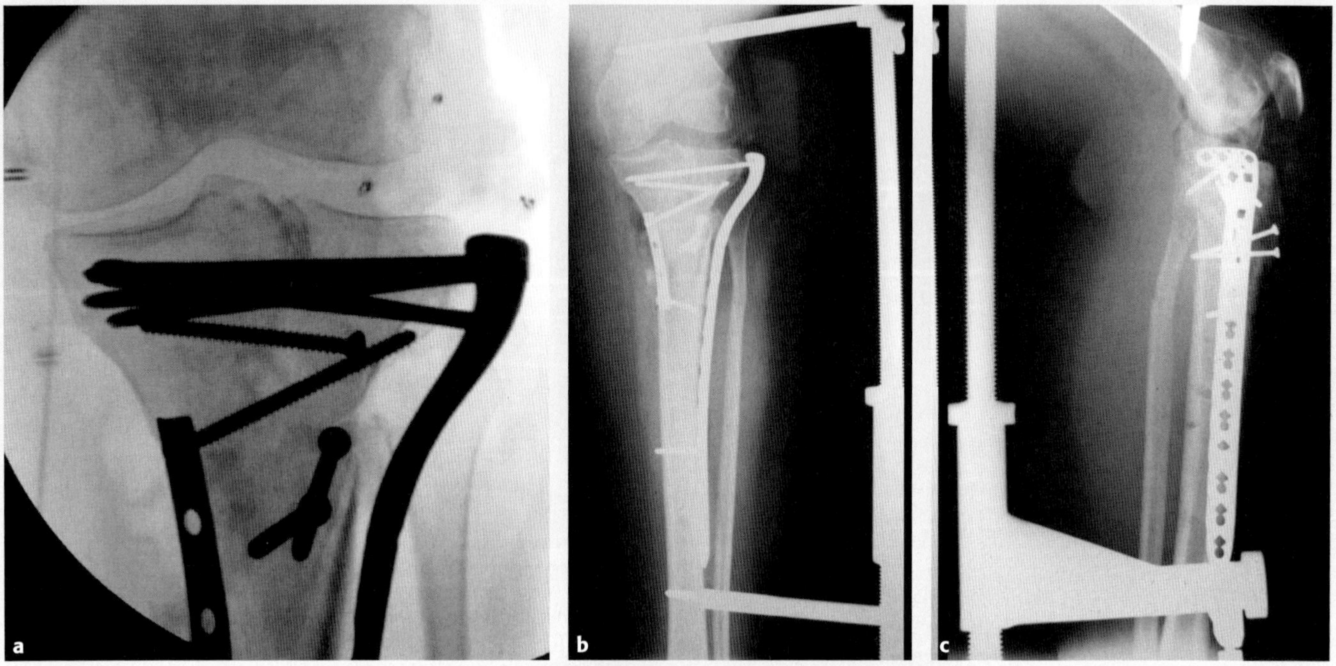

Fig 2.2-6a–c X-rays of the reduction and stabilization taken during the refixation.
a Intraoperative x-ray obtained with the image intensifier of the reconstruction.
b–c Radiographic aspect of the reconstruction in AP and lateral views.

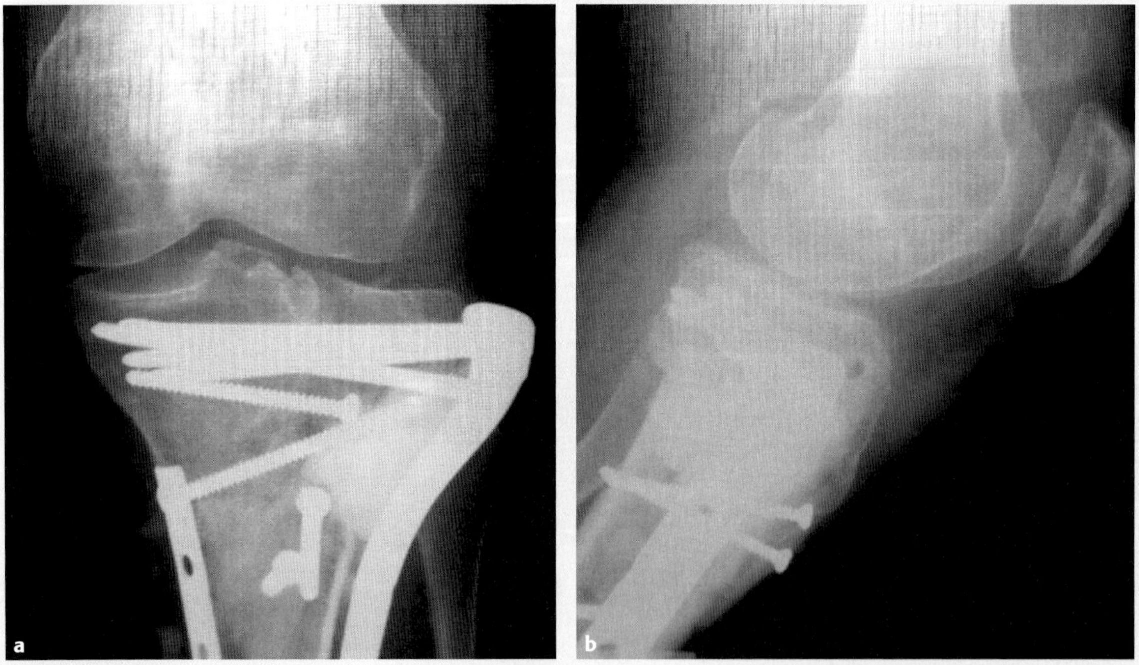

Fig 2.2-7a–d Postoperative AP and lateral control x-rays during the period of partial weight bearing.
a–b X-ray checks of the joint region during the postoperative period.

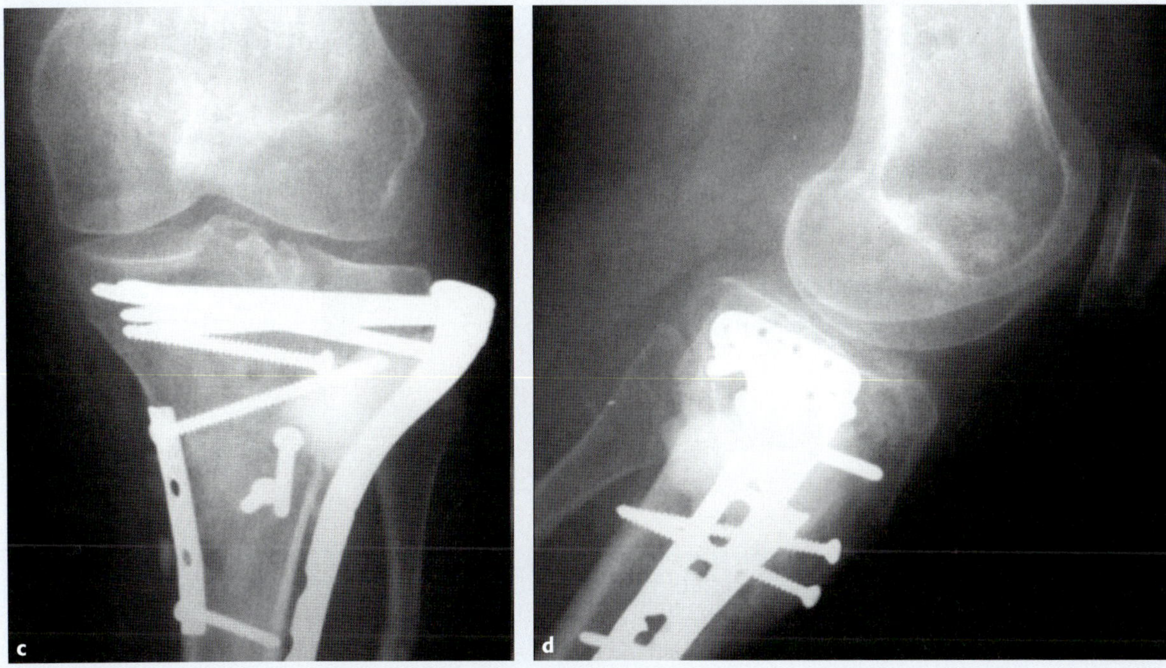

Fig 2.2-7a–d (cont) Postoperative AP and lateral control x-rays during the period of partial weight bearing.
c–d X-ray checks of the osteosynthesis in AP and lateral views during the postoperative period.

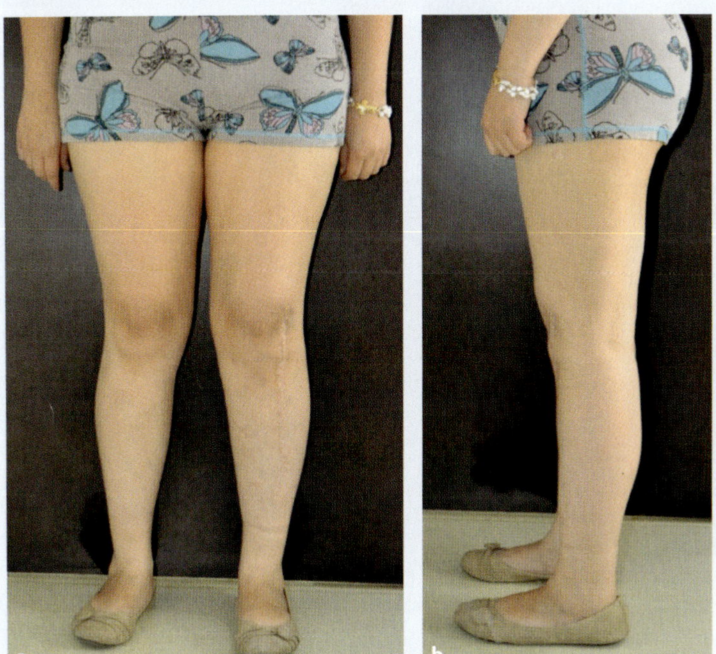

Fig 2.2-8a–h Final postoperative AP and lateral clinical and x-ray controls.
a–b Final appearance of the lower limbs in AP and lateral views. Complete extension of the joint.

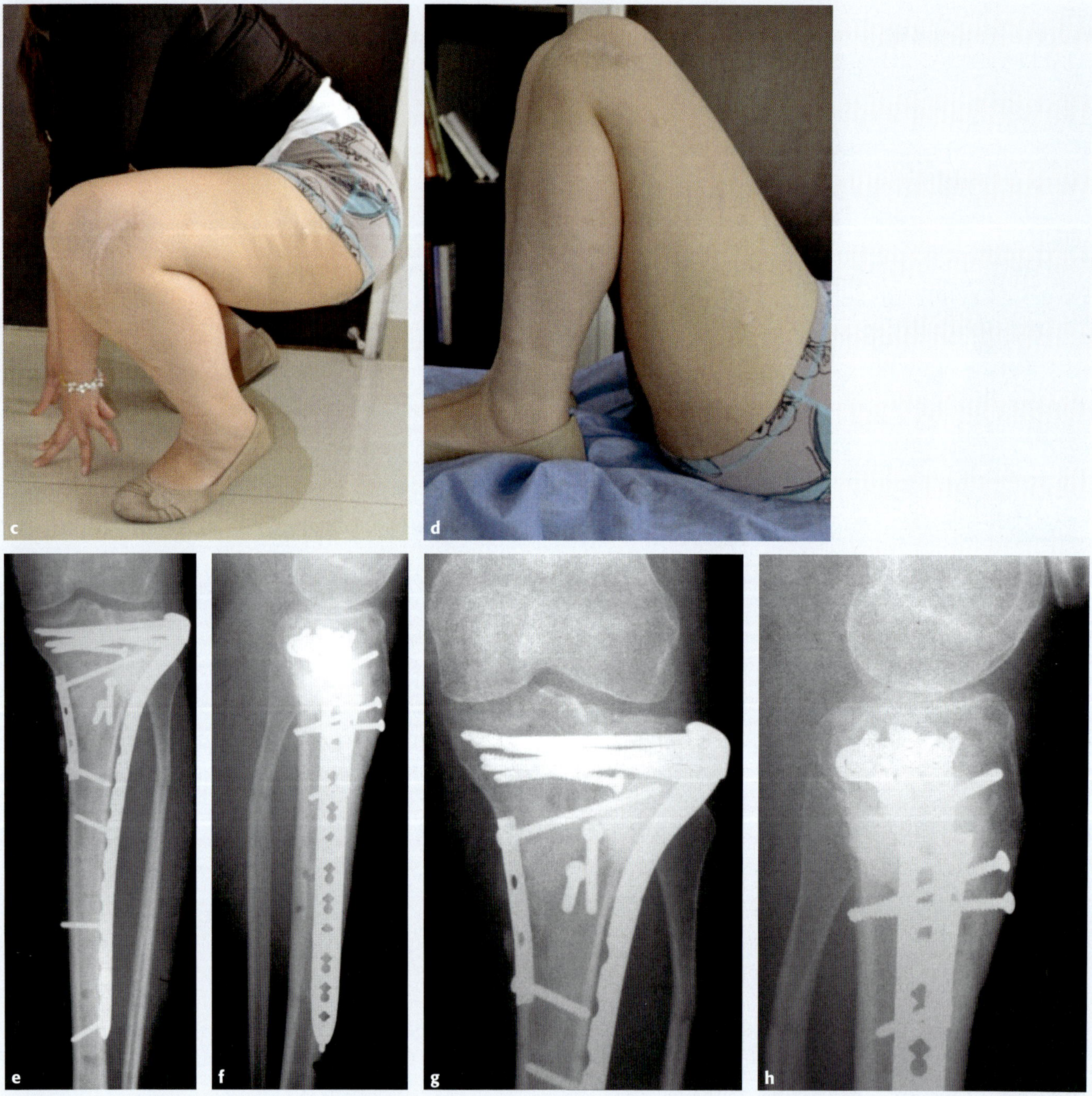

Fig 2.2-8a–h (cont) Final postoperative AP and lateral clinical and x-ray controls.
c–d Mobility in flexion obtained at the final follow-up.
e–f Final control x-rays of the reconstruction and of the osteosynthesis performed.
g–h Detail of the joint region and of the proximal tibial metaphysis.

Case description

A 54-year-old woman suffered a ski accident and presented with a pertrochanteric fracture of the left hip (AO/OTA 31A1) (**Fig 2.2-9**) without other traumatic injuries.

A trochanteric nail was planned, using a hip fracture nail system that combines the principles of a compression hip screw with an intramedullary nail. The postoperative control x-ray showed a lack of reduction at the fracture site and rotation of the proximal fragment, but the surgeon decided to trust the implant and continue with the planned fracture treatment (**Fig 2.2-10**).

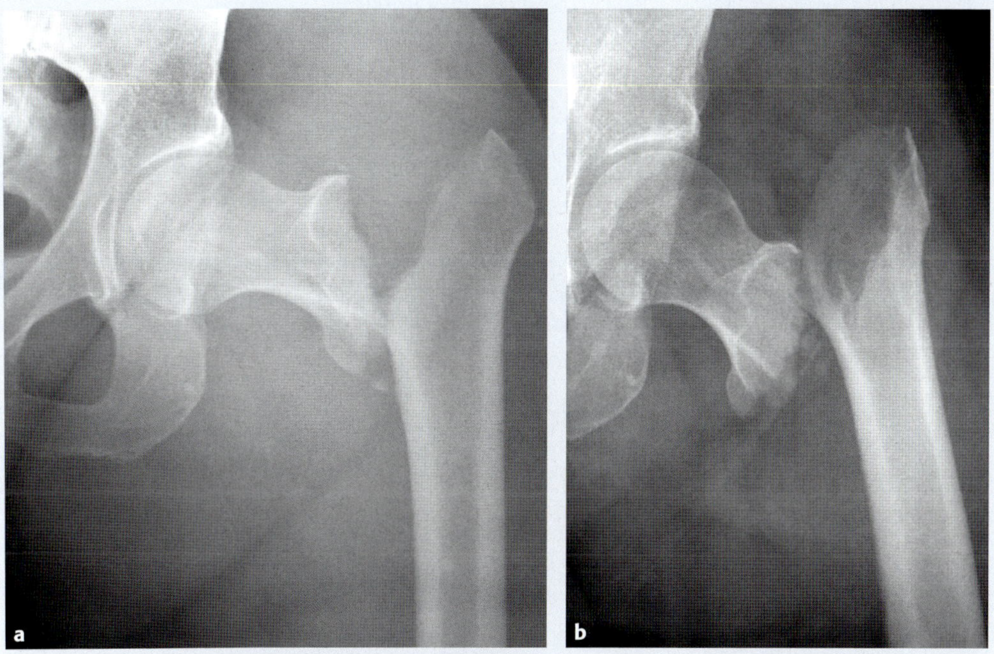

Fig 2.2-9a–b Preoperative x-rays showing a simple trochanteric fracture with a rare fracture pattern that indicates a high-energy trauma despite it being a simple trochanteric fracture.

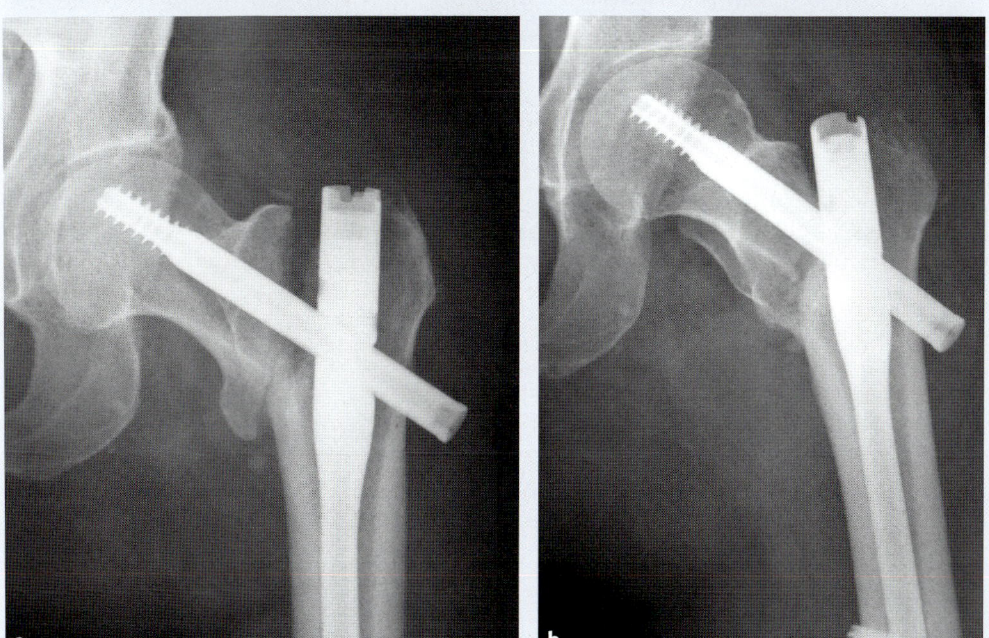

Fig 2.2-10a–b Postoperative x-rays at 2 months.

Analysis of failure and reflection

We cannot expect an implant that bears all the weight to improve the reduction of a fracture that we have not managed to achieve by either indirect or direct reduction maneuvers.

When a right femur is treated, torque maneuvers in a clockwise direction of the screw situated in the femoral head cause anterior rotation and flexion of the femoral neck; the secondary displacement occurs in extension and in posterior rotation. The topographic anatomy of the proximal femur causes a rotational displacement of the head and neck of the left femur (**Fig 2.2-11**). In the right femur, clockwise torque causes a rotation and a subsequent extension that contribute to the impaction and reduction of the fracture **[Mohan et al, 2000]**.

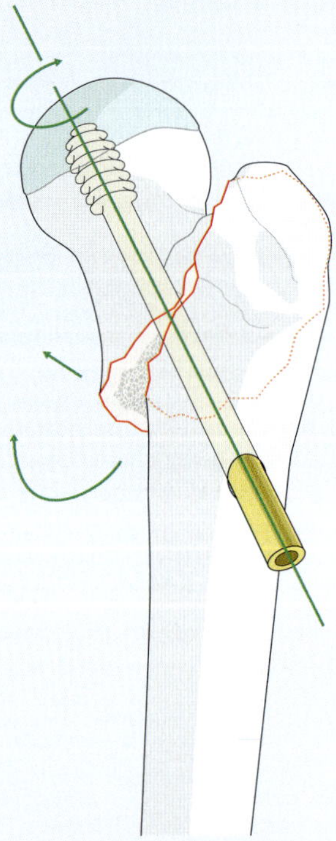

Fig 2.2-11 In the left femur, clockwise torque maneuvers of the screw situated in the femoral head cause anterior rotation and flexion of the femoral head.

Final outcome

One year after the fracture, no cut-out has taken place despite the lysis phenomena around the femoral head screw and the proximal migration at the femoral head and neck. In the fracture healing process, the still poor callus formation has stabilized the fracture. Despite a reduced quality of life, the patient is able to walk with crutches (**Fig 2.2-12**). Eventually, the patient will be able to walk without crutches.

"Patients heal despite the surgeon."

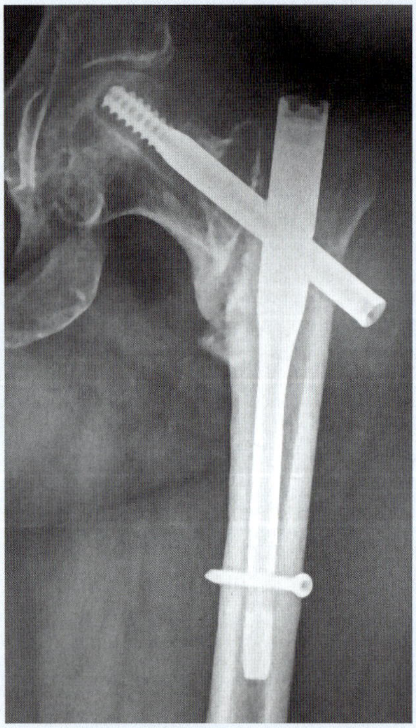

Fig 2.2-12 Postoperative x-ray check at 1 year after the fracture. Although the fracture presents poor callus formation, bone resorption exists around the femoral head screw but there is no cut-out.

Case description

A 75-year-old woman presented after falling from standing height on a public road. She did not present with any other traumatic symptoms (ie, the assessment of the patient being checked for airway, breathing, circulation, disability, exposure/examination (ABCDE) following advanced trauma life support was fine). X-rays taken upon admission showed an intertrochanteric fracture of the left hip (AO/OTA 31A2) (**Fig 2.2-13**).

The surgeon decided on a sliding hip screw system (eg, dynamic hip screw [DHS]) with a stabilizing plate and performed the intervention with trust in the implant (**Fig 2.2-14**).

Three months after the intervention, the patient was allowed to bear weight and ambulate using forearm crutches; clinically, the pain was remitting (**Fig 2.2-15**). The control x-ray showed impaction of the fracture with the implant acting with dynamic stability driving the impact through it. The radiographic signs of consolidation had started when the fracture impacted with a certain valgus position that was beneficial to its stability.

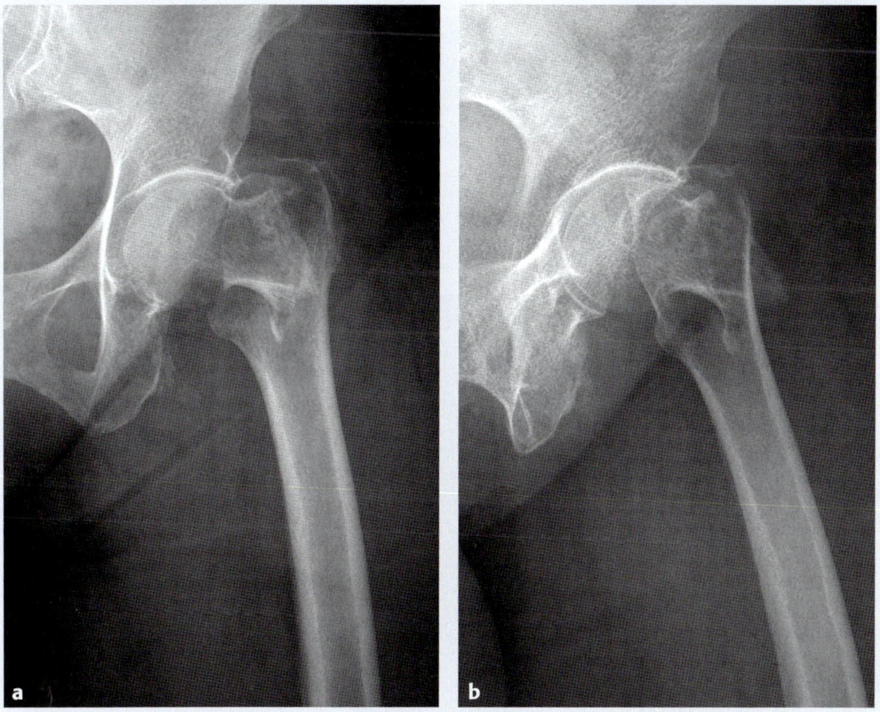

Fig 2.2-13a–b Preoperative x-rays in AP and axial views showing a simple intertrochanteric fracture.

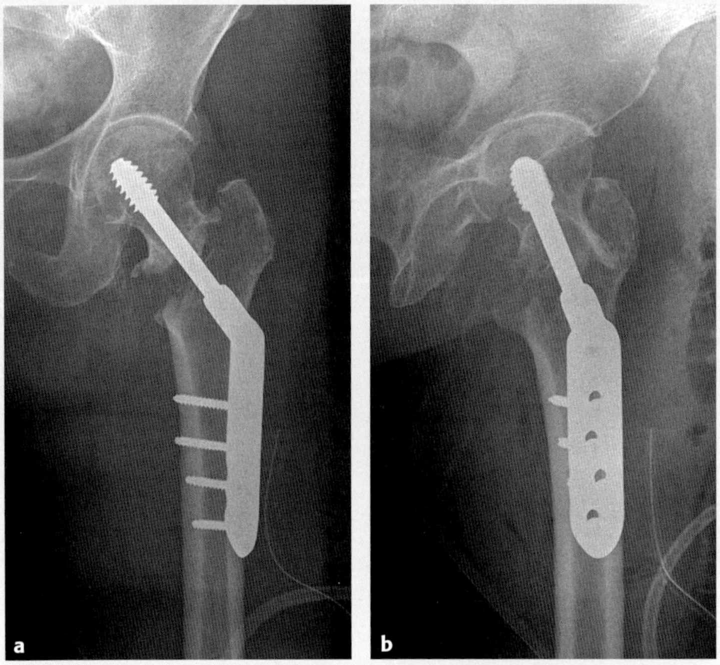

Fig 2.2-14a–b Postoperative x-rays in AP and axial views showing the unreduced fracture. Despite the lack of reduction, the surgeon decided to leave the implant in place.

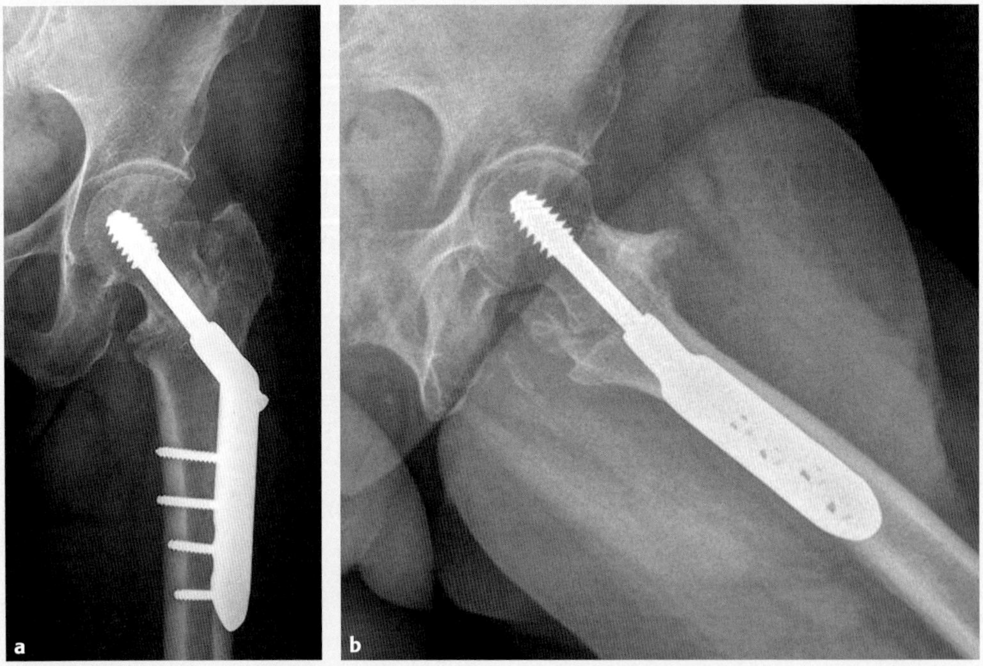

Fig 2.2-15a–b Postoperative control x-ray at 3 months. The fracture shows an incipient callus with impaction of the fracture. No weakening of the implant is observed, which together with the valgus position of the proximal end of the fracture ultimately enabled healing.

Analysis of failure and reflection

As seen in Case 2 where the fracture was treated with an intramedullary nail, the topographic anatomy of the proximal femur causes a rotational displacement of the femoral head and neck segment. In the left femur, torque maneuvers in a clockwise direction applied to the screw situated in the femoral head cause an anterior rotation and flexion of the femoral neck. In the right femur, the secondary displacement causes subsequent extension and rotation **[Mohan et al, 2000]**.

This case demonstrates how the effect caused does not depend on the implant being extra- or intramedullary. The effect is caused by the clockwise rotational movement as the head and neck screw enters. An impacted blade would not cause this effect with the same intensity.

Final outcome

Three months after the fracture, no weakening of the implant is observed. This and the valgus position of the proximal end of the fracture in the metaphyseal area led to healing.

"Patients can heal despite the surgeon."

CASE 4

Case description

A 47-year-old woman with a history of high blood pressure, venous insufficiency of the lower limbs, and obesity fell onto the shoulder girdle sustaining a proximal humeral fracture (AO/OTA 11C3) (**Fig 2.2-16**).

Four days later, osteosynthesis was performed using a minimally invasive plate osteosynthesis (MIPO) technique with an angular stability plate. The surgery was laborious with an acceptable intraoperative imaging result. At the postoperative x-ray control, migration of the osteosynthesis material with intraarticular screws was visible along with a loss of reduction in the fracture (**Fig 2.2-17**).

The patient underwent reoperation 48 hours after the first intervention using a longitudinal extended deltoid-split approach and respecting the axillary neurovascular bundle. The material from the previous osteosynthesis was then removed. An open reduction was performed with a larger PHILOS plate and reanchoring of tuberosities to the plate using nonabsorbable sutures (**Fig 2.2-18**).

The injured limb was kept immobilized for 3 weeks, but active-assisted exercises were started from that point onwards with a progressively increasing demand under the supervision of a rehabilitation therapist. In the third postoperative month, the patient could manage active elevation of 90° and passive elevation of 120°. At the clinical check-up at 6 months, pain persisted especially at night and during physical activity. The active mobilization of the shoulder was 90° elevation, 90° abduction, and 20° external rotation and internal rotation hand-buttocks. The fracture was consolidated, with signs of necrosis of the humeral head (**Fig 2.2-19**).

One year after the reintervention, the patient felt no pain at rest but during physical activity, which limited her activity at work. A hypertrophic scar was observed in the proximal area with atrophy of the deltoid musculature. There was no sensitivity deficit in the axillary area. Elevation of 130°, abduction of 160° without claudication, external rotation of 15° against elastic resistance, internal rotation of the hand was L4. Radiologically, the implant was in situ, with no signs of necrosis of the humeral head and consolidation of the fracture (**Fig 2.2-20**).

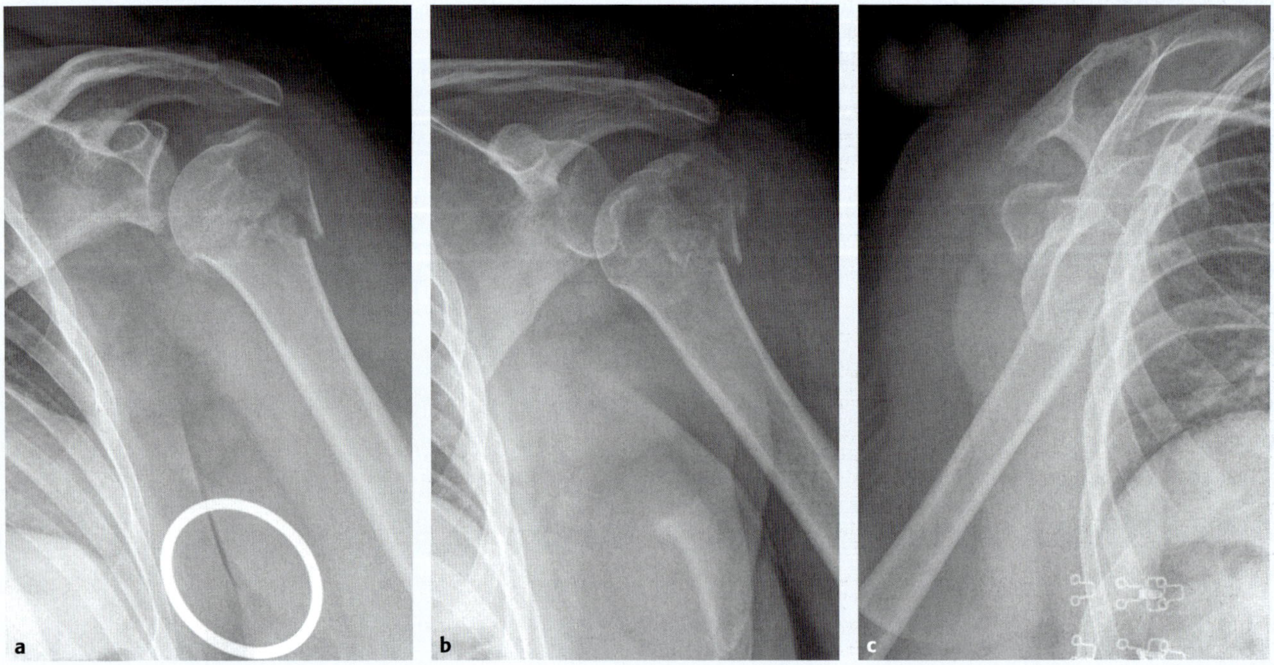

Fig 2.2-16a–c Preoperative x-rays of the left humeral fracture in AP view (**a–b**) and Velpeau view (**c**).

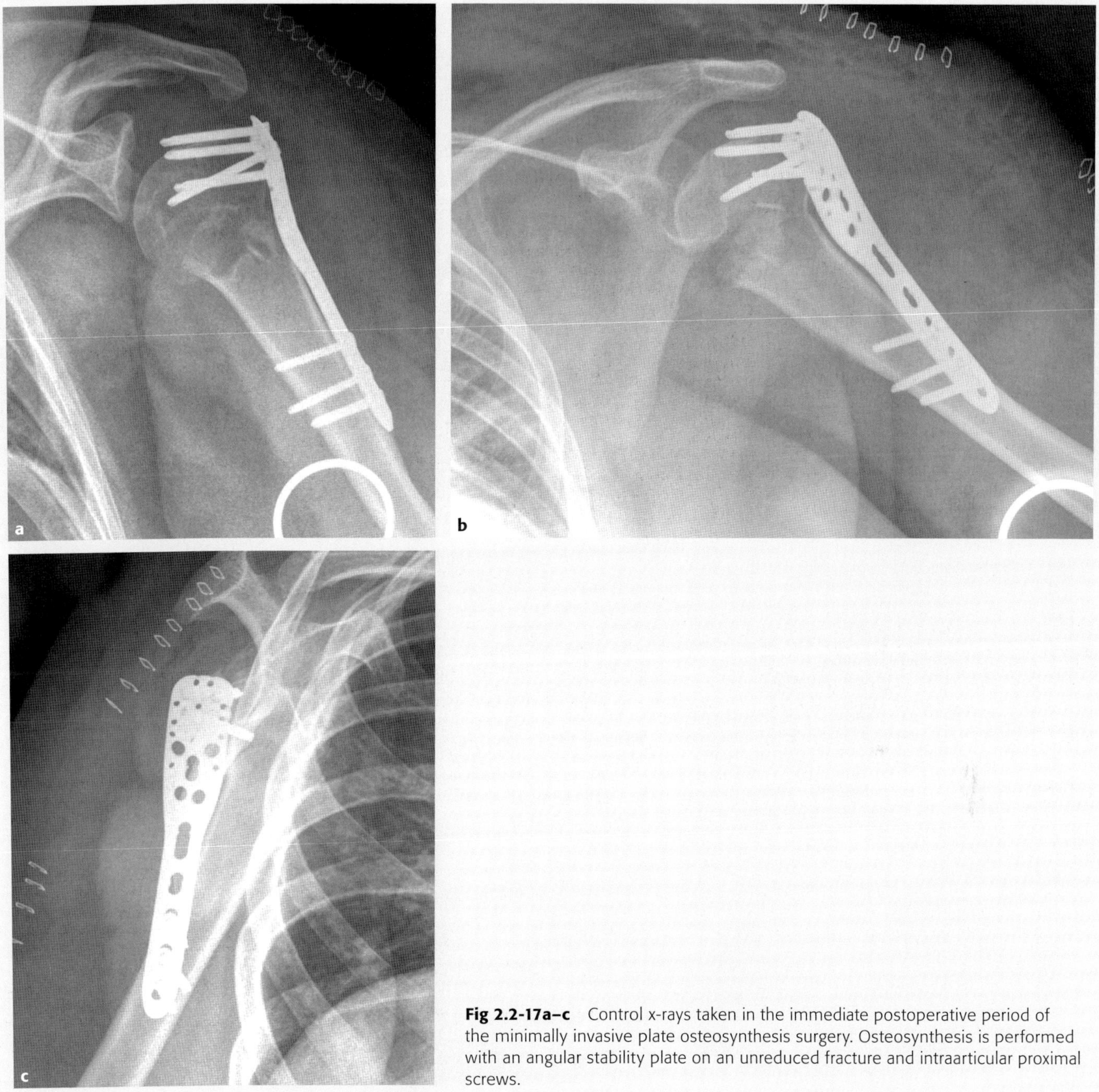

Fig 2.2-17a–c Control x-rays taken in the immediate postoperative period of the minimally invasive plate osteosynthesis surgery. Osteosynthesis is performed with an angular stability plate on an unreduced fracture and intraarticular proximal screws.

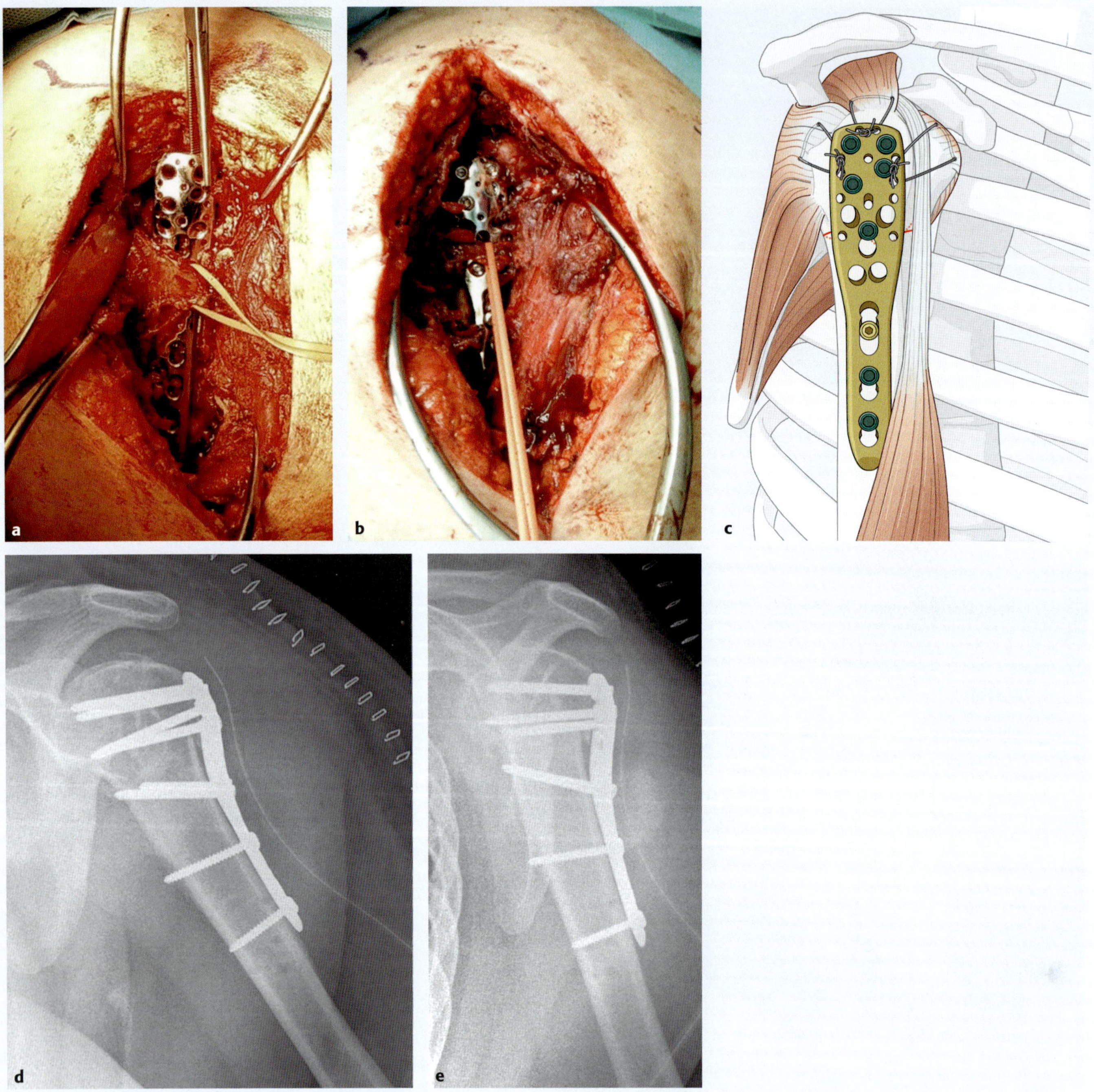

Fig 2.2-18a–e Situation of the definitive implant and anatomical relationships.

a–b Intraoperative photographs. Extraction of the previous plate through an extended transdeltoid splitting approach and insertion of the new PHILOS plate. The anatomical relationship with the axillary nerve, which is identified, can be observed.

c Bone sutures are used to reanchor the rotator cuff tendons to the plate.

d–e Immediate postoperative control x-rays taken after reintervention showing fixation with definitive angular stability plate.

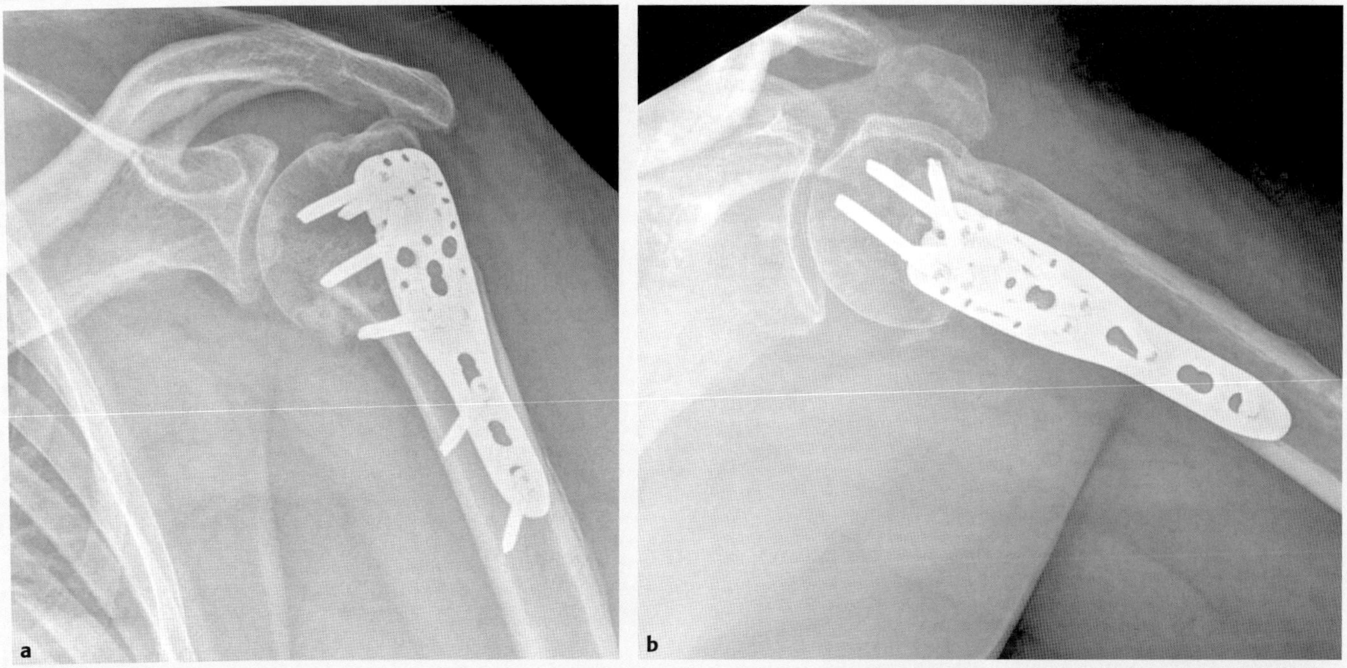

Fig 2.2-19a–b Control x-rays at 6 months after the reintervention showing the consolidated fracture in AP view (**a**) and axial view (**b**).

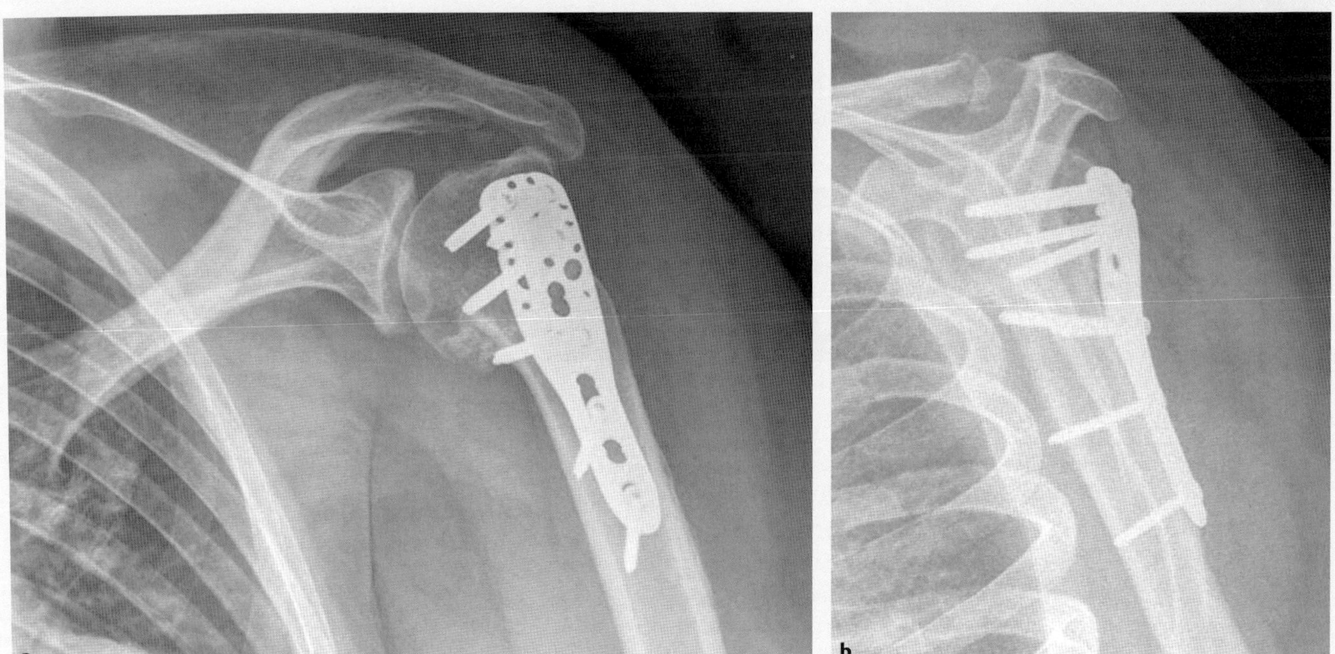

Fig 2.2-20a–e Radiographic and clinical evaluation of the result obtained 1 year after the reintervention.
a–b Control x-ray 1 year after the reintervention showing the consolidated fracture.

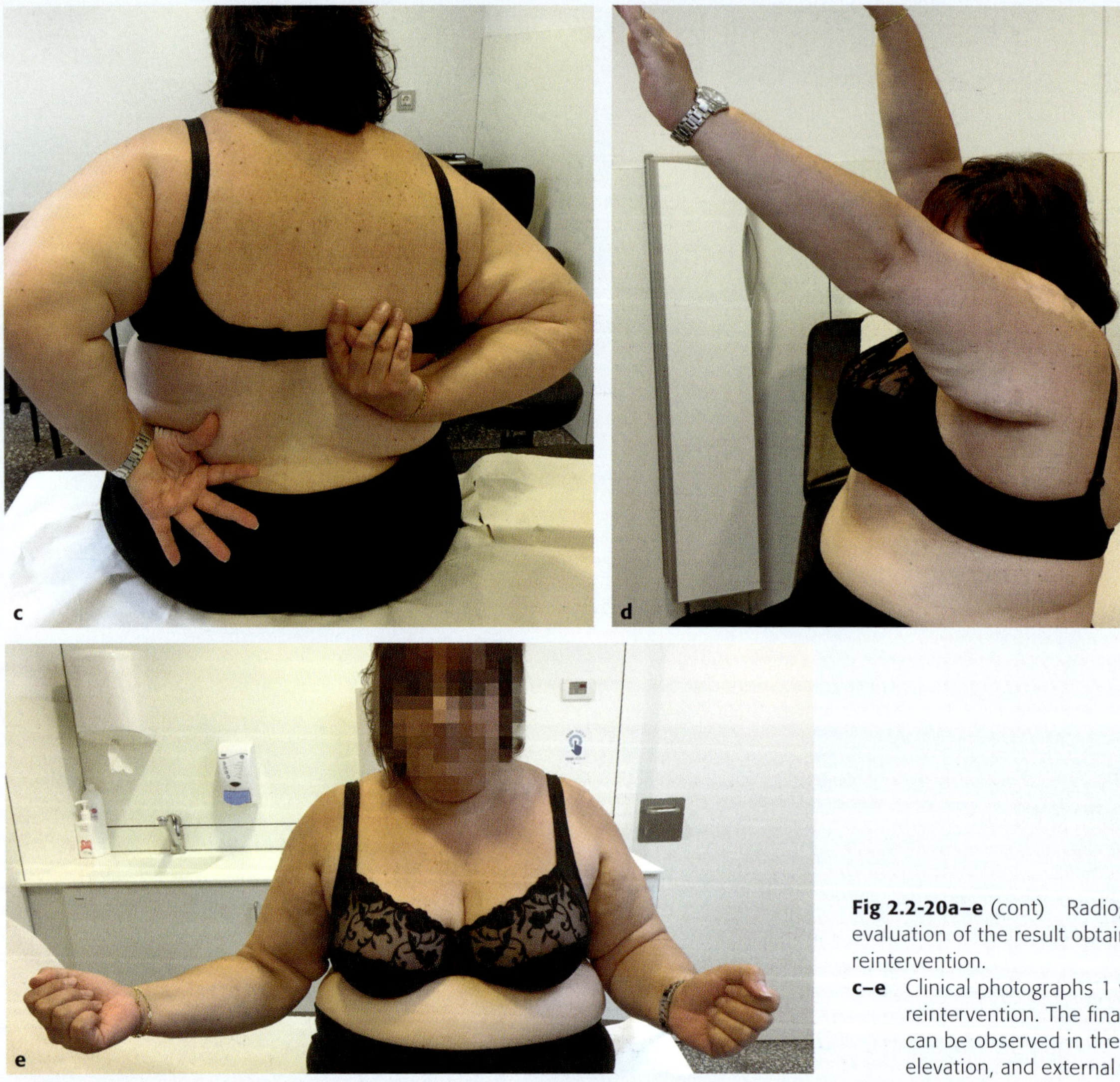

Fig 2.2-20a–e (cont) Radiographic and clinical evaluation of the result obtained 1 year after the reintervention.
c–e Clinical photographs 1 year after the reintervention. The final articular balance can be observed in the internal rotation, elevation, and external rotation.

Analysis of failure and reflection

The failure in this patient's treatment may be associated with preoperative planning, insufficient reduction, and incorrect fixation. We believe that the choice of a preshaped proximal humeral angular stable plate was correct. The reason for the failure may have been the choice of surgical approach, and not having taken into account the patient's obesity which is likely to have made correct reduction of the fracture and fixation with MIPO technique more difficult. Choosing a deltopectoral approach would probably have been more appropriate. The surgeon must ensure that the fracture reduction is correct and the fixation stable by checking it through various intraoperative radiological views. Osteosynthesis implants without adequate fracture reduction may result in serious complications that require a new surgical intervention and increase the healthcare costs considerably.

Final outcome

After two surgical interventions, immobilization, and a long and painful rehabilitation period, consolidation of the humeral fracture was achieved. The result included muscle atrophy and certain functional restrictions. The patient has recovered an articular range that allows her to continue with her activities of daily living within certain limitations. Pain has prevented her from returning to her previous job and she is currently undergoing disability assessment procedures due to sequelae.

Case description

A 69-year-old man and heavy smoker with a history of atrial flutter with pacemaker, dyslipidemia, ulcerative proctitis, and prostatism fell from a horse onto his back resulting in an unstable pelvic fracture (AO/OTA 61C1.3) and a trochanteric fracture of the left femur (AO/OTA 31A2.3) (**Fig 2.2-21**–**Fig 2.2-26**).

He was taken to a local hospital where the injury was stabilized. Before being transferred to the university hospital, it was decided to perform an osteosynthesis of the trochanteric fracture. A trochanteric intramedullary nail was used (130°, 180 mm long, 11 mm diameter) but since the fracture was not reduced, it resulted in a malunion (**Fig 2.2-27** and **Fig 2.2-28**).

Eleven days after the accident, after the inflammatory phase during which the transfusion of six units of red blood cell concentrate was required, stabilization surgery of the pelvis was performed with two sacroiliac screws, and anterior closure with a reconstruction plate and screw, isolated on the left iliopubic branch (**Fig 2.2-29** and **Fig 2.2-30**). One week after pelvic surgery, the patient was discharged from hospital and transferred to his home.

Revision surgery of the malunion of the proximal femur was not performed after the pelvic surgery due to the expressed will of his family. After 21 days he suffered a urinary sepsis with orchitis, which further delayed the planned rescue surgery of the malunion by another 3 weeks.

Finally, the surgeon proceeded to remove the trochanteric nail, by performing an osteotomy through the fracture callus, to re-reduce and stabilize the fracture using a new trochanteric nail (eg, trochanteric femoral nail advanced, which is a proximal femoral nailing system). This surgery was carried out with general anesthesia, on a radiolucent table, without applying axial traction, with the help of pointed clamps, collinear clamps, and temporary K-wires (**Fig 2.2-31**–**Fig 2.2-36**). No weight bearing was allowed for 12 weeks after pelvic surgery, but the patient was allowed to sit as well as perform passive and assisted mobilizations.

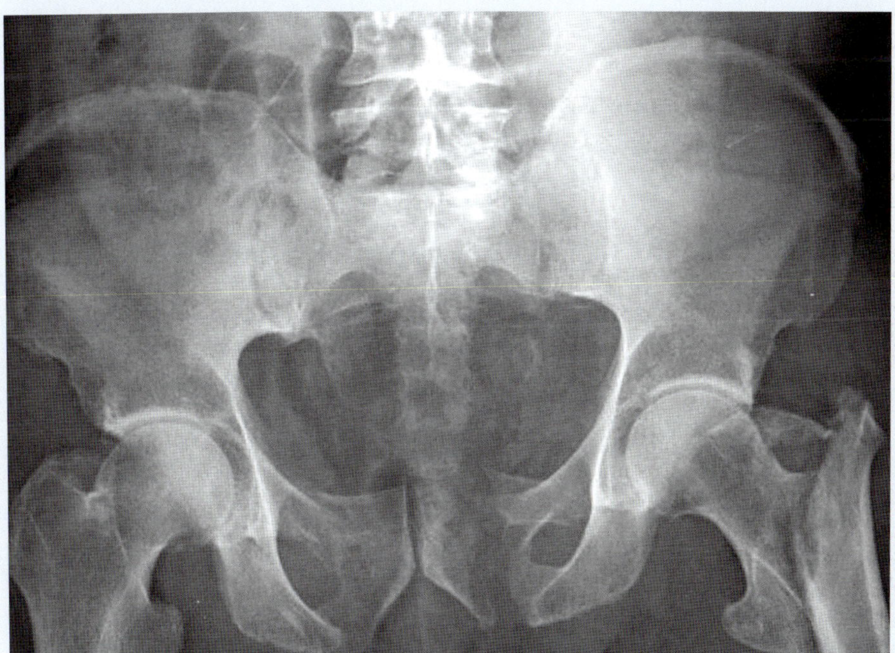

Fig 2.2-21 Plain x-ray of the pelvic fracture and left trochanteric fracture.

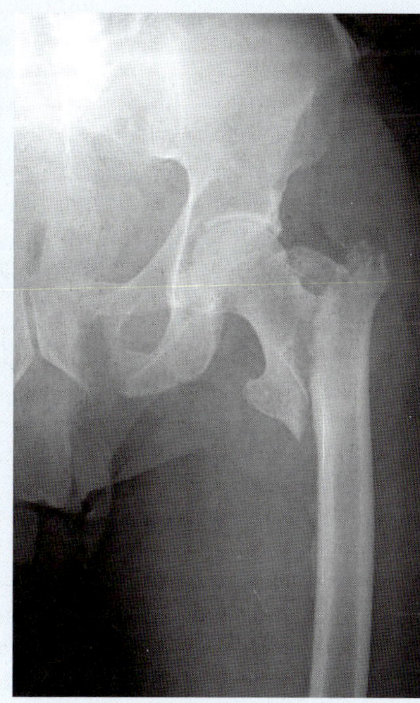

Fig 2.2-22 Judet oblique view of the left hip. Note that the patient's left obturator foramen is not closed, as is usual in this view. This is because of the combined deformity of the unstable fracture of the pelvic ring plus the trochanteric displaced fracture.

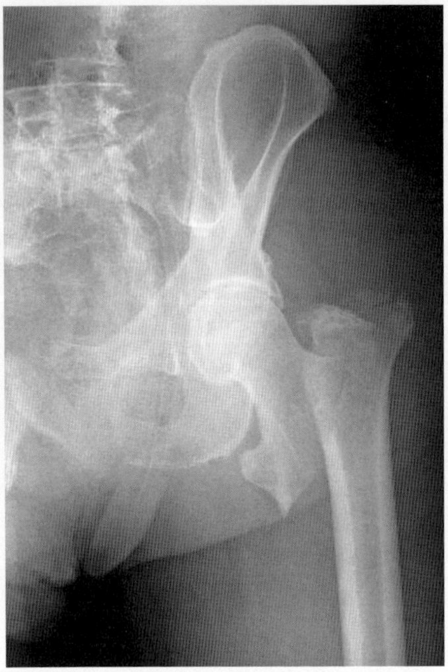

Fig 2.2-23 Judet left oblique view of the left hip. Note that the patient's left obturator foramen is "open" in this view, despite the combined severe deformity of the unstable pelvic ring fracture plus the trochanteric displaced fracture.

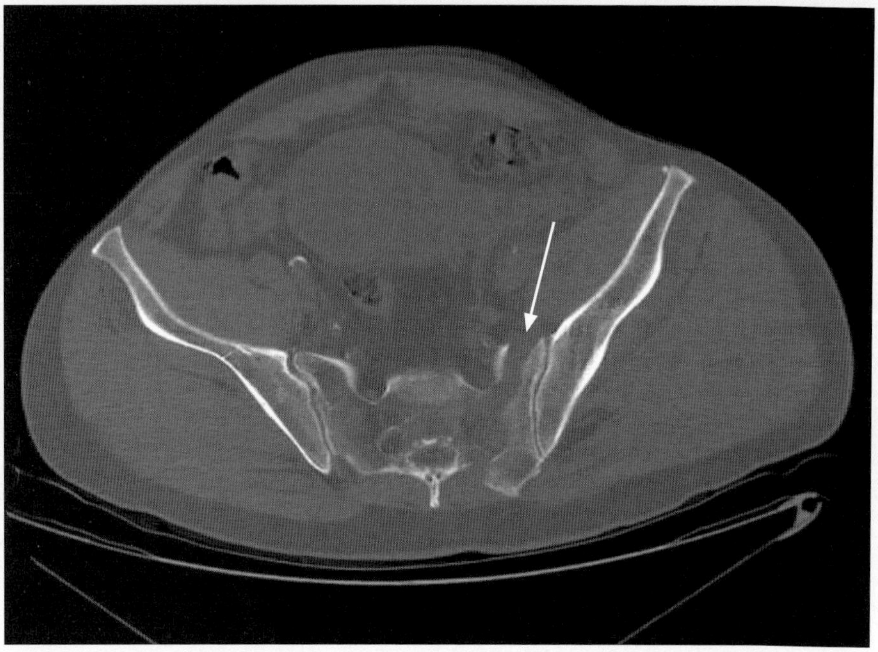

Fig 2.2-24 Two-dimensional computed tomographic (CT) scan showing an axial view of the pelvis. The arrow points to the left sacral fracture.

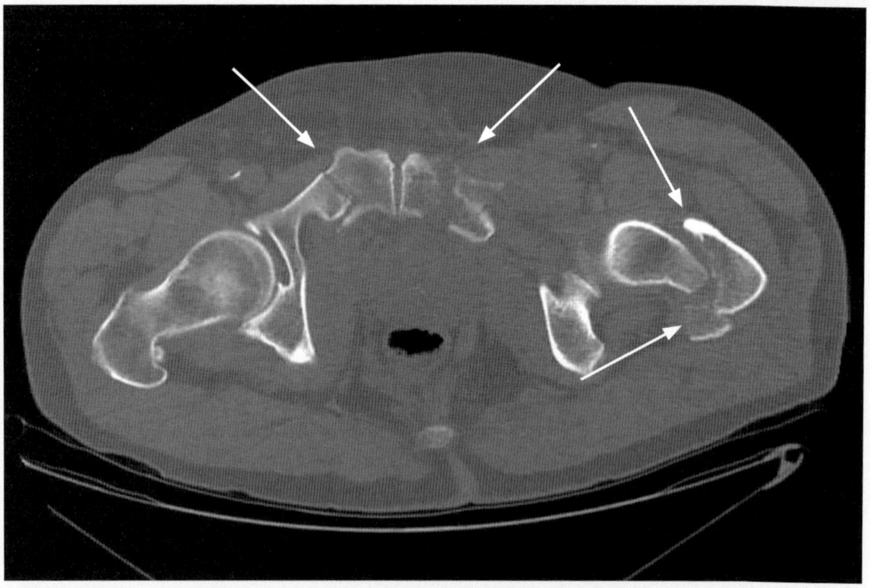

Fig 2.2-25 Two-dimensional computed tomographic (CT) scan showing an axial view of the pelvis. The arrows point to the fractures in both pelvic branches and the comminuted fracture of the lateral trochanteric wall.

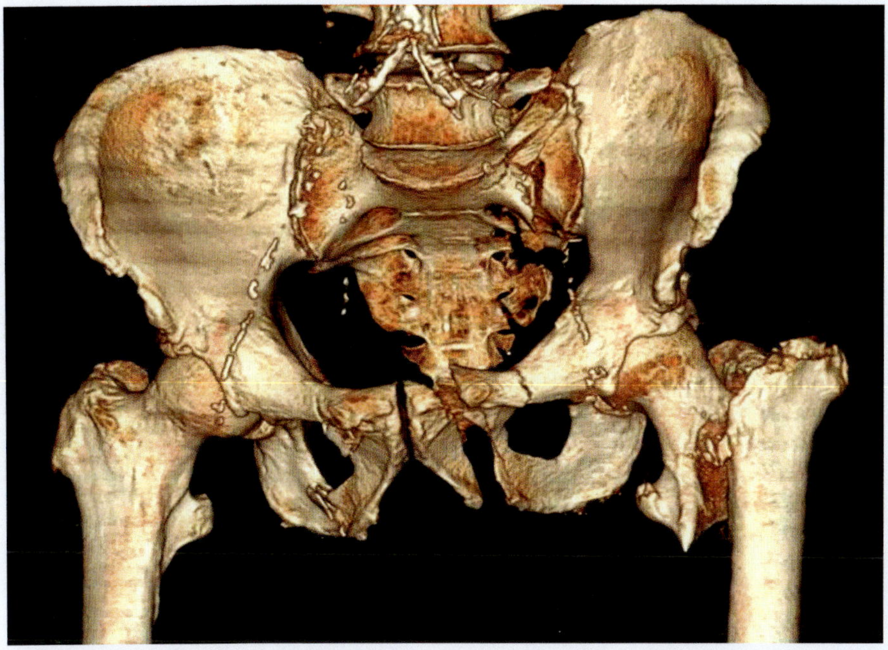

Fig 2.2-26 Three-dimensional computed tomographic scan of the pelvis showing the complex combination of an unstable pelvic ring fracture plus trochanteric fracture with comminution of the trochanteric lateral wall.

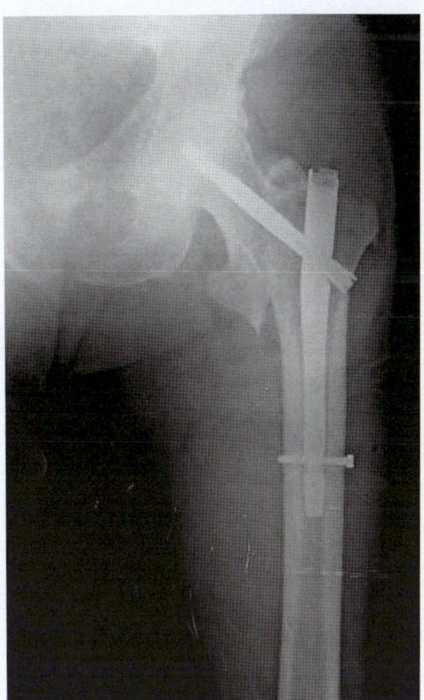

Fig 2.2-27 Postoperative AP x-ray of the first trochanteric intramedullary nail. Note that the fracture is not properly reduced with shortening and extra external rotation, and the neck offset is altered.

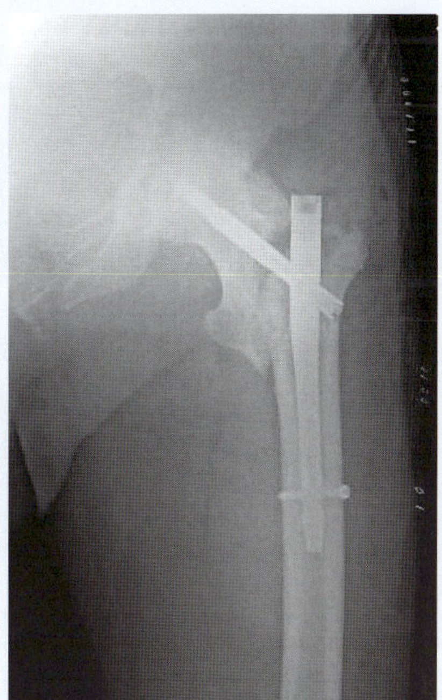

Fig 2.2-28 Postoperative oblique view of the first trochanteric intramedullary nail. Note that the fracture is not properly reduced with a wide fracture gap and the femoral neck rotated and slightly flexed, which indicates that the two main fragments are fixed in different planes.

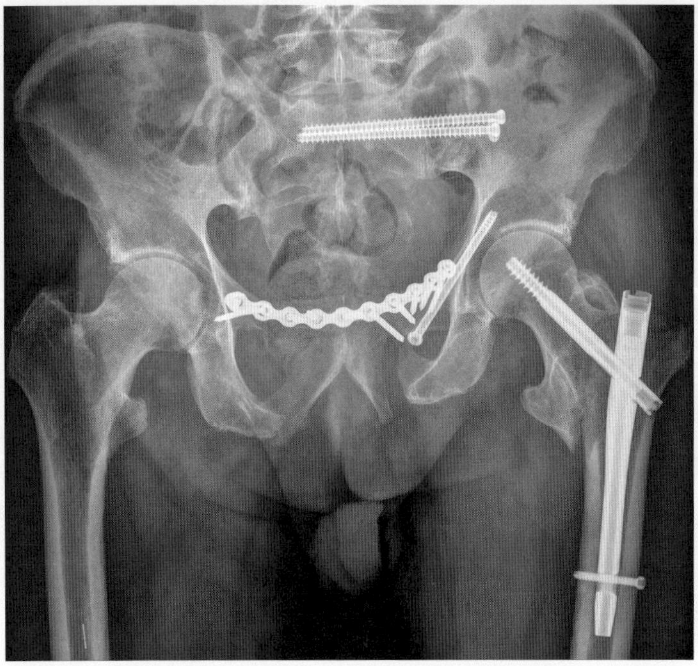

Fig 2.2-29 Postoperative AP view of the pelvic internal fixation: two sacroiliac screws, anterior reconstruction plate to close the "open book", and an isolated cannulated screw in the left iliopubic branch.

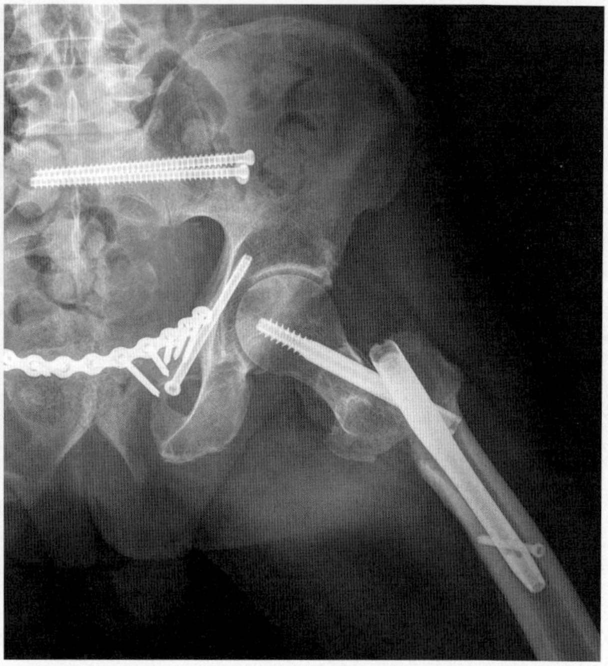

Fig 2.2-30 Axial view of the left hemipelvis and left proximal femur, showing a correct osteosynthesis of the fractures of the pelvic ring and an absence of reduction of the trochanteric fracture where the femoral neck is in a different plane to the trochanteric zone and the femoral shaft.

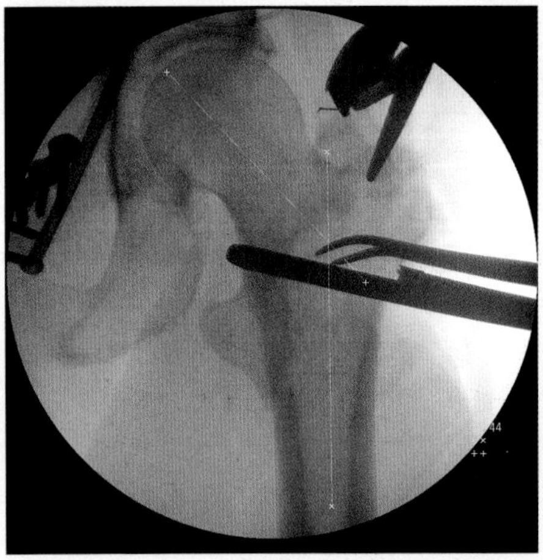

Fig 2.2-31 C-arm control AP view after achieving an open reduction using pointed clamps and a collinear clamp. The angle of the intramedullary trochanteric nail is calculated on the C-arm screen.

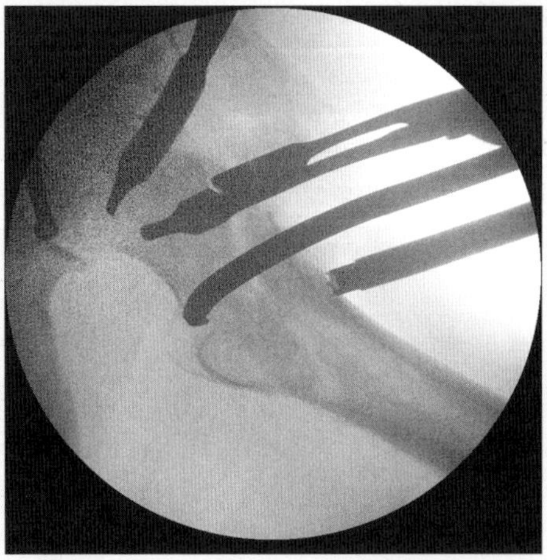

Fig 2.2-32 C-arm control axial view after achieving an open reduction using pointed and collinear clamps. The femoral neck axis is in line with the femoral shaft. This stable situation technically helps the introduction of the implant.

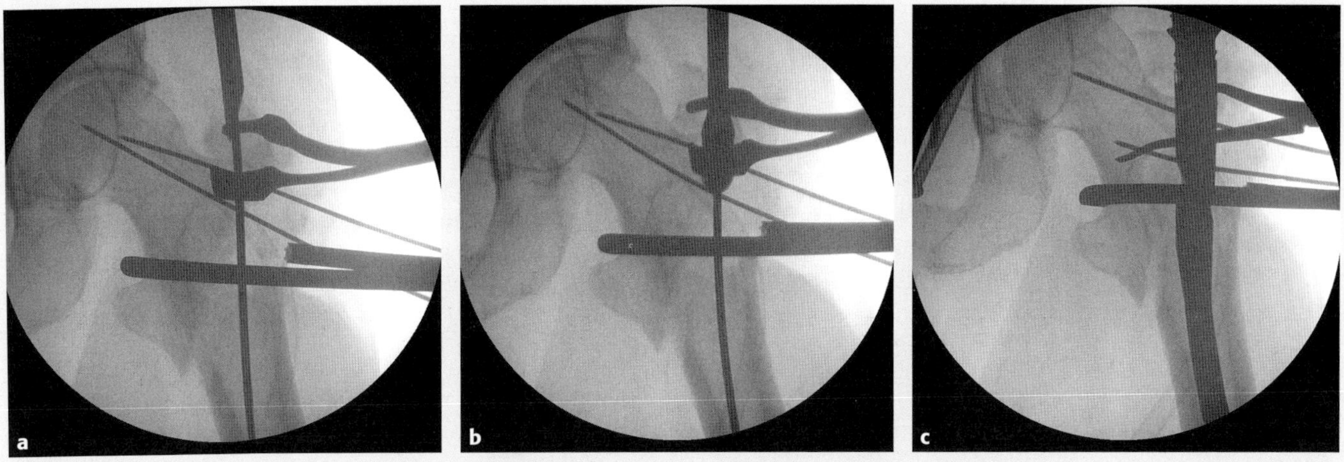

Fig 2.2-33a–c During the drilling–reaming process and the introduction of the nail, it could be necessary to fix the main fracture fragments with temporary K-wires to avoid the loss of reduction. Reaming and hammering should be done with gentle movements, taking care not to lose reduction or to damage instruments or temporary K-wires in each technical step.

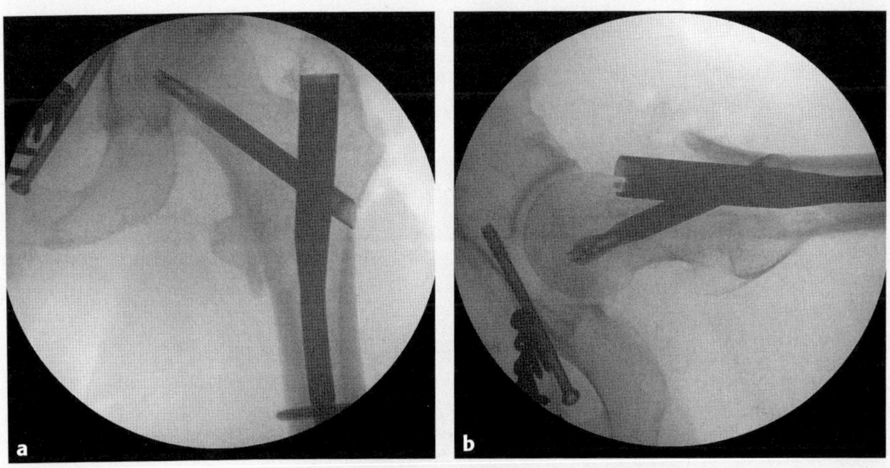

Fig 2.2-34a–b AP (**a**) and axial (**b**) C-arm view of the final intraoperative result. The shortening and malrotation have been corrected.

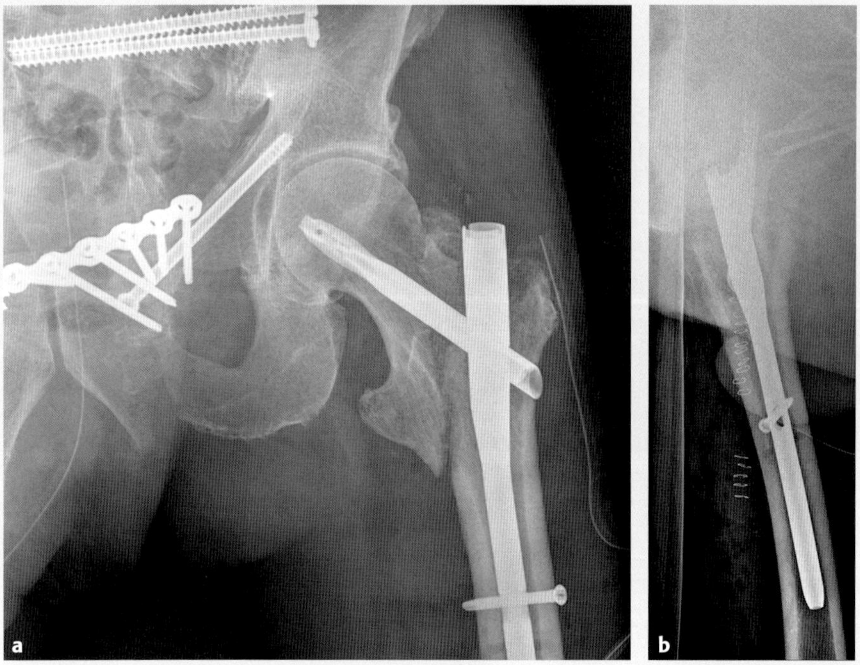

Fig 2.2-35a–b Postoperative AP (**a**) and axial (**b**) control x-rays.

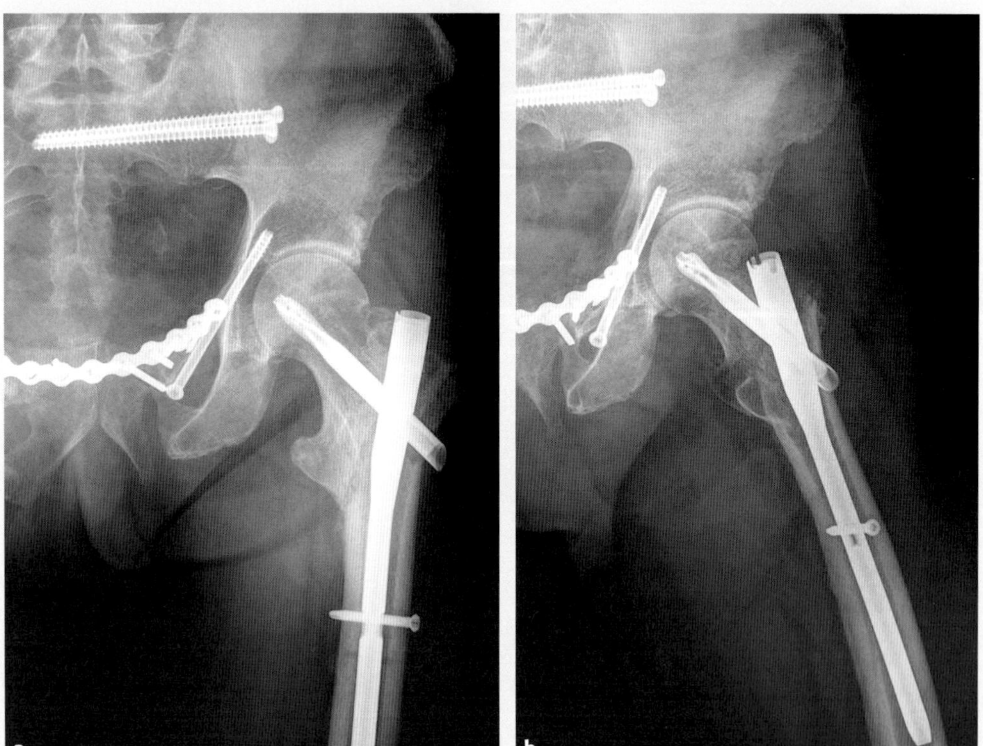

Fig 2.2-36a–b AP (**a**) and axial (**b**) control x-rays at 3 months showing the consolidation of the trochanteric fracture.

Analysis of failure and reflection

The first doubt that arises when analyzing this case is the order of actions. Once the patient is stabilized, which fracture should be treated surgically first? The pelvic ring or the proximal femoral fracture?

Confronted with a polytrauma patient with unstable pelvic fracture, minimal retroperitoneal hemorrhage, and a high-energy trochanteric fracture, what is the best and safest surgical schedule?

It is correct to make a good diagnosis and stabilize the patient knowing that the pelvic injury needs to be treated at another hospital, involving transfer. However, is it then correct to perform surgery on the proximal femoral fracture before the transfer?

This floating hip has great challenges with the choice of a surgical table or the traction strategy to align and reduce the proximal femoral fracture.

To achieve a good reduction without a traction table, the surgeon and surgical team must be technically experienced and very skilled. The surgical team needs to know how to manage this kind of fracture on a radiolucent table, and it also needs to know technical tricks for reduction using reduction tools like pointed clamps, bone clamps, and collinear clamps.

Once the failure or the problem has been detected, rescue surgery should be carried out as quickly as possible to minimize the potential local and systemic complications and to avoid a fracture healing in malunion.

Final outcome

Both fractures have made good progress and are healing. Load bearing with assisted weight started at 12 weeks after the pelvic ring surgery. The surgical wounds evolved correctly. The patient sustained mild and sporadic pain, which is controlled with low-level painkillers.

Key points to remember

- The reduction of the fracture creates stability until consolidation by favoring load transmission more uniformly over the whole bone-implant structure rather than just over the healthy bone.
- A fracture must be properly reduced.
- Mechanical needs are different in fractures depending on whether they occur in the diaphysis or joint.
- Not all fractures require a strictly anatomical reduction to achieve adequate function; the concept of anatomical reduction therefore evolves into functional reduction.
- In compression fractures, compressed anatomical reduction and osteosynthesis with absolute stability are essential.
- Diaphyseal fractures require a functional reduction while respecting the vascularization, with correct alignment of the bone and limb, recovery of bone length, and avoiding axial displacement and rotation.

References and suggested reading

Afsari A, Liporace F, Lindvall E, et al. Clamp-assisted reduction of high subtrochanteric fractures of the femur: surgical technique. *J Bone Joint Surg Am.* 2010 Sep;92 Suppl 1 Pt 2:217–225.
Brunner A, Thormann S, Babst R. Minimally invasive percutaneous plating of proximal humeral shaft fractures with the Proximal Humerus Internal Locking System (PHILOS). *J Shoulder Elbow Surg.* 2012 Aug;21(8):1056–1063.
Carr JB. The anterior and medial reduction of intertrochanteric fractures: a simple method to obtain a stable reduction. *J Orthop Trauma.* 2007 Aug;21(7):485–489.
Furman BD, Olson SA, Guilak F. The development of posttraumatic arthritis after articular fracture. *J Orthop Trauma.* 2006 Nov-Dec;20(10):719–725.
Mast J, Jakob R, Ganz R. *Planning and Reduction Technique in Fracture Surgery.* Berlin Heidelberg: Springer-Verlag; 1989.
Mohan R, Karthikeyan R, Sonanis SV. Dynamic hip screw: does side make a difference? Effects of clockwise torque on right and left DHS. *Injury.* 2000 Nov;31(9):697–699.
Pape HC, Tarkin IS. Intraoperative reduction techniques for difficult femoral fractures. *J Orthop Trauma.* 2009 May–Jun;23(5 Suppl):S6–11.
Park J, Yang KH. Correction of malalignment in proximal femoral nailing — Reduction technique of displaced proximal fragment. *Injury.* 2010 Jun;41(6):634–638.
Peters AC, Lafferty PM, Jacobson AR, et al. The Effect of Articular Reduction After Fractures on Posttraumatic Degenerative Arthritis: A Critical Analysis Review. *JBJS Rev.* 2013 Dec 24;1(2).
Schatzker J. Intra-articular Fractures. In: Schatzker J, Tile M, ed. *The Rationale of Operative Fracture Care.* 3rd ed. Berlin Heidelberg: Springer-Verlag; 2005:33–43.
Schenker ML, Mauck RL, Ahn J, et al. Pathogenesis and prevention of posttraumatic osteoarthritis after intra-articular fracture. *J Am Acad Orthop Surg.* 2014 Jan;22(1):20–28.

2.3 Principles of stability, selection of implants, and the combination of absolute and relative stability

Reto Babst, Frank Beeres, Jaroslaw Brudnicki, Matej Cimerman, Joan Girós Torres, Björn Link, Roberto Rivero Sosa, J Miquel Sales Pérez, Matevž Tomaževič, Miquel Videla Cés

Man is always disposed to deny everything that is incomprehensible to him.

Blaise Pascal

Osteosynthesis is the surgical procedure used to stabilize bone fragments through use of implants, taking into account the rules of both biology and mechanics. The surgical technique is demanding and essential for achieving the aim of osteosynthesis, ie, to restore the bone's anatomy, achieve sufficient and lasting stability between bone fragments while the healing callus forms, and enable immediate pain-free function.

Stability is the fracture's capacity to resist functional weight bearing. A stable osteosynthesis enables fixation of the bone fragments during the time necessary for the consolidation of the fracture. Surgeons must account for the mechanical aspects of the internal fixation according to its stability.

Principles of stability

Absolute stability: Absolute stability is the absence of mobility on the surfaces of the fracture when subjected to functional weight bearing. It requires anatomical reduction without diastasis at the site. This is only achieved if interfragmentary compression is performed using traction screws or a prestressed plate with axial compression effects. This stimulates vascular proliferation across the fracture site that may heal by direct consolidation with osteonal remodeling, without a periosteal callus, thus achieving direct consolidation. Direct consolidation is a consequence of the biomechanical conditions that exist and not in itself an objective.

Absolute stability requires a balance between fracture stabilization and biological aggression, ie, damage to biology. It needs the correct indication, anatomical reduction, and interfragmentary compression. It requires a demanding surgical technique with minimal vascular injury. Absolute stability has positive effects on vascularization because in conditions of stability the blood vessels can cross the fracture site more easily.

Absolute mechanical stability evolves towards direct, intercortical, vascular, Haversian consolidation with a primary intention callus of an intramembranous type without x-ray imaging.

Relative stability: In diaphyseal fractures the concept of stability has evolved to recommend relative stability especially for multifragmentary fractures. The evolution of the principles for the treatment of diaphyseal fractures has led us to not demand strict anatomical reductions that cause manipulation of the fragments with additional bone devascularization. In diaphyseal fractures of the long bones, the aim of reduction is to recover the length of the bone, correct alignment of the axis, and avoid axial rotations, which should be maintained during mobilization. Vascularization must be preserved and with this, functionality recovered.

In relative stability, a controlled movement exists between the bone fragments. Sufficient movement must exist to stimulate tissue differentiation, but always below critical strain levels (over 5% but below 30%).

Relative stability produces indirect consolidation by secondary intention, stimulating the formation of fibrocartilaginous callus which is substituted secondarily by radiographically visible bone tissue. The callus formation depends on the size of the interfragmentary movements.

Indications of stability

Absolute stability: in joint fractures, in forearm fractures, and in diaphyseal fractures with a simple pattern when intramedullary osteosynthesis is not indicated.

Relative stability: in multifragmentary metaphyseal and diaphyseal fractures.

Combined stability: in joint fractures with multifragmentary diaphyseal impact, requiring anatomical reduction and absolute stability in the joint area and the application of relative stability in the multifragmentary metaphyseal and diaphyseal areas.

Nowadays, opinions on the use of combined stability in simple fractures of the metaphysis and/or diaphysis are divided. Absolute *or* relative stability can be used when applied judiciously.

Implant selection

As for selection of the implant, surgeons must remember that no implant is rigid. All have some degree of elasticity and flexibility, depending on their dimensions. It is important to make the most of implant characteristics to achieve optimum mechanical performance and to secure the best adaptation between bone and implant. On occasion, implants will have to be prebent before placement if they are not already shaped or do not fit the specific anatomy of each case. With simple diaphyseal fractures, plates that are straight before use should be bent in slight flexion to exercise better compression on the opposite cortex. At the tibial diaphysis they should also be bent in torsion to adapt better to the bone. The insertion of screws must be performed in a judicious and ordered way to facilitate adaptation to the anatomy and permit adequate distribution between fixation and elasticity. Repeated manipulations of the implants must be avoided to prevent erosion of the external layer of the metal that may weaken the material or encourage corrosion.

Intramedullary nails are not very elastic so they are manufactured to cater to the needs of their specific placement or adaptation to the bone, and their indications must be respected. It is also important to bear in mind these characteristics when planning their placement following reaming and/or locking.

For the placement of implants, it is essential to have perfect knowledge of both the instruments to be used and the congruency between the implants that make up the whole ensemble.

Case description

A 38-year-old woman, with no history of medical issues of interest, suffered a horse-riding accident while on holiday. The initial x-rays showed a complete fracture of the tibial plateau of the right knee (AO/OTA 41C3.1; Schatzker type V fracture, depression/flexion/ varus). The fracture affects the lateral, medial, and posterior columns in accordance with the Luo classification (**Fig 2.3-1**) [Luo, 2010; Schatzker, 1979].

After the local inflammation reduced, the knee was operated on in the holiday locality. Five weeks after surgical treatment, she presented at our clinic. Her leg was immobilized with a plaster cast and she was walking with crutches but without bearing weight. The postoperative x-rays and computed tomographic scans are shown in **Fig 2.3-2**.

The patient underwent a reintervention 6 weeks following the initial operation. With a medial approach (**Fig 2.3-3a**), the articular fracture of the medial tibial plateau was reduced (**Fig 2.3-3b**). The posterior column was reinforced with a posterior tibial locking compression plate (LCP), and a one-third tube-type plate functioning like an anterior tension band was used to stabilize the medial column (**Fig 2.3-3c–h**).

The lateral side was reduced through the initial incision that was extended proximally and distally (**Fig 2.3-4a**). The anterior tibial compartment was opened and the fibula exposed after marking the peroneal nerve (**Fig 2.3-4b**). An osteotomy of the fibular head was performed (**Fig 2.3-4c**) and of Gerdy's tubercle with the attached iliotibial band (**Fig 2.3-4d**).

Additional osteotomy of the lateral tibial platform was performed to approach the impacted intraarticular part of the external tibial plateau (**Fig 2.3-5a**) and reconstruction of the plateau, including the posterior margin, which was reinforced from the posterior part with a one-third tubular plate (**Fig 2.3-5b**). The impacted subchondral area was filled with porous bone graft material and hydroxyapatite.

Subsequently, the external tibial plateau was reduced and a proximal tibial LCP was adapted to support the lateral column (**Fig 2.3-6**). The head of the fibula was fixed with a 3.5 mm screw. The meniscus was joined once more to the capsule and the meniscotibial (coronary) ligament and sutured to the plate. Postoperative passive mobilization began on the first postoperative day. A partial weight of 15 kg was allowed during the first 12 postoperative weeks, after which the load was progressively increased to full weight bearing.

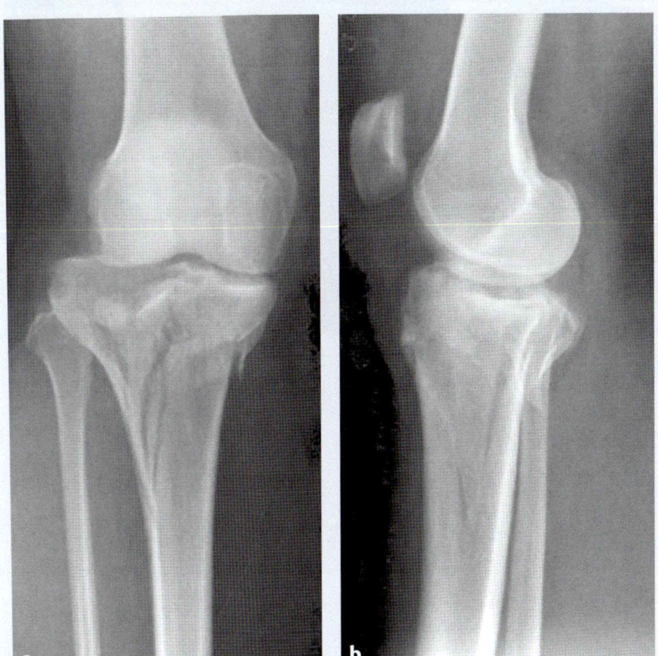

Fig 2.3-1a–b Preoperative AP and lateral x-rays of the fractured right knee.

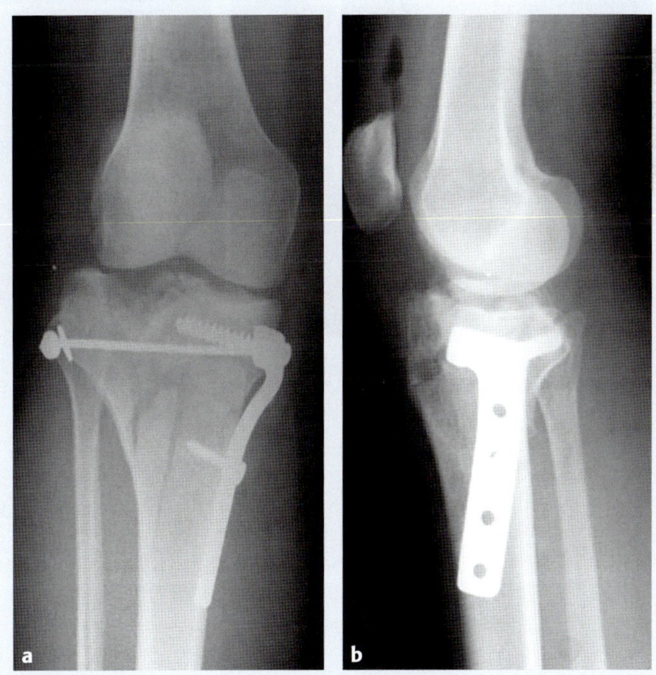

Fig 2.3-2a–h X-rays and computed tomographic (CT) scans after initial surgery.
a–b Postoperative AP and profile lateral x-rays.

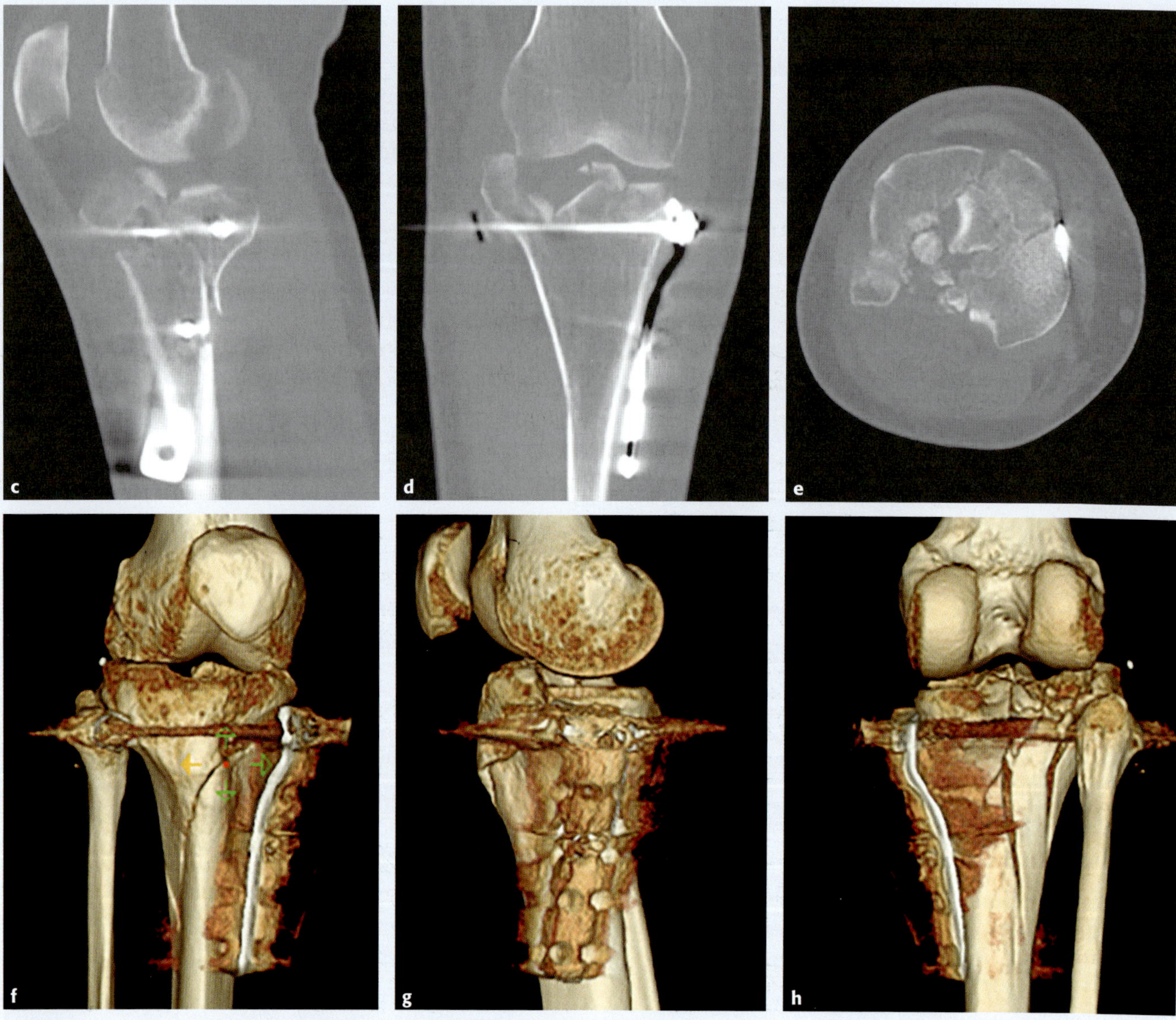

Fig 2.3-2a–h (cont) X-rays and computed tomographic (CT) scans after initial surgery.
c–h Computed tomographic scan 5 weeks after osteosynthesis. The CT image shows a reduction failure in the medial plateau and of the lateral plateau. The posterior column is not corrected either.

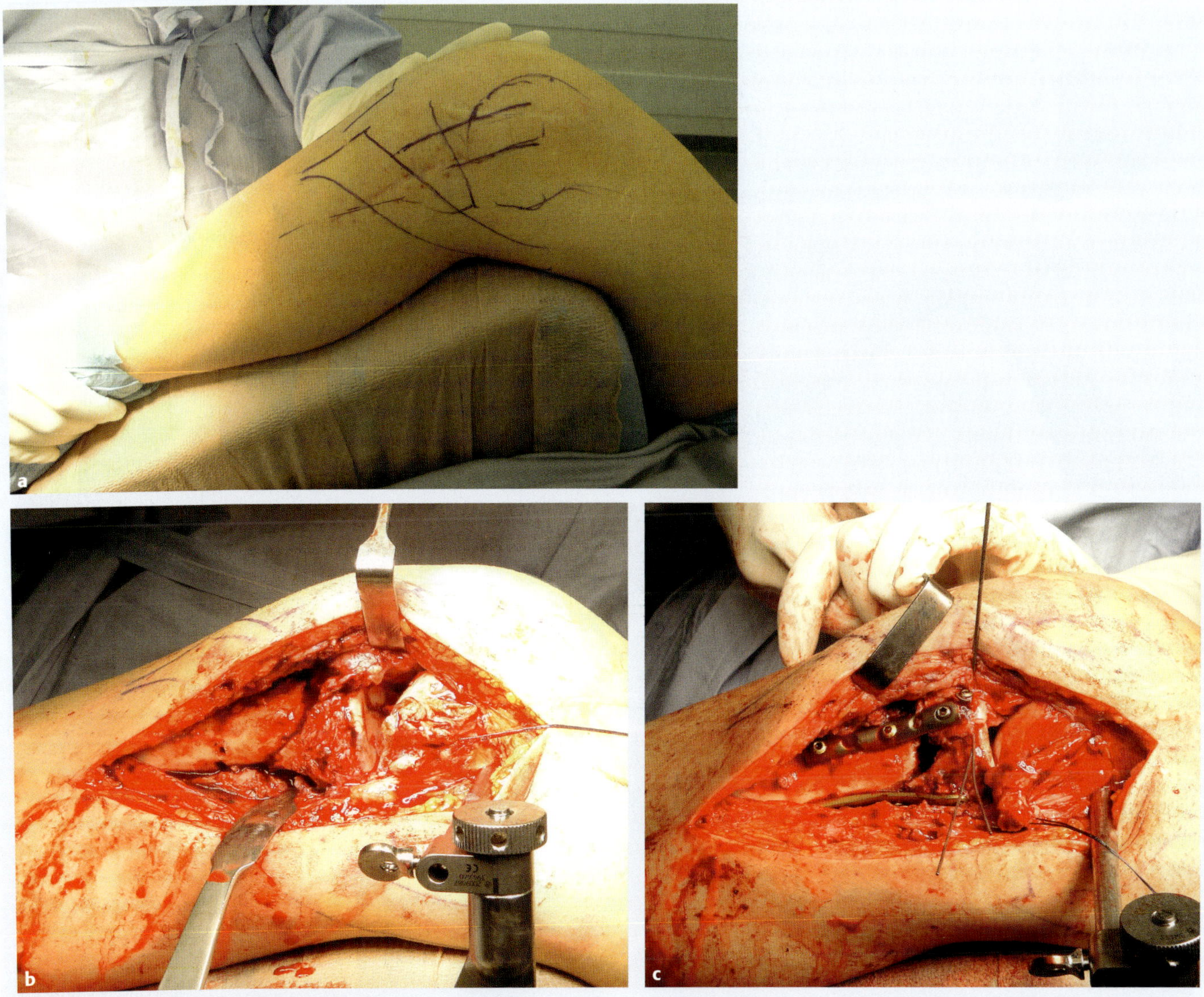

Fig 2.3-3a–c Intraoperative photographs of the surgical reintervention on the medial side.

a Reference points on the medial side.

b Medial tibial plateau with intraarticular fracture and posterior column fracture using a distractor to help the reduction.

c Medial tibial plateau reduced with a posterior locking compression plate, sustaining plate, and a plate functioning like an anterior tension band.

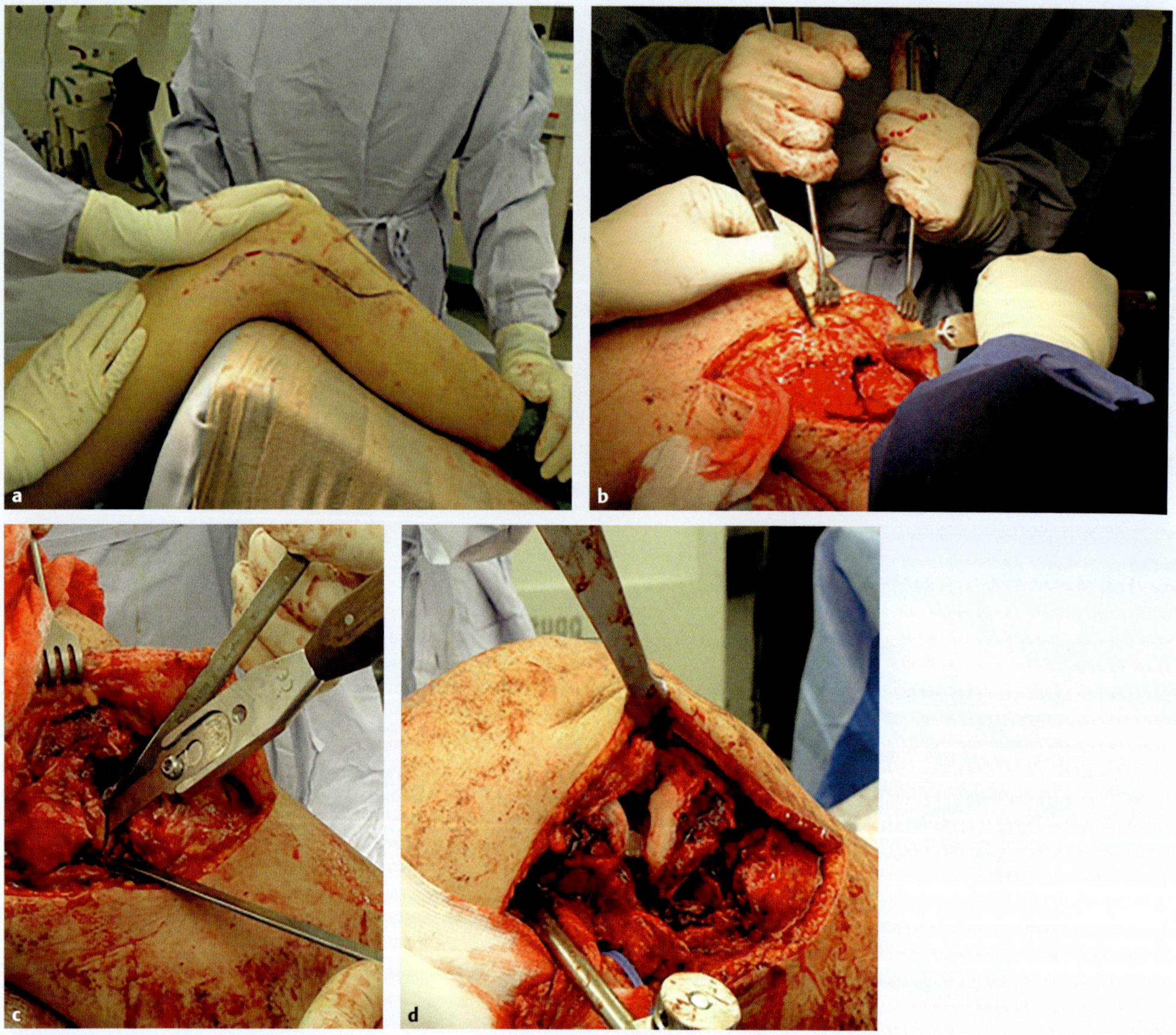

Fig 2.3-4a–d Intraoperative photographs of the surgical reintervention on the lateral side.
a Reference points for the lateral extended incision.
b Incision of the anterior compartment and marking of the peroneal nerve.
c Fibular head osteotomy.
d Gerdy's tubercle osteotomy and direct view of the external tibial plateau.

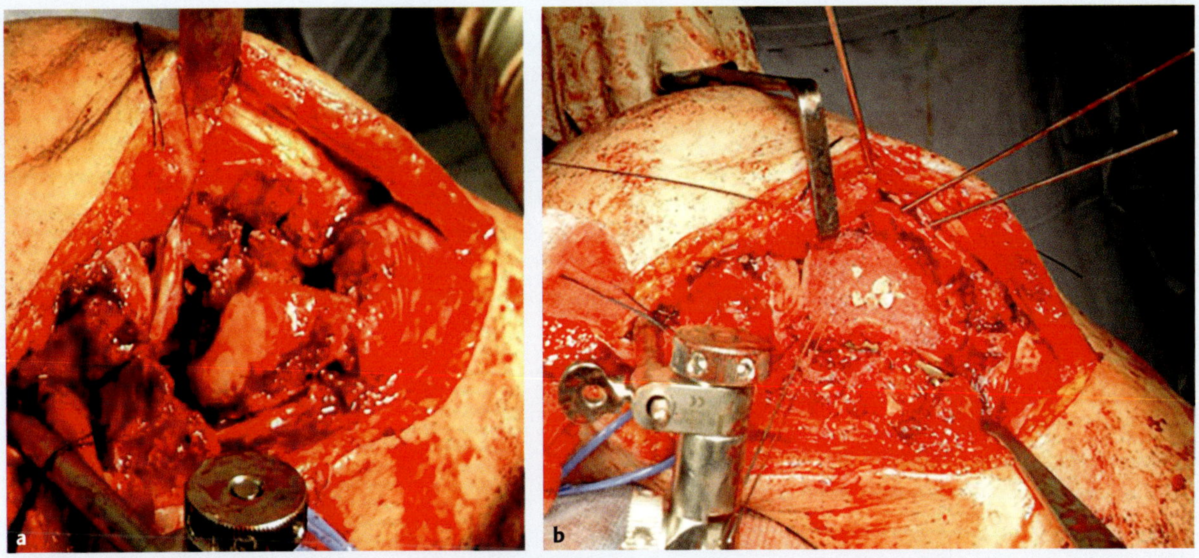

Fig 2.3-5a–b Intraoperative photographs of the osteotomy, reduction, and grafting of the external tibial plateau.
a Anterior osteotomy of the lateral tibial plateau with articular fracture and area including the posterior column.
b Reduction of the intraarticular fracture and filling with porous bone graft.

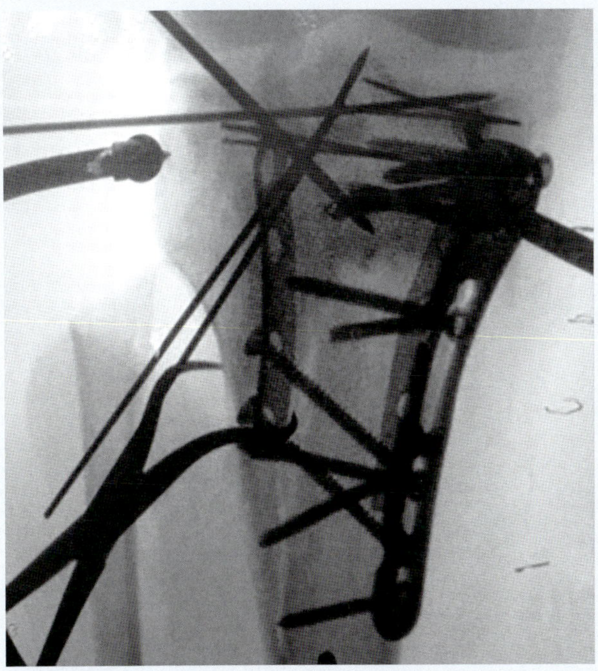

Fig 2.3-6 Intraoperative C-arm control of the lateral reconstruction.

Analysis of failure and reflection

There was inadequate preoperative planning, without a CT scan, probably due to a lack of resources.

The fracture was treated adequately on the medial side, reinforcing the medial column, as a reference for the lateral column. However, the stability of the medial construction using two short screws on the articulation block and a single unicortical screw on the diaphysis did not allow adequate stability. The medial articular region was not reduced.

The posterior column was not treated. The flexion forces were therefore not neutralized and the lateral articular line was not reduced. Compression was applied between the medial and lateral columns with an interfragmentary compression screw to reduce the width of the tibial platform. The lateral column was neither approached nor stabilized with a supporting plate. The flexion forces on the anterior side were not neutralized.

This case shows an open internal fixation without any fracture reduction, an inadequate choice of implants due to poor planning, a lack of stability, and poor execution technique.

If the adequate resources were not available, the patient should have been transferred to another institution with adequate facilities capable of providing good treatment for complex fractures of this type. However, the patient was also partly responsible because she did not want to return to her place of residence before the end of her holidays.

Final outcome

After 2.5 years, the implants were removed due to pain in the distal end of the lateral plate. Five years after the operation the patient is working part-time (50%) as a midwife. She takes no medication and is able to perform her activities of daily living independently. Her ambulatory capacity is 3–4 hours due to knee pain and water on the knee (knee effusion). She has a stable knee and a range of motion of 0–0–110° (**Fig 2.3-7**).

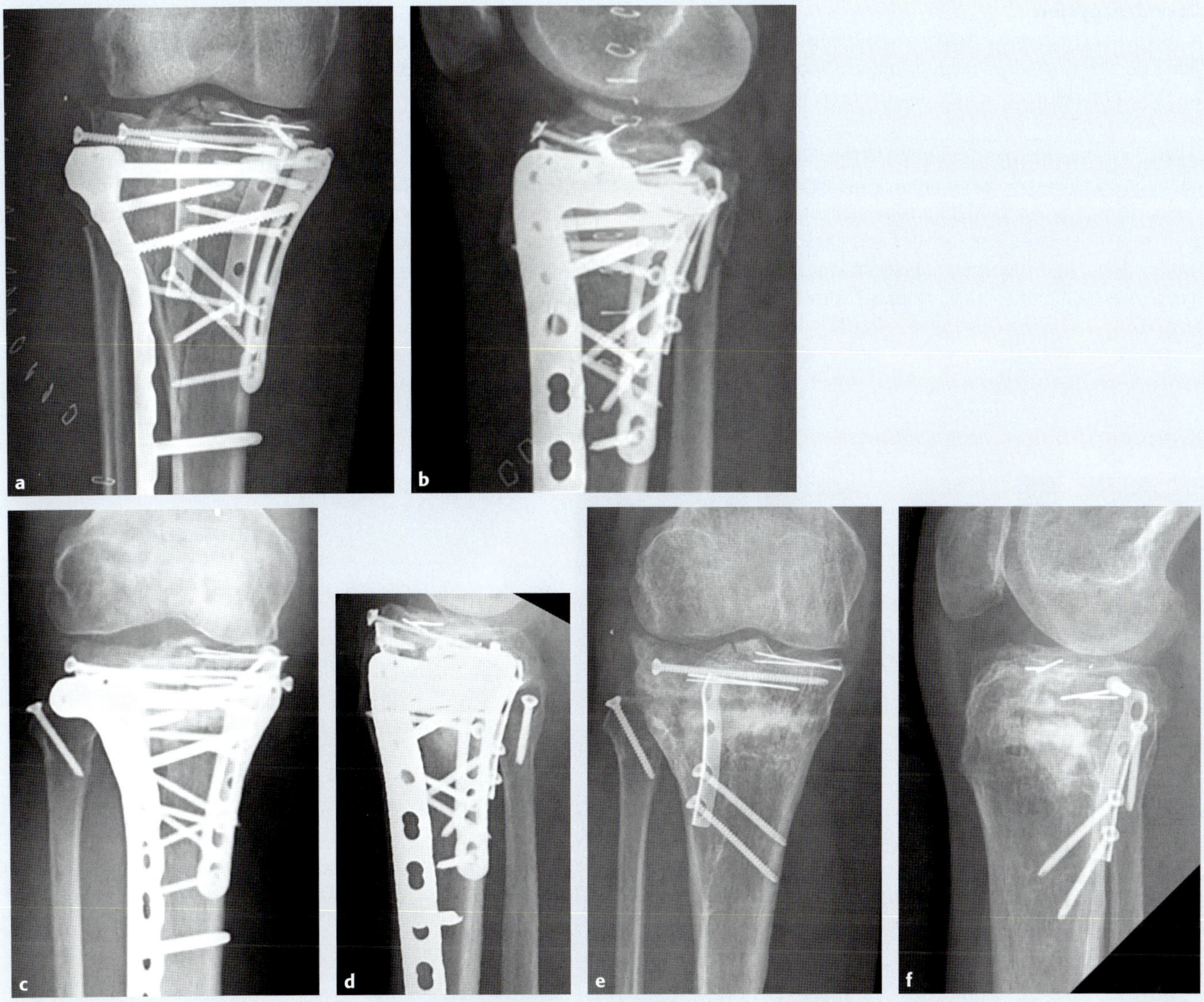

Fig 2.3-7a–f Final x-rays.
a–b Postoperative x-rays.
c–d Postoperative control x-rays at 1 year.
e–f Control x-rays 5 years after the operation following removal of the osteosynthesis material.

CASE 2

Case description

A 46-year-old man with a history of motorbike accidents presented with a possibly multifragmentary diaphyseal fracture of the left femur with two or three intermediate fragments (AO/OTA 32C3).

Surgical intervention was performed to stabilize the fracture, using an intramedullary nail. Subsequent reinterventions were required due to delayed union, in which an iliac crest bone graft plus a bone graft substitute composed of demineralized bone matrix, nail dynamization, and subsequent replacement of the intramedullary nail plus bone morphogenetic protein-2 were performed.

The patient consulted the surgeon because of "mechanical" pain in the left thigh and discomfort in the region of the trochanter and knee. Notable in the physical examination was his stature: 178 cm tall and weighed 105 kg. Hip and knee were able to move freely without pain and the thighs were very muscular. There was a leg-length discrepancy of 3 cm. Visible on the x-ray was a bone callus on the fracture site suggestive of partial union with possible pseudarthrosis, narrow cortices, and a nail of appropriate diameter. A computed tomographic scan showed partial union. Blood tests showed 7,300 leukocytes, an erythrocyte sedimentation rate of 7, and C-reactive protein of 1.10 mg/L. Bone scintigraphy showed persistent bone remodeling suggestive of pseudarthrosis in the middle third of the left femur (**Fig 2.3-8**).

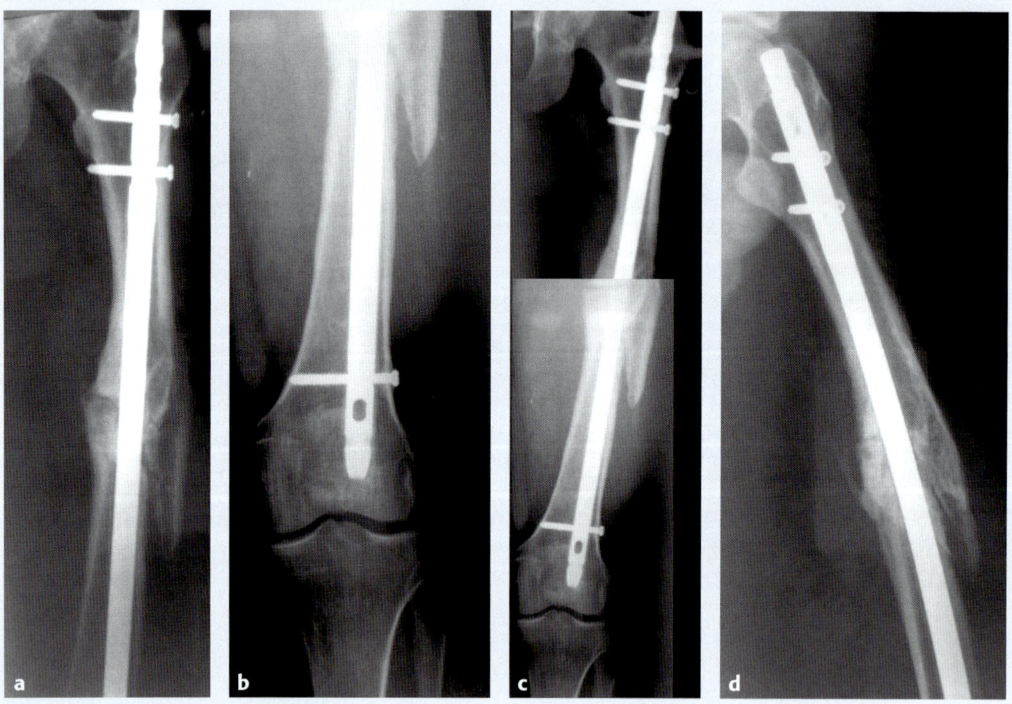

Fig 2.3-8a–u Preoperative images taken for case evaluation.
a–d X-rays showing AP and lateral views of the femur.

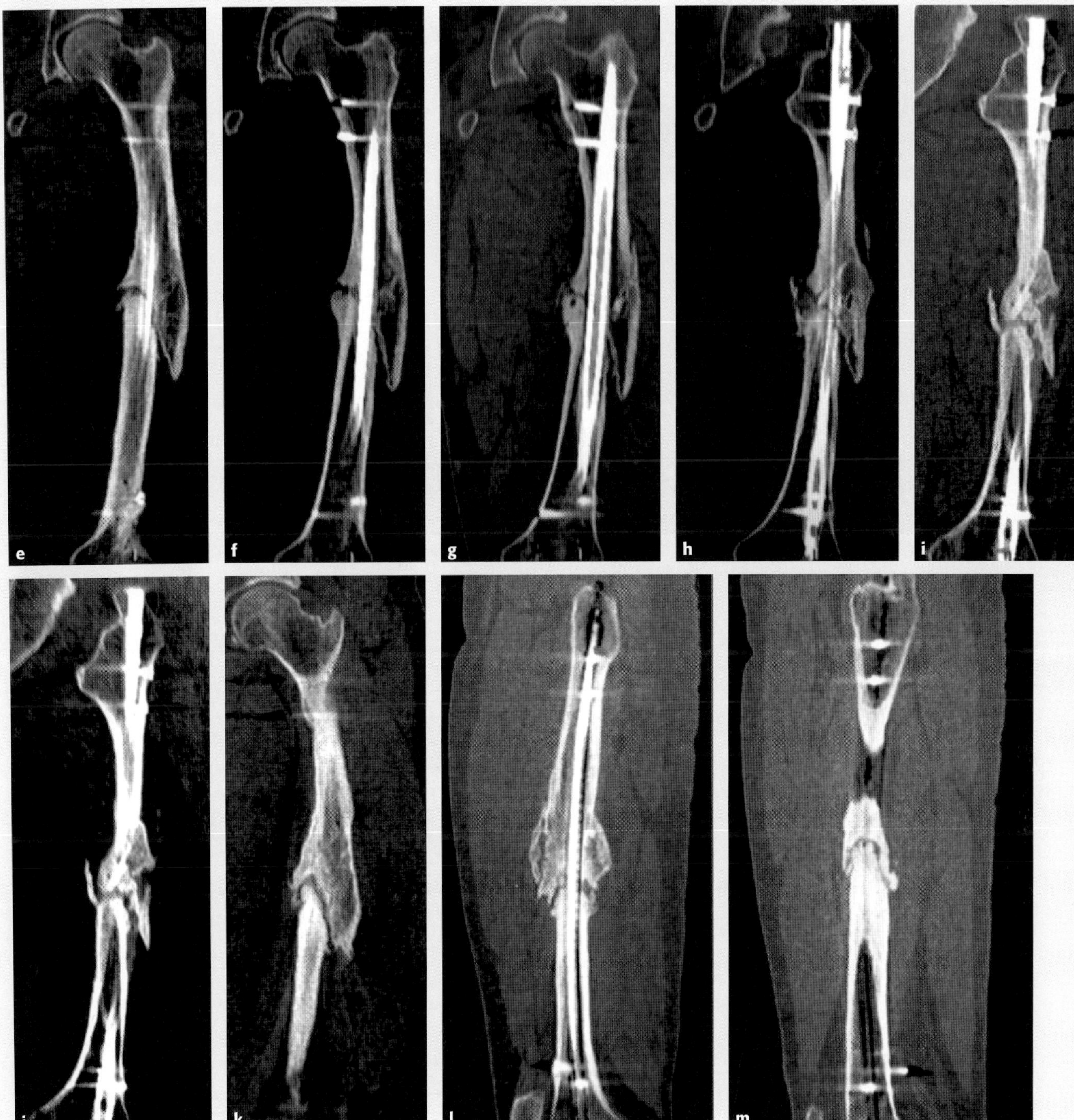

Fig 2.3-8a–u (cont) Preoperative images taken for case evaluation.
e–k Study of the femoral pseudarthrosis through computed tomographic (CT) scan in AP views.
l–m Study of the femoral pseudarthrosis through CT scan in lateral view.

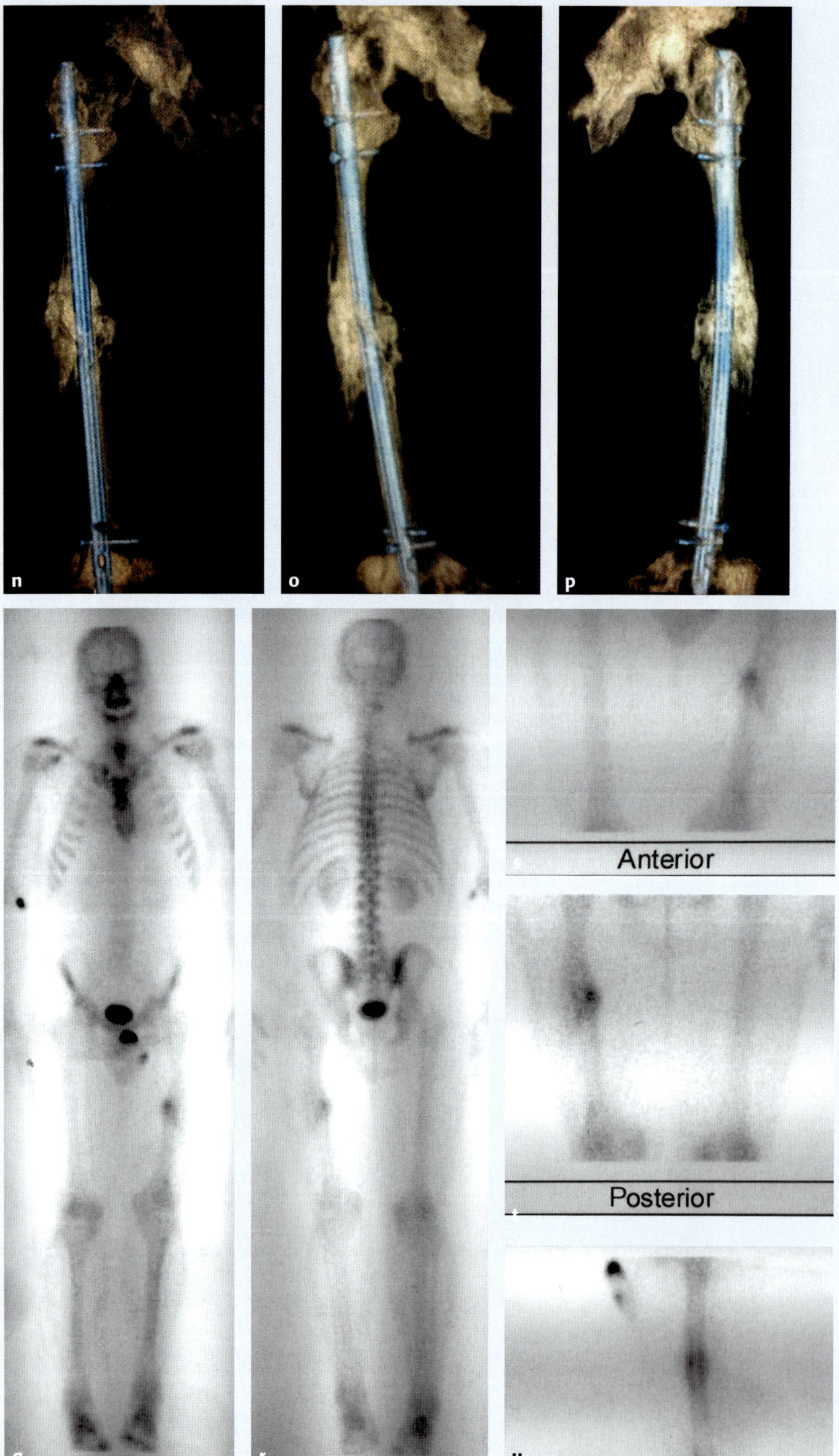

Fig 2.3-8a–u (cont) Preoperative images taken for case evaluation.
n–p Study of the femoral pseudarthrosis through 3D CT scan reconstruction.
q–u Study of the femoral pseudarthrosis through bone scintigraphy.

Analysis of failure and reflection

Both mechanical and biological factors play a key role in the fracture consolidation process. The two types are not mutually exclusive but they must meet sufficient conditions to favor fracture healing. On occasion, even well planned and technically well executed interventions can result in nonunion, which means that the patient does not recover as expected.

In this particular case, repeated interventions have tried to favor the biological (ie, bone grafting and use of growth factors) and mechanical (ie, nail dynamization and its exchange with another reamed larger diameter nail) factors but have not managed to provide sufficient stability and biology to achieve complete consolidation of the fracture site.

In these cases, the surgeons must reflect on the reasons behind the nonunion. Repeating techniques have proven not to achieve the expected results. The surgeons must determine the factors that may negatively affect the fracture to try to better stabilize the forces that counteract stability and give biological feasibility to a site which has been operated on previously.

Final outcome

Given the clinical data and test results that rule out infection, a new intervention is proposed to heal the pseudarthrosis while the leg-length dissymmetry must be accepted. Through decortication, keeping the nailing and additional stabilization with a locking compression plate (used as a protection or augmentation plate) joined to the femoral plate through proximal and distal locking-attachment plates (LAP), greater stability against rotational loads and flexion is provided. A generous decortication will bring biology to the consolidation process (**Fig 2.3-9a–q**).

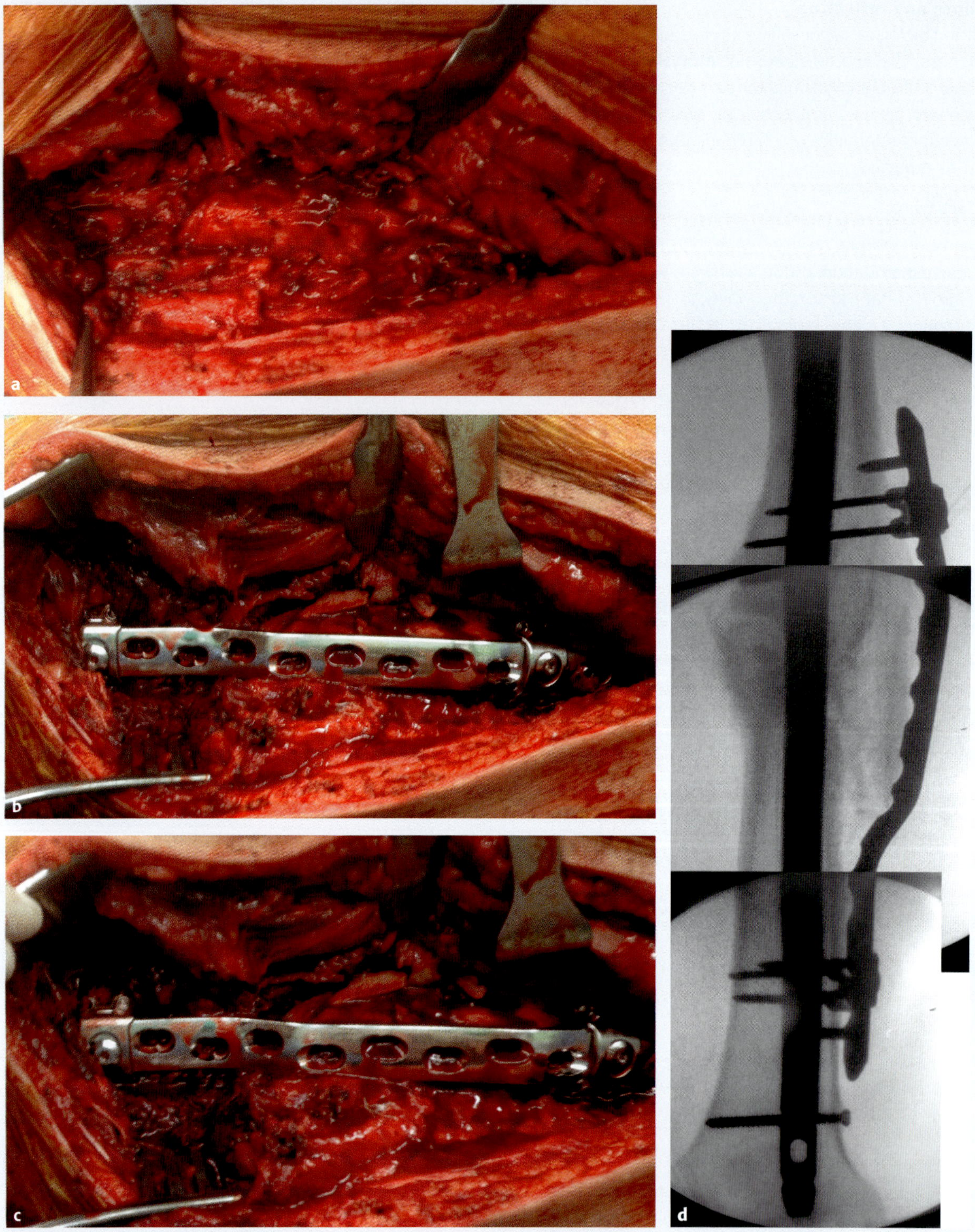

Fig 2.3-9a–q Clinical photographs and x-rays obtained up until consolidation of the fracture.
a–c Intraoperative photographs of the surgical intervention for decortication, bone graft, and stabilization with locking compression wave plate and locking-attachment plate.
d Intraoperative control x-ray taken with an image intensifier.

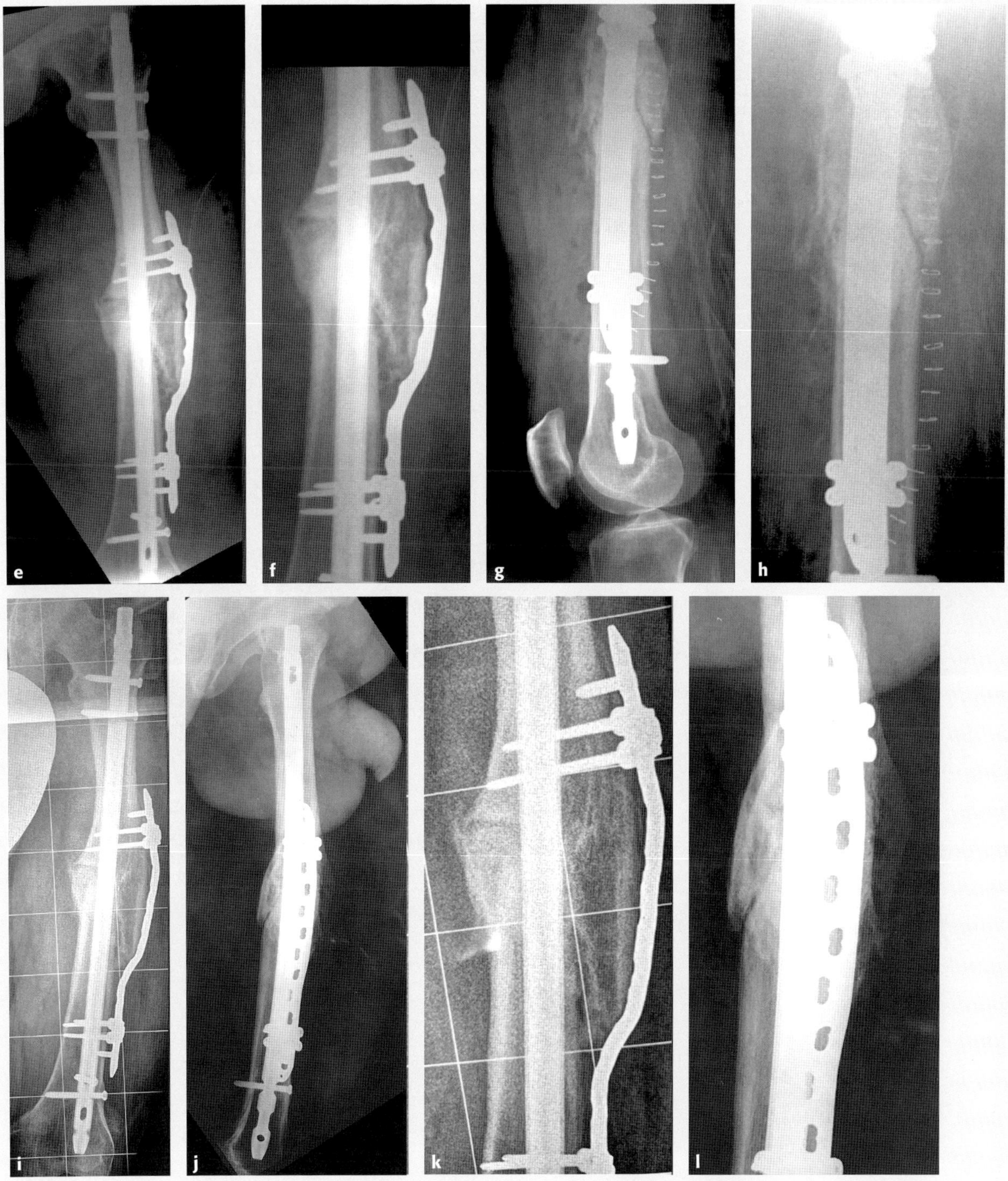

Fig 2.3-9a–q (cont) Clinical photographs and x-rays obtained up until consolidation of the fracture.
e–h Immediate postoperative control x-rays showing detail of the decorticated and stabilized pseudarthrosis in AP and lateral views.
i–l Control x-rays 1 month after the intervention and detail of the pseudarthrosis site in AP and lateral views.

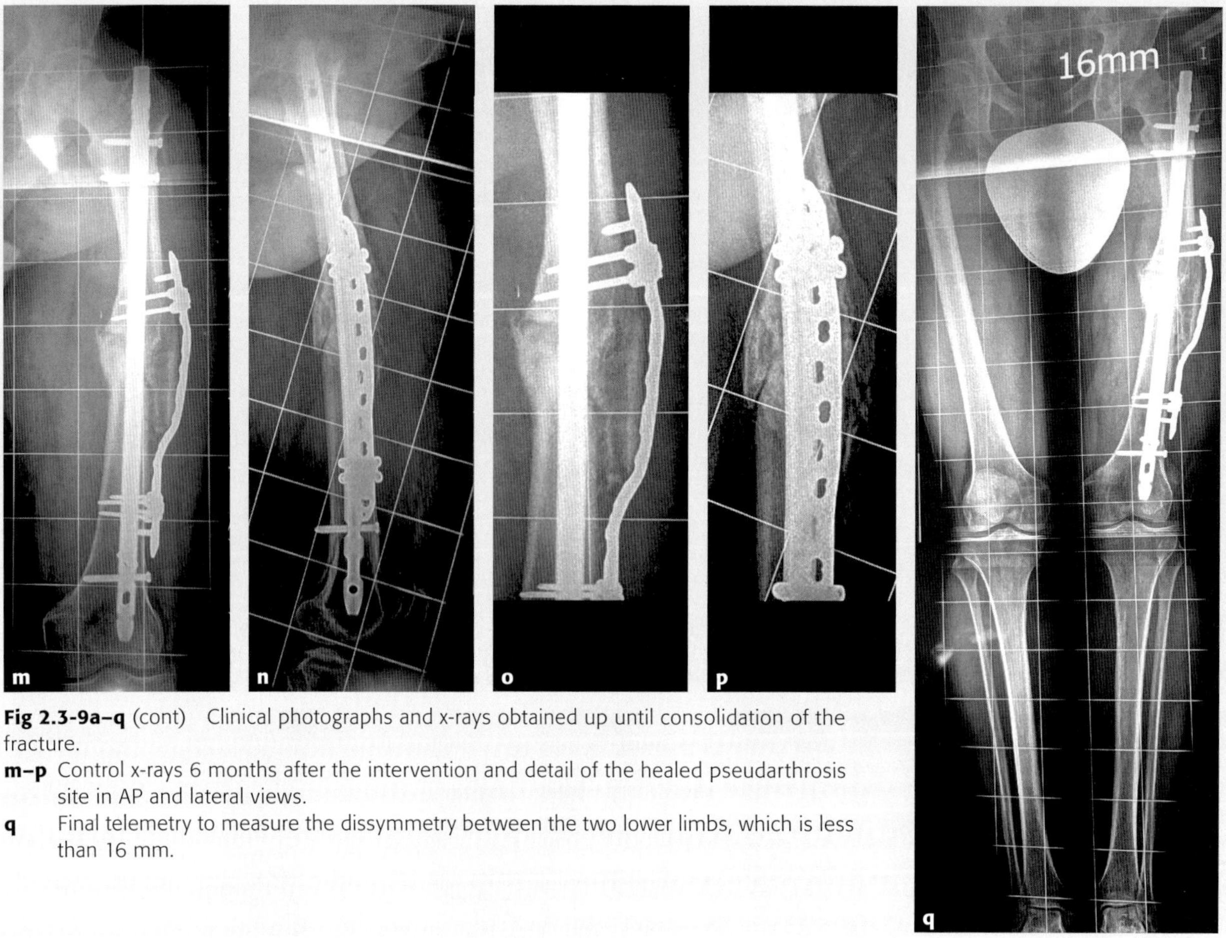

Fig 2.3-9a–q (cont) Clinical photographs and x-rays obtained up until consolidation of the fracture.
m–p Control x-rays 6 months after the intervention and detail of the healed pseudarthrosis site in AP and lateral views.
q Final telemetry to measure the dissymmetry between the two lower limbs, which is less than 16 mm.

Reto Babst, Frank Beeres, Jaroslaw Brudnicki, Matej Cimerman, Joan Girós Torres, Björn Link, Roberto Rivero Sosa, J Miquel Sales Pérez, Matevž Tomaževič, Miquel Videla Cés

Case description

A 67-year-old woman, who used to walk unaided, was uncooperative in the postoperative period following total replacement of the right knee (**Fig 2.3-10**). She had a fall in the hospital at night, sustaining a fracture in the femoral diaphysis proximal to the knee prosthesis (AO/OTA 32A1) (**Fig 2.3-11**). The x-ray confirmed the fracture and the patient underwent temporary immobilization with traction. The stabilization of the fracture with interfragmentary compression screws and a distal femoral locking compression plate (LCP) was performed the following day (**Fig 2.3-12**). The patient was discharged 5 days later, but she reported pain and was seen at an outpatient clinic 5 days after hospital discharge. The control x-ray revealed breakage of the plate (**Fig 2.3-13**). The patient was readmitted to hospital and operated 3 days later using a distal femoral LCP and a different distribution of the screws. The compression screws used previously were removed (**Fig 2.3-14**).

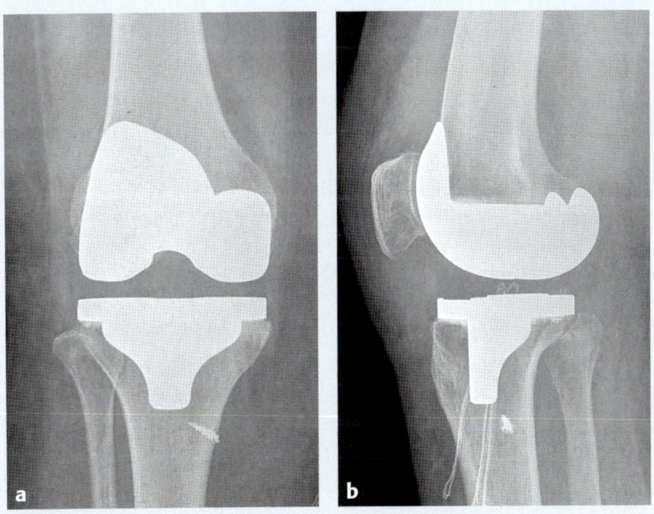

Fig 2.3-10a–b Control x-rays of the patient's right knee in AP (**a**) and lateral (**b**) views 1 week after total knee arthroplasty and before her fall at the hospital.

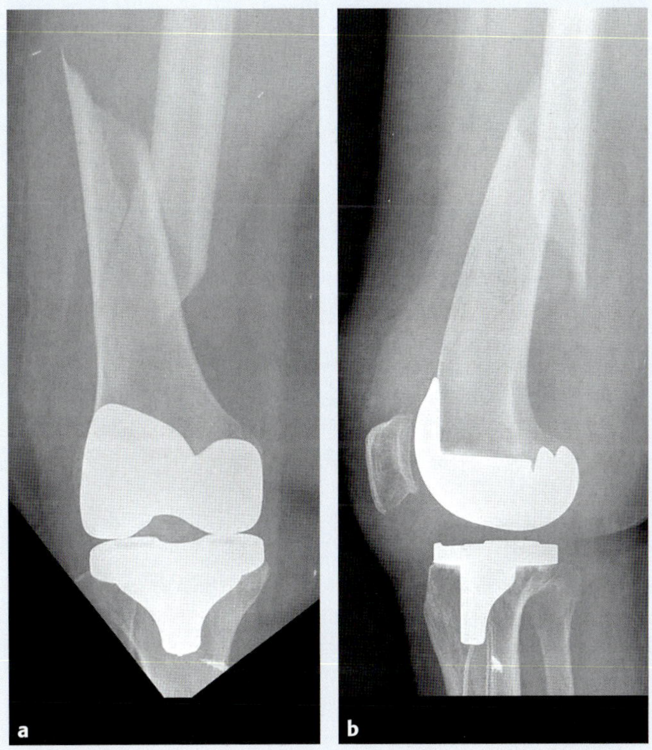

Fig 2.3-11a–b AP (**a**) and lateral (**b**) views of the femoral diaphyseal fracture following a fall at the hospital.

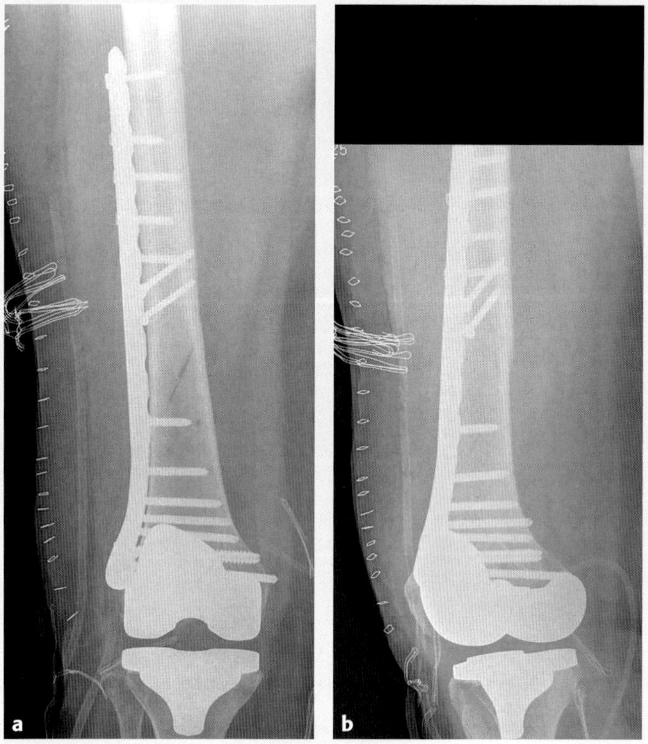

Fig 2.3-12a–b Postoperative AP (**a**) and lateral (**b**) x-rays after internal fixation of the fracture with interfragmentary compression screws and a distal femoral locking compression plate.

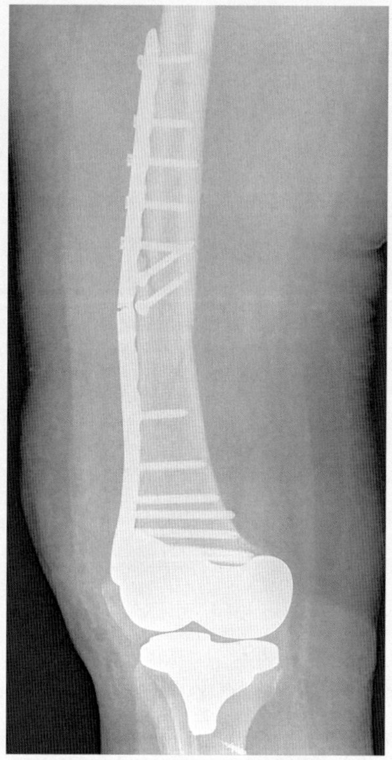

Fig 2.3-13 The outpatient control x-ray 5 weeks after osteosynthesis showing plate breakage.

Analysis of failure and reflection

There were several mistakes in the case presented. Firstly, the principle of stability for the fixation of the fractures was confused, mixing up absolute and relative stability. Using absolute stability in the case of an osteoporotic bone must be avoided, even in the case of simple fractures where absolute stability is recommended. It is almost impossible to achieve absolute stability with interfragmentary compression in osteoporotic bone. In this case, two traction screws and a distal femoral LCP in the form of a bridge were used. The excessive proximity of the screws to the fracture site caused a high degree of stiffness with a high concentration of tensions in a limited area of the plate, which due to fatigue, led to its breaking. To avoid this complication, the entire treatment concept must be changed.

If the decision is taken to use a bridging plate, a much longer plate must be used with a completely different distribution of screws, applying it far from the fracture site to permit elasticity. Such a distribution of the screws will favor the tension forces being distributed in a safer way across a greater expanse of the plate capable of load bearing. If it is decided to use a plate to stabilize the femoral fracture, it must be remembered that tension and pressure concentrate on the implant. If the plate is short, it may cause a fracture of the bone above the proximal end of the plate. If the site is excessively rigid because of screws, the tension concentrates at one point and breakage of the material may occur.

Another possible error is to perform excessive periosteal stripping at the fracture site to place the screws, affecting the vascularization of the area, which delays healing so the implant must bear weight for a longer time and may fail due to fatigue before union occurs.

Final outcome

Immediately after x-ray control at the check-up in the outpatient clinic, the patient was admitted to hospital and operated on 3 days later.

The concept of fracture fixation was completely changed. The traction screws were removed and the broken plate was replaced with a much longer less invasive stabilization system (LISS) plate with a different distribution of screws. This new distribution of screws created a much better situation biomechanically. The plate used to treat the fracture was sufficiently long to achieve a more secure distribution of the tension forces as shown in the postoperative x-ray (**Fig 2.3-14**). The patient was discharged from the hospital and sent home after 5 days. The cutaneous suture was removed after 12 days during her visit to an outpatient clinic and healing was achieved without further incident.

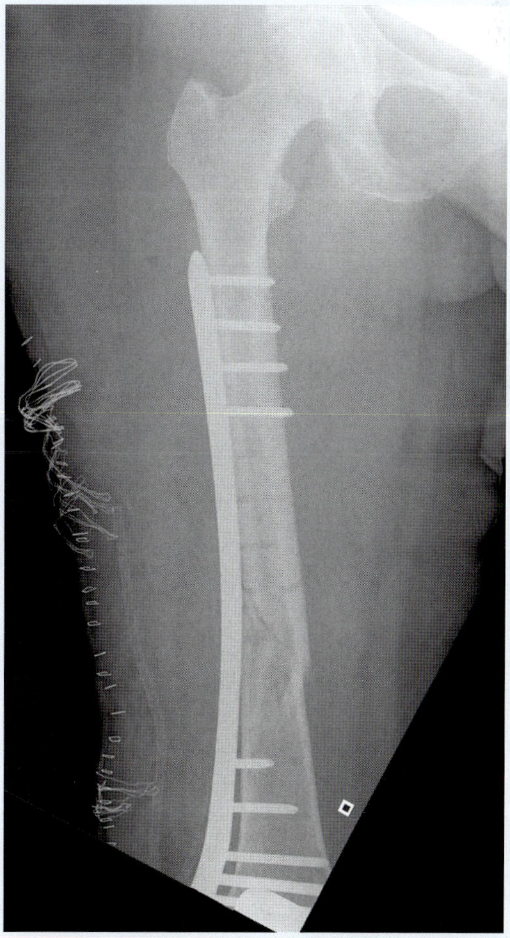

Fig 2.3-14 Postoperative x-ray taken after reintervention with a longer plate and different distribution of the screws.

CASE 4

Case description

A healthy 38-year-old woman was hit by a car while jogging. She presented with polytrauma, a fracture dislocation of the right hip ("Pipkin II"), a fracture of the thoracic vertebrae, and an intraarticular fracture of the proximal tibia associated with a segmental fracture of the tibial diaphysis (AO/OTA 41B1.1 and AO/OTA 42C2) (**Fig 2.3-15**) [Pipkin, 1957].

Initially, damage control treatment involved a reduction of the dislocated hip and application of an external fixator to stabilize the tibia. After the inflammation had improved, osteosynthesis was performed on the Pipkin fracture with surgical dislocation of the hip. The external fixator was removed, osteosynthesis of the proximal tibia performed, and the fracture of the tibial diaphysis fixed with a lateral angular stable plate (**Fig 2.3-16**).

After 9 months, the pseudarthrosis of the proximal tibial fracture was evident (**Fig 2.3-17**).

Due to continuous pain, the position screw was extracted from the lateral side and additionally stabilized using a straight plate on the medial side (**Fig 2.3-18**). The fracture was completely healed after 6 weeks.

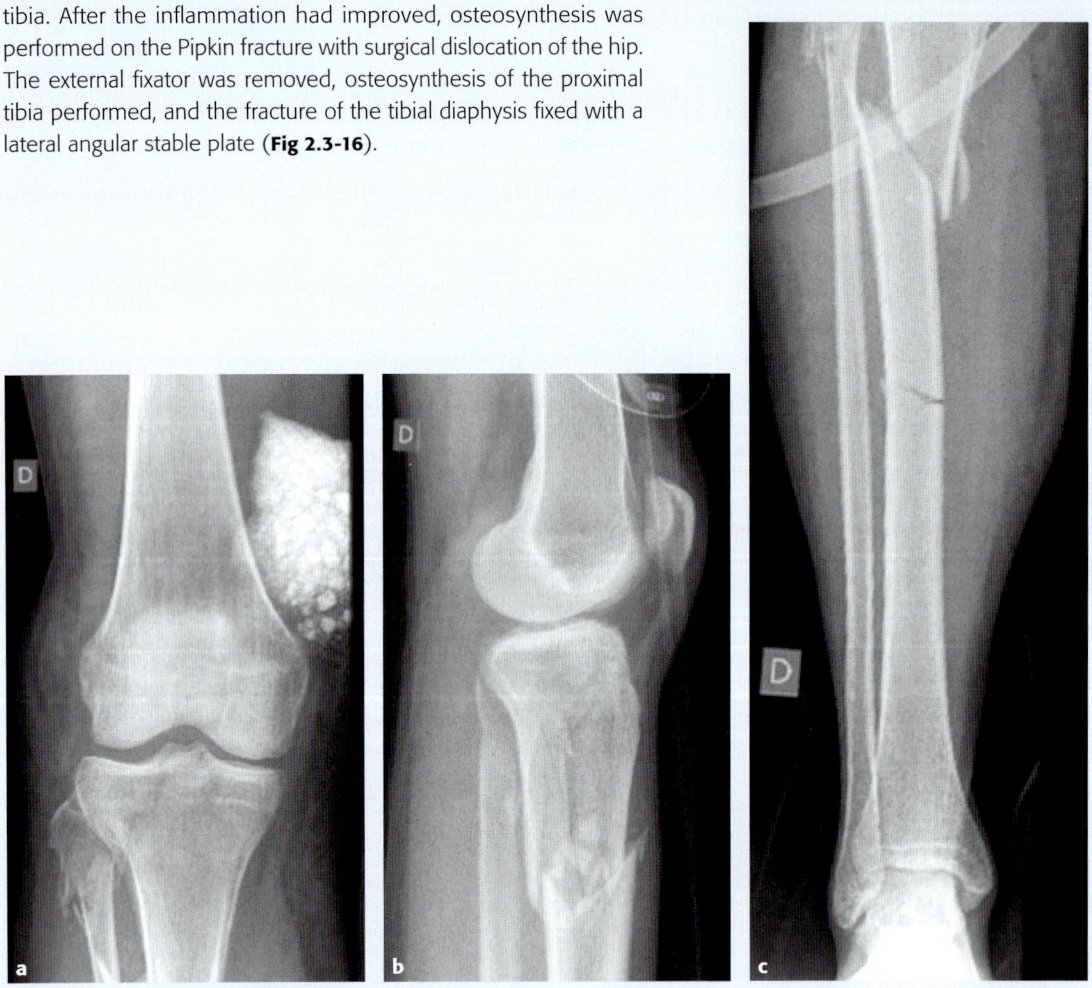

Fig 2.3-15a–c X-rays of the tibial fractures.
a–b X-ray with AP and lateral views of the knee showing the tibial plateau fracture.
c AP x-ray of the tibia showing the segmental fracture of the tibial diaphysis.

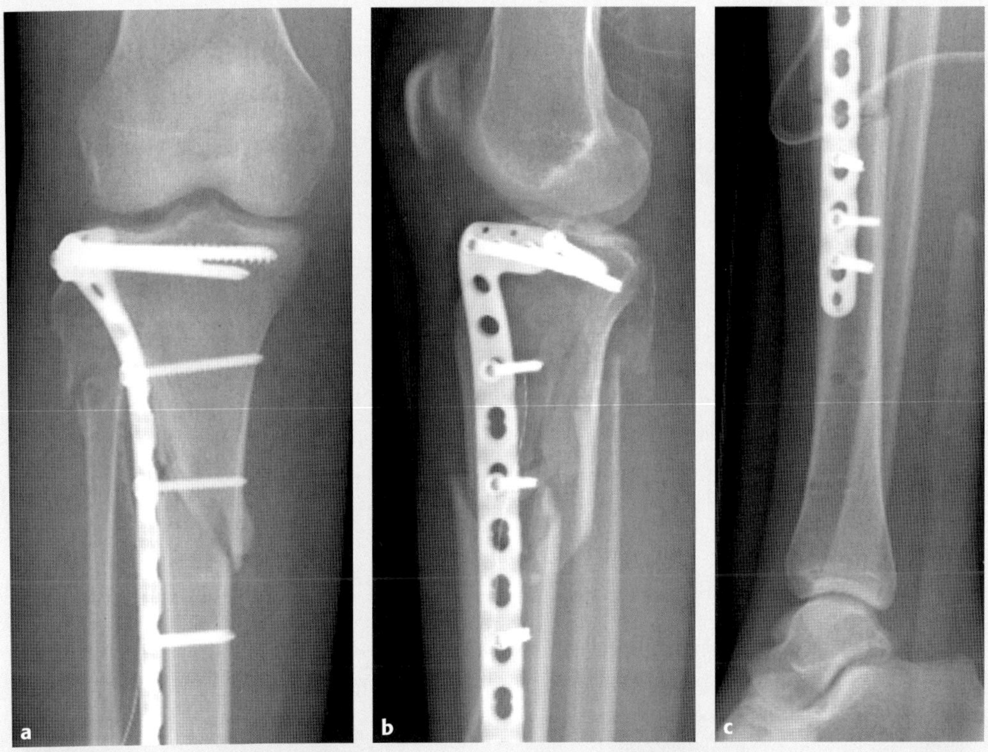

Fig 2.3-16a–c X-rays of the osteosynthesis of both tibial fractures.
a–b X-ray in AP and lateral views showing osteosynthesis of the proximal tibia.
c X-ray showing the profile of the distal segment of the tibial diaphyseal fracture.

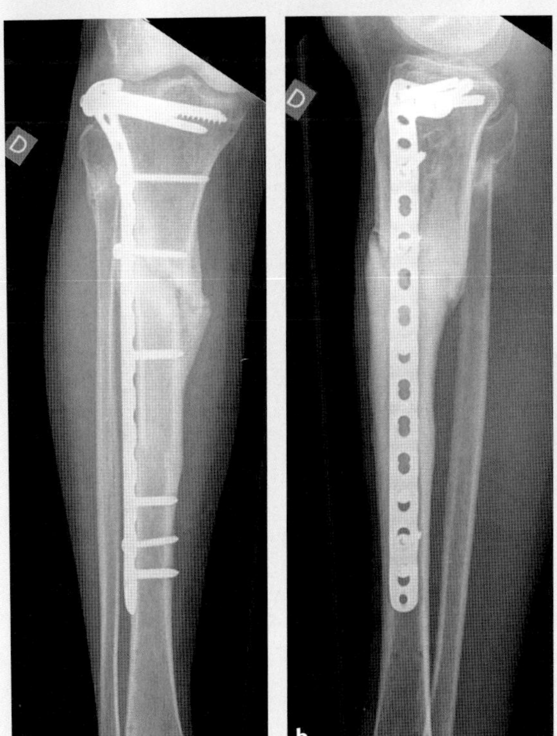

Fig 2.3-17a–b AP and lateral views showing pseudarthrosis of the proximal oblique pattern of the segmental tibial diaphyseal fracture.

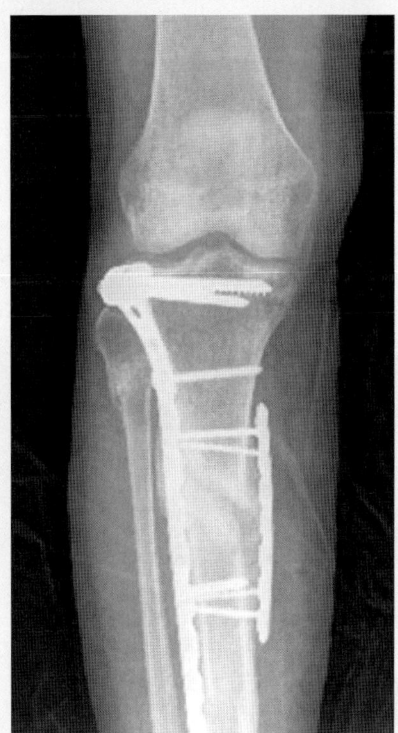

Fig 2.3-18 Healing of the pseudarthrosis after additional stabilization with the plate on the medial side.

Analysis of failure and reflection

According to the first treatment plan, compression of the tibial plateau fracture was performed using a traction screw, which bridged this fracture to the tibial diaphysis. Due to the polytrauma, the tibia was stabilized with an external fixator, but sufficient reduction was not achieved because the proximal fragment was shortened and angulated and only traction was used. To maintain the proximal fragment in its place, a positional screw was also used to reduce and avoid valgus deformity of the proximal fragment.

After consolidation of the metaphysis, articular fragments, and distal site of the diaphyseal segment, a pseudarthrosis appeared at the level of the diaphyseal-metaphyseal union. The pseudarthrosis was resolved using two methods: firstly, extraction of the position screw and secondly, additional stabilization with a plate on the medial side. Following the second operation, the fracture healed completely after 6 weeks.

The tibial plateau fracture was treated with a traction screw. This screw provided compression on the side of the lateral fracture of the tibial plateau. The angular stability plate and proximal screws were used as support beams for the tibial plateau; they achieved sufficient stability at the articular surface, enabling the joint to be mobilized immediately. Due to the insufficient reduction of the proximal site of the segmental fracture, a positioning screw was used for the reduction and to minimize injury to the soft tissues. Using a medial approach limited to the medial part of the fracture and placing a small buttress plate would have been better. With this plate additional stabilization and better reduction could have been achieved. The union of the proximal construction with the distal diaphyseal fragment would have been possible if it had been performed in the same way as the first time.

Final outcome

The pseudarthrosis was resolved using two methods: firstly, extraction of the positioning screw and secondly, additional stabilization on the medial side. With the removal of the positioning screw in the proximal tibia, the surgeons eliminated that part of the osteosynthesis where a mixture of principles was used. By using the reinforcement plate as additional support on the medial side, stability was restored sufficiently to enable healing of the pseudarthrosis. With the decortication and perforation at the pseudarthrosis site, bone biology, new bone formation, and blood supply were improved, and the patient was able to resume her normal sporting activities (**Fig 2.3-19**).

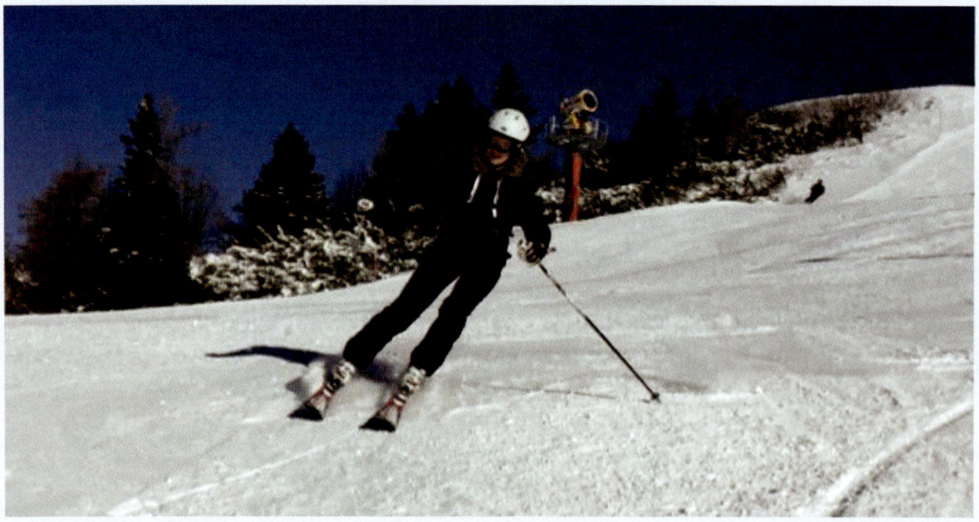

Fig 2.3-19 The patient returned to her sporting activities.

Reto Babst, Frank Beeres, Jaroslaw Brudnicki, Matej Cimerman, Joan Girós Torres, Björn Link, Roberto Rivero Sosa, J Miquel Sales Pérez, Matevž Tomaževič, Miquel Videla Cés

Key points to remember

Stability is the ability of the fracture to resist functional loads:

- Absolute stability is the absence of mobility on the surfaces of the fracture when subjected to a functional load.
- Relative stability allows a controlled movement between the bone fragments, always below critical levels of tension, offering a stimulus to tissue differentiation.
- Confusing the principles of absolute and relative stability must be avoided.
- When selecting implants, we must consider what stability we need and which implant can perform that specific function long enough for healing. The selection of the implant is influenced according to the fracture type, the fracture location, and the bone quality.
- Implants must achieve optimal mechanical performance, and the best adaptation to bone must be achieved.
- The instruments for and technique of placing the implants must be prepared beforehand.
- Type of stability is indicated for the following fractures:
  - Absolute stability: in joint fractures, in forearm fractures, and in diaphyseal fractures with a simple pattern when intramedullary osteosynthesis is not indicated.
  - Relative stability: in multifragmentary metaphyseal and diaphyseal fractures.
  - Combined stability: in joint fractures with multifragmentary diaphyseal impact, requiring anatomical reduction and absolute stability in the joint area and the application of relative stability in the multifragmentary metaphyseal and diaphyseal areas.

References and suggested reading

Bonyun M, Nauth A, Egol KA, et al. Hot topics in biomechanically directed fracture fixation. *J Orthop Trauma.* 2014;28 Suppl 1:S32–35.
Claes L. Biomechanical principles and mechanobiologic aspects of flexible and locked plating. *J Orthop Trauma.* 2011 Feb;25 Suppl 1:S4–7.
Gautier E. Bridge plating. *AO Dialogue.* 2009 (2):24–27.
Hunt SB, Buckley RE. Locking plates: a current concepts review of technique and indications for use. *Acta Chir Orthop Traumatol Cech.* 2013;80(3):185–191.
Krettek C, Miclau T, Grun O, et al. Intraoperative control of axes, rotation and length in femoral and tibial fractures. Technical note. *Injury.* 1998;29 Suppl 3:C29–39.
Luo CF, Sun H, Zhang B, et al. Three-column fixation for complex tibial plateau fractures. *J Orthop Trauma.* 2010 Nov;24(11):683–692.
Pauwels F. *Biomechanics of the locomotor apparatus: contributions on the functional anatomy of the locomotor apparatus.* Maquet P, Furlong R, trans-rev. Berlin New York: Springer-Verlag; 1980.
Perren SM. The biomechanics and biology of internal fixation using plates and nails. *Orthopedics.* 1989 Jan;12(1):21–34.
Perren SM. Minimally invasive internal fixation history, essence and potential of a new approach. *Injury.* 2001 May;32 Suppl 1:Sa1–3.
Perren SM. Evolution of the internal fixation of long bone fractures. The scientific basis of biological internal fixation: choosing a new balance between stability and biology. *J Bone Joint Surg Br.* 2002 Nov;84(8):1093–1110.
Pipkin G. Treatment of grade IV fracture-dislocation of the hip. *J Bone Joint Surg Am.* 1957 Oct;39-a(5):1027–1042 passim.
Ricci WM. Use of Locking Plates in Orthopaedic Trauma Surgery. *JBJS Rev.* 2015 Mar 17;3(3).
Schatzker J, McBroom R, Bruce D. The tibial plateau fracture. The Toronto experience 1968–1975. *Clin Orthop Relat Res.* 1979 Jan–Feb(138):94–104.
Stoffel K, Lorenz KU, Kuster MS. Biomechanical considerations in plate osteosynthesis: the effect of plate-to-bone compression with and without angular screw stability. *J Orthop Trauma.* 2007 Jul;21(6):362–368.
Wagner M, Frigg R. *Internal Fixators—Concepts and Cases Using LCP and LISS.* New York: Thieme; 2006.

2.4 Biology management (including soft-tissue management)

Jordi Bertrán, Jaroslaw Brudnicki, Joan Girós Torres, Roberto Rivero Sosa, J Miquel Sales Pérez, Miquel Videla Cés

We cannot direct the wind but we can adjust the sails.

Anonymous

Initially, the alteration of the blood supply to the bone occurs due to the fracture and its displacement, which interrupts the vascularization and causes necrosis at the ends of the fracture. The soft tissues are affected by the traumatic event and this also alters the periosteal circulation. Subsequently, the biological conditions of the bone are also affected by contact with the implant used in the treatment, so the negative effects must be weighed against the benefits.

The vascularization enables cellular function to be maintained in the fracture site which determines the formation and quality of the healing callus. Respect for the biology enables the formation, destruction, and differentiation of the tissues (elimination and substitution of the necrotic area). The biology, together with the mechanics, permits consolidation. Depending on the type of reduction and the mechanical conditions (stability), the biology permits the healing of the fracture by direct or indirect union.

Open surgical treatment in the process of performing osteosynthesis must preserve the vascularization to avoid damaging the bone and the surrounding soft tissues.

The devitalization of the bone fragments leads to bone necrosis and an increase in instability due to resorption by the site and/or bone necrosis. Therefore, preserving the vascularization of the bone fragments is a biological necessity and also has mechanical implications.

One violation to the fracture biology that must be avoided is devascularization caused by interventions with untimely reduction maneuvers, with exaggerated periosteal stripping, and in which the surrounding soft tissues are not respected during the stabilization maneuvers.

Surgeons must remember that necrotic bone does not form a union. When the fracture is properly reduced and stabilized, the optimal conditions are in place for obtaining union through the formation of a healing callus (by primary or secondary intention).

Considering the biological need of conservation, the authors include in this book those osteosyntheses that require special attention due to the quality of the bone on which they occur (patients with diabetes, circulatory insufficiency, open fractures, etc). In addition, today the increased life expectancy of the population means that many fractures are sustained by elderly people with marked osteoporosis.

CASE 1

Case description

A 73-year-old woman with osteoporosis had undergone a total knee arthroplasty 2 years earlier with good evolution. She had a fall at home, sustaining a fracture of the femoral diaphysis above the knee prosthesis (AO/OTA 32B3) (**Fig 2.4-1**).

The plan was to reduce and perform osteosynthesis with a less invasive stabilization system (LISS) plate. Following the recommended initial technique, the monocortical screws were locked to the plate. The total knee prosthesis was not loosened. The surgery proceeded without incident and the patient was discharged from hospital after 5 days (**Fig 2.4-2**).

Five weeks following intervention, the patient was readmitted to hospital due to pain, inability to walk, and deformity in the thigh after tripping in her bedroom. A new x-ray detected a subtrochanteric fracture of the femur just above the proximal end of the LISS plate that was bridging the fracture (**Fig 2.4-3**).

As the union of the periprosthetic fracture was delayed given the evolution time, the extraction of the LISS plate was not taken into consideration. It was planned to remove the proximal screw of the LISS plate and stabilize the subtrochanteric fracture with a short intramedullary proximal femoral nail (PFN) (**Fig 2.4-4**).

The patient was discharged 4 days after surgery. At the outpatient follow-up visit at 7 weeks, the patient reported pain when trying to bear weight and difficulties with walking. The x-rays revealed destabilization of the fracture and breakage of the intramedullary nail at the level of the upper distal locking hole (**Fig 2.4-5**).

In a new intervention, the broken implant was removed and the fracture was again stabilized with an intramedullary PFN nail with bone graft placed around the fracture space (**Fig 2.4-6**).

Two months later, the patient returned for an outpatient follow-up with the second PFN broken at the same level as the first. Since she only had discomfort and a large callus around the fracture site had formed, the angular deformity was accepted and no further surgical procedures were performed on this patient (**Fig 2.4-7**).

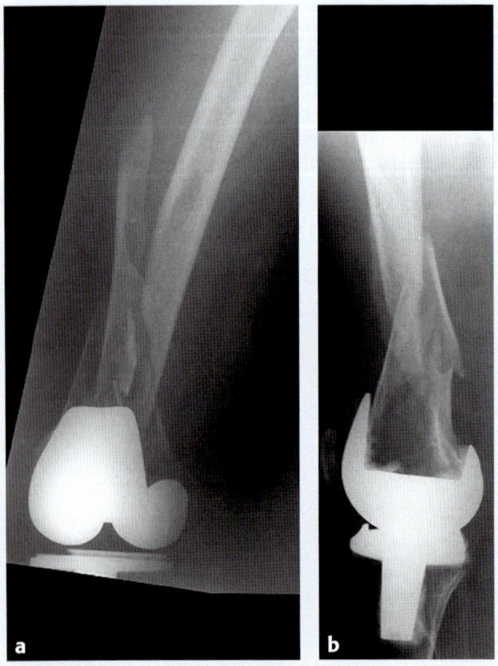

Fig 2.4-1a–b Initial x-rays in AP (**a**) and lateral (**b**) views showing the periprosthetic fracture of the right femur.

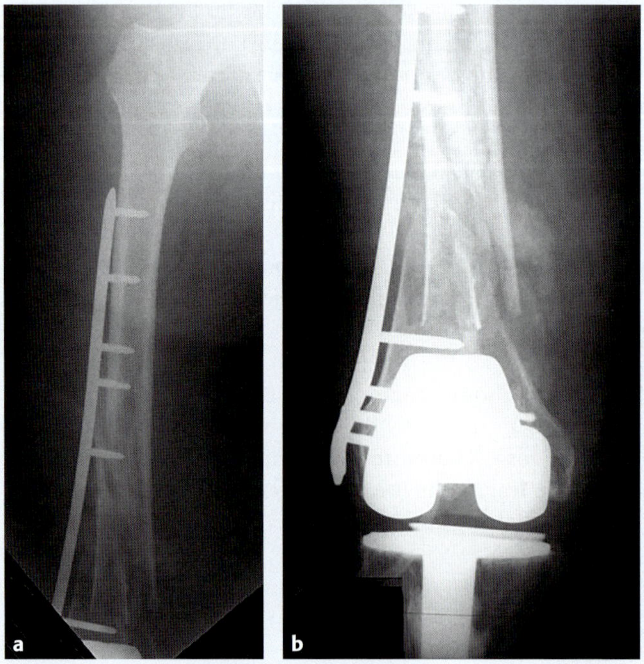

Fig 2.4-2a–b Postoperative x-rays of the periprosthetic fracture stabilized with the less invasive stabilization system plate.
a AP view of the femur.
b View of the center of the knee.

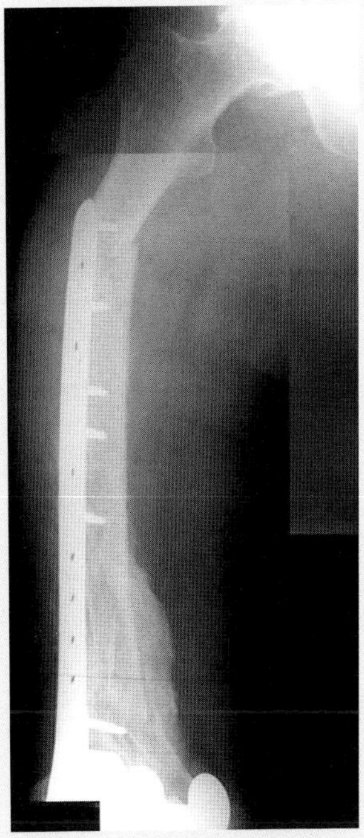

Fig 2.4-3 X-ray of the femur showing a subtrochanteric fracture at the level of the proximal end of the less invasive stabilization system plate.

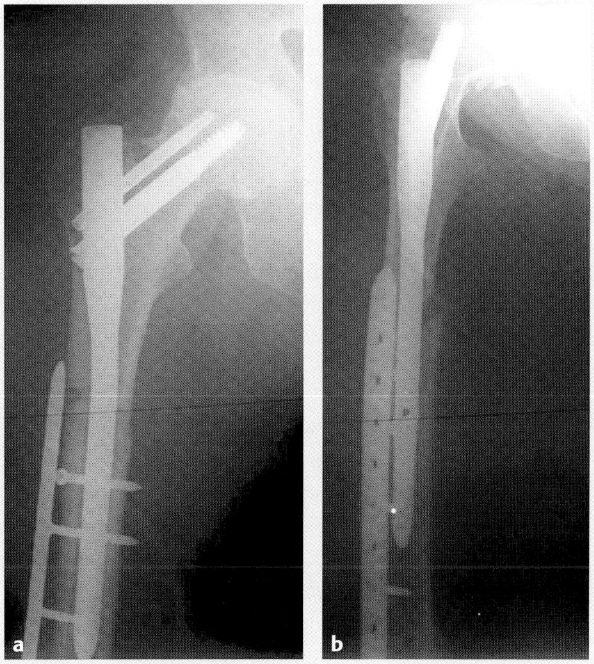

Fig 2.4-4a–b X-rays with AP (a) and axial (b) views of the subtrochanteric fracture stabilized with a short proximal femoral nail.

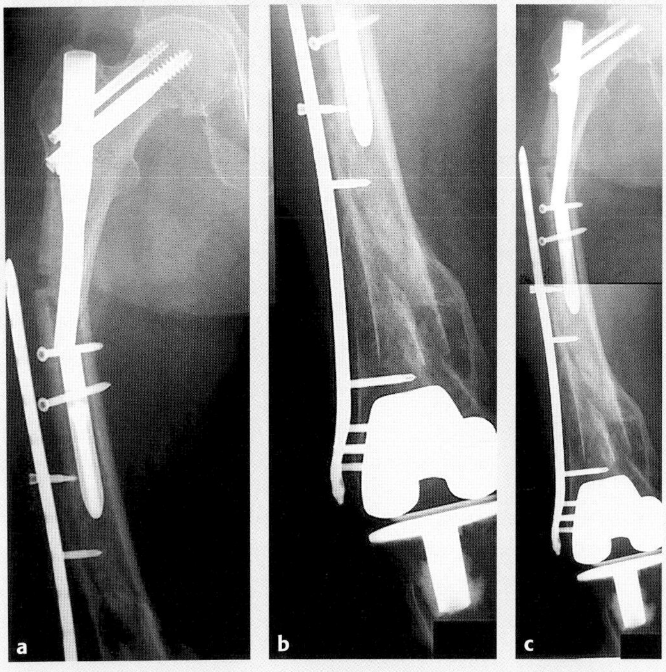

Fig 2.4-5a–c X-rays showing the breakage of the nail 7 weeks following intervention (a–b). Initial callus formation around the subtrochanteric fracture can be observed (c).

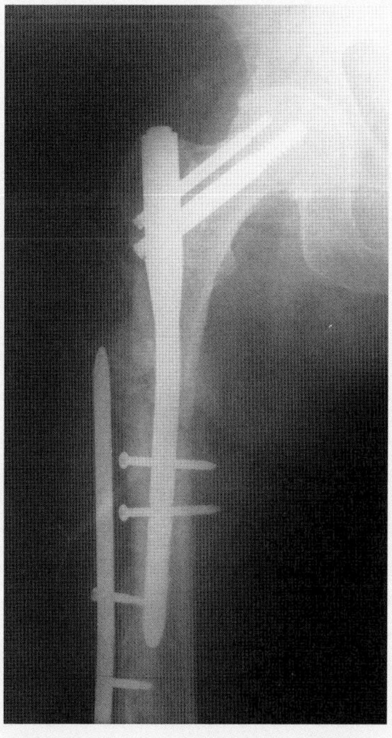

Fig 2.4-6 Postoperative x-ray after the second osteosynthesis with a short proximal femoral nail and bone graft around the fracture site.

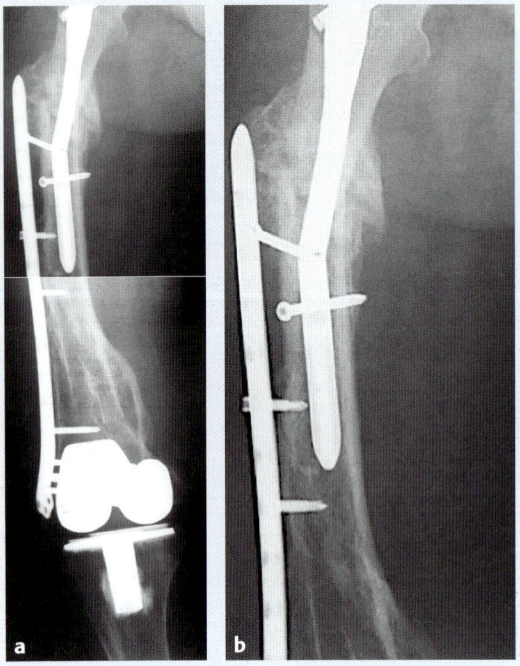

Fig 2.4-7a–b Breakage of the second proximal femoral nail at the same level as the first one (ie, upper distal locking hole) (**a**). Massive callus formation around the subtrochanteric and periprosthetic fractures (**b**).

Analysis of failure and reflection

The case presented here is an example of an accumulation of errors. The idea of fixing the periprosthetic fracture of the distal femur with the LISS plate was correct. Another option would have been retrograde intramedullary nailing if the patient had had a knee prosthesis model allowing this. When treating the femoral fracture, we must remember that any implant applied to the femur will increase tension. In this case, the LISS plate was too short, which was the reason why the subtrochanteric fracture occurred just at the proximal end of the plate in the osteoporotic bone with diminished resistance. Longer plates must be used to protect the bone and to better distribute the stresses.

The fixation of the subtrochanteric fracture was another problem. Extraction of the plate was not considered, as union of the periprosthetic fracture was not yet complete 7 weeks after fixation. The short PFN is an implant designed for fixing trochanteric but not subtrochanteric fractures. For the fixation of these fractures, a long nail should be chosen.

The incorrect choice of implant size was the reason for the next failure. After breakage of the first short nail, several errors were committed. At that moment, the bony union of the periprosthetic fracture was sufficiently visible to permit the removal of the plate and repair the subtrochanteric fracture with a long trochanteric nail. Choosing a short nail again was simply a repeated error. However, the use of bone graft caused a massive callus formation around the subtrochanteric fracture. The second breakage of the short PFN caused an angular deformation of the femur in the presence of massive callus formation.

Final outcome

Due to limited discomfort tolerated by the patient and the massive bone callus formation in both fractures, the angular deformity was accepted and no further surgical treatments were performed. The patient was operated on three times as a consequence of the periprosthetic fracture. Based on the final x-ray, the surgeons decided not to operate again. Some surgeons refer to this acceptance of an imperfect result as a John Lennon and Paul McCartney "Let it be ..." procedure.

Case description

A 59-year-old man who fell on his right ankle from 1 m, presented with a suprasyndesmotic fracture dislocation of the ankles (AO/OTA 44C1) (**Fig 2.4-8**).

Osteosynthesis was performed on the day of admission. The surgeon chose an external approach with a longitudinal incision, slightly curved posteriorly in the distal area (posterior hockey stick incision). The plate was placed on the anterior surface of the fibula and the syndesmosis was fixed with a peroneal intertibial positioning screw directly from the fibula without direct repair of the anterior syndesmosis (**Fig 2.4-9**).

Three weeks after surgery, the patient was readmitted due to necrosis and a superficial infection of the wound; negative-pressure wound therapy (eg, vacuum-assisted wound closure) was administered (**Fig 2.4-10**).

At 8 weeks postoperatively the peroneal intertibial screw was removed without extracting the washer (**Fig 2.4-11**). Fortunately, the ankle joint showed good articular congruity without signs of dystrophy.

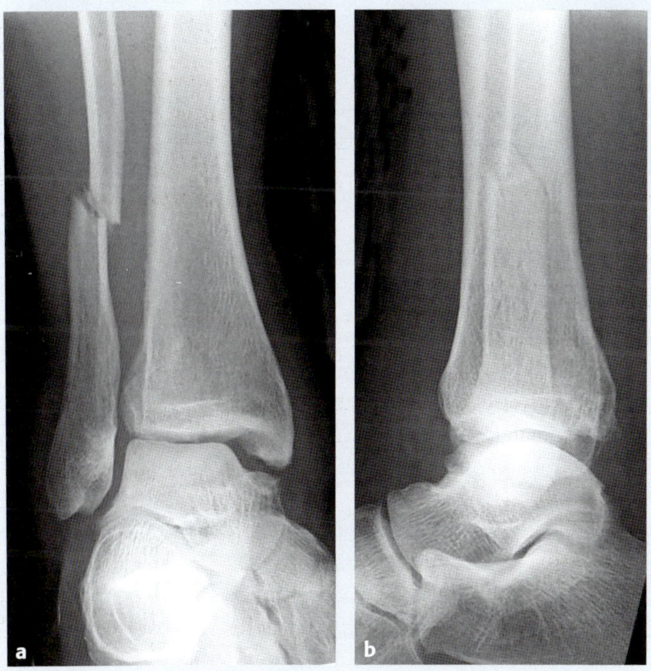

Fig 2.4-8a–b Preoperative x-rays of the suprasyndesmotic bimalleolar fracture.

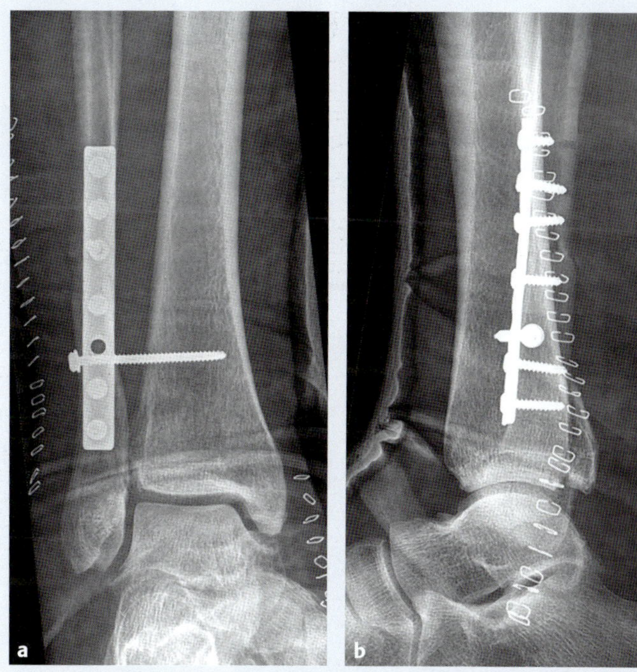

Fig 2.4-9a–b X-ray of the osteosynthesis performed in the immediate postoperative period.

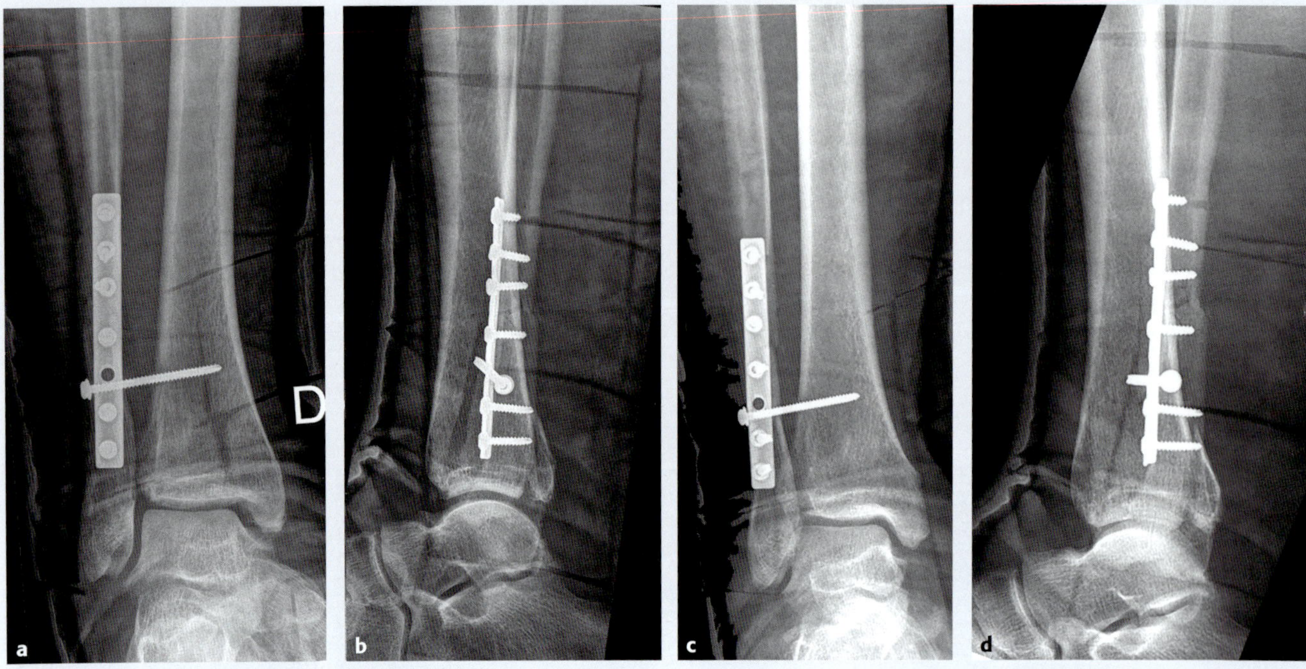

Fig 2.4-10a–d Ambulatory follow-up control x-rays.
a–b X-rays at 3 weeks.
c–d X-rays 1 month following the intervention.

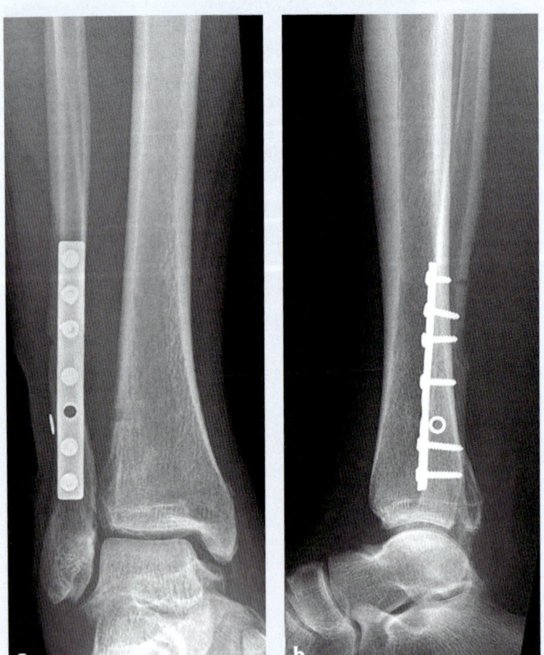

Fig 2.4-11a–b X-rays 8 weeks after the removal of the peroneal intertibial screw.

Analysis of failure and reflection

Despite having a good radiographic diagnosis from the emergency department, we must first evaluate the soft tissues and choose the best approach depending on the skin condition, swelling, and pathological anatomy of the fracture.

Performing an osteosynthesis on the anterior surface of the fibula through a posterolateral approach increases tension on the soft tissues when putting the plate in. This may result in skin necrosis and wound problems. The adequate surgical approach for tackling, reducing, and stabilizing the bone injury and the suprasyndesmotic injury should have been selected more carefully.

Emergency treatment should also be well planned and the osteosynthesis must be performed using an atraumatic surgical technique. Care of the soft tissues should respect vascularization and avoid necrosis of the tissues and infection. It is preferable to wait for the support of an expert surgeon, as this both benefits the patient and helps the practicing surgeons to improve their knowledge and experience.

Final outcome

The immobilization was maintained with a cast splint for 4 weeks and with no weight bearing for 6 weeks following surgery. The patient started rehabilitation and was able to return to work 14 weeks after the initial surgery.

Case description

A 79-year-old woman with insulin-dependent type 1 diabetes and high blood pressure suffered a low-energy fall in the street, causing trauma and a sprain of the left ankle. In the emergency department the injury was classified as a bimalleolar fracture, and it was decided to perform urgent surgery using open reduction and internal fixation (AO/OTA 44B3.2) (**Fig 2.4-12**).

In the postoperative control x-ray poor articular reduction was observed (**Fig 2.4-13**). A plaster boot was applied with windows for controlling the surgical wounds. The immobilization was maintained for 5 weeks (**Fig 2.4-14**).

The surgical wounds evolved to ischemia and subsequent cutaneous necrosis, leaving the tendons exposed and developing an infection due to methicillin-resistant *Staphylococcus aureus* with a poor response to systemic antibiotic treatment and local measures (**Fig 2.4-15**).

Due to a general worsening of the patient's condition, it was decided to perfom an amputation below the knee (**Fig 2.4-16**).

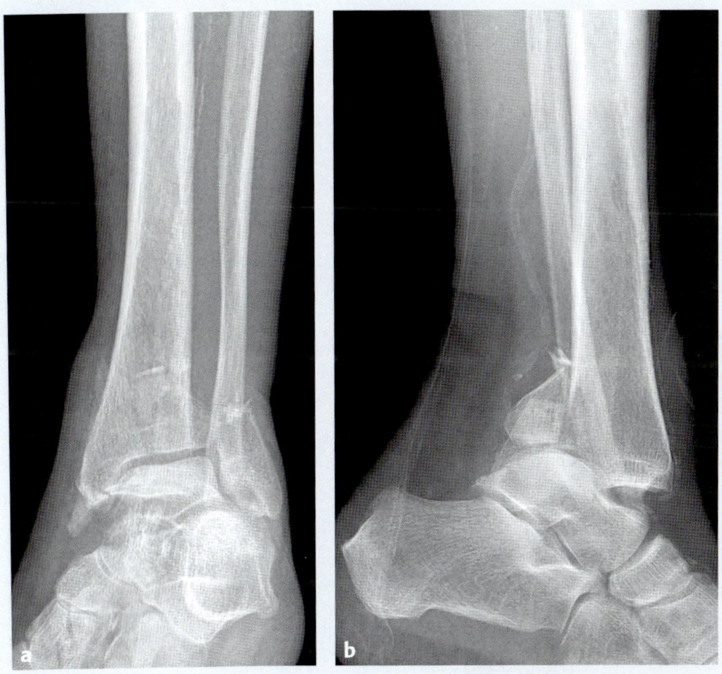

Fig 2.4-12a–b Preoperative AP (**a**) and lateral (**b**) x-rays of the fracture. The size of the Volkmann posterior malleolar fragment is large and affects the articular weight-bearing surface. Evident in both views are the calcified arteries, frequent in diabetic patients leading to a reduced distal vitality.

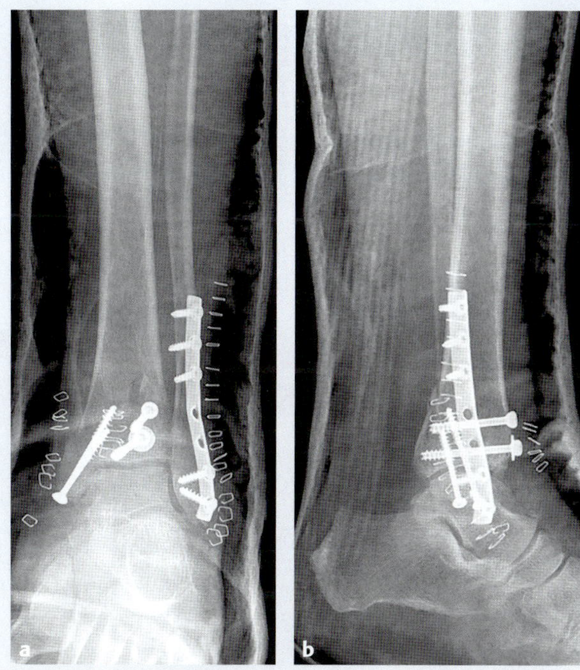

Fig 2.4-13a–b Postoperative control x-rays in which a precarious reduction of the posteromedial component of the fracture can be observed.

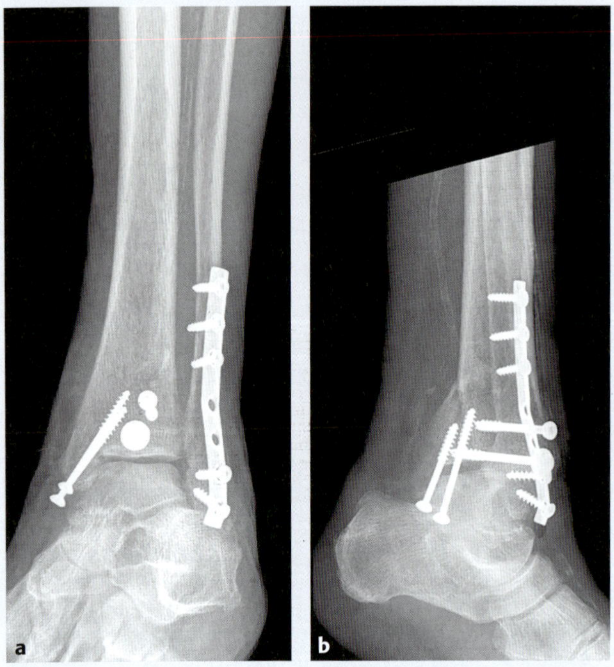

Fig 2.4-14a–b Control x-rays at 6 weeks in which a suboptimal reduction can be observed. This led to the precarious situation of the soft tissues being covered.

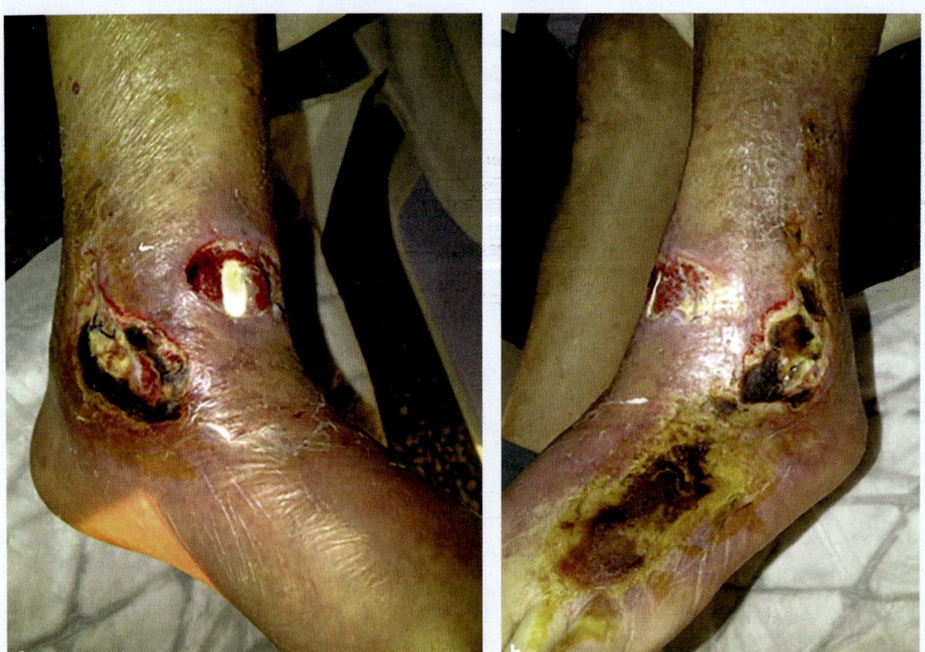

Fig 2.4-15a–b Appearance of the ulcers superinfected with methicillin-resistant *Staphylococcus aureus*, and tendinous exposure around an ischemic and diabetic ankle.

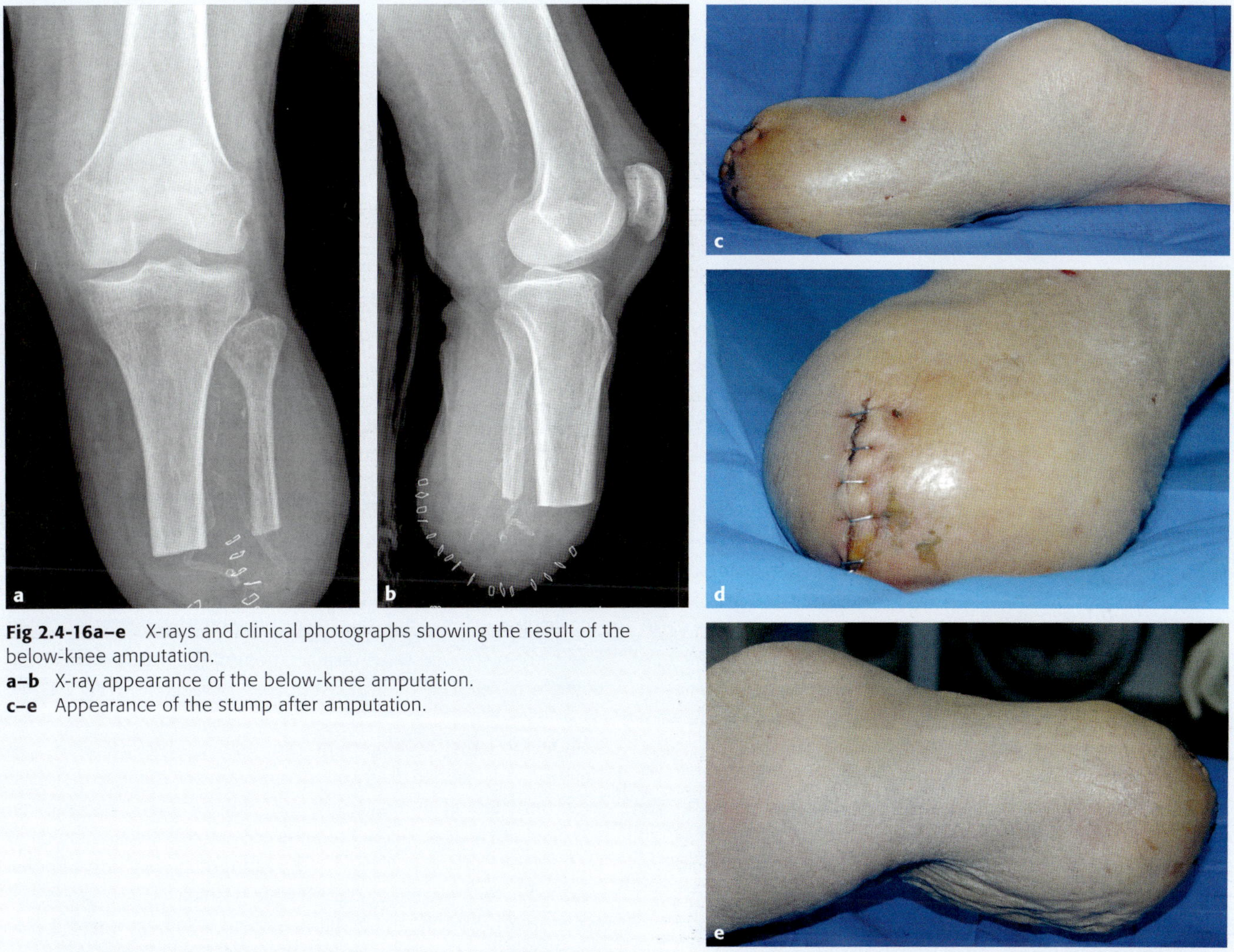

Fig 2.4-16a–e X-rays and clinical photographs showing the result of the below-knee amputation.
a–b X-ray appearance of the below-knee amputation.
c–e Appearance of the stump after amputation.

Analysis of failure and reflection

It is necessary to carry out a thorough examination of the pathological anatomy of the fracture. If evaluation and classification of the fracture based on the x-rays taken in the emergency department is not possible, surgeons should request more imaging tests. In joint fractures, it is necessary to perform a computed tomographic scan to reconstruct and assemble the articular surface. In this case, the injury was misinterpreted and categorized as a bimalleolar fracture instead of an articular tibial pilon fracture.

The state of the soft tissues and the occurrence of any comorbidities will determine the pace of the therapeutic action. During the first 12 hours, the swelling is caused by the fracture hematoma and the limb shortening effect. After those 12 hours, the swelling is due to intradermal edema, which increases the probability of wound problems.

In elderly diabetic patients, the management of the soft tissues must be handled extremely carefully. It is important to avoid large dissections with major detachments.

Wrongly diagnosing the bone injury will most certainly also lead the surgeons to choose the wrong approach, causing greater dissection, attrition, and suffering of the soft tissues, as seen in this case.

Final outcome

The patient's age, comorbidities, and poor compliance have led to a poor adaptation to the prosthesis; therefore, she is now wheelchair-bound and dependent on help.

CASE 4

Case description

A 72-year-old woman suffered a casual fall and presented with a fracture in the subtrochanteric region of the right femur. She sustained a multifragmentary diaphyseal fracture of the proximal femur with two intermediate fragments. Once the fracture was reduced, no contact existed between the proximal and distal fragments (AO/OTA 32B3) (**Fig 2.4-17**).

The recommendation of the surgeon was fixation with a long intramedullary nail with anchorage in the proximal head and neck area of the femur and locked in the distal area.

During the intervention and through a surgical anatomical approach with anterior retraction of the external vastus muscle (subvastus approach), reduction of the intermediate fragments was performed using metallic wires to then insert the nail. An approximate reduction of the fragments was achieved with correct stabilization owing to an intramedullary nail (**Fig 2.4-18**).

The postoperative period was uneventful, allowing early ambulation with crutches and full weight bearing. The postoperative x-ray follow-ups showed partial union of the intermediate fragments with a pattern of vital atrophic pseudarthrosis in the frontal plane at the fracture site level. Given the patient's lack of pain and normal activities of daily living, no therapeutic measures for the pseudarthrosis site were chosen, relying on the strength of the implant (**Fig 2.4-19**).

The patient returned after 13 months due to sudden pain in the thigh and functional impairment. The x-rays showed a breakage of the implant due to fatigue at the level of the pseudarthrosis site (**Fig 2.4-20**).

A new intervention was planned to stabilize and improve the compression and the biological capacity of the pseudarthrosis that union achieves. In the intervention, begun with obtaining iliac crest bone graft on the same side and removing the distal rods, the prior surgical approach was repeated. The bone was assessed via direct osteoperiosteal decortication to see if the cerclage wires and the broken nail could be removed, which was difficult in the distal fragment.

The reduction of the pseudarthrosis site was successfully achieved by using forceps, and a traction screw was inserted. The complete screw was exchanged except for the distal rods to permit the additional compression of the site. As an additional implant, an impacted hook plate was used with an associated compressor to add axial compression to the entire ensemble. This was followed by careful closure, adding the obtained iliac crest bone fragments as a graft (**Fig 2.4-21**).

An uneventful postoperative period was followed by good evolution of the surgical wound and the start of ambulation with crutches (**Fig 2.4-22**).

Despite the nail exchange, the removal of the cerclage wires, the decortication, and the additional stability of the hook plate with axial compression effect and the compressor, the patient presented once more with a broken intramedullary nail but without associated trauma, 9 months after the reintervention (**Fig 2.4-23**).

The decision was taken to wait and trust in the stability provided by the hook plate. Days later the patient had increased pain and the x-rays taken showed varus displacement of the proximal fragment of the femur with the hook plate becoming unanchored (**Fig 2.4-24**).

Due to the latest development, the case was reconsidered. The decision was taken to diagnose the problem and plan the definitive treatment taking into account the biological and mechanical conditioning factors. Given the possibility of nonaffiliated infection and before carrying out any other treatment, biopsy and samples were taken for microbiology which were positive for *Staphylococcus epidermidis*. Specific antibiotic treatment was begun and it was decided to remove all the osteosynthesis material and necrotic bone and provide temporary stabilization with a new intramedullary nail (ie, proximal femoral nail antirotation) coated in antibiotics (ie, gentamycin and vancomycin) to which the microorganism was sensitive.

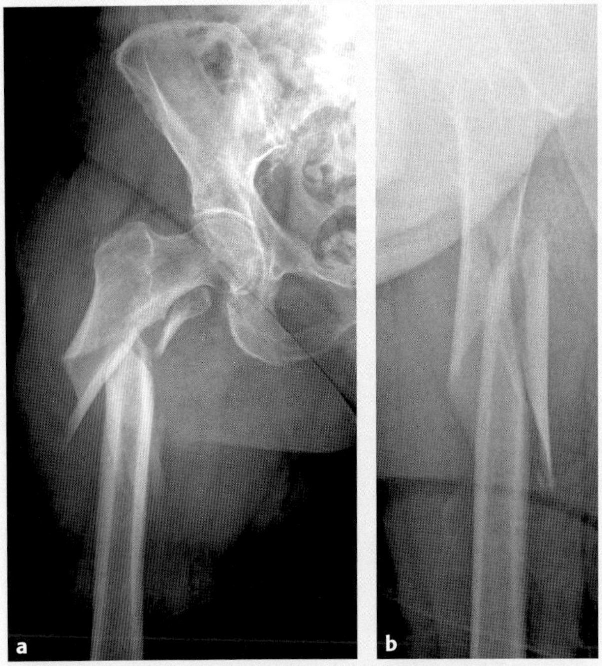

Fig 2.4-17a–b X-rays in AP (**a**) and axial (**b**) views of the fracture.

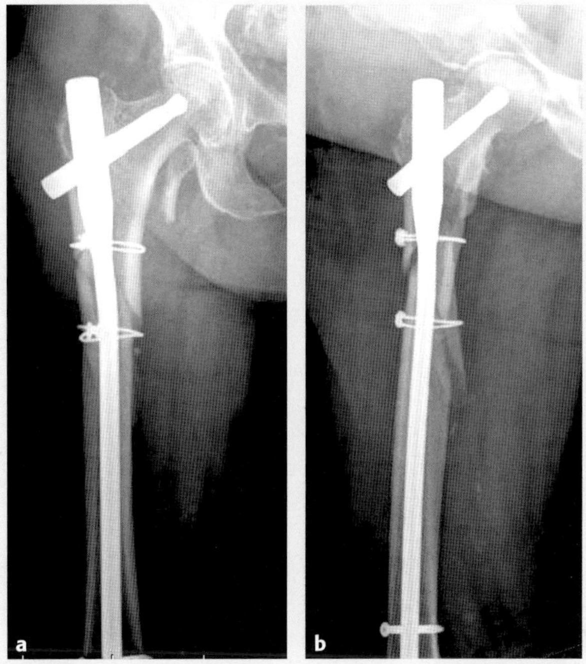

Fig 2.4-18a–b Immediate postoperative x-rays with AP (**a**) and axial (**b**) views.

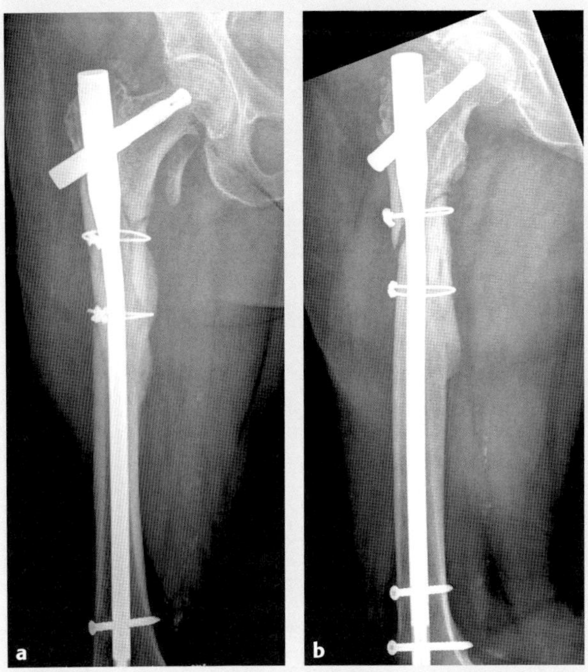

Fig 2.4-19a–b Control x-rays 1 year after the fracture in AP (**a**) and axial (**b**) views. The nonunion pattern (ie, pseudarthrosis) can be observed.

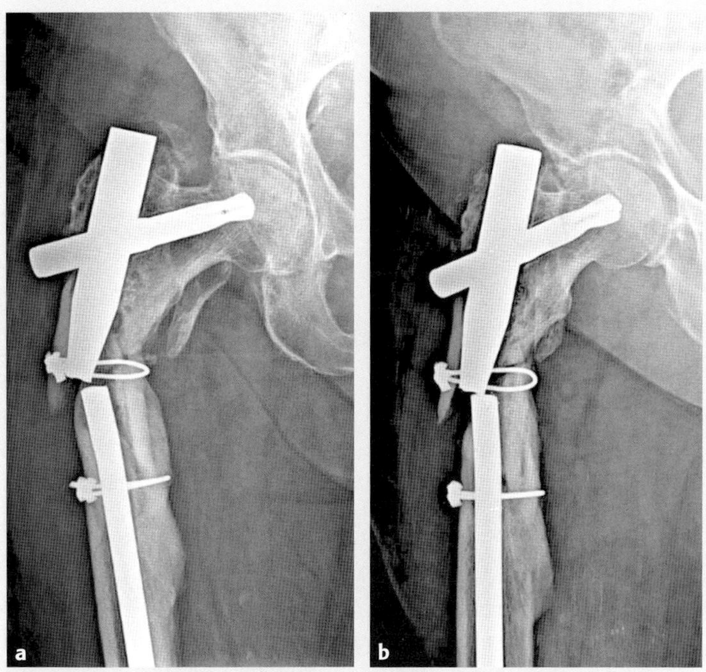

Fig 2.4-20a–b X-rays in AP (**a**) and axial (**b**) views showing breakage of the nail due to fatigue of the material 13 months postoperatively.

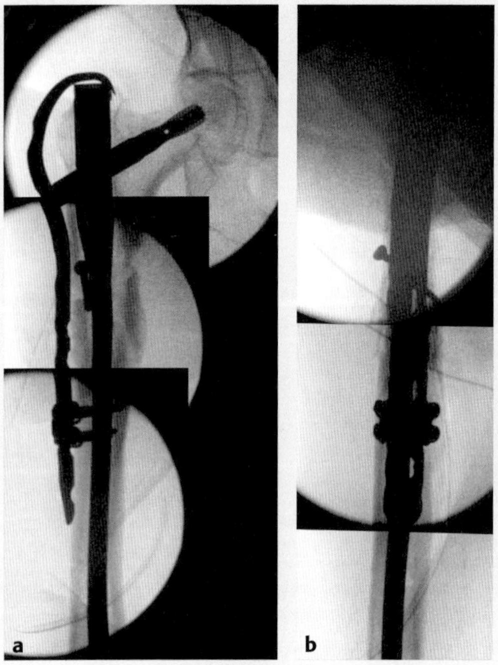

Fig 2.4-21a–b Montage of intraoperative control x-rays in AP (**a**) and axial (**b**) views.

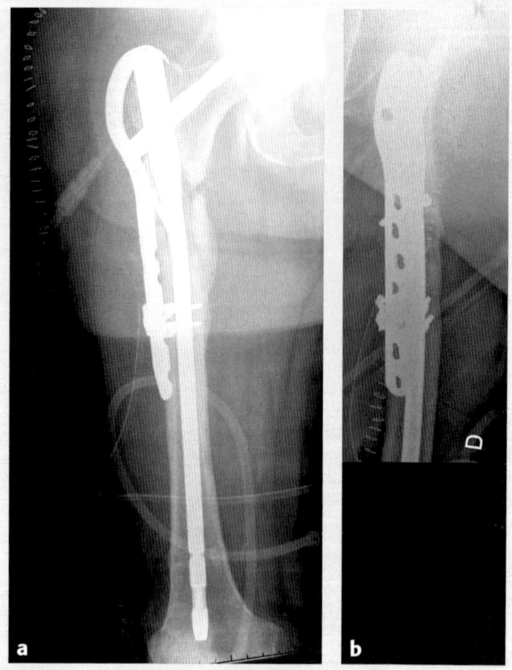

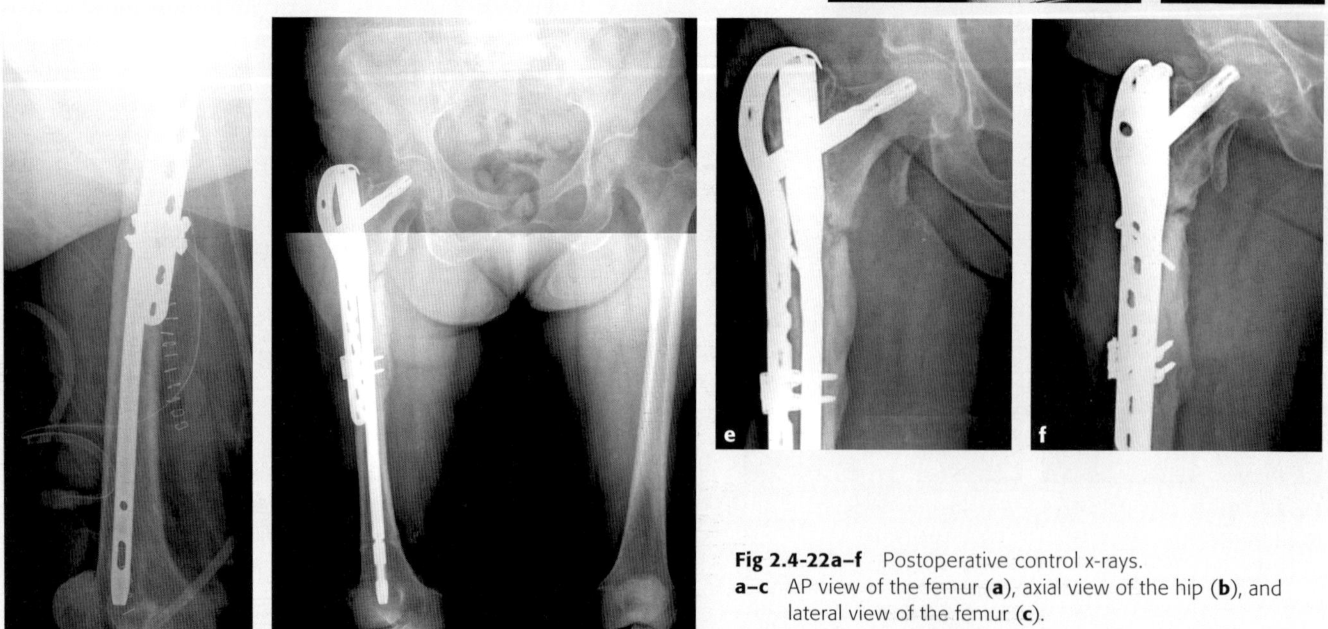

Fig 2.4-22a–f Postoperative control x-rays.

a–c AP view of the femur (**a**), axial view of the hip (**b**), and lateral view of the femur (**c**).

d–f AP (**d**) and axial (**e–f**) views taken 4 and 7 months after the reintervention.

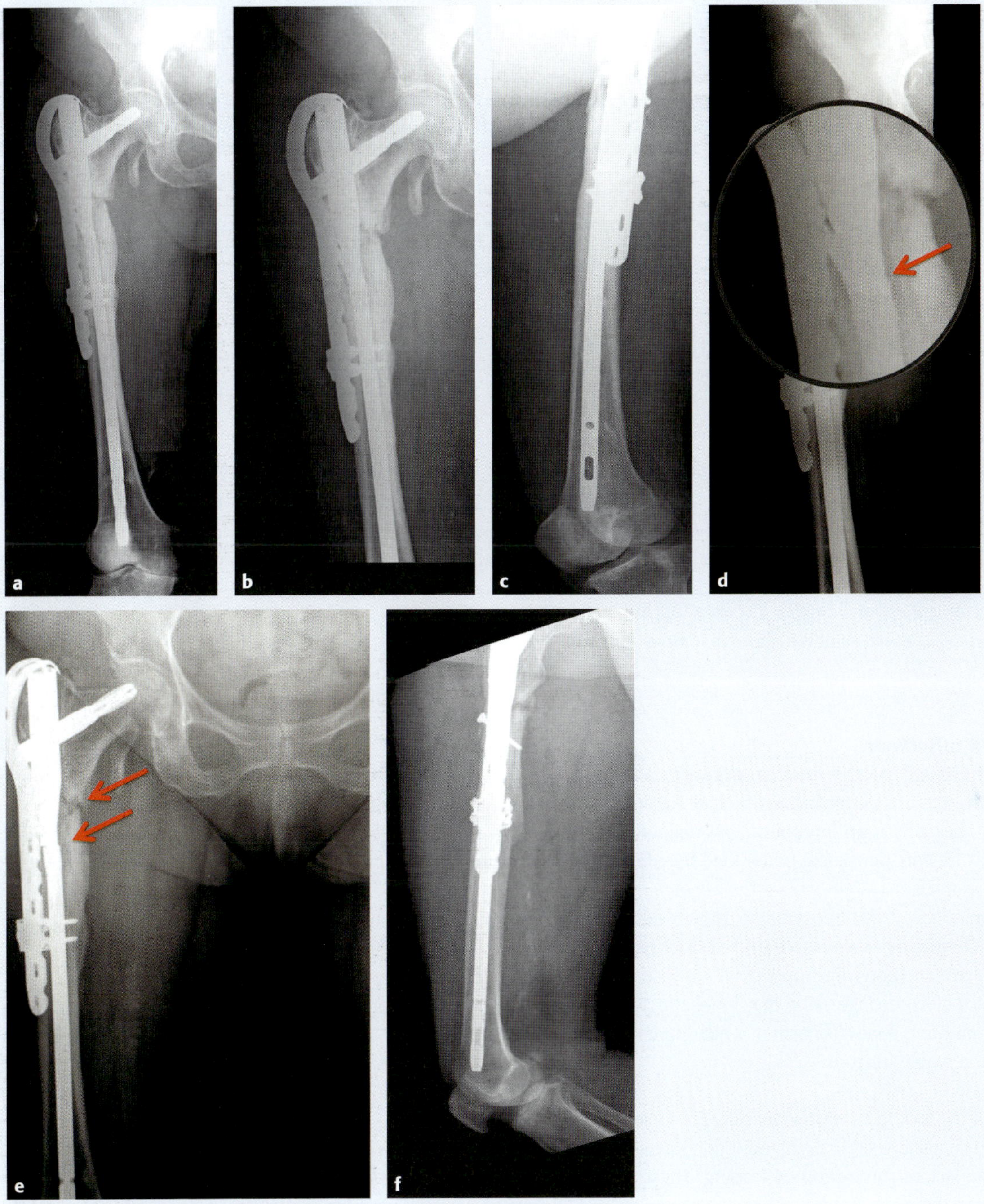

Fig 2.4-23a–f Control x-rays at 9 months following reintervention. In the first x-rays (**a–c**), it was not clear if the nail was broken, but the enlargements (**d–e**) confirmed this together with the unhealed pseudarthrosis x-ray (**f**).

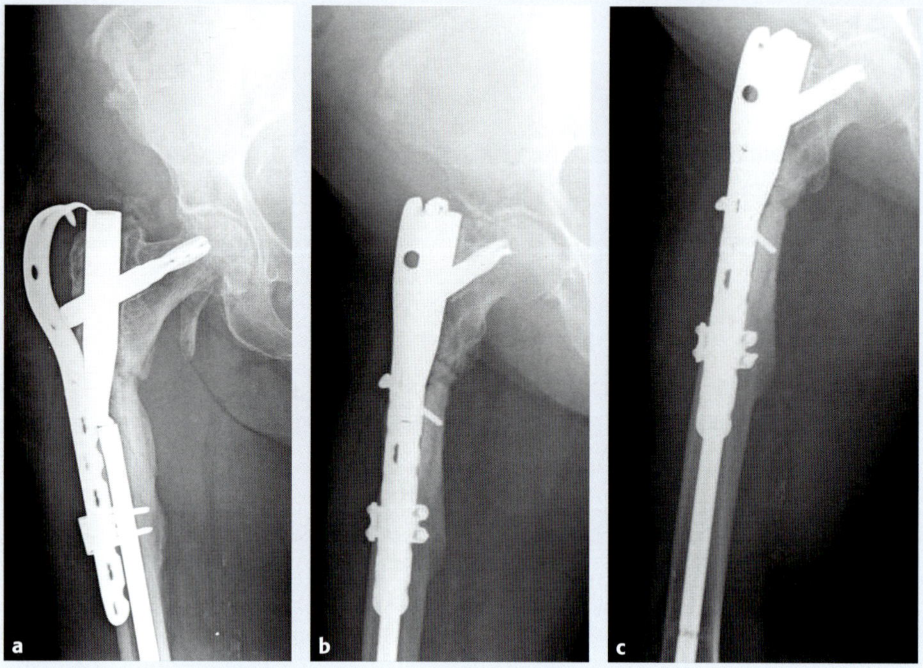

Fig 2.4-24a–c Control x-rays showing the unanchored hook plate after the breakage of the intramedullary nail and varus displacement of the proximal femoral fragment.

Analysis of failure and reflection

Reduction and osteosynthesis with intra- or extramedullary implants was indicated. Due to the patient's age and for biomechanical reasons, the implant of choice was an intramedullary nail, with associated head and neck fixation, permitting better load transfer.

Due to the fracture comminution, it was necessary to open the site to reduce the fragments. Despite using a suitable surgical approach to fully respect the biological conditions, the approximate reduction of the fragments and associated cerclage wires may have affected the biological conditions of bone revascularization, which partially prevented the union of the whole fracture.

In this case, the rigidity of the locked assembly possibly prevented the consolidation of the main fracture site, causing evolution towards pseudarthrosis due to the lack of stimulation by loading. The two cerclage wires were placed too close to each other and may also have compromised the vascularization at the fracture site.

If complete fracture union does not occur, the bone cannot participate in weight bearing. It is the implant that absorbs all the strain and breaks due to material fatigue, a fact corroborated by studies published on material fatigue especially 12–18 months postoperatively. After this time and if no measures have been taken previously to heal the pseudarthrosis, failure of the fixation may appear before the physiological demand for weight bearing.

Final outcome

The clinical course was good; the patient presented at subsequent outpatient check-ups with improvement of pain and a reduction in the analytical markers for inflammation. She also started to walk without pain. The control x-rays showed signs of union (**Fig 2.4-25**).

The clinical course in this case confirms that septic complication can occur, which can delay healing. It is always necessary to think about the possibility of a septic process when faced with situations of poor evolution that are difficult to explain.

If no infection presents, we should reconsider the biological and mechanical conditioning factors. It would be possible to plan an addition of autogenous graft, extracted by the reaming, irrigation, and aspiration system from the contralateral femur, and new decortication and osteosynthesis which can be performed using a 95° plate or dynamic condylar screw with axial compression through the use of an articulated compressor. A pharmacological treatment with teriparatide could also help with bone formation.

In cases without final fracture consolidation, prosthetic substitution of the proximal femur by hip arthroplasty with diaphyseal anchorage or after tumor resections should be considered.

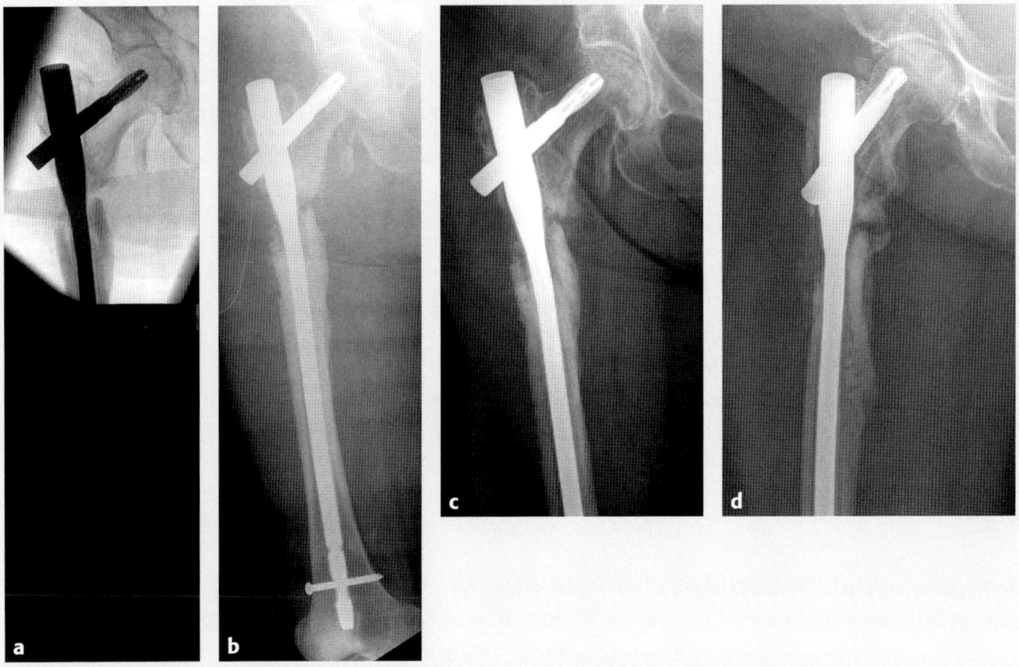

Fig 2.4-25a–d Postoperative control x-rays 3 months after the reintervention with signs of incipient union.

CASE 5

Case description

A 46-year-old woman without significant medical conditions had a motorcycle accident. She sustained an open fracture of the right femur (AO/OTA IO1; Gustilo type I) and a fracture of the right clavicle where nonoperative treatment was indicated. There was also a transverse fracture of the femoral diaphysis, with a bending wedge fragment (AO/OTA 32B2).

Osteosynthesis was performed through proximal and distal locking intramedullary nailing without opening the fracture site. The immediate postoperative control x-ray revealed contact of the main proximal and distal fragments along the lateral cortex (**Fig 2.4-26**). An ultrasound scan revealed the wedge fragment remained close to the fracture site but with anterior looseness and incarceration of the soft tissues (muscle and skin). The patient reported pain on the interior side of the thigh where the muscle was incarcerated, which exacerbated pain during ambulation.

Reintervention was performed to release the soft tissues, stabilizing the intermediate fragment with two cerclage wires (**Fig 2.4-27**).

Subsequently, dynamization of the proximal nail was done at 3 months to achieve the axial compression of the site, as the fracture was not presenting signs of union (**Fig 2.4-28**).

Six months later there were still no signs of callus formation and the pain at the fracture site during ambulation persisted. The nail was replaced with a reamed nail with a greater diameter (9–14 mm). The cerclage wires were removed, the bone was decorticated, and autogenous bone graft originating from the iliac crest was applied (**Fig 2.4-29**).

Four weeks after replacing the nail, the control x-ray showed the start of bone callus formation at the level of the decortication and the added bone graft material. Clinically, no rotational defects or limb shortening existed; although the pain and functional impairment persisted when walking, she continued using crutches (**Fig 2.4-30**).

The patient received alternative therapies and at 18 months presented with resorption of the graft and viable hypotrophic pseudarthrosis (**Fig 2.4-31**).

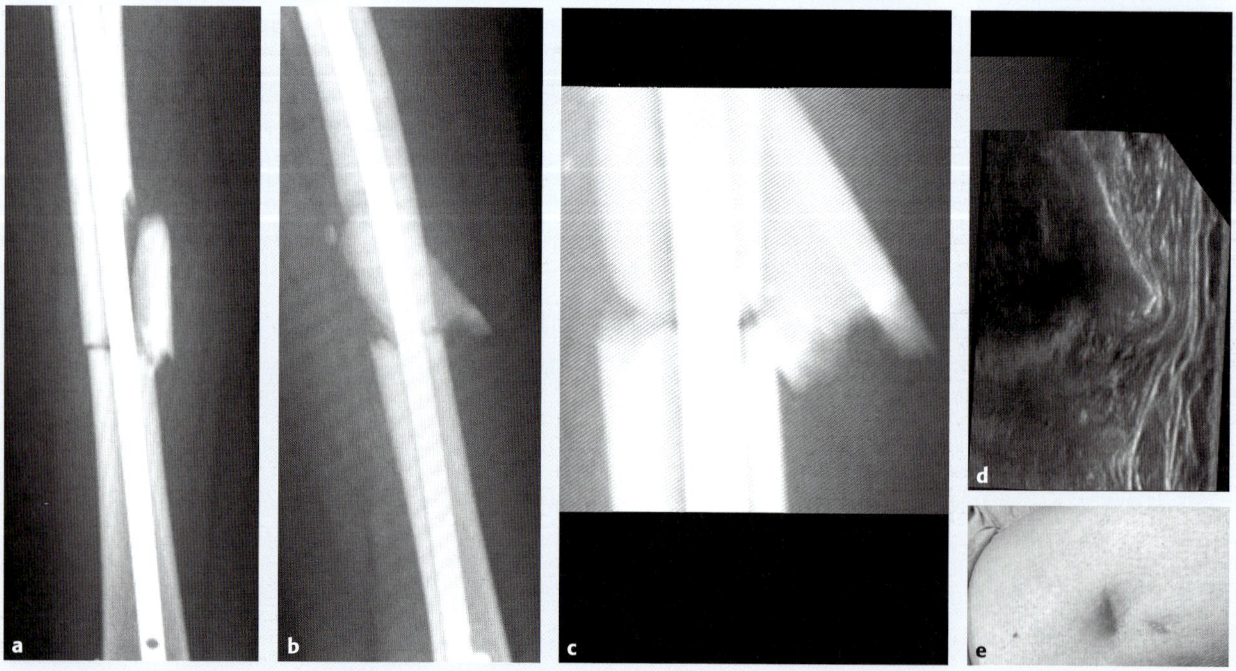

Fig 2.4-26a–e Control x-rays in AP and lateral views at 1 month following surgical intervention for the diaphyseal femoral fracture (**a–b**). The third unreduced fragment can be seen and the detail of the ultrasound imaging shows the incarceration of the soft tissues (**c–d**). Clinical photograph (**e**) showing the incarceration at the cutaneous level.

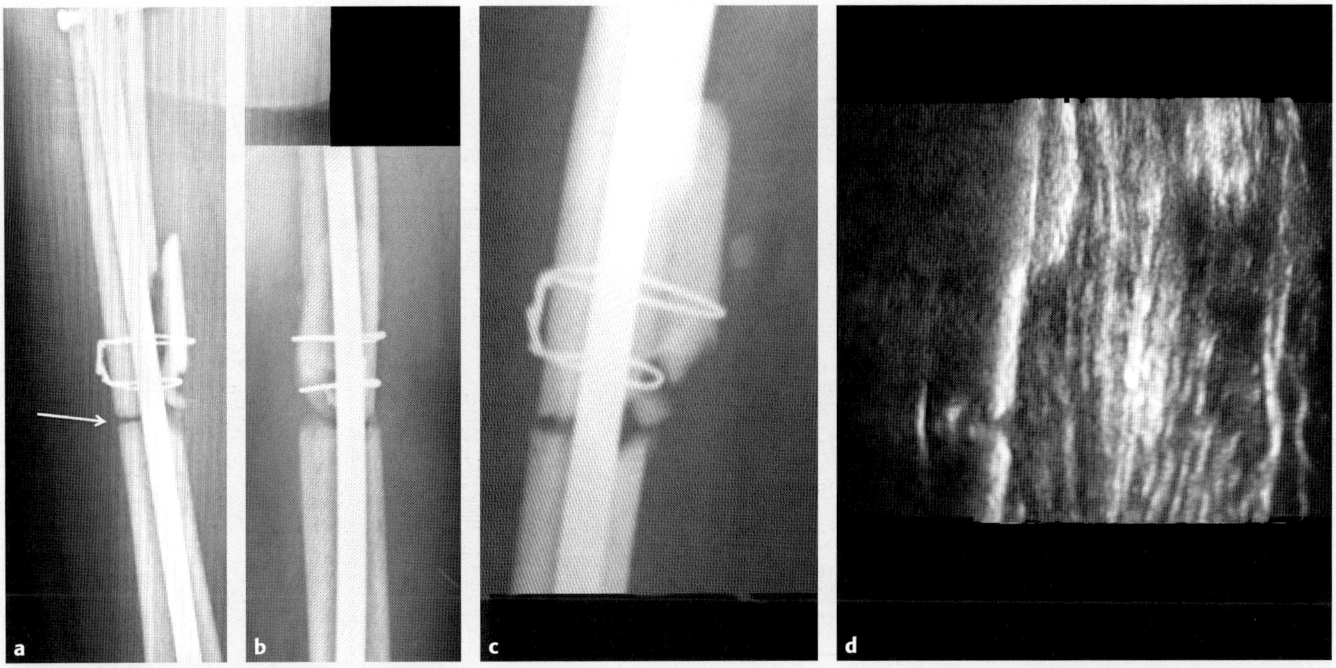

Fig 2.4-27a–d Postoperative control x-rays after reintervention to release the soft tissues, reduce the third bone fragment, and stabilize the intermediate fragment with two cerclage wires (**a–c**). Ultrasound imaging showing detail of the soft tissues released at the fracture site level (**d**).

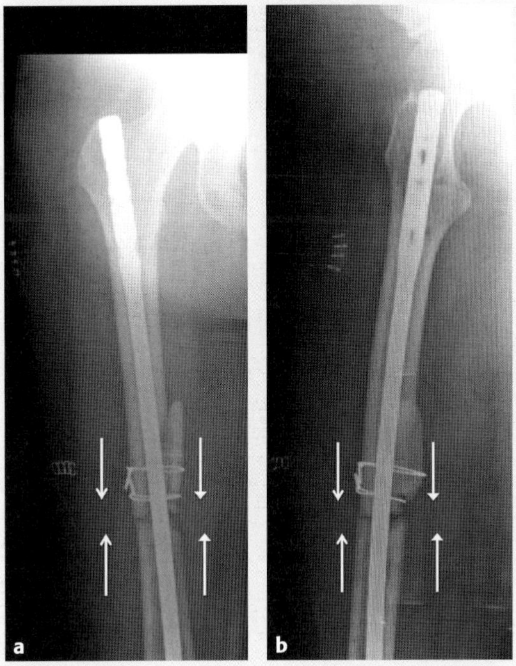

Fig 2.4-28a–b Postoperative control x-rays of the dynamization of the intramedullary nail for the axial compression (arrows) of the fracture site.

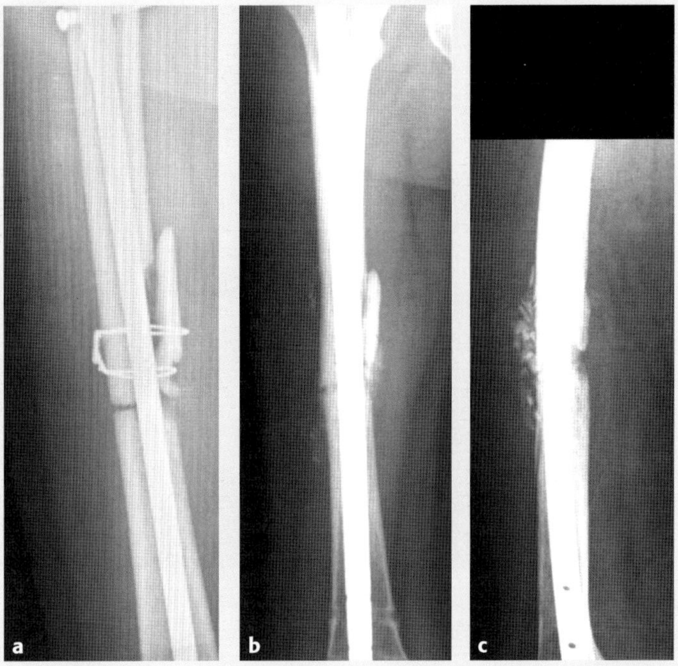

Fig 2.4-29a–c Control x-ray of the new intervention undertaken to exchange the intramedullary nail and add bone graft material at the fracture site.

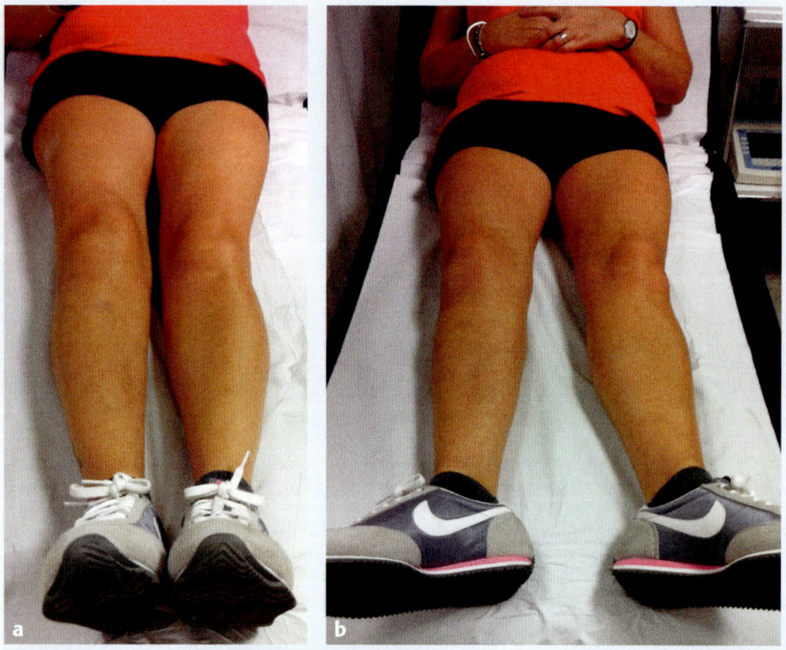

Fig 2.4-30a–b The limbs showing good alignment.

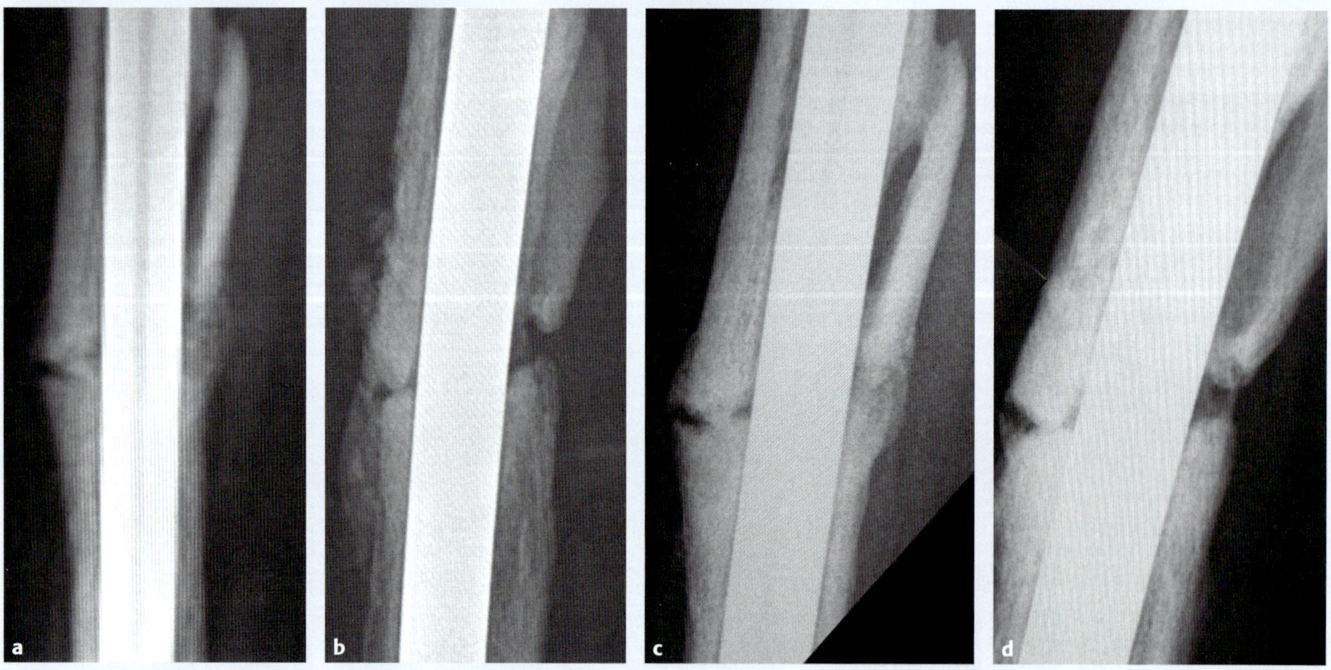

Fig 2.4-31a–k X-rays and computed tomographic (CT) scans of the pseudarthrosis of the femoral diaphysis.
a–d X-rays showing the evolution of the pseudarthrosis site.

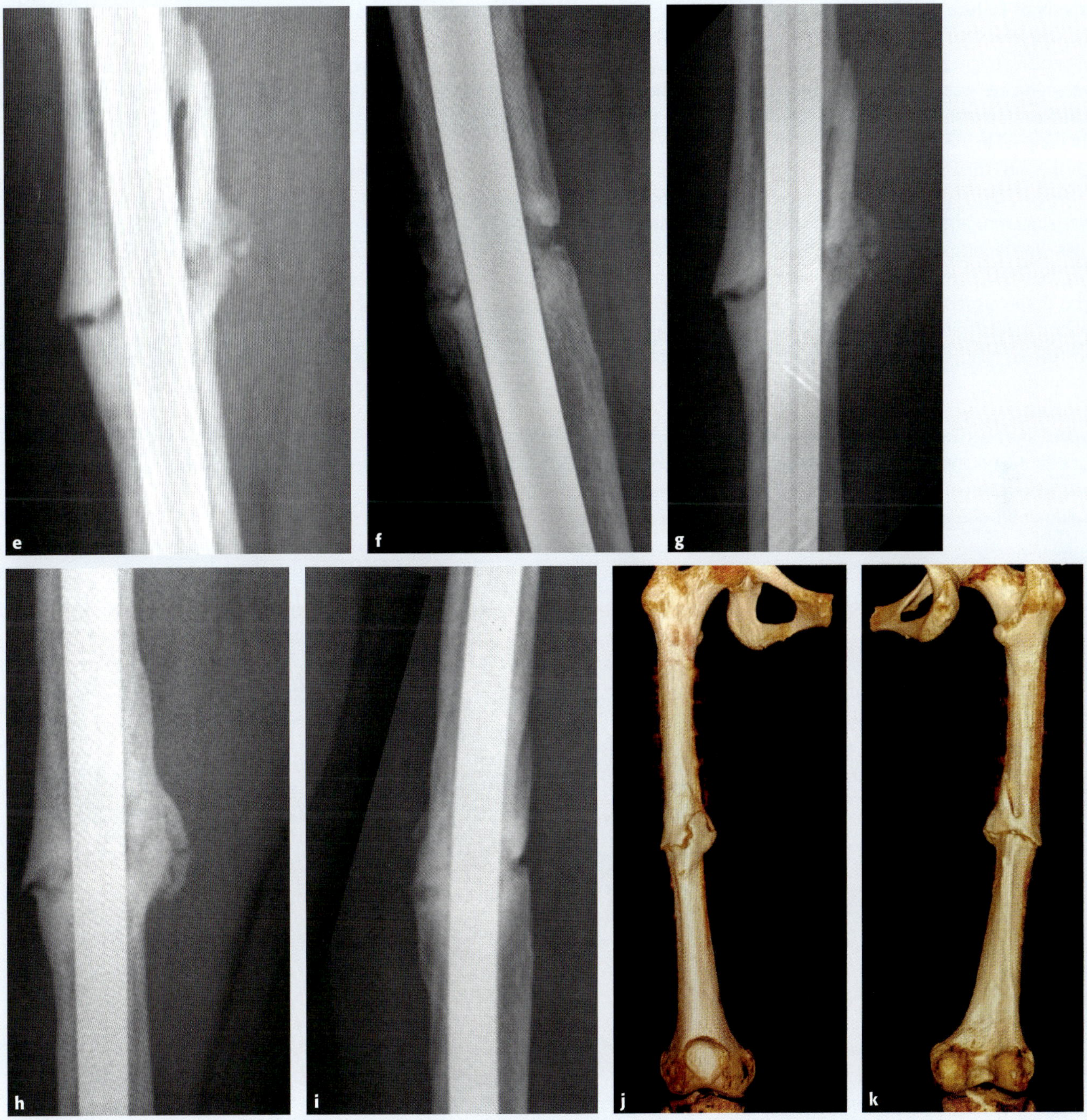

Fig 2.4-31a–k (cont) X-rays and computed tomographic (CT) scans of the pseudarthrosis of the femoral diaphysis.
e–i X-rays showing the evolution of the pseudarthrosis site.
j–k A 3D CT scan reconstruction showing the anterior and posterior aspects of the pseudarthrosis.

Analysis of failure and reflection

In the case of a transverse fracture of the femoral diaphysis with a third bending fragment, osteosynthesis with nailing is indicated. In this case the nail was reamed and locked distally since the fracture was in the zone of the femoral distal isthmus where the intramedullary cavity of the femur starts to widen. Sometimes, the need to open the site for correct reduction of the fragments must be evaluated, especially in situations where the interposition of the musculature may affect union and normal muscular contraction. In this case, the reduction of the intermediate fragment was overlooked during the emergency department intervention and at reintervention. Maybe the intermediate fragment was excessively devitalized by positioning cerclage wires too close together, thus altering the periosteal vascularization. Replacing the nail with one with a larger diameter that provides greater stability after reaming the medullary cavity, decorticating, and applying bone graft is a reasonable option; however, in this patient the evolution was not satisfactory. The causes for the poor evolution may be multifactorial and sometimes it may occur even after a correct action. In this case, the reamed nail did not provide enough stability to the fracture site.

Final outcome

Given the nonunion and lack of clinical healing, the decision was taken to perform a new intervention to have greater biological and biomechanical options. A new Judet-type decortication was planned and performed. The musculature was lifted through a direct decortication to approach the cortex, obtain the bone fragments with the muscular soft-tissue insertions, and thus preserve the existing vascularization (**Fig 2.4-32**).

A straight locking compression plate was prebent and applied with axial compression; it was joined to the femur with two locking attachment plates before carefully closing the surgical access (**Fig 2.4-33**).

The properly performed decortication favored the biological healing of the pseudarthrosis also due to the additional stability provided by the extramedullary plate that counteracted the rotational forces (ie, neutralization, protection, or augmentative plate) (**Fig 2.4-34**).

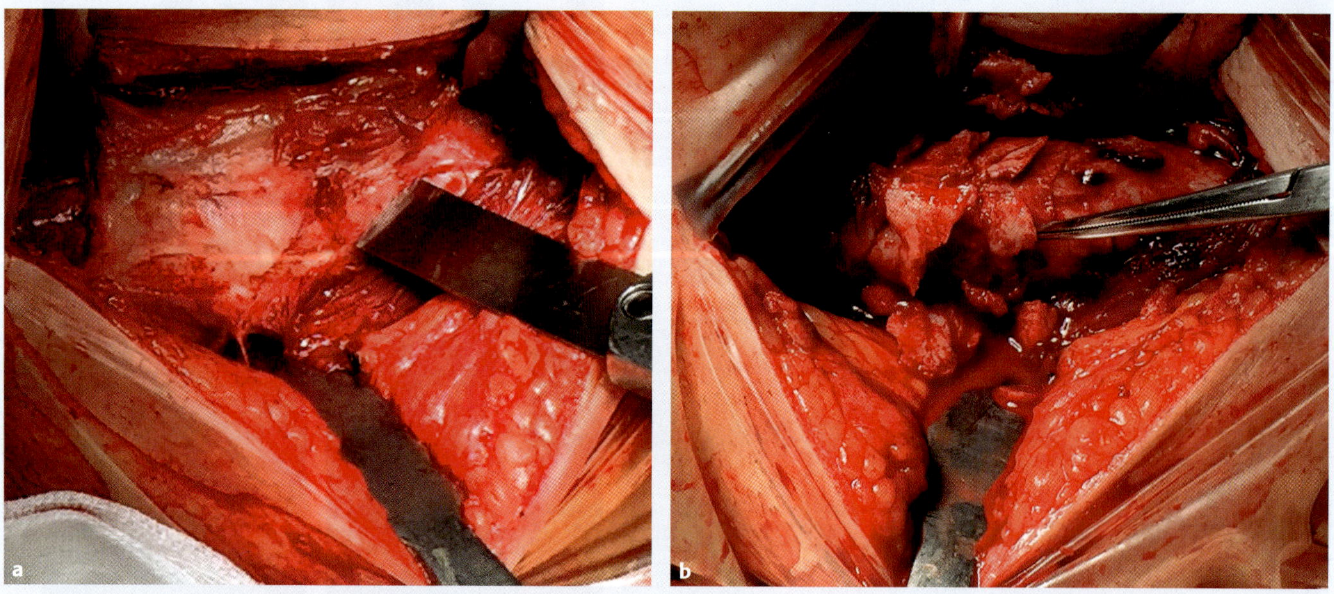

Fig 2.4-32a–b Osteoperiosteal decortication at the level of the pseudarthrosis site.

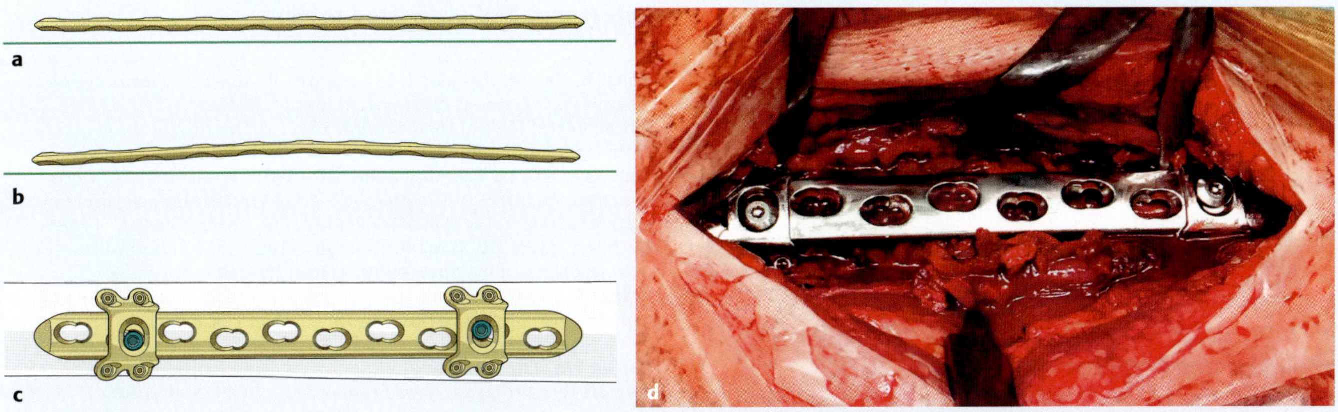

Fig 2.4-33a–d Straight plate (**a**) should be prebent (**b**) before applying it to the fracture. Placing of the straight locking compression plate fixed to the femur with two locking attachment plates (**c**). The decortication and bone graft can be seen (**d**).

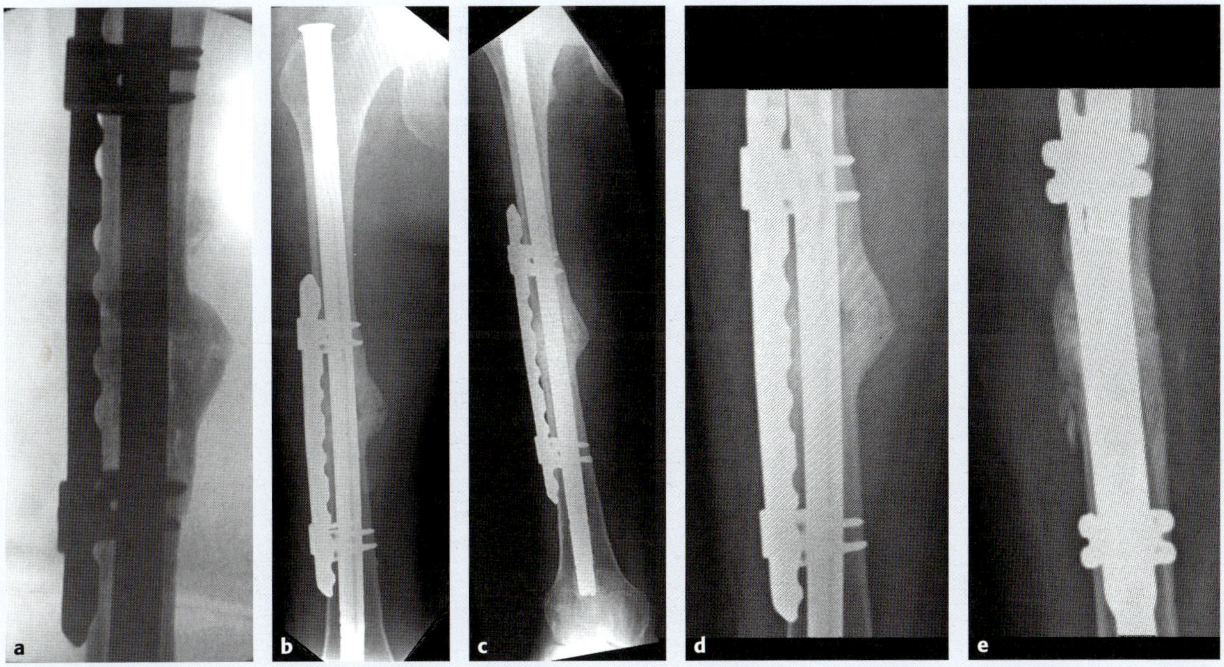

Fig 2.4-34a–e Intraoperative, postoperative, and final control x-rays of reintervention.
a–b Intraoperative and immediate postoperative control x-rays showing the application of the augmentative plate.
c–e Final control x-rays in AP and lateral views of the consolidated pseudarthrosis site.

Key points to remember

- Biology together with mechanics allows consolidation.
- Vascularization allows cellular function to be maintained in the area of the fracture, which determines the formation and quality of the bone healing.
- Depending on the type of reduction and the stability achieved, the biology allows fracture healing by direct (primary) or indirect (secondary) healing.
- Preservation of vascularization is a biological necessity and has mechanical implications.
- Knowledge of the vascular changes in the bone and the soft tissue as a result of the fracture has led to the evolution of concepts both in surgical technique and in surgical access routes.
- Biological conditions of bone healing are also affected by contact with the implant.

References and suggested reading

Babst R, Bavonratanavech S, Pesantez R. *Minimally invasive plate osteosynthesis.* 2nd ed. Stuttgart: Thieme; 2012.
Baumgaertel F, Buhl M, Rahn BA. Fracture healing in biological plate osteosynthesis. *Injury.* 1998;29 Suppl 3:C3–6.
Casstevens C, Le T, Archdeacon MT, et al. Management of extra-articular fractures of the distal tibia: intramedullary nailing versus plate fixation. *J Am Acad Orthop Surg.* 2012 Nov;20(11):675–683.
Gerber C, Mast JW, Ganz R. Biological internal fixation of fractures. *Arch Orthop Trauma Surg.* 1990;109(6):295–303.
Judet PR, Patel A. Muscle pedicle bone grafting of long bones by osteoperiosteal decortication. *Clin Orthop Relat Res.* 1972 Sep;87:74–80.
Perren SM. The concept of biological plating using the limited contact-dynamic compression plate (LC-DCP). Scientific background, design and application. *Injury.* 1991;22 Suppl 1:1–41.
Perren SM. Minimally invasive internal fixation history, essence and potential of a new approach. *Injury.* 2001 May;32 Suppl 1:Sa1–3.
Perren SM, Klaue K, Pohler O, et al. The limited contact dynamic compression plate (LC-DCP). *Arch Orthop Trauma Surg.* 1990;109(6):304–310.
Sirkin M, Sanders R, DiPasquale T, et al. A staged protocol for soft tissue management in the treatment of complex pilon fractures. *J Orthop Trauma.* 1999 Feb;13(2):78–84.
Tscherne H, Oestern HJ. [A new classification of soft-tissue damage in open and closed fractures (author's transl)]. *Unfallheilkunde.* 1982 Mar;85(3):111–115. Germna.
Volgas DA, Harder Y. *Manual of Soft-Tissue Management in Orthopaedic Trauma.* Stuttgart: Thieme; 2011.

Section 3
Implant-related issues

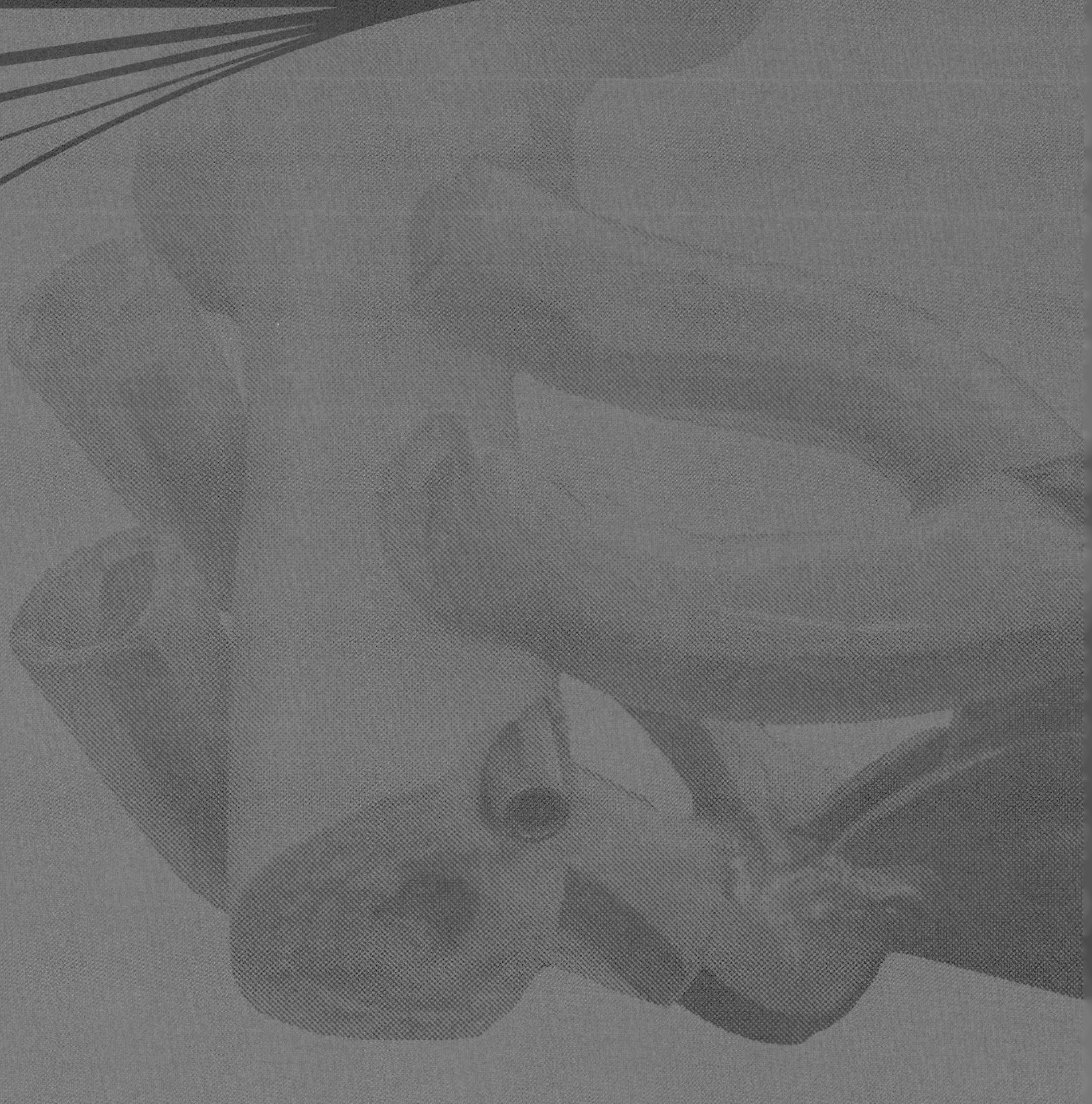

Section 3
Implant-related issues

3.1 Implant selection issues

Miquel Videla Cés
Joan Girós Torres, Roberto Rivero Sosa, J Miquel Sales Pérez

Doubt is the beginning of wisdom.
Aristotle

The four founding AO principles of fracture fixation were:

- Anatomical reduction
- Stable internal fixation
- Preservation of blood supply
- Early active pain-free mobilization

Strict compliance with these principles often pushed the surgeon treating a fracture to ignore biology in favor of perfect anatomical restoration achieved by absolute stability.

The AO philosophy has evolved and now advocates that except in the case of intraarticular fractures, perfect anatomical reduction can be deleterious to bone healing due to the disrespect for biology. Anatomical reduction should only be attempted in cases of simple 2-part fractures. In all other fractures, the aim should be to align and stabilize the two main fragments without disturbing the biology. When the soft tissue surrounding and giving vitality to the fracture and the blood supply to the fractured bone are not disturbed, fracture healing proceeds more rapidly. Minimal damage occurs by aiming to achieve functional instead of anatomical reduction of shaft fractures.

Internal fracture fixation provides mechanical stability to the fractured bone allowing weight bearing and early use of the limb, which facilitates rapid bone healing.

The use of devices for internal fixation modifies the biomechanics of the fracture. Although the ultimate goal of fracture treatment is bone healing and restoration of the functional limb, there are constraints and variables that can influence surgeons' decision making.

In preoperative planning, the patient's age, functional requirements, fracture location, and the morphological and biological status of the bone play an important role in the choice of technique and implant. The choice of treatment depends not only on the patient and the fracture, but also on the surgeon's experience and skills, the hospital environment, and the means available to the surgeon.

With an increase in the longevity over the past decades, there has been a demographic shift toward a growing aging, yet active global population, especially in Western countries; this has led to a rise in the number of osteoporotic fractures that trauma surgeons have to deal with. Such fragility fractures will be one of the future epidemics.

The World Health Organization (WHO) defines osteoporosis according to measurements of bone mineral density (BMD) using dual-energy x-ray absorptiometry (DEXA).

There are three key elements to be considered when defining osteoporosis:

- Bone mass (ie, how much is still left)
- Loss of bone mass (ie, how much is lost)
- Microstructural changes (ie, how the bone is structured)

The bone structure and mechanical resistance may not be expressed only as a BMD value. It is a well-known and proven fact that aging humans lose a substantial amount of bone mass after the age of 25 years. It is also well documented that after the age of 40, women lose more bone and at a faster rate than men.

The pattern of age-related cortical bone loss involves thinning of long-bone cortices or loss of cortical thickness with concomitant increase in medullary diameter. Osteoporosis then influences strength and stiffness of bone, both of which decrease with age and degree of demineralization.

This is true for cortical and cancellous bone [Thompson, 1980]. In osteoporotic bone we therefore see changes in both cortical and cancellous bone.

Cortical bone: The thinned cortex is also poorer quality because of lacunae (ie, Haversian canal areas). The more of these minute cavities that exist, the more porous the bone. The normal Haversian system of bone is dense and compact and is very well organized into a lamellar structure. Normal bone is anisotropic with different properties that depend on the direction of load applied in relation to the orientation of the Haversian system.

Cancellous bone: The change in bone structure is due to decreasing trabecular thickness, interruption of the trabecular network, reduction of trabecular number, and reduction of trabecular connectivity. The overall ratio of cancellous bone to cortical bone is increased. The thinner layer of cortex is weaker and is predisposed to low-energy or fragility fractures.

The decreased cortical thickness greatly affects the holding capacity of screws and also causes an increase in the diameter of the medullary shaft canal, so the anchorage and primary stability of the intramedullary nails are also affected. The nailing technique therefore offers different options depending on whether it is a young or an old bone affected by osteoporosis.

An ever-increasing implant selection is available, which occasionally makes the choice difficult. The commercial pressure of new products should never be greater and valued more highly than the biological and biomechanical criteria; neither should new trends in treatment influence the choice of the most suitable implant for a given fracture. However, we must emphasize that the surgeon's experience and skills can influence decision making, especially when the scientific evidence does not clearly differentiate between the most appropriate techniques and implants for fracture fixation.

The majority of cases in which an implant loosens from the bone or a modular implant appears to be unlocked are likely attributable to a defect in the fixation technique: This is especially true for reduction techniques in which primary stability is not achieved by the fracture itself, so the load is borne by the implant only, leading to material fatigue and causing either loss of locking system in the modular implants or the fracture of the nail, even breakage of the plate or screws.

In a few cases, it is the implant that fails. Although it is difficult to predict the failure, we must suspect it when the locking systems of the spiral blades or the screw locking threads attached to the plate or to the bone show even minimal irregularities in the embossing of the implant.

Miquel Videla Cés
Joan Girós Torres, Roberto Rivero Sosa, J Miquel Sales Pérez

Case description

An 87-year-old woman without severe comorbidities fell at home from standing height and sustained a pertrochanteric fracture (AO/OTA 31A2). Treatment with a proximal femoral nail antirotation (PFNA) was planned (**Fig 3.1-1**).

The postoperative control x-ray showed that the spiral blade was placed in a center–center position but it appeared not to be completely blocked (**Fig 3.1-2**). However, the rotational forces in the femoral neck conflicted with the spiral blade, as the blade could have moved into the bone, causing bone loss and loosening and leading to the cut-out.

At the 6-week follow-up control, the blade was clearly unlocked and an initial loosening of the spiral blade could be seen, which allowed the blade to freely rotate in the mobile part of the spiral blade. This movement did not stop the intrinsic rotational movement of the femoral neck and so this unstable situation in the proximal femur caused a fracture in the lateral cortex.

The patient was reoperated 3 months after the first surgery, after the cut-out had occurred (**Fig 3.1-3**). The absence of bone (ie, bone loss) in the femoral neck and head as well as calcar and lesser trochanter led the surgeon to plan rescue surgery with a total hip prosthesis (**Fig 3.1-4**). Considering the age and functionality of the patient, the surgeon chose a cemented arthroplasty. The patient was authorized to walk with full weight bearing in the immediate postoperative period after the second surgery.

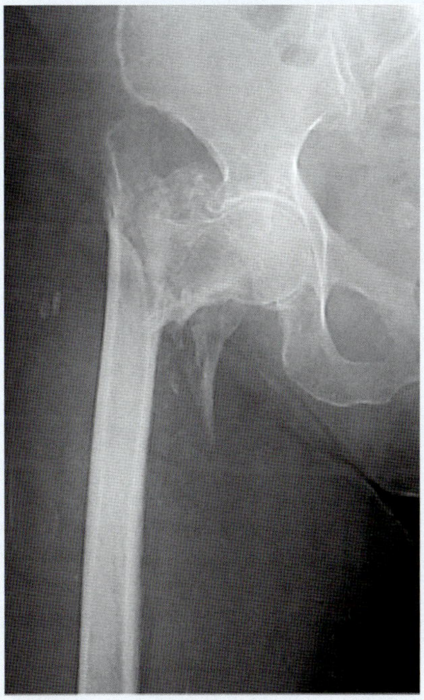

Fig 3.1-1 X-ray of the pertrochanteric right femoral fracture.

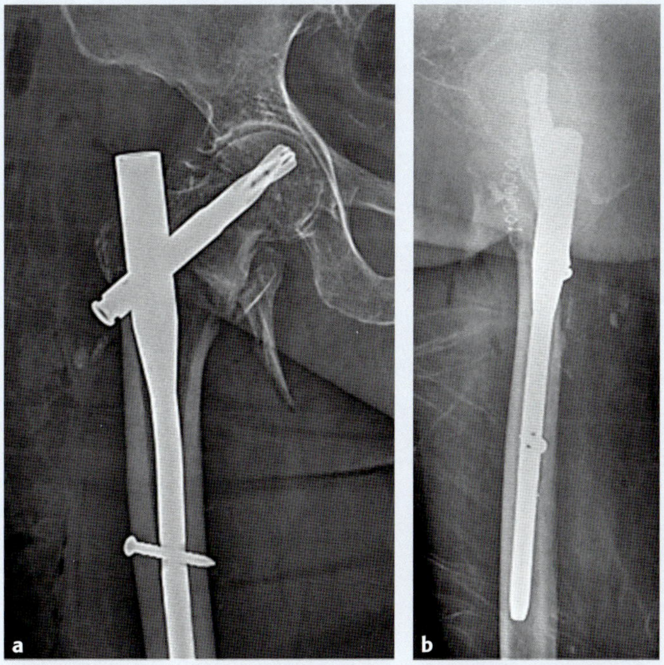

Fig 3.1-2a–b Postoperative control x-rays showing the spiral blade in center–center position but apparently not completely blocked. A double contour is seen at the distal end of the spiral blade that appears to be unlocked. Normally, this double contour should not be visible when the blade is locked.

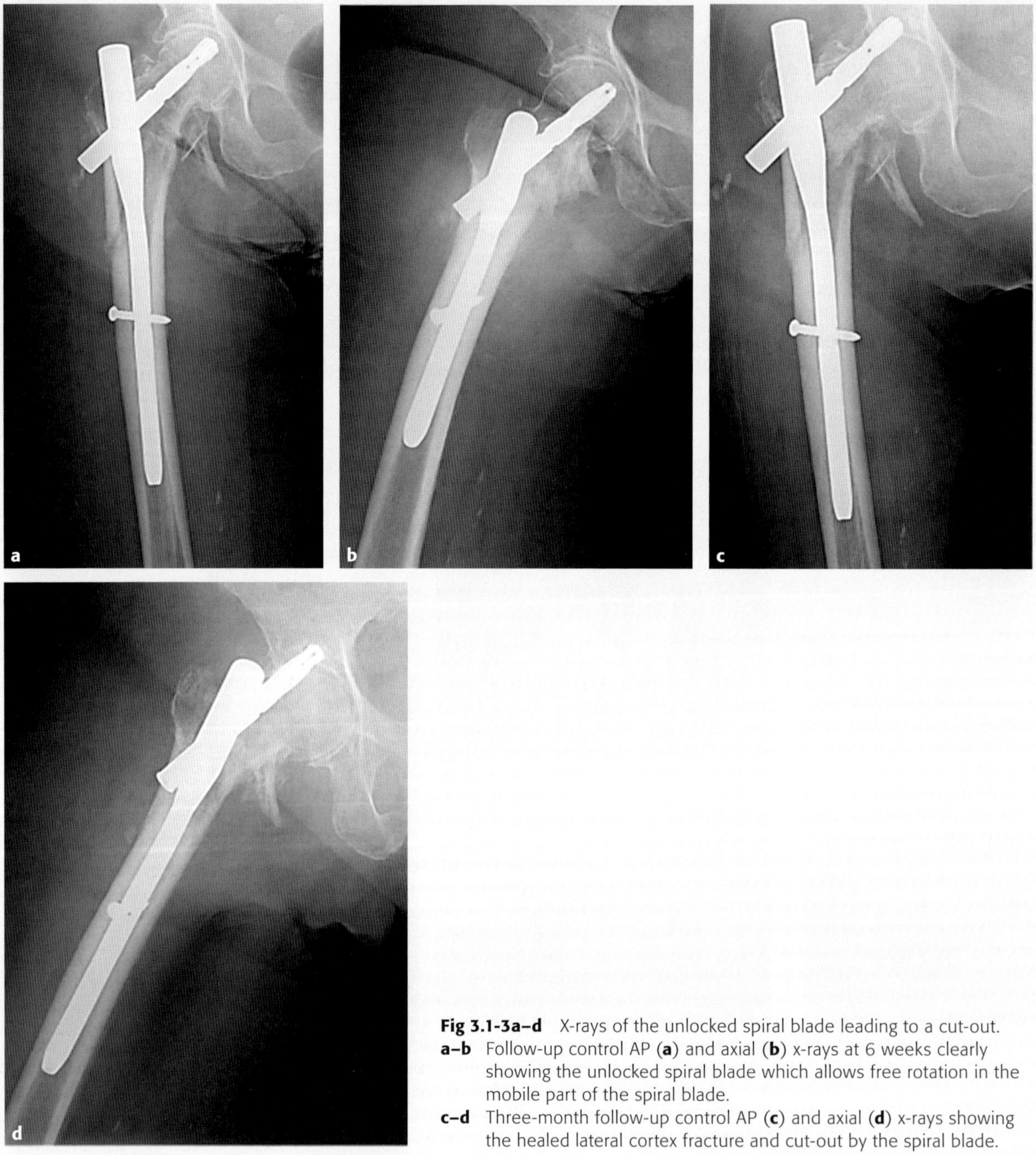

Fig 3.1-3a–d X-rays of the unlocked spiral blade leading to a cut-out.
a–b Follow-up control AP (**a**) and axial (**b**) x-rays at 6 weeks clearly showing the unlocked spiral blade which allows free rotation in the mobile part of the spiral blade.
c–d Three-month follow-up control AP (**c**) and axial (**d**) x-rays showing the healed lateral cortex fracture and cut-out by the spiral blade.

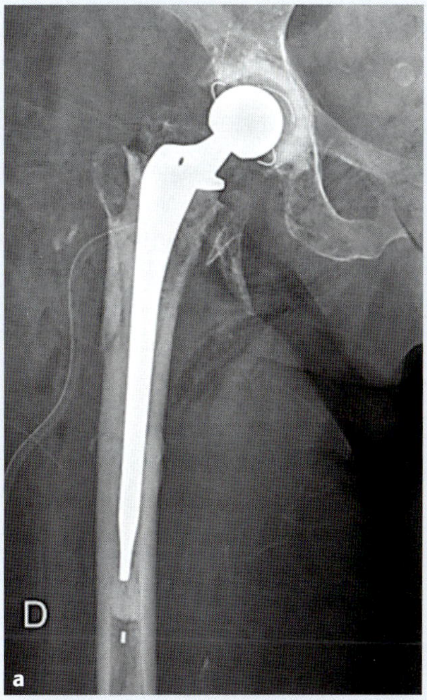

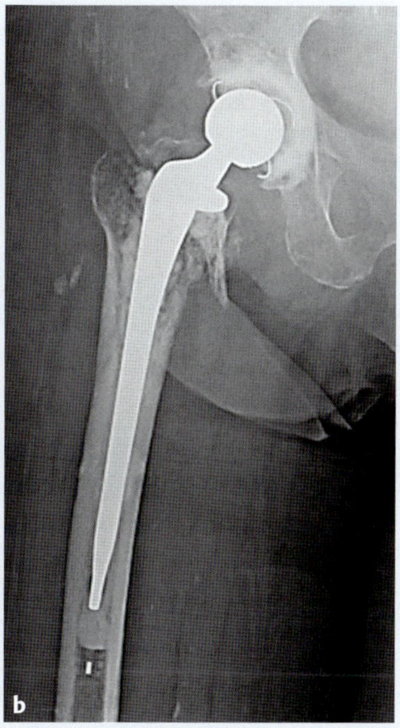

Fig 3.1-4a–b X-rays after the rescue surgery was performed, ie, removal of the proximal femoral nail antirotation and the application of a total hip prosthesis that was cemented because of the patient's age and functional status.

Analysis of failure and reflection

Although good preoperative imaging and a good biomechanical device in the intertrochanteric nail were available, the surgical team probably failed to properly check the connections between the PFNA blade and the impactor. The surgeon should have checked the C-arm images and also the locked system of the spiral blade because a blocked blade is easily seen by looking at the images on the screen.

If, in the first weeks, changes like an unlocked PFNA blade or lateral and cranial migration of the PFNA blade are observed in the x-ray, reoperation should be considered, as it is a better choice than a cut-out. Time will not improve an adverse situation once it has been detected.

Final outcome

Some functional recovery was achieved. Although the patient recovered the ability to walk with crutches, she had lost quality of life 1 year postfracture. It is well known that elderly people who sustain a proximal femoral fracture lose some physical ability after the fracture and surgery. Two or more surgeries add morbidity to her or his biological frailty.

Key points to remember

- Anatomical reduction should only be attempted in articular fractures and in cases of simple 2-part fractures.
- When an extramedullary fixation is planned in osteoporotic bone with decreased cortical thickness, angular stable screws with a larger diameter core should be chosen to improve their holding capacity.
- To increase the anchorage and primary stability of the endomedullary nails in the wide canal of an osteoporotic shaft, nails with a large diameter should be used.
- The commercial pressure of new brands and implants should never be considered more important than the biological and biomechanical criteria; nor should new trends in treatment influence the choice of the best or most appropriate implant for a given fracture.
- Fracture reduction must be aimed at ensuring that the primary stability is achieved by the fracture itself, avoiding gaps and axial alterations that lead to implant fatigue due to overload.

References and suggested reading

Thompson DD. Age changes in bone mineralization, cortical thickness, and haversian canal area. *Calcif Tissue Int.* 1980;31(1):5–11.

3.2 Type of implant related to biomechanical principles

Joan Girós Torres, Christian Kammerlander, Roberto Rivero Sosa, Bianka Rubenbauer, J Miguel Sales Pérez, Fabian Sommer, Miquel Videla Cés

Few see what we are, but everyone sees what we look like.

Niccolò Machiavelli

The term "stability" is widely used by surgeons, but its meaning differs from that used in engineering. The surgeon uses the word "stability" to express the degree of displacement at the fracture site induced by load.

Fracture fixation with absolute stability means that there is no micromotion at the fracture site under physiological load, nor is there an increase in the rigidity of the fixation of the bone implant, because this would indicate a stress riser in the implant–bone interface, generating a zone of weakness and a starting point for periimplant fractures.

With relative stability, the bone fragments are displaced relative to each other when physiological load is applied to the fracture. Displacement increases with the applied load and decreases with the rigidity of the fixation device. A fixation method is considered flexible if it allows controlled interfragmentary movement under physiological load. Therefore, all fixation methods with the exception of compression techniques may be seen as flexible fixations that provide relative stability. The degree of flexibility can vary; this is determined by how the surgeon applies the device and how it is loaded [Ito et al, 2007].

Planning the treatment of a fracture should not only take into account the morphology of the fracture and its location in a certain bone segment but also the patient's age, cognitive status, comorbidity, and commitment as well as discipline in the postoperative period. These play an important role in surgical decision making and in the choice of implant and technique.

The long bones have a tension/traction side and a compression side. The biomechanical principle of the tension band is based on the fact that tensile forces are transformed into compression forces.

In engineering, the biomechanical principle of the tension band consists in placing a rigid attachment on the surface tension of a structure to provide reinforcement and avoid falls or breakage. In traumatology, this principle was introduced by Friedrich Pauwels [Pauwels, 1935; Hak et al, 2007] and applied to treatment in bone surgery.

All bone subjected to an eccentric load works under flexion forces [Pauwels, 1935]. The typical distribution in external tensile and internal compression forces causes distraction of the fracture line on the tension side resulting in external angulation of the bone. If these stresses are absorbed by an implant and internal compression efforts are supported by the bone, the load capacity of the bone is restored. As a result, axial interfragmentary compression will be achieved during loading.

This principle is evident when any implant is applied to the tension side of the bone. Although cerclage wiring is the best example of a tension band, any implant placed on the tension side of the bone will demonstrate this principle [Rüedi et al, 2007; Browner et al, 2008].

In the early stage of healing when mainly soft tissue is still present, the fracture tolerates a greater deformation or higher tissue strain than at a later stage when the callus contains mainly calcified tissue. The manner in which mechanical factors influence fracture healing is explained by Perren's strain theory (**Fig/Animation 3.2-1– Fig/Animation 3.2-4**) [Buckley et al, 2017].

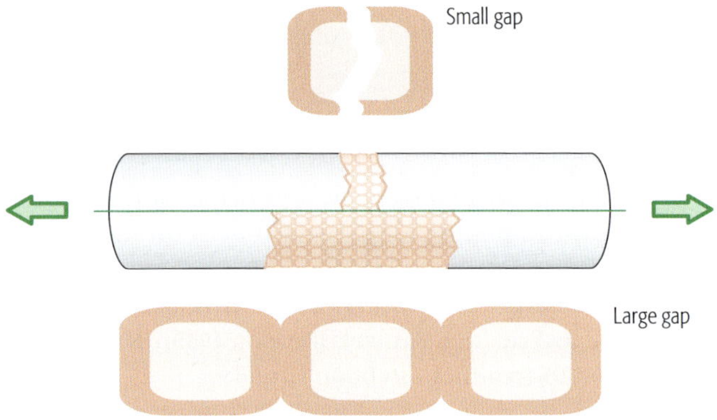

Fig/Animation 3.2-1 Perren's strain theory. Motion at the fracture results in deformation producing strain in the granulation tissue at the fracture site.

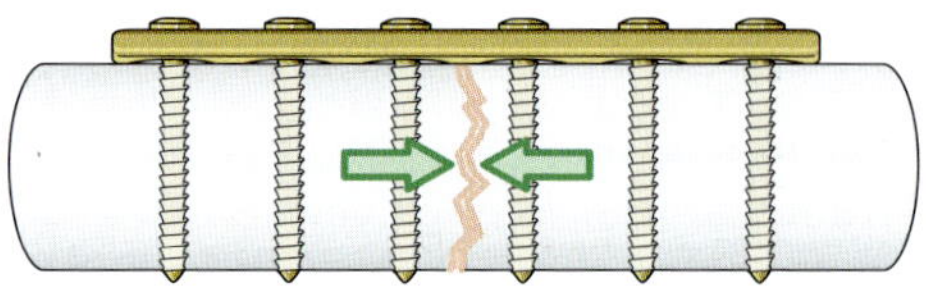

Fig/Animation 3.2-2 Perren's strain theory. A perfectly reduced simple fracture (small gap) stabilized under compression (absolute stability and low strain) heals without external callus (direct healing).

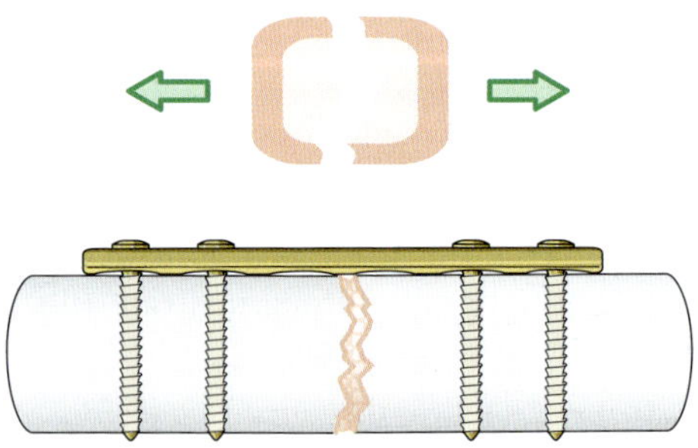

Fig/Animation 3.2-3 Perren's strain theory. A simple fracture (small gap) fixed with a bridging plate (relative stability) is exposed to movement (high strain). Fracture healing is delayed or will not occur at all. The plate will eventually fail.

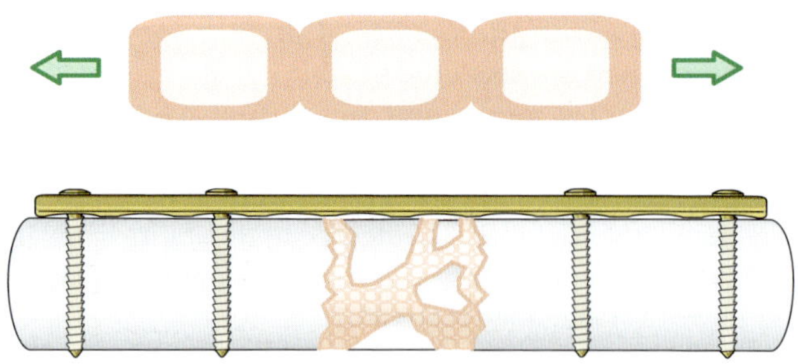

Fig/Animation 3.2-4 Perren's strain theory. In a multifragmentary fracture (large gap) fixed with a bridging plate (relative stability) the strain will be low despite movement, and fracture healing will occur with callus formation (indirect bone healing).

According to Perren's strain theory, strain is the relative deformation of a material (eg, granulation tissue within a gap) when a given force is applied. Normal strain is the change in length (Δ l) in comparison to original length (l) when a given load is applied, ie, Δ l/l. Thus, it has no dimensions and is often expressed as a percentage. The amount of deformation that a tissue can tolerate and still function varies greatly. Intact bone has a normal strain tolerance of 2% (before it fractures), whereas granulation tissue has a strain tolerance of 100%. Bony bridging between the distal and proximal callus can only occur when local strain (ie, deformation) is less than the woven bone forming in the gap can tolerate. Thus, hard callus will not bridge a fracture gap when the movement between the fracture ends is too great [Perren et al, 1980]. Nature deals with this problem by expanding the volume of soft callus. This results in a decrease in the local tissue strain to a level that allows bony bridging. This adaptive mechanism is not effective when the fracture gap has been considerably narrowed so that most of the interfragmentary movement occurs at the gap, producing a high-strain environment. Thus, overloading the fracture with too much interfragmentary movement later in the healing process is not well tolerated [Claes et al, 1999].

At the cellular level, where the fundamental process of bone regeneration and tissue differentiation occurs, the situation is more complex. The biomechanical conditions, such as strain and fluid pressure, have an inhomogeneous distribution within the callus. The mechanoregulation of callus cells is a feedback loop in which the signals are created by the applied load and modulated by the callus tissue. Mechanical loading of the callus tissue produces local biophysical stimuli that are sensed by the cells. This may regulate cell phenotype, proliferation, apoptosis, and metabolic activities. With alteration of the extracellular matrix, and the associated changes in tissue properties, the biophysical stimuli caused by mechanical loading are modulated, producing different biophysical signals even with the same load. In normal fracture healing this feedback process reaches a steady state when the callus has ossified and the original cortex has regenerated. The biophysical signals themselves and the way they interact to produce the biological response are still being investigated. Several mechanoregulation algorithms have been postulated and have been shown to be consistent with some aspects of fracture healing, but they require further corroboration. Transduction of these stimuli into intracellular and extracellular messenger systems are being investigated; so both physical and molecular methods of treatment may be developed to treat delayed union and nonunion [Perren et al, 1980].

When fractures are splinted, movement of the fragments in relation to each other depends on the:

- Amount of external loading
- Stiffness of the splints
- Stiffness of the tissues bridging the fracture

This explains why multifragmentary fractures are more tolerant to instability than simple fracture lines. However, when choosing an initially somewhat larger gap width, the strain can be kept low in simple gaps as well.

CASE 1

Case description

A 77-year-old man suffering from ankylosing spondylitis and osteoporosis fell on the ground during a bout of excessive alcohol consumption. The initial computed tomographic (CT) scan (**Fig 3.2-5a–b**) and magnetic resonance imaging (**Fig 3.2-5c**) showed a dislocated and entangled facet joint in the cervical vertebrae between C6 and C7 (AO/OTA 51.F4.C) without neurological symptoms. The patient was immediately treated operatively with corpectomy of C7 and ventral stabilization from C6 to T1 with a cervical spine locking plate with 16 mm screws and a bone graft from the iliac crest. Postoperative x-rays showed a correct implant placement and an accurate anatomical reduction (**Fig 3.2-6**). Further treatment was immobilization by a rigid cervical collar. Almost 1 week later the patient presented a complete quadriplegia after mobilizing in the ward. A CT scan was performed and a failure of the distal screws was diagnosed combined with an almost complete diversion of the spinal cord due to a ventral dislocation of C7 (**Fig 3.2-7**). The patient was immediately reoperated, using the

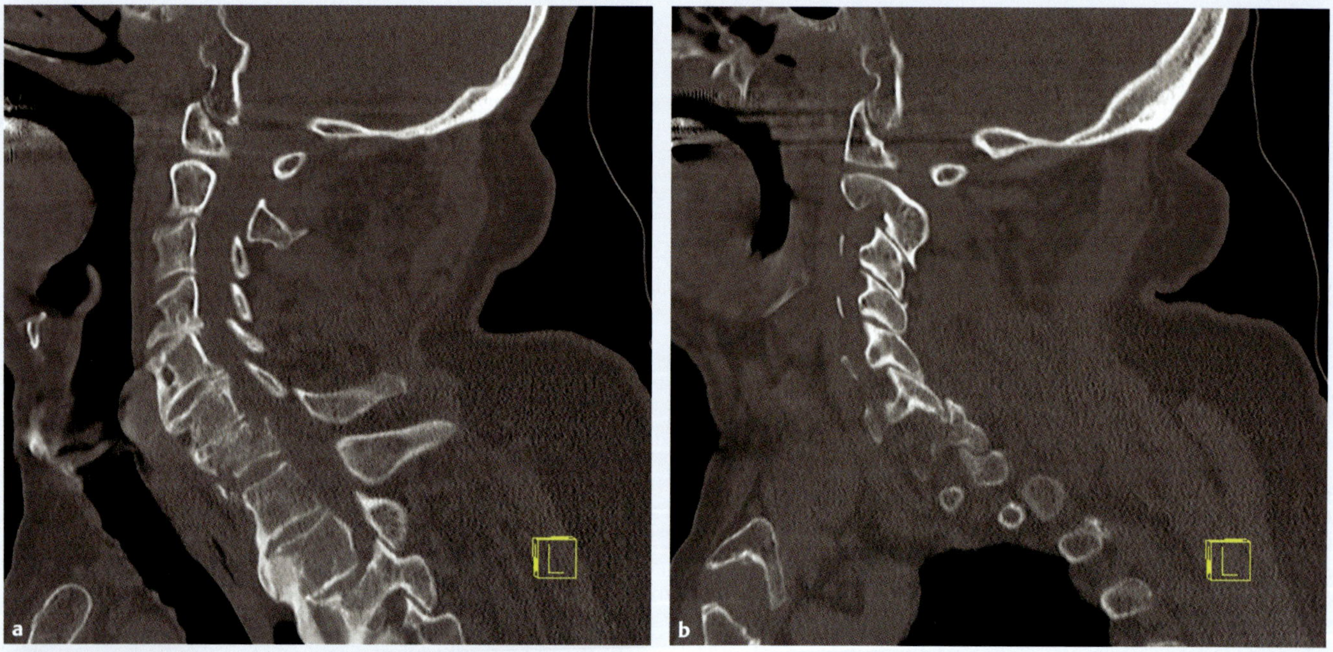

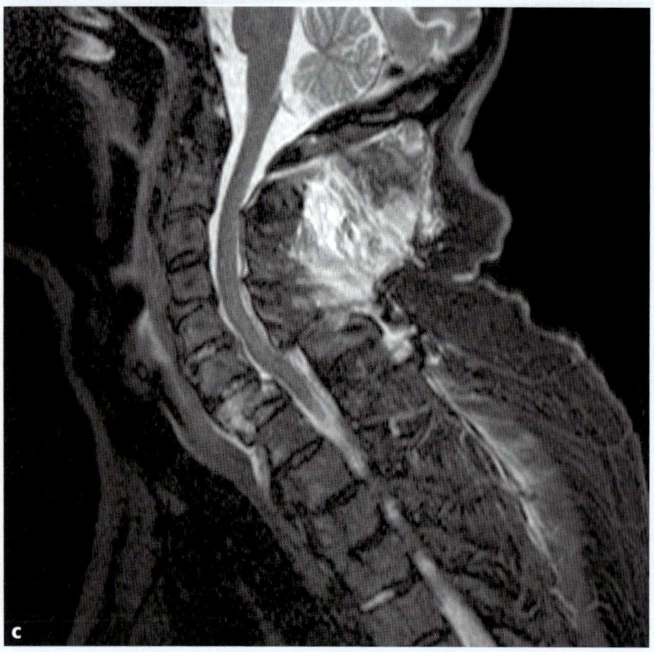

Fig 3.2-5a–c Initial computed tomographic scans (**a–b**) and magnetic resonance imaging (**c**) showing a dislocated and entangled facet joint between the sixth and seventh cervical vertebrae without neurological symptoms.

existing ventral approach to remove the screws, plate, and bone graft. Because of the damage to the C6 end plate, a corpectomy of the whole vertebra had to be performed. For the vertebral replacement of C6 and C7, a metal spacer was implanted and stabilized using a ventral plate from C5 to T1 (**Fig 3.2-8**). The plate was fixed with 16 mm and 18 mm angular stable direct locking screws. Reduction and fixation were checked with an intraoperative three-dimensional x-ray scan.

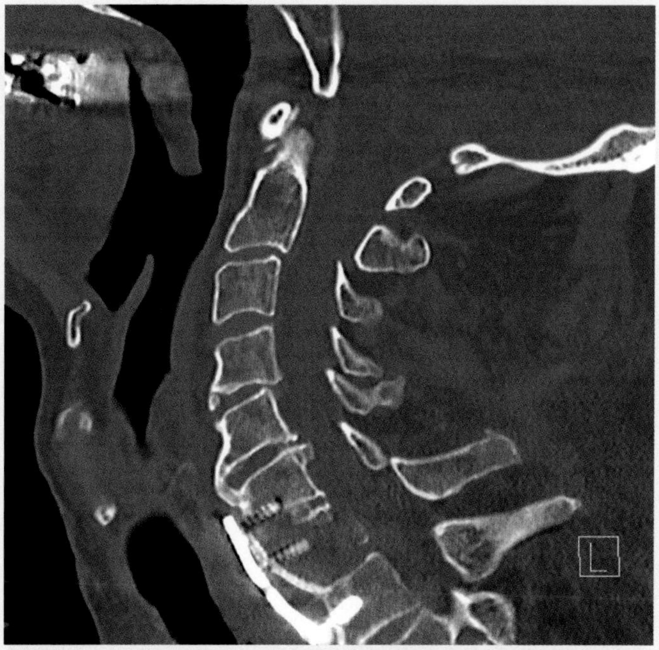

Fig 3.2-6 Postoperative control x-ray showing treatment with corpectomy of C7 and ventral stabilization from C6 to T1 with a cervical spine locking plate and bone autograft from the iliac crest.

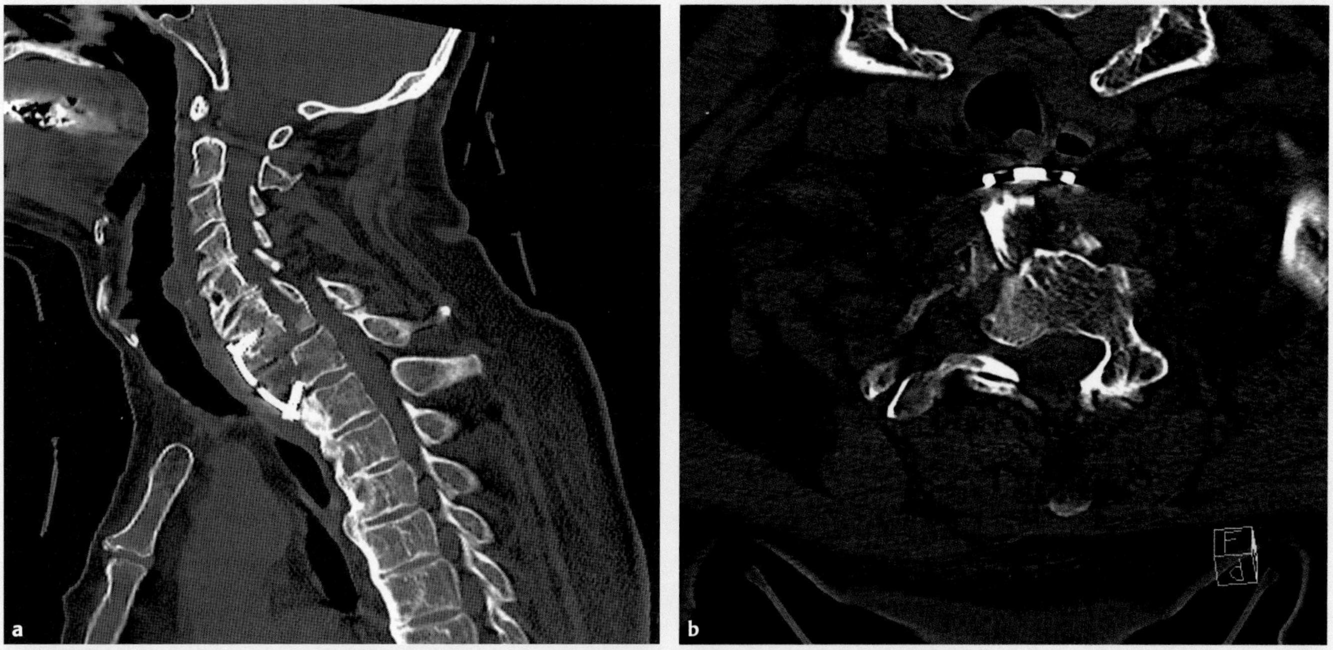

Fig 3.2-7a–b Computed tomographic scans performed 1 week after the surgery show a ventral dislocation of C7 (**a**) secondary to the failure of the distal screws combined with an almost complete diversion of the spinal cord (**b**).

Analysis of failure and reflection

The reduction and fixation of the fracture was adequate for a healthy patient, but in this case the patient was suffering from ankylosing spondylitis and osteoporosis. The selected implant allowed only expansion head screws with a maximum length of 16 mm to be used, without a direct interlocking mechanism.

Due to the ankylosing spondylitis, the leverage on the spinal column was increased, especially in the transition area between the flexible cervical and the more rigid thoracic spine. Furthermore, the screws could not provide the stability expected of the osteosynthesis in the osteoporotic bone. During the initial operation, the forces loading the implant in the ankylosing spondylitis were underestimated and the bone quality was overestimated.

In cases with unknown or poor bone quality and/or signs of increased leverage on the implant, the implants of choice should be plates with the possibility of angle-stable screw locking and a large selection of screw lengths. Also, additional dorsal stabilization should be considered earlier. Another option is the extension of initial stabilization to more vertebral levels. For patients suffering from ankylosing spondylitis, a ventral extension of the stabilization is possible without replacement of the intervertebral discs because of their ossification.

Final outcome

The postoperative treatment was similar to that after the first operation, ie, immobilization with a rigid cervical collar. Immediately after the last operation, the neurological symptoms were decreasing and the quadriparesis had almost disappeared.

In addition to the emergency ventral restabilization, a planned dorsal stabilization of C4/5 to T3 was performed 5 days later (**Fig 3.2-9**). Nine days after the dorsal stabilization, the patient could leave the intensive care unit and was mobilized with physiotherapy. The neurological symptoms almost completely disappeared. Only a lesion of the C7 and C8 spinal nerve with paresis of the radial nerve occurred. In this condition the patient could be transferred to a rehabilitation center.

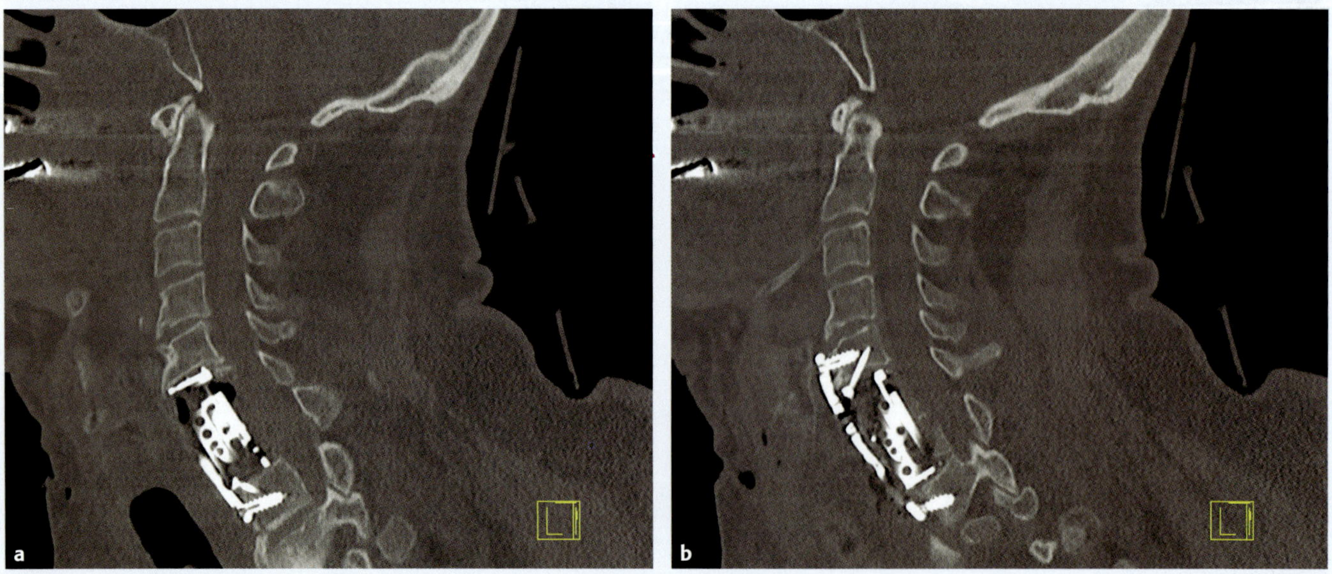

Fig 3.2-8a–b Computed tomographic scans of the emergency ventral restabilization.

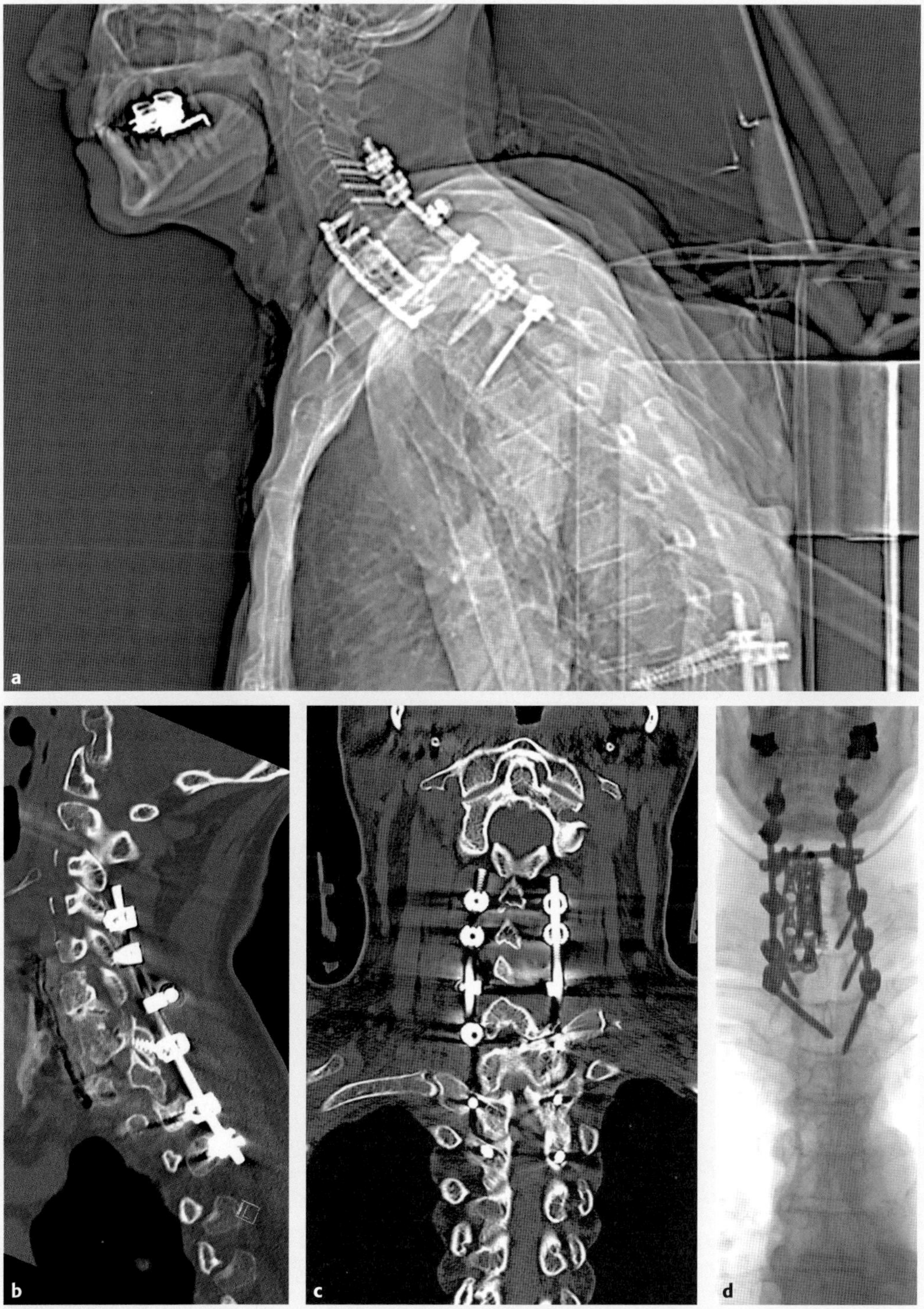

Fig 3.2-9a–d Images of the dorsal stabilization and complete arthrodesis.
a–c Computed tomographic scans showing the dorsal stabilization of C4/5–T3 that was performed 5 days later.
d Intraoperative C-arm view of the complete arthrodesis of C4–T3.

CASE 2

Case description

An 84-year-old woman stumbled and fell at home. Her airway, breathing, circulation, disability, and exposure/examination (ABCDE) following advanced trauma life support were fine, but she sustained a simple spiral fracture of the right distal femoral shaft (AO/OTA 32A1) (**Fig 3.2-10**). Surgery with an angle-stable side plate (ie, reversed distal femoral less invasive stabilization system [LISS DF]) was planned, and the surgeon decided to use a first-generation LISS plate (with only round holes as combi-holes did not exist) but lacked hands-on training.

The result of the first surgery led the authors to believe that marketing criteria had won out over the stability criteria, mixing the principles of absolute stability and relative stability in the first surgery (**Fig 3.2-11** and **Fig 3.2-12**). The first rescue surgery was planned and performed. The same implant was used but absolute stability criteria were followed with excess stiffness that caused a weak stress zone between the elasticity of the osteopenic bone and the rigidity of the proximal end of the LISS plate, which was attached to the bone with too many screws and cerclage wires leading to the second failure (**Fig 3.2-13**). Thus, a predictable periimplant fracture in the stress zone was the next failure. Finally, the hardware was removed and an intramedullary internal fixation was performed in a second rescue surgery.

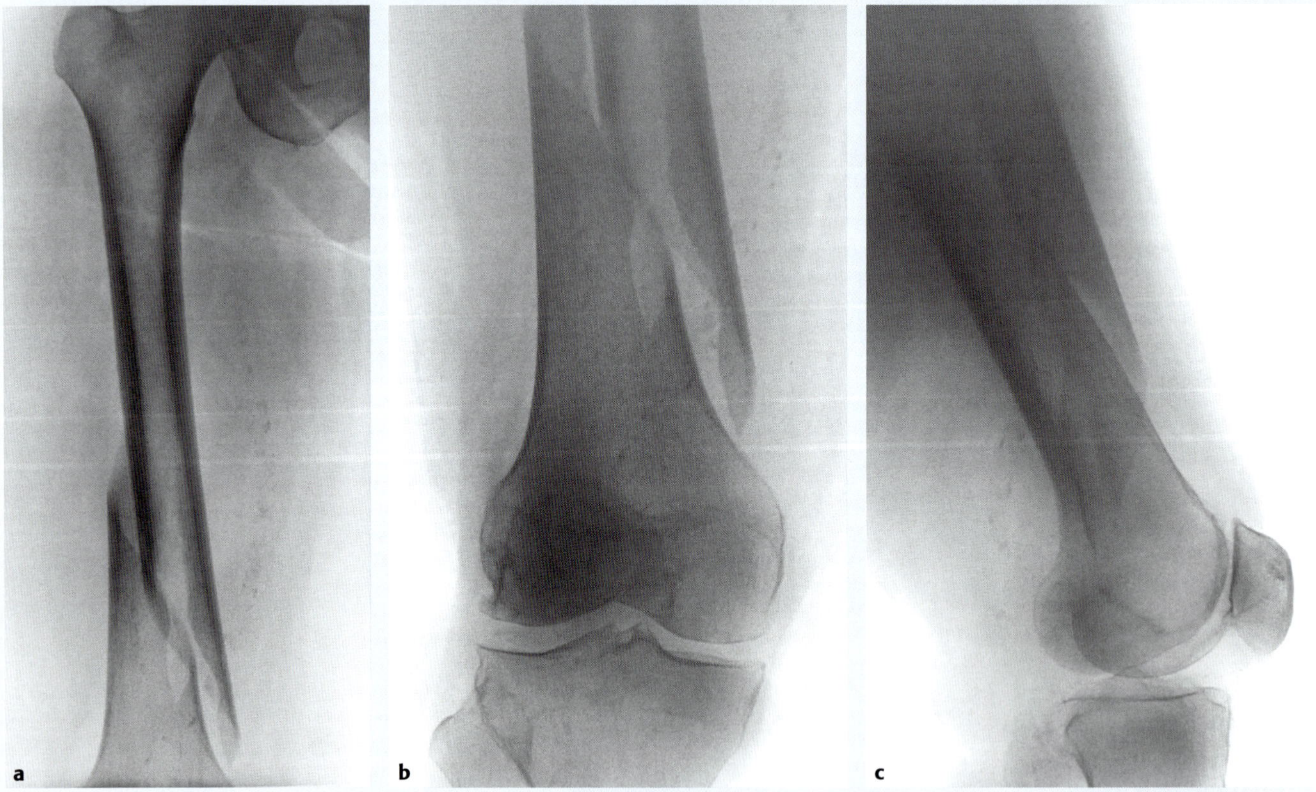

Fig 3.2-10a–c X-rays showing a simple spiral distal femoral shaft fracture.

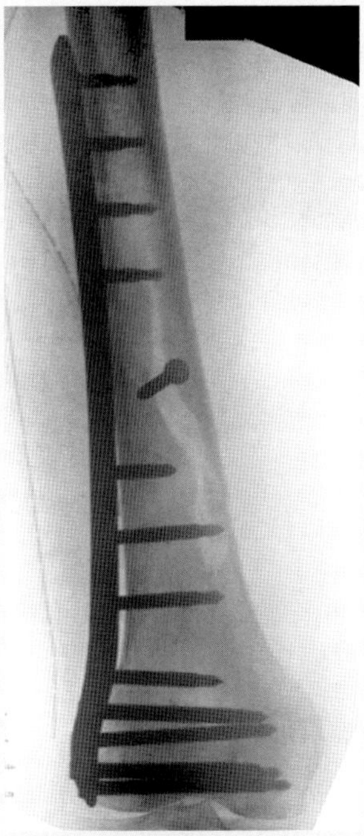

Fig 3.2-11 Postoperative x-ray showing the malreduction of the trochanteric fracture. The distal locking screw is placed outside the distal locking hole of the nail, probably due to an incorrect assembly of the aiming device for the nail.

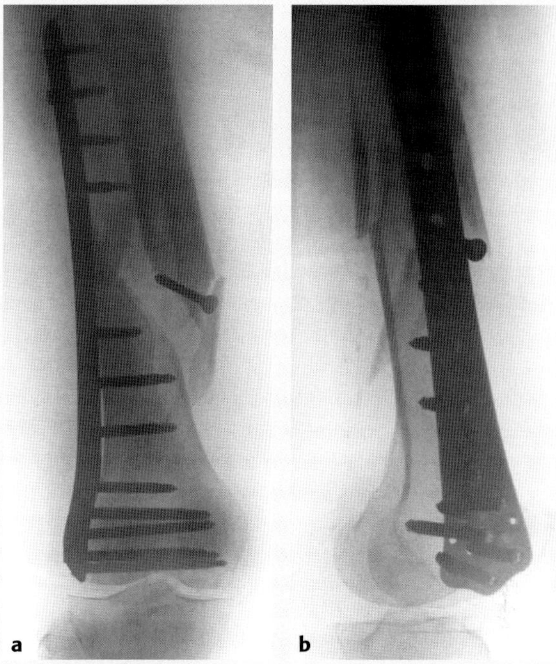

Fig 3.2-12a–b Instability caused by poor anatomical reduction, incorrect interfragmentary compression, and insufficient plate length caused loss of reduction and fracture alignment in the first postoperative days.

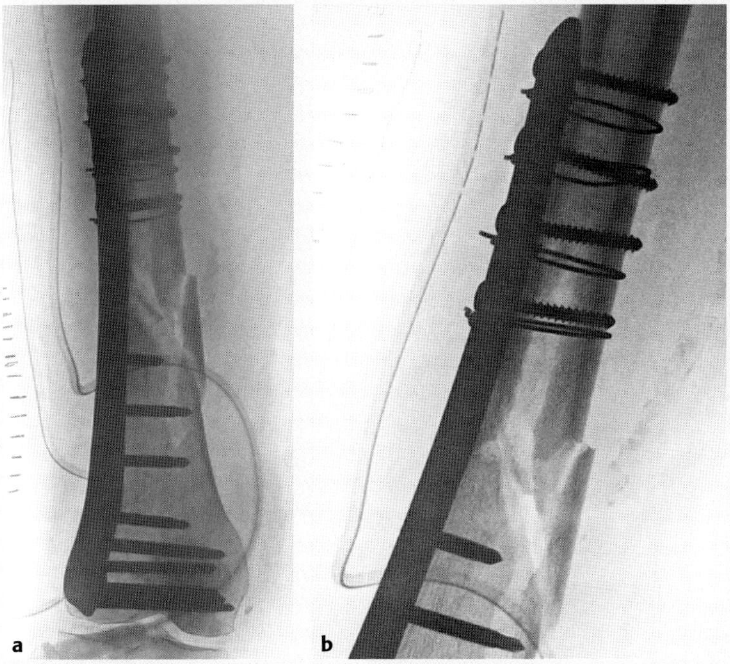

Fig 3.2-13a–b X-rays after the first rescue surgery.

a Reattachment of plate with cortex screws and cerclage wires. The same implant was used but absolute stability criteria with excess stiffness were followed as can be seen in the distal femoral less invasive stabilization system (LISS DF) plate.

b At the proximal end of the plate the excess hardware creates a zone of stress riser at the tip of the plate by the sudden transition from the rigid assembly to the elasticity of the osteopenic femur.

Analysis of failure and reflection

The x-rays of the first surgery show an insufficient reduction according to the criteria of absolute stability, with the interfragmentary compression screw having no function. The plate length appears to be short so that it is difficult to apply relative stability criteria, which results in a highly unstable assembly causing the loss of the reduction to the minimum load.

In recent years, monocortical screws have been proven to be ineffective; in fact, they are nowadays no longer used, and self-drilling screws with a drill bit tip have been removed in many countries.

If the first failure was due to the instability of the internal fixation, the second fracture in this chain of failures was a consequence of an overemphasized absolute stability criteria with excess stiffness, which caused a weak stress zone between the elasticity of the osteopenic bone and the rigidity of the proximal end of the LISS plate attached to the bone with too many screws and cerclage wires. This in turn led to the second failure: a predicted periimplant fracture in the stress zone (**Fig 3.2-14**).

Intramedullary nailing, which was chosen for the third intervention, should probably have been the first choice, as it is the gold standard in the treatment of femoral shaft fractures and would have avoided iatrogenic morbidity and mortality (**Fig 3.2-15**).

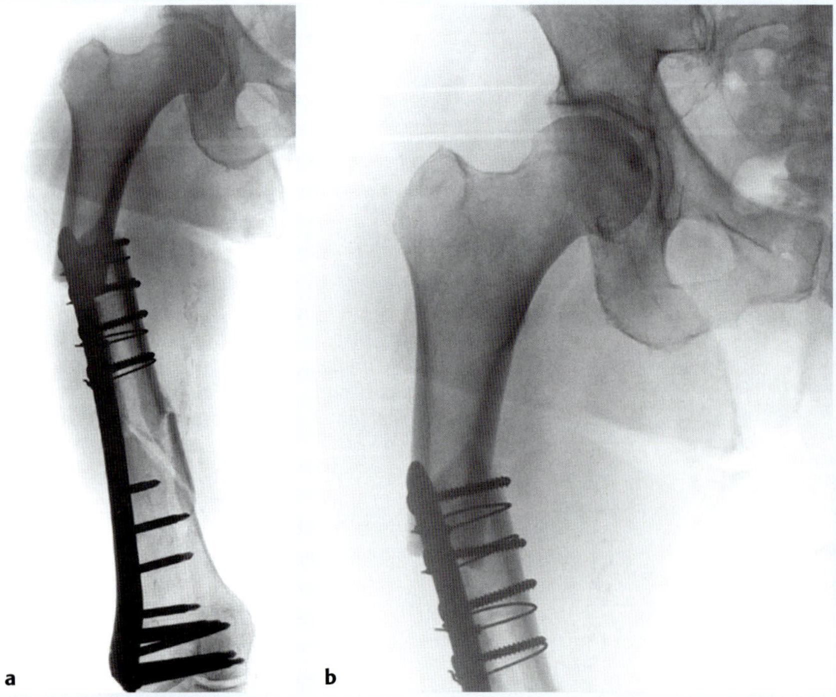

a b

Fig 3.2-14a–b Second failure: The fracture occurred as predicted, resulting in a periimplant fracture in the stress zone at the tip of the plate.

Final outcome

The patient remained handicapped and unable to walk for a long time. Rest and the use of a wheelchair caused sarcopenia (ie, reduced muscle mass with limited mobility); the biological impact on the femoral fracture site and the three previous surgeries had a negative impact on the overall functionality of this frail and elderly woman, who could eventually ambulate with a walker.

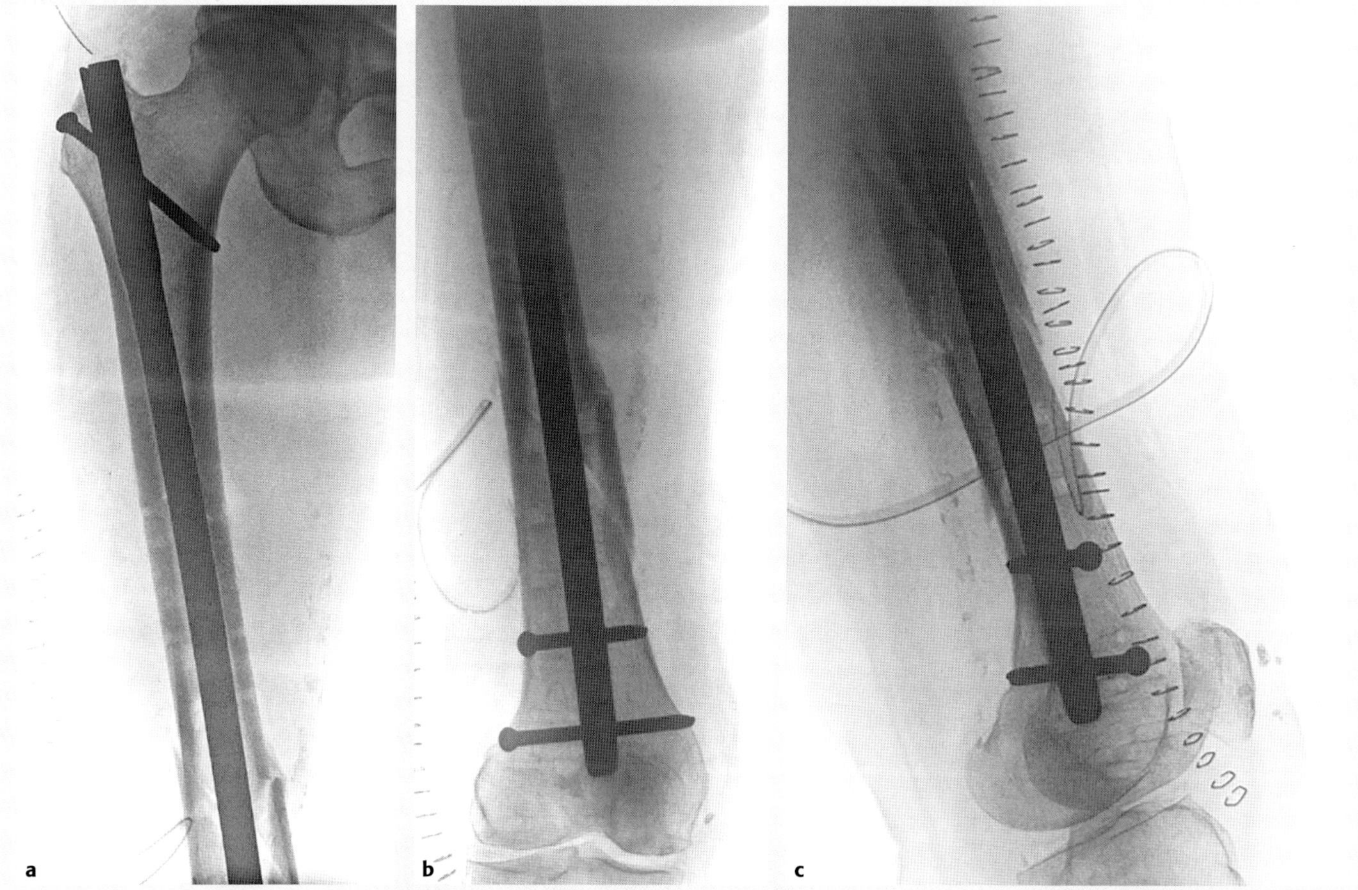

Fig 3.2-15a–c Second rescue surgery: X-rays show intramedullary nailing performed as a third surgery.

CASE 3

Case description

A 36-year-old man with a history of anxiety-depressive disorder, suicide attempts, excessive smoking, excessive use of alcohol, and tranquilizer dependence presented with a fracture of the left tibia and fibula (AO/OTA 42A2) after being hit by a car in a road traffic accident (**Fig 3.2-16**).

Initially, surgery with intramedullary nailing was planned, but due to the surgeon's poor choice of entry point for the introduction of the nail, satisfactory nail placement was not possible. The surgical team decided to perform an osteosynthesis with a plate as a second option, without having planned this in advance, which resulted in insufficient and poor fixation of the plate (**Fig 3.2-17** and **Fig 3.2-18**).

The patient neither followed the nonweight-bearing orders in the postoperative period nor took necessary care of the surgical wound, which resulted in the failure of the precarious osteosynthesis and wound infection (**Fig 3.2-19**). Due to the failure and infection, a reintervention was performed 6 weeks later (**Fig 3.2-20**). The implant material was removed and the soft tissues were debrided. After initial intravenous and then oral antibiotic treatment and once the biochemical inflammatory parameters had normalized at 6 months, intramedullary nailing was performed (**Fig 3.2-21**).

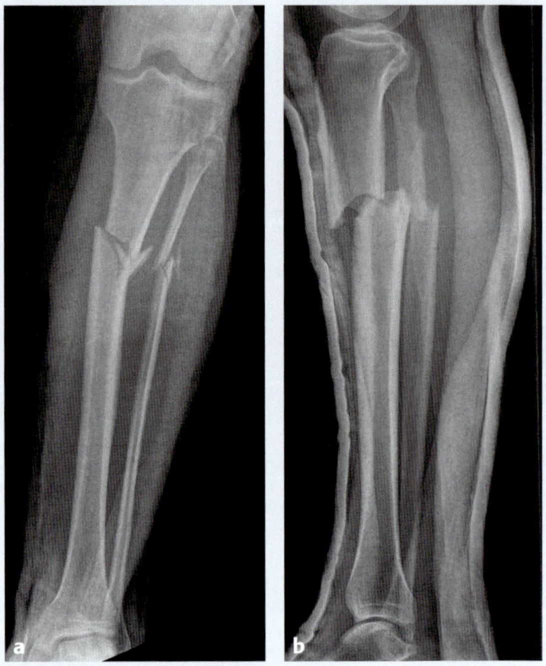

Fig 3.2-16a–b Preoperative AP (**a**) and lateral (**b**) x-rays of the left tibial and fibular fractures.

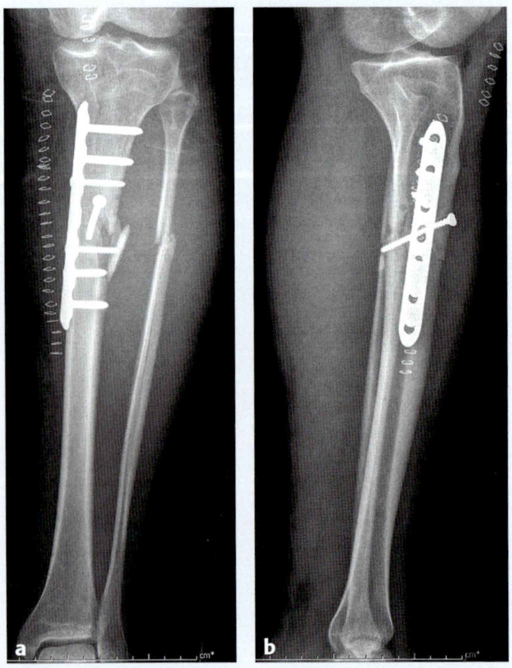

Fig 3.2-17a–b Immediate postoperative AP (**a**) and lateral (**b**) x-rays.

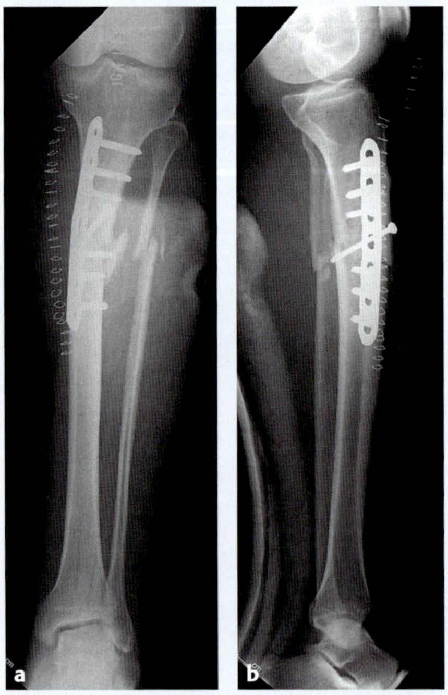

Fig 3.2-18a–b Two-week postoperative x-rays.

- **a** The AP view shows the plate slightly bent maintaining the fracture acceptably aligned.
- **b** Lateral view.

Failure analysis and reflection

The treatment failure in this case was multifactorial. There was a lack of preoperative planning and there was no plan B. In addition, the surgery was performed by a surgeon with little experience who chose a wrong entry point for the nail, which prevented fracture alignment. Osteosynthesis (ie, internal fixation) with the plate was insufficient.

These technical errors and the noncompliance of the patient in the postoperative period (neither following the nonweight-bearing protocol as indicated nor taking care of the surgical wound) led to the failure.

Final outcome

Although the final implant was not ideal because of its lack of rigidity, an acceptable reduction and stability of the fracture were achieved after 3 years (**Fig 3.2-22**). The fracture consolidated with a moderate valgus deformity of the tibia, which is clinically well tolerated by the patient.

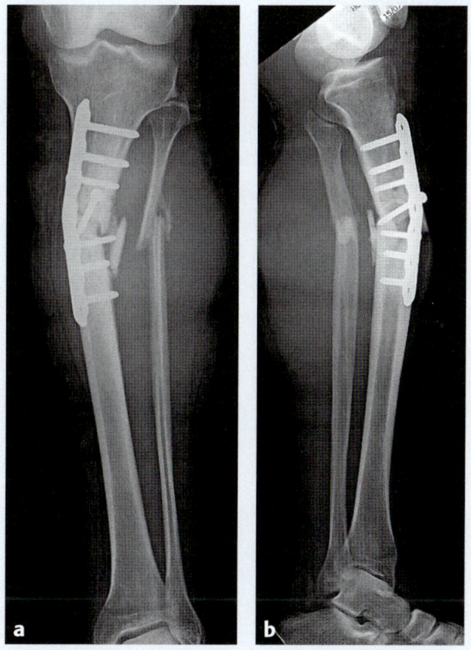

Fig 3.2-19a–b Postoperative x-rays at 6 weeks.
a AP view showing the osteosynthesis failure.
b Lateral view.

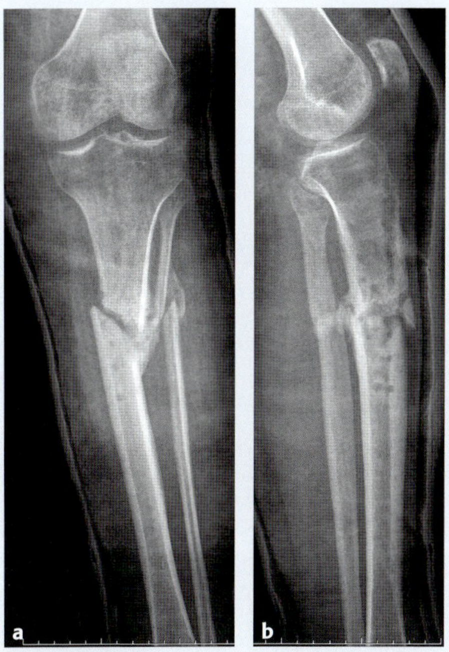

Fig 3.2-20a–b X-rays of the reintervention with the osteosynthesis material removed.
a AP view.
b Lateral view.

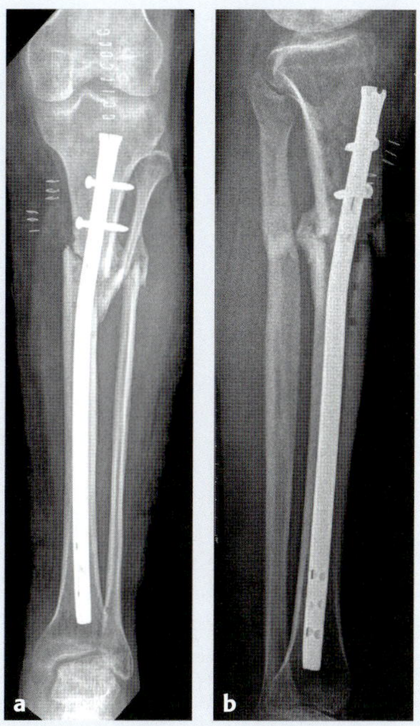

Fig 3.2-21a–b Immediate postoperative x-ray of the reintervention with intramedullary nailing.
a AP view.
b Lateral view.

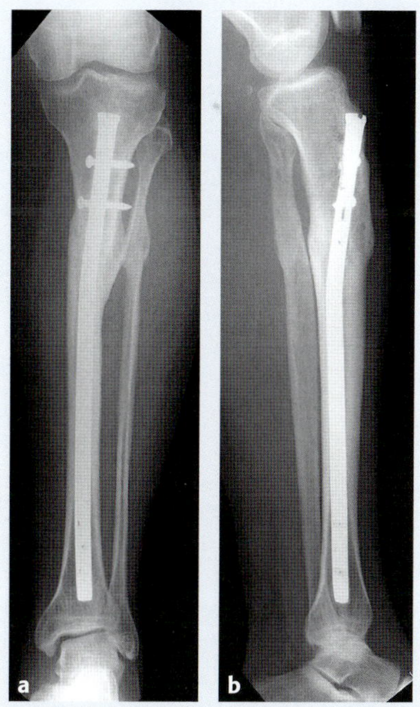

Fig 3.2-22a–b X-rays of the final outcome at 3 years, showing a consolidated fracture with valgus deformity.
a AP view.
b Lateral view.

Key points to remember

- Fracture fixation with absolute stability means that there is no micromotion at the fracture site under physiological load nor an increase in the rigidity of the implant fixation in the bone.
- When planning the treatment of a fracture, surgeons should not only take into account the morphology of the fracture itself and its location in a certain bone segment but also the patient's age, cognitive status, comorbidity, as well as commitment and discipline in the postoperative period, as these also play an important role.
- Plates should be placed on the external tensile side to neutralize the eccentric loading forces in flexion.
- Overloading the fracture with too much interfragmentary movement delays the healing process and is not well tolerated.
- When fractures are splinted, movement of the fragments in relation to each other depends on the amount of external loading, stiffness of the splints, stiffness of the tissues bridging the fracture. That is the reason why multifragmentary fractures are more tolerant to instability than simple fractures.

References and suggested reading

Baumgaertel F. Bridge plating. In: Buckley RE, Moran CG, Apivatthakakul T, eds. *AO Principles of Fracture Management.* 3rd ed. Stuttgart New York: Thieme; 2017:241–252.
Browner B, Levine A, Jupiter JB, et al. *Skeletal Trauma.* 4th ed. Edinburgh: Elsevier; 2008:215–217, 219.
Claes LE, Heigele CA. Magnitudes of local stress and strain along bony surfaces predict the course and type of fracture healing. *J Biomech.* 1999 Mar;32(3):255–266.
Hak DJ, Stewart RL. Tension band principle. In: Rüedi TP, Buckley R, Moran C, eds. *AO Principles of Fracture Management.* 2nd ed. Davos: AO Publishing; 2007:249–254.
Ito K, Perren SM. Biology and biomechanics in bone healing. In: Rüedi TP, Buckley R, Moran C, eds. *AO Principles of Fracture Management.* 2nd ed. Davos: AO Publishing; 2007:9–31.
Pauwels F. Der Schenkelhalsbruch— ein mechanisches Problem: Grundlagen des Heilungsvorganges, Prognose und kausale Therapie. *Beilageheft zur Zeitschrift für Orthopädische Chirurgie.* 1935;63. German.
Perren SM. The concept of biological plating using the limited contact-dynamic compression plate (LC-DCP). Scientific background, design and application. *Injury.* 1991;22 Suppl 1:1–41.
Perren SM, Cordey J. The concept of interfragmentary strain. In: Uhthoff HK, Stahl E, eds. *Current Concepts of Internal Fixation of Fractures.* Berlin Heidelberg New York: Springer-Verlag; 1980. 63–77.
Rüedi T, Buckley R, Moran C. *AO Principles of Fracture Management.* 2nd ed. Stuttgart New York: Thieme Verlag; 2007.

3.3 Implant size, prebending, molding, and shape adapted to the fractured bone

Reto Babst, Frank Beeres, Joan Girós Torres, Björn Link, Roberto Rivero Sosa, J Miquel Sales Pérez, Miquel Videla Cés

Diseases desperate grown
By desperate appliance are relieved,
Or not at all.
William Shakespeare

Implant size

Once the appropriate implant model has been chosen for each fracture, its proper size and length must be chosen. However, the wrong implant dimension is often selected. Although we may think that this error typically occurs during a surgeon's training and learning period, it frequently happens to (more) experienced surgeons. Failing to choose the correct size and length of the implant can generate serious complications and we have seen this happen with both intramedullary nails and extramedullary plates.

In the case of intramedullary nails, surgeons often select the wrong length and thickness. Nails of excessive length can penetrate the joint causing irreversible joint injuries and/or damage while nails, if too short, can cause instability and alter the healing process. Too thick nails require overreaming with subsequent cortical weakening while too thin nails do not fill the canal and lose the primary stability effect.

When using trochanteric nails, there may be a discrepancy between the radius of nail curvature and the physiological curvature of the femur, causing impingement of the anterior cortex of the distal femur or "tip effect", which can lead to a periimplant fracture.

Generally, there are two basic principles of internal fracture fixation: interfragmentary compression and splinting. Both are useful and the orthopedic trauma surgeon should be capable of performing both techniques. Compression is a safe, high-rigidity method of fixation suitable for simple fracture patterns in each segment of a bone. Splinting is the more flexible fixation method that should be used mainly in multifragmentary or comminuted fractures of the meta- and diaphyseal segments of a long bone [Gautier et al, 2003].

When using minimally invasive techniques for indirect reduction, subcutaneous or submuscular plate insertion, and splinting as a stabilization concept, the selected plate can be very long without the need of additional soft-tissue section and devascularization. Theoretically, the plate can equal the whole length of the broken bone, but the minimal length of the internal plate can be determined by the plate span width and plate-screw density. Plate span width is defined as the quotient of plate length and overall fracture length. Empirically we find that the plate length should be 2–3 times higher than the overall fracture length in comminuted fractures and 8–10 times higher in simple fractures (**Fig 3.3-1**). The other factor is the plate-screw density which is the quotient of the number of screws inserted and the total number of plate holes. Empirically we recommend values below 0.5, indicating that less than half of the plate holes are occupied by screws.

From a mechanical point of view, two (monocortical or bicortical) screws on each main fragment is the minimum number of screws needed to keep the plate-bone construction stable. Unfortunately, such a construction will fail if one screw breaks due to overload or when the interface between bone cortex and screw is threatened due to bone resorption with subsequent screw loosening. Thus, for safety reasons we recommend a minimum of three screws in both the proximal and distal main fragments. When adjusting the plate-screw density to a maximum value of 0.5, the plate length chosen should not be less than a 12-hole plate for treatment of a diaphyseal fracture. But to increase the leverage of the screws, the use of a 14–22-hole plate would be better.

Depending on the length of the plate and the position of the screws, the loading conditions of the screws change. Increasing the length of the plate decreases the pull-out force acting on the screw due to an improvement of the active lever arm of each screw. This argument supports the use of longer plates [Gautier, 2009].

Prebending, molding, and shape adapted to the fractured bone

To stabilize the straight segment of a diaphysis, a straight internal fixator can be used. In such a situation all screws have the same direction and the screw loading is identical. However, this can be dangerous in osteoporotic bone. To avoid identical screw directions for all the screws, slight bending (in multiple waves back and forth) of the internal fixator offers an advantage because it results in divergent and convergent screw direction, thereby enhancing the pull-out strength of the screws. This slight shaping can be used in "eggshell bone" (ie, strong but inflexible and brittle) in cases of severe osteoporosis. Other bone segments, such as the olecranon, need a bent plate from the beginning, as shaping the plate avoids the screws being parallel to each other [Gautier et al, 2003].

When planning to use a locking compression plate (LCP), surgeons need to decide whether to use it as an internal fixator, a conventional plate, or a combination of the two. If the LCP is used as a conventional plate, the implant must be contoured precisely to match the shape of the bone, which helps to reduce the fracture against the plate. When, on the other hand, the LCP is applied as an internal fixator, exact contouring is not required, but the fracture has to be reduced first before the plate can be applied (**Fig 3.3-2**) [Gautier et al, 2007].

Fernández Dell'Oca published an article in 2002 entitled *The principle of helical implants* that gives a new perspective on internal fixation of fractures, both from the point of view of extramedullary fixation and intramedullary fixation, with clinical results that are very encouraging. A helical nail allows more freedom when choosing an entry point. With a helical periosteal device, it is possible to position an implant on different regions of bone (ie, lateral at the proximal end and anterior in the distal third). These options have proven particularly useful when attempting to avoid damage to the neurovascular system while using minimally invasive plate osteosynthesis (MIPO) for bridge plating [Fernández Dell'Oca, 2002].

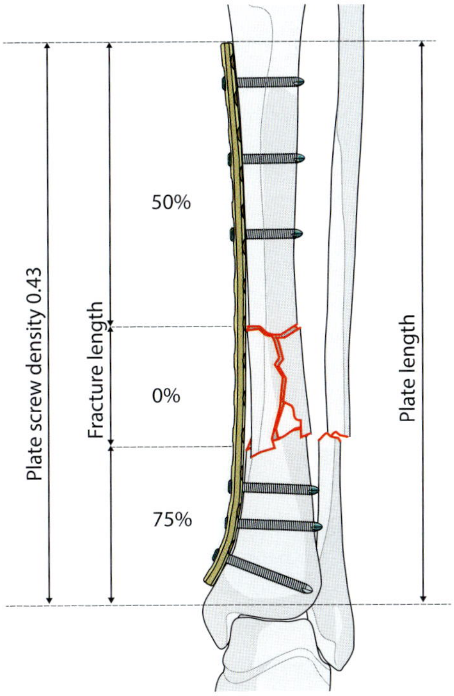

Fig 3.3-1 Plate span ratio $= \frac{\text{plate length}}{\text{fracture length}}$

The plate length should be 2–3 times higher than the overall fracture length in comminuted fractures and 8–10 times higher in simple fractures.

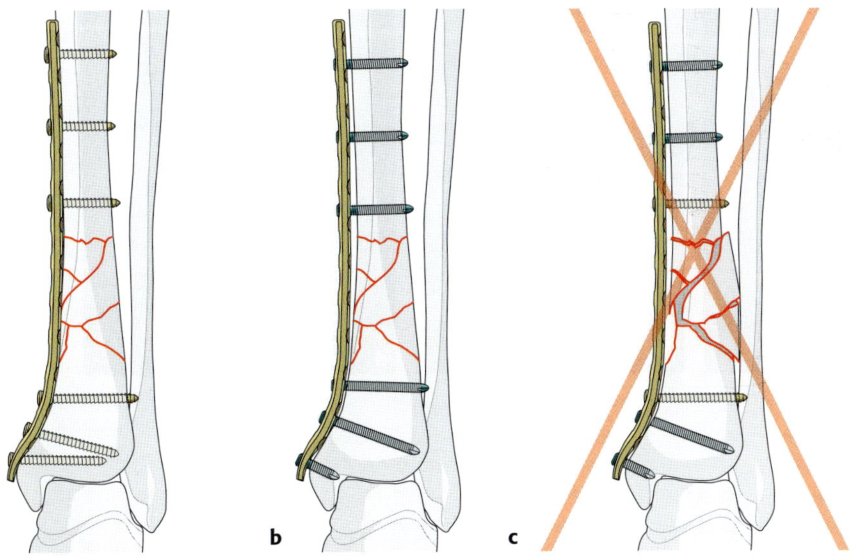

Fig 3.3-2a–c How (not) to use locking compression plates with screws.

a When used with conventional screws, the locking compression plate (LCP) must be contoured precisely to the shape of the bone.

b An LCP used as an internal fixator will bridge the fracture. The plate does not require exact contouring.

c If conventional screws are added, the plate will either be bent or more probably the fracture fragments will be pulled towards the plate and rotational malalignment might result. If conventional screws and locking head screws are used in the same bone segment, the order of screw insertion is important and must always start with conventional screws.

CASE 1

Case description

A 25-year-old man presented at the emergency department after a fall from height. A moderate head trauma (according to advanced trauma life support [ATLS]) **[American College of Surgeons, 2013]** and a Gustilo type I multifragmentary distal femoral fracture (AO/OTA 33C2) were diagnosed with a full-body computed tomographic (CT) scan (**Fig 3.3-3**). The patient's neurovascular status was normal. After applying a temporary external fixator, definitive fracture treatment was achieved with minimally invasive plate osteosynthesis on day 5 (**Fig 3.3-4**). Clinical course and further recovery were uneventful.

After 6 months, walking with full weight bearing was not possible due to pain. Plain x-rays and a single-photon emission computed tomography showed nonunion, a nonvital bone fragment, and no signs of infection (**Fig 3.3-5**).

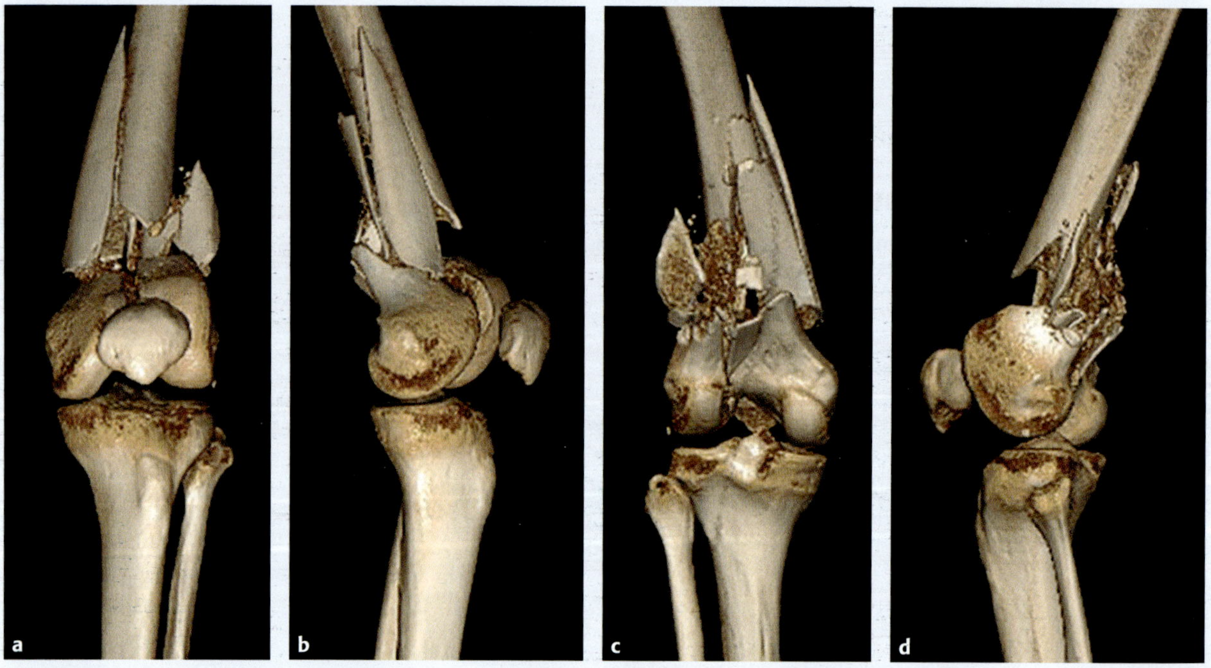

Fig 3.3-3a–d Three-dimensional reconstructions of the multifragmentary distal femoral fracture.

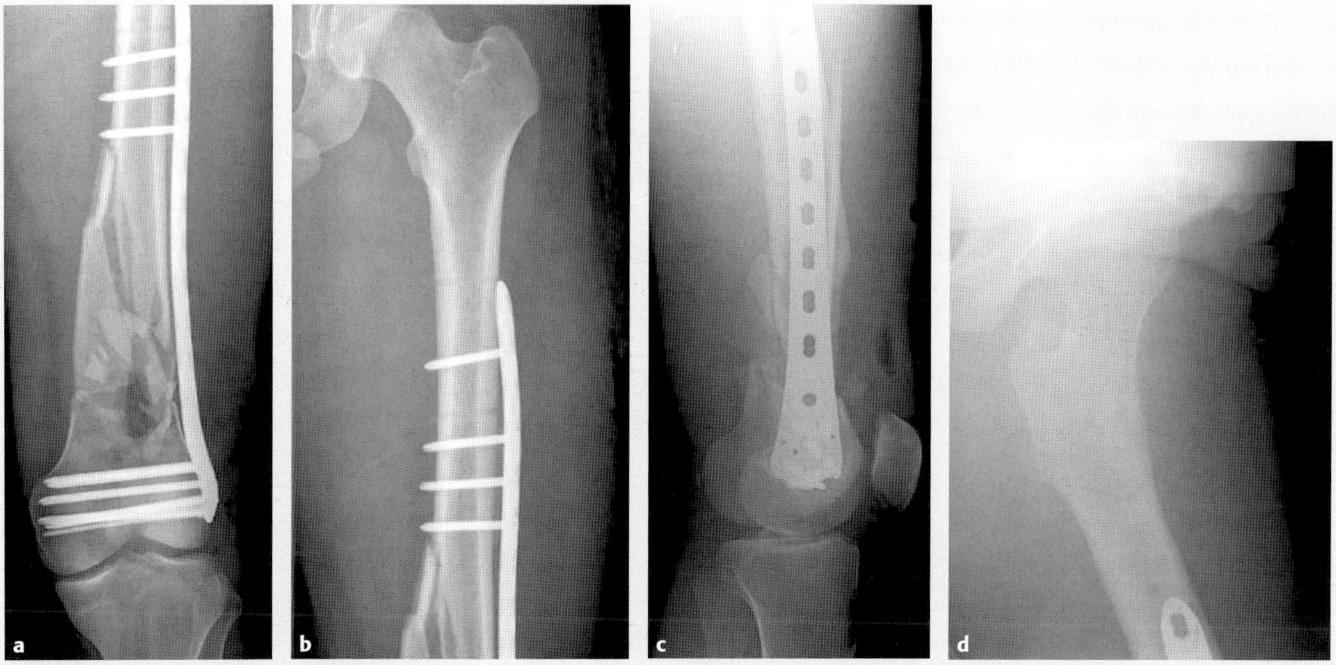

Fig 3.3-4a–d Definitive fracture fixation 5 days after trauma with a minimally invasive distal femoral plate.

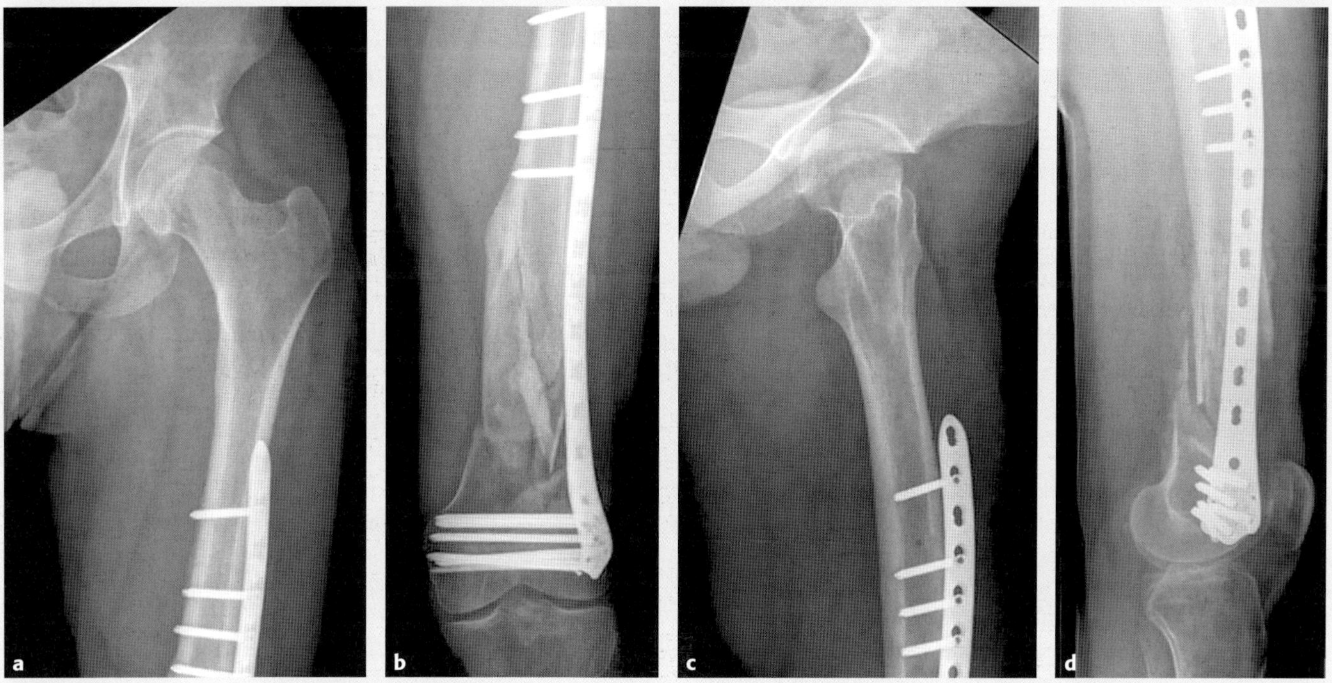

Fig 3.3-5a–h Nonunion and fracture without activity.
a–d X-rays 6 months after trauma showing a nonunion.

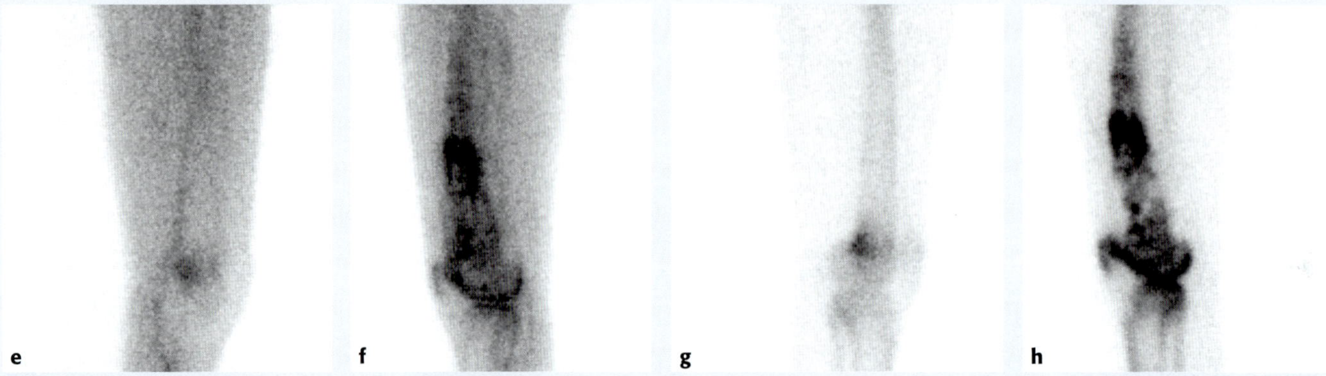

Fig 3.3-5a–h (cont) Nonunion and fracture without activity.
e–h Single-photon emission computed tomography 6 months after trauma showing no activity in the fracture and a nonvital bone fragment.

Analysis of failure and reflection

The first revision surgery was performed: the plate and sequester were removed, the fracture debrided and decorticated, a cement spacer implanted, and a reosteosynthesis performed (**Fig 3.3-6**). In one of six cultures a few *Propionibacterium acnes* colonies were found. Sonication was negative. The positive culture was interpreted as contamination.

Two weeks later the spacer was exchanged for cancellous bone autograft (obtained from the iliac crest) and additional stability was provided by adding three screws (**Fig 3.3-7**). Based on the initial cultures, antibiotics (ie, amoxicillin and rifampin) were administered for 6 weeks. The following two issues that arose at that time should be pointed out:

- Interpreting the results of the cultures as contamination and performing an early reosteosynthesis after 2 weeks is risky as it could lead to infection despite administering antibiotic treatment for 6 weeks.
- Adding three screws does not provide enough additional stability in highly multifragmentary fractures.

After 15 months a persistent nonunion was present with no signs of infection either clinically or on the CT scan. In a third reoperation the fracture was debrided again, the implant removed, and a new cement spacer implanted (**Fig 3.3-8**). Cultures showed growth of *P. acnes* and antibiotics were administered for 3 months. The following point arising at that time needs to be mentioned here:

- No stability (eg, external fixator) was provided as the fracture was interpreted as clinically stable, and the patient was mobilized in a brace.

Eighteen months after the initial trauma, a fourth reoperation was performed in which a 95° blade plate and a minimally invasive helical locking compression plate (LCP) 4.5 were inserted to provide maximal stability (**Fig 3.3-9**). Cancellous bone autograft obtained from the iliac crest was added. The cultures remained negative. One point regarding the last operation needs to be discussed:

- The helical plate was fixed proximally on the lateral side of the femur. In the scarce literature on this topic, the plate is often fixed proximally on the ventral side to obtain a fixation in three directions **[Fernandez Dell'Oca, 2002; Regazzoni et al, 2016]**. In this case a lateral fixation was chosen to use the same incision as used for the 95° blade plate.

Final outcome

Twelve months after the final operation (and 30 months after the initial trauma), a CT scan indicated fracture union (**Fig 3.3-10**).

Lessons to be learned from this case:

- Interpreting cultures as contaminated should be done with care.
- Adding stability with additional screws does not provide absolute stability in comminuted fractures.
- Augmenting distal femoral fractures with a second (helical) plate inserted with a minimally invasive technique, provides sufficient additional stability.

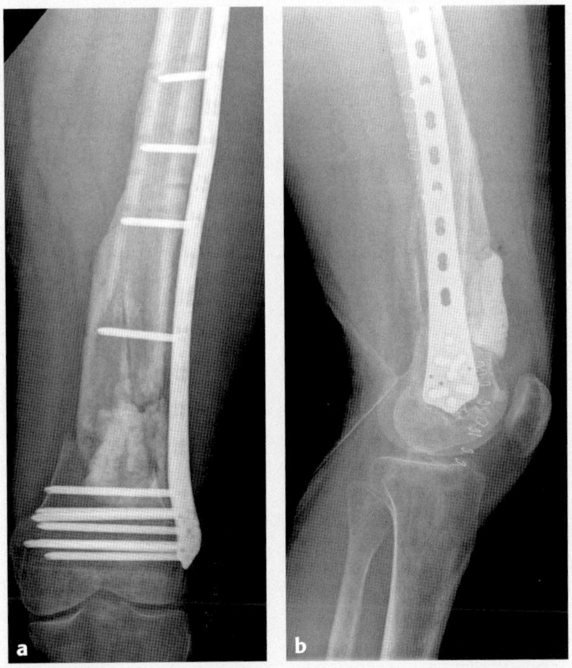

Fig 3.3-6a–b Reosteosynthesis after approximately 7 months with a new distal femoral plate and a cement spacer in situ.

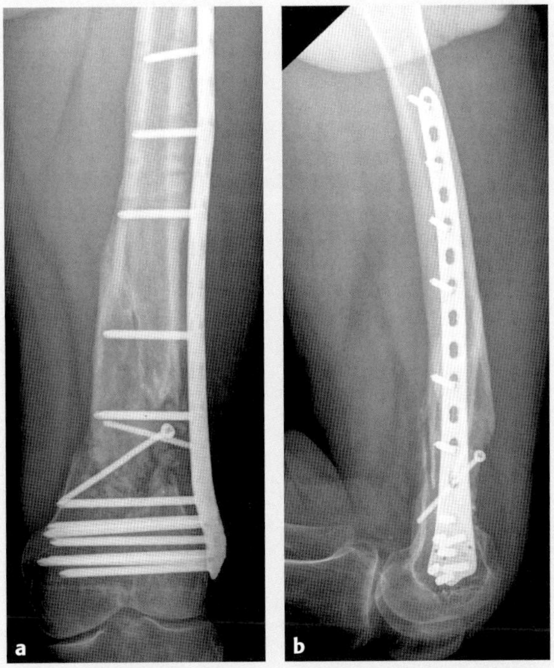

Fig 3.3-7a–b The spacer was replaced with cancellous bone autograft from the iliac crest and three additional screws were inserted to add stability.

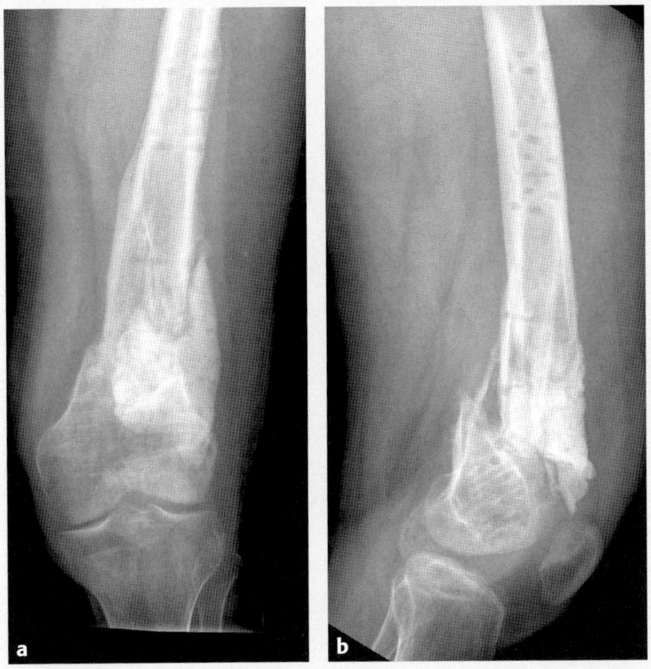

Fig 3.3-8a–b X-rays taken approximately 15 months after the initial trauma showing a persistent nonunion.

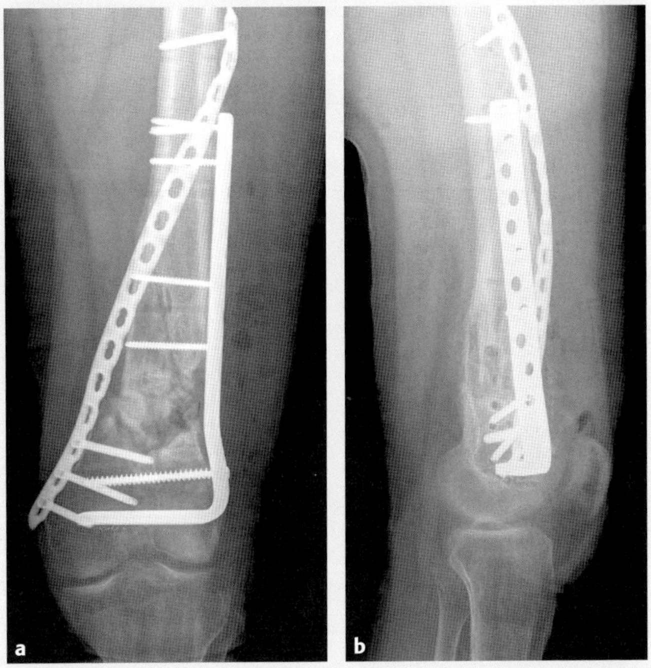

Fig 3.3-9a–b X-rays of the reosteosynthesis at 18 months after the trauma showing the inserted 95° blade plate and a minimally invasive helical locking compression plate 4.5.

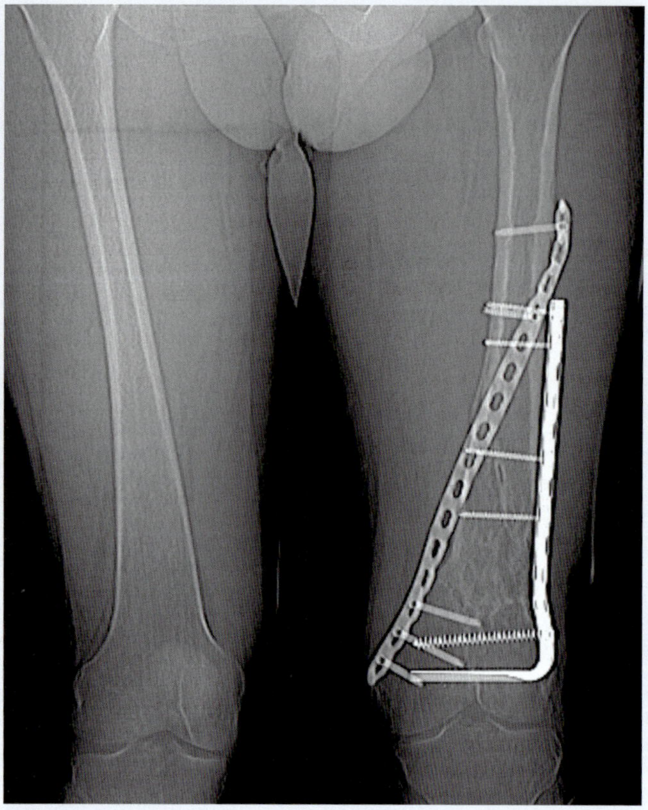

Fig 3.3-10 Computed tomographic scan showing the fracture union 30 months after trauma.

Case description

A 77-year-old woman without severe comorbidity except for high blood pressure fell at home from standing height and sustained an intertrochanteric fracture (AO/OTA 31A3.3). Fracture treatment with a trochanteric nail system (170 mm long) was planned (**Fig 3.3-11**).

In the postoperative control x-ray, a fracture extension was seen near the tip of the nail (**Fig 3.3-12**). The surgical team decided to wait and see and allow mobilization without weight bearing.

At the 2-week follow-up control, loosening of the locking screw was noticed (**Fig 3.3-13**). The patient was reoperated 2 weeks after the first surgery and the nail replaced with a longer one (**Fig 3.3-14**). She was authorized to walk with full weight bearing in the fourth week after the second surgery (**Fig 3.3-15**).

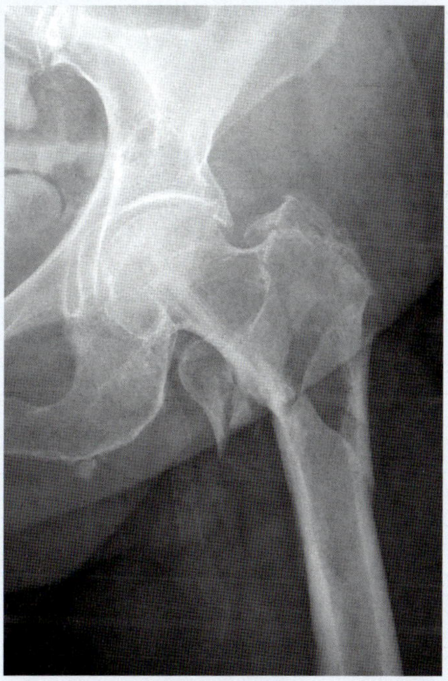

Fig 3.3-11 X-ray of an intertrochanteric left femoral fracture.

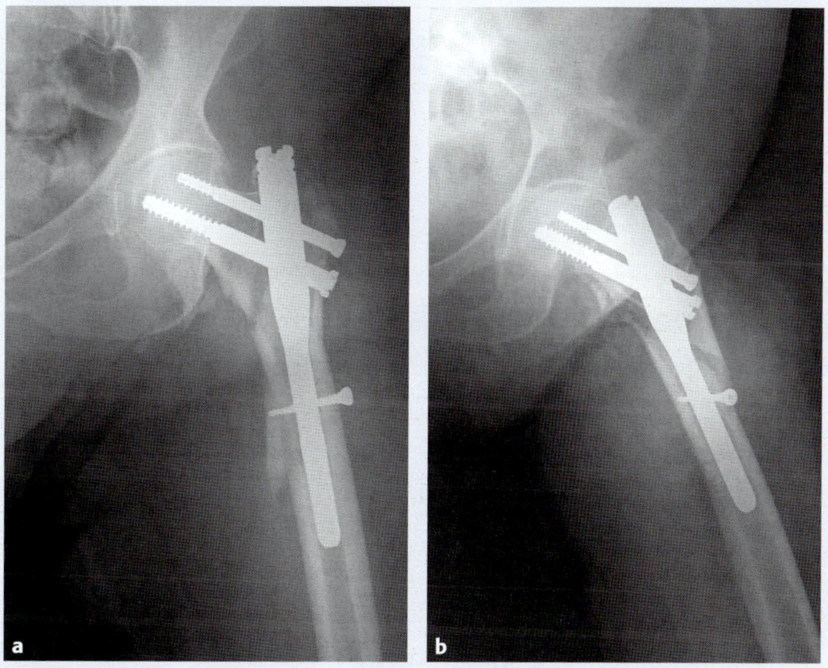

Fig 3.3-12a–b Postoperative control x-ray showing the intertrochanteric fracture after being treated with a trochanteric nail system (170 mm long). A subtrochanteric fracture extension can be seen at the level of the locking bolt, near the tip of the nail (**b**).

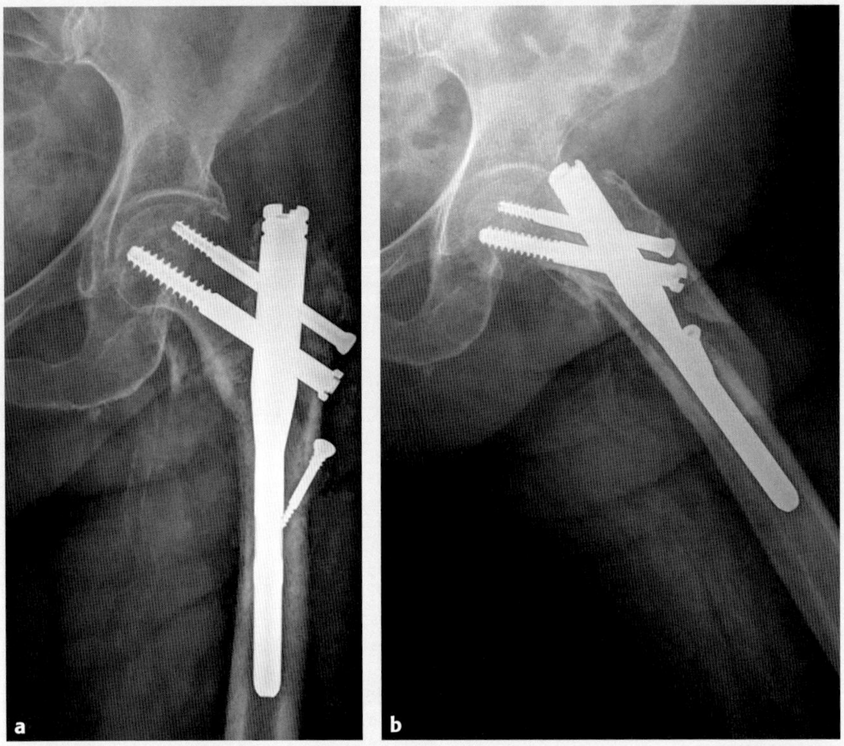

Fig 3.3-13a–b Two-week follow-up control x-rays showing the loosened locking screw.

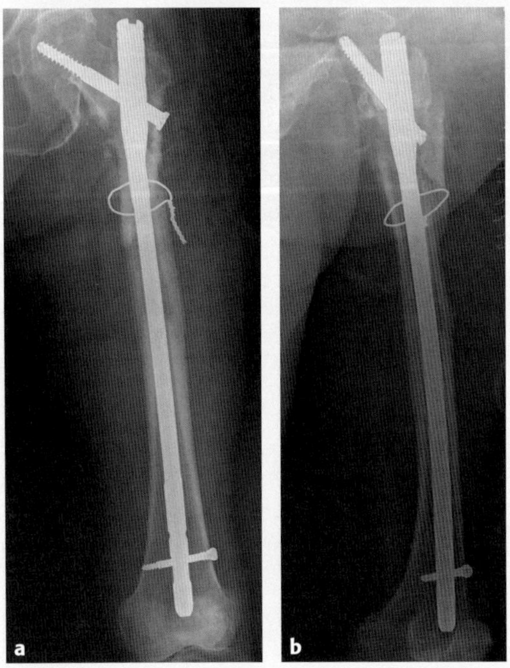

Fig 3.3-14a–b Postoperative AP (**a**) and axial (**b**) x-ray views of the reoperation.

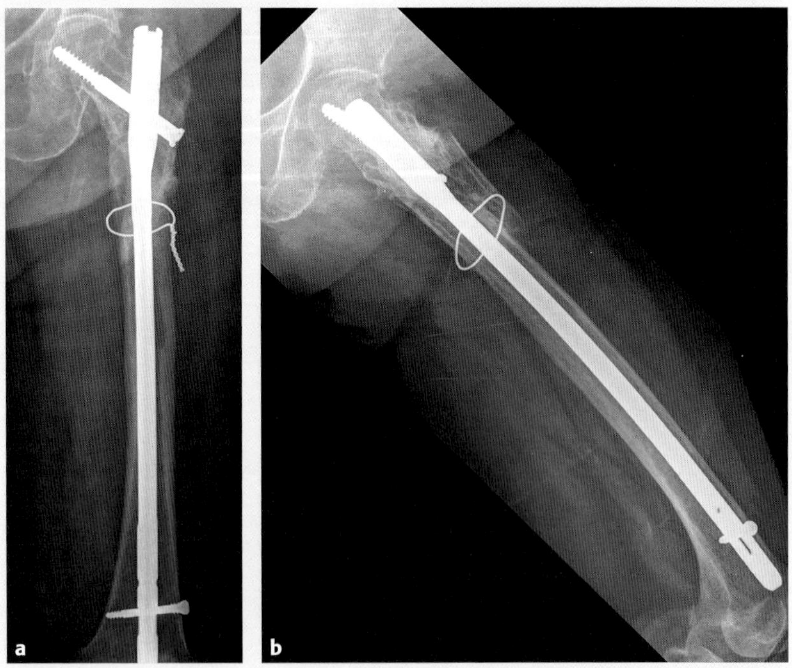

Fig 3.3-15a–b AP (**a**) and axial (**b**) x-rays at the 1-year follow-up show complete healing and bone remodeling.

Analysis of failure and reflection

The poor bone quality in the proximal third of the femur and the lack of preoperative planning may have been the cause of the failure. The trochanteric nail needs to be inserted in a reduced fracture and the working length of the implant has to be large enough to achieve the stability needed for weight bearing.

Waiting to see the outcome without load bearing does not facilitate fracture healing and is biologically harmful in fragile patients.

The implant itself cannot make up for the surgeon's poor technique (ie, technical skills are needed to avoid possible mistakes). To have an alternative plan (ie, plan B) does not mean to increase morbidity. Time will not improve an adverse situation after it has been detected.

Final outcome

The fracture healed and the patient was eventually able to walk without crutches. She recovered complete functionality and quality of life 1 year after the fracture.

Case description

A 99-year-old woman with a fracture of the right femur (AO/OTA 31A3) after a casual fall (**Fig 3.3-16**).

During the intervention, the surgeon used more force than necessary when inserting the spiral blade through the nail and it became blocked (**Fig 3.3-17**). Subsequently, she or he realized that trying to insert a spiral blade into a 130° nail with a guide wire of 125° was not working. This nail was removed and a 125° nail was inserted placing the spiral blade within the corresponding guide wire. Since the control x-rays were satisfactory, weight bearing was authorized in the post-operative period (**Fig 3.3-18**).

A few days later the patient complained of great pain in the right hip. A new control x-ray was then taken which revealed the presence of a cut-in. Reintervention to remove the spiral blade and insert another shorter spiral blade was planned for the following week (**Fig 3.3-19**).

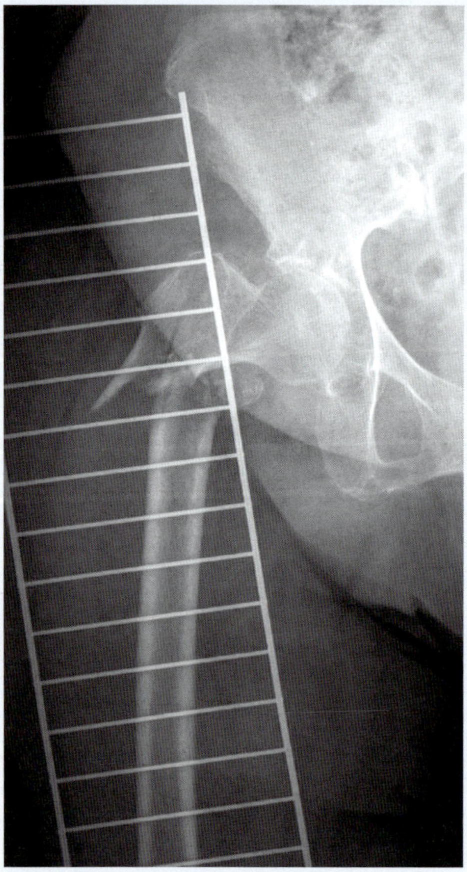

Fig 3.3-16 Preoperative AP x-ray of the right femoral fracture.

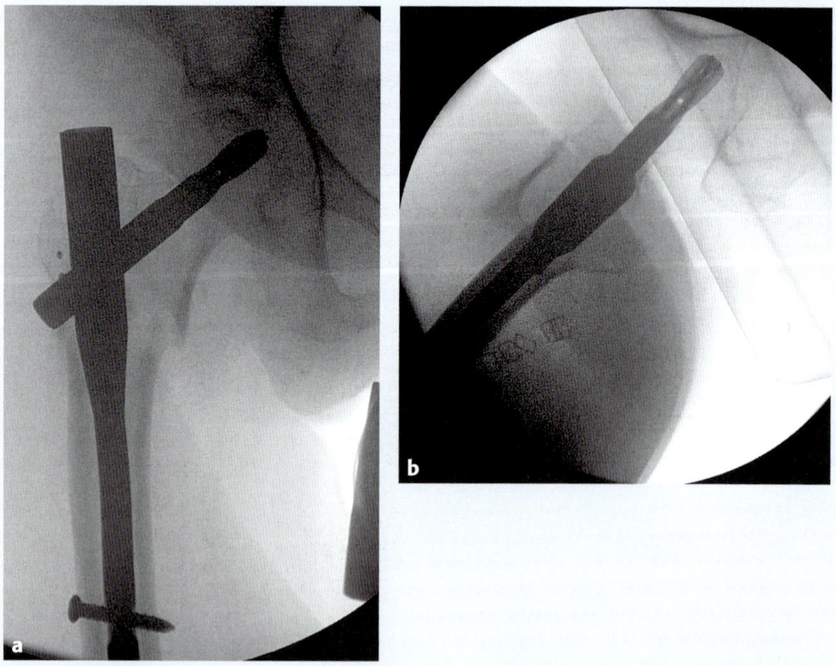

Fig 3.3-17a–b Intraoperative C-arm images.
a AP view showing a metallic fragment in the area where the spiral blade was inserted into the nail.
b Axial view.

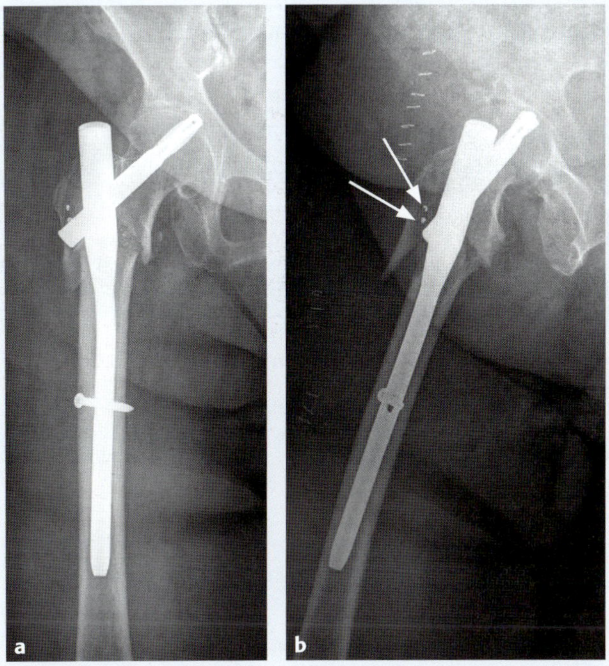

Fig 3.3-18a–b Postoperative x-rays at 1 week.
a AP view.
b Axial view revealing a metallic fragment where the spiral blade was inserted into the nail (arrows).

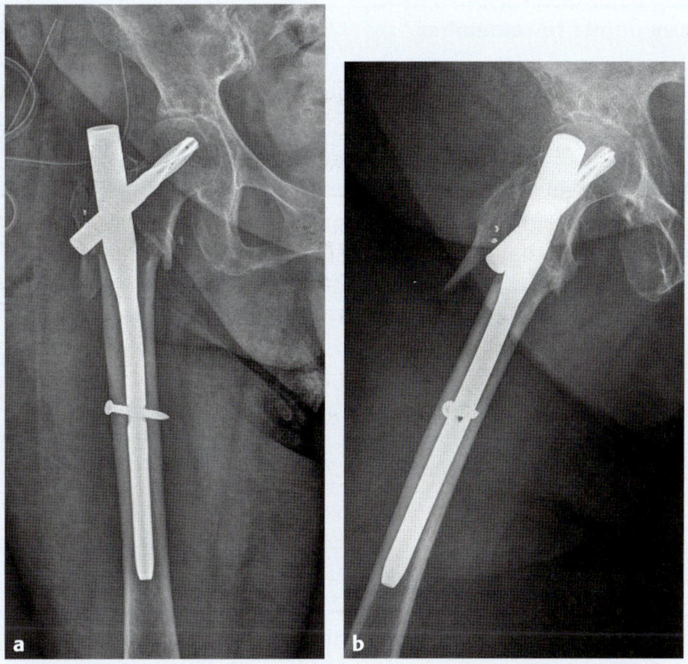

Fig 3.3-19a–b Reintervention in which the original spiral blade was replaced with a shorter one.
a AP view.
b Axial view.

Failure analysis and reflection

During surgery the operating room personnel used guide wire that did not correspond to the angulation of the nail chosen for the intervention. Combined with the surgeon's failure to check, this meant that insertion of the spiral blade was traumatic, further weakening the bone of the 99-year-old woman and resulting in the cut-in. A new surgical intervention to change the spiral blade was necessary for this already fragile patient.

Final outcome

The patient underwent two surgical interventions, the first to treat the initial fracture and the second to change the spiral blade for another shorter blade. Following this reintervention, the patient continued with uneventful healing of the fracture, but she died a few months later due to a urological disease.

Key points to remember

- Compression is a safe, high-rigidity method of fixation suitable for simple fracture patterns in each segment of a bone and in articular fractures. Splinting is the more flexible method of fixation that should be used mainly in multifragmentary or comminuted fractures of the meta- and diaphyseal segments of a long bone.
- Care must be taken when choosing intramedullary nails because mistakes are often made in the choice of length and thickness.
- Nails with excess length can penetrate the joint causing irreversible joint injuries while nails that are short can cause instability.
- Too thick nails require overreaming with consequent cortical weakening or breakage while too thin nails do not fill the canal and loose the primary stability effect.
- The plate should be long enough based on the fracture pattern. The plate should be 2–3 times longer than the overall fracture length in comminuted fractures and 8–10 times longer than in simple fractures.
- The recommended values for plate–screw density are below 0.5, indicating that less than half of the plate holes can be occupied by screws. Not every plate hole needs to be filled.
- The length of the plate and the position of the screws modify the loading conditions of the screws. Increasing the length of the plate decreases the pullout force acting on the screw because the active lever arm of each screw is better.
- In osteoporotic bone it is mandatory to avoid identical screw directions for all the screws. Especially in "eggshell" bone (in severe osteoporosis), screws should not face the same direction.
- When planning to use a locking compression plate (LCP) as a conventional plate, the implant must be contoured to precisely match the shape of the bone. This helps to reduce the fracture.
- When planning to use an LCP as an internal fixator, exact contouring is not required, but the fracture must be reduced before applying the plate.
- The use of helical implants has proven particularly useful in preventing damage to the neurovascular system during MIPO bridge plating.

References and suggested reading

American College of Surgeons' Committee on Trauma. Advanced trauma life support (ATLS(R)): the ninth edition. *J Trauma Acute Care Surg.* 2013 May;74(5):1363–1366.
Fernandez Dell'Oca AA. The principle of helical implants. Unusual ideas worth considering. *Injury.* 2002 Apr;33 Suppl 1:Sa1–27.
Gautier E. Bridge plating. *AO Dialogue.* 2009(2):24–27.
Gautier E, Pesantez R. Surgical reduction. In: Rüedi T, Buckley R, Moran C, eds. *AO Principles of fracture management.* 2nd ed. Stuttgart New York: Thieme; 2007: 165–187.
Gautier E, Sommer C. Guidelines for the clinical application of the LCP. *Injury.* 2003 Nov;34 Suppl 2:B63–76.
Regazzoni P, Perren S, Fernández A. Fatigue resistance. 2016 Apr. *ICUC One-Page Paper.* Available at: www.icuc.net/multimedia/#papers. Accessed May 2019.

3.4 Anatomical implants: ready-to-wear versus custom-fit

Joan Girós Torres, Roberto Rivero Sosa, J Miquel Sales Pérez, Miquel Videla Cés

Failure is simply the opportunity to begin again, this time more intelligently.

Henry Ford

With the development and widespread use of minimally invasive surgical methods and implants for fracture fixation, it has become increasingly important that the available implants are precontoured to the specific anatomical location for which they are designed [Perren, 2001; Wagner, 2003]. However, significant differences in the bone morphology, bone size and shape, are related to factors as patient age, gender, ethnicity, and region of origin. These differences are a great challenge when designing well-fitting anatomical plates that can be used for the entire human population [White et al, 2005]. The current fixation plates fit most patients of Asian-Pacific origin neither well nor poorly, because the implants were designed to fit the 50th percentile of the Caucasian population [Schmutz et al, 2008].

From the biomechanical point of view, the plate is not necessarily a perfect fit for the bone if it is used as an internal fixator with angular stability criteria. The locking fixation technique achieves stable fracture fixation without the need for compression of the plate to the bone surface. According to basic mechanics of fixed-angle locking plates load transfer is optimal when the plate–screw interface is closest to the near cortex. An increase in the distance between the plate and bone leads to an increase of the moment of flexion at the level of the screw–plate unit.

Clinically, an anatomically well-fitted plate can greatly facilitate the process of reduction in terms of axial and rotational alignment of the main fragments. The protrusion caused by a poor fit of the plate to the bone can cause soft-tissue impingement and/or irritation, especially in subcutaneous areas such as the medial malleolus, medial side of the proximal tibia, lateral femoral epicondyle, and proximal humerus. Schmutz et al [2008] found in their study that only 19% of the cases achieved an anatomical fit. Soft-tissue irritation can be seen where an anatomical plate does not perfectly fit the bone, requiring the surgeon to make smooth adjustments in the molding of the implant with the bending press and twisting irons.

The experience of the surgeon is essential when determining the degree of molding required to optimally fit the plate. Molding the plate at the level of fixed-angle and variable-angle threaded holes should be avoided because it can deform the thread. The thread must always be protected by putting it in the threaded sleeve. In periarticular threaded holes, the locking screws should always be placed parallel to the articular surface.

A wrong location of the locking screws in the epiphyseal area changes the axis of the plate, so that often the plate no longer correctly fits the cortical bone, resulting in deformation and loss of fracture reduction. As much time as is needed should be spent on mastering this milestone of the surgical technique; it is not a waste of time in surgery but absolutely necessary.

CASE 1

Case description

A 47-year-old man with a medical history of alcohol addiction and diabetes fell from a roof while manipulating an antenna and sustained a Gustilo type II pilon fracture **[Gustilo, 1984]**. It was a complete articular multifragmentary fracture of the left distal tibia with a simple fracture of the distal fibula (AO/OTA 43C3,4F3A) (**Fig 3.4-1**).

Due to the open wound and soft-tissue swelling when he presented in the emergency department, surgery was planned. The aim of the first surgical treatment was to clean the open wound, restore the fibular length and rotation through an open reduction and internal fixation, providing a stable lateral column, and immobilize the ankle using an ankle-spanning temporary external fixator (**Fig 3.4-2**).

The second surgery to restore the articular pilon surface and to fix the medial component was performed only 5 days after the first surgery. The surgeon planned, for the first time in his career, to use an anterolateral distal tibial locking compression plate (LCP); frozen allograft was also used to fill the bone defect in the epiphyseal-metaphyseal zone (**Fig 3.4-3** and **Fig 3.4-4**). The postoperative control x-ray showed poor reduction of the ankle surface and poor fracture alignment (**Fig 3.4-3**). The anterolateral plate was placed at the posteromedial aspect of the distal tibia.

One month after hospital discharge, the patient complained of pain and suppuration through the surgical wound of the tibial pilon began, evolving to cutaneous necrosis that required surgical cleaning and the application of negative-pressure wound therapy (eg, vacuum-assisted wound therapy). Later control x-rays showed metaphyseal collapse with a loss of reduction and distal displacement of the plate causing a soft-tissue disorder (**Fig 3.4-4**).

Removal of the internal fixation and debridement was done 4 months after the first surgery (**Fig 3.4-5**). Penicillin-sensitive *Staphylococcus aureus* was isolated and amoxicillin-clavulanic acid therapy was initiated until normalization of the inflammatory parameters. One month later, the external fixator was removed and a plaster cast was applied and retained until bone healing was achieved.

At the 18-month follow-up control after the third surgery, the patient had regained the ability to ambulate but had some limping due to a loss of ankle range-of-motion and posttraumatic swelling. The control x-ray showed sclerotic fracture callus formation and a recurvatum malunion of the distal tibia (**Fig 3.4-6**).

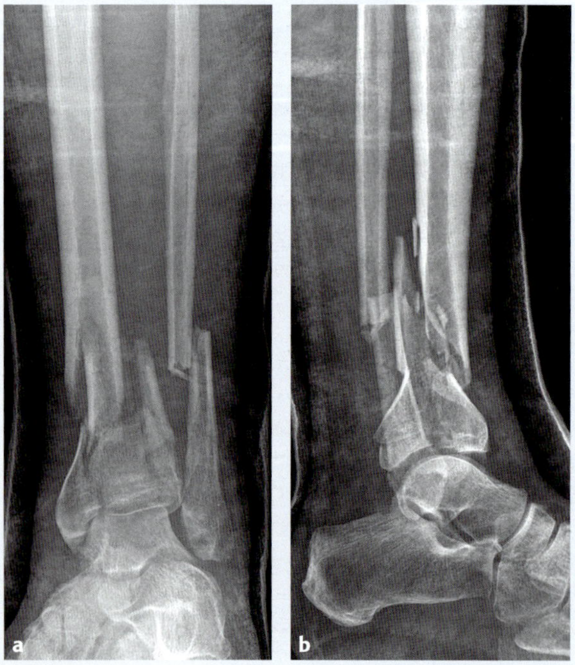

Fig 3.4-1a–b AP (**a**) and sagittal (**b**) views of the articular fracture.

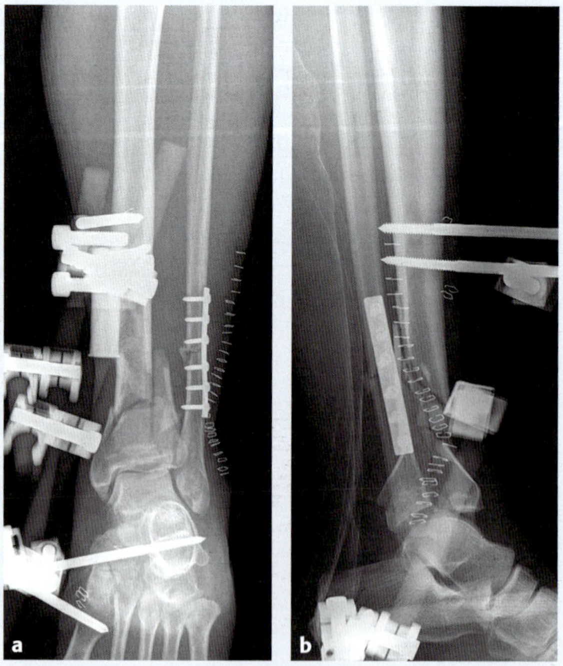

Fig 3.4-2a–b AP (**a**) and sagittal (**b**) views of the first surgery: open reduction and internal fixation of the fibula and application of an external fixator. Only length was restored, but the articular surface was unreduced, as seen in the sagittal view (**b**).

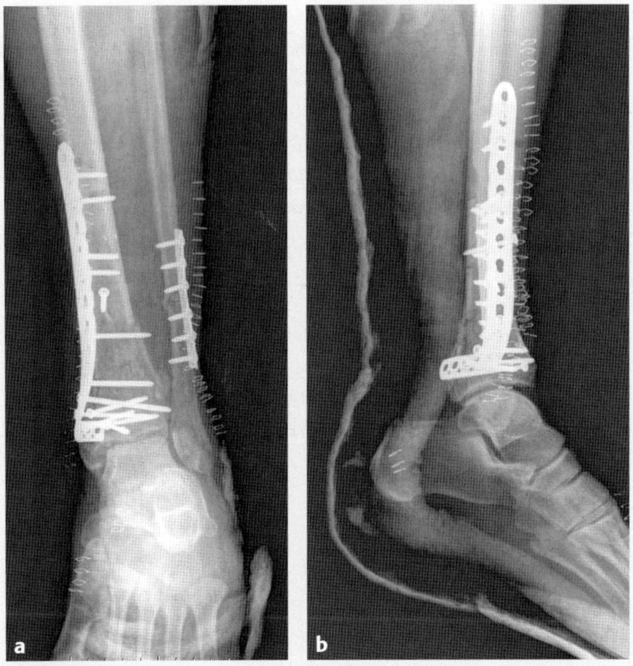

Fig 3.4-3a–b Postoperative AP (**a**) and sagittal (**b**) views of the second surgery: open reduction and internal fixation of the medial component, placing the anterolateral plate in a wrong position, ie, the posteromedial position, which could lead to a difficult dissection with soft-tissue injury.

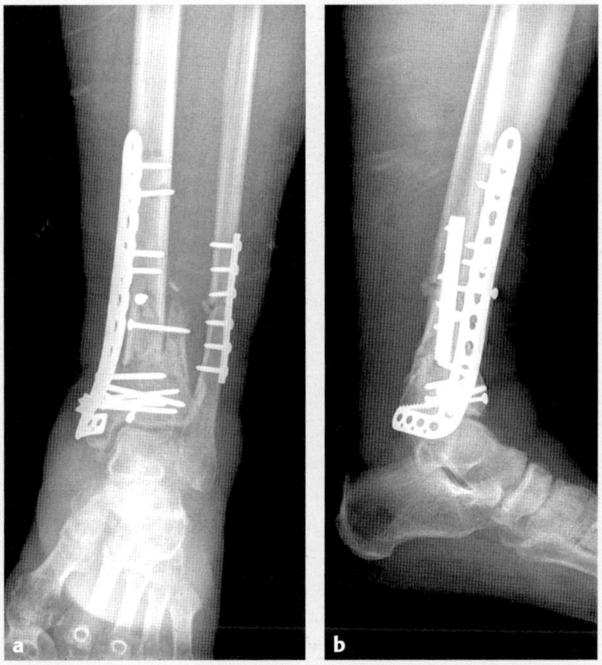

Fig 3.4-4a–b Four-month follow-up x-rays after the second surgery: not every plate hole needs be filled, but to avoid a collapse, the distal end of the plate must be fixed to the epiphysis with at least one or two screws. The collapse seen in the present case was due to the lack of periarticular fixation.

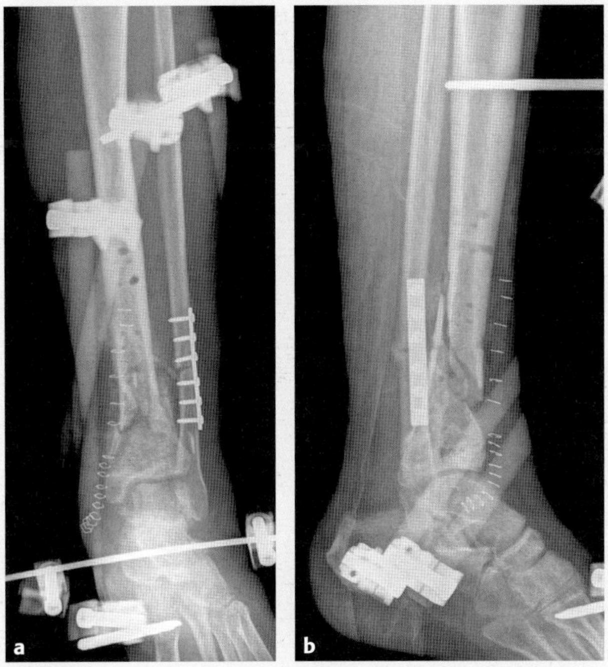

Fig 3.4-5a–b AP (**a**) and sagittal (**b**) views of the third surgery: hardware removal, debridement, and application of an ankle-spanning temporary external fixator.

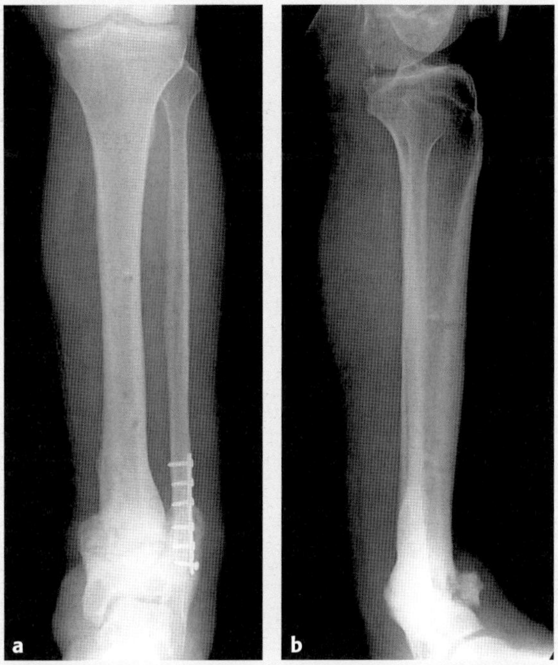

Fig 3.4-6a–b X-rays of the final result at 18 months showing the fracture healed in malunion (**a**), and in varus and recurvatum (**b**).

Analysis of failure and reflection

"Pilon fracture surgery is not for beginners and not for the middle of the night. Emergency surgery should be performed only under optimal overall conditions" [Rüedi, 1991].

Open and high-energy pilon fractures require careful preoperative planning of the incision placement and the timing of surgery. In accordance with the traditional principles of open fracture management, devitalized tissue, including devitalized bone fragments, require removal. If a defect persists after debridement, placement of antibiotic spacers should be considered until the time of definitive fixation.

Five days between the first surgery and the definitive internal fixation seems too little time to achieve the best condition for soft-tissue regeneration. This could be one reason for failure.

An LCP anterolateral distal tibial plate can never adapt in the posteromedial corner of the pilon. Anatomical variants related to the different bone morphologies can cause a lack of adaptation of the preformed implant to the bone, and extra molding for a correct adaptation may occasionally have to be performed. If the anatomical plates are applied in a position on the bone for which it has not been designed, greater dissection is certainly needed, generating ischemic zones. These lead to damaged skin or poor skin conditions that facilitate infection.

It is mandatory for surgeons to practice new techniques with the appropriate devices and tools in workshops before the definitive surgery rather than in the operating room, as seems to have happened in the present case. Not every plate hole has to be filled with a screw, but to prevent a collapse, the distal end of the plate must be fixed to the epiphysis with at least one or two screws. Lack of periarticular fixation may have caused the collapse in the present case.

Final outcome

Eighteen months after the third surgery, the patient was able to walk with some limping due to a loss of ankle range-of-motion and post-traumatic swelling. The x-rays showed hypertrophic and sclerotic callus formation and malunion in the recurvatum of the distal tibia (**Fig 3.4-6**).

Cases 2 and 3

The following two cases are not "complete" cases in the sense that they have no case description, clinical follow-up, and final outcome. However, the editors have decided to include them because they clearly show that anatomical implants were used that either do not fit and adapt to the bone or have been wrongly used and placed.

Case 2

A large, supposedly anatomical plate was applied without any correction to a small femur, which caused the plate to detach from the femur and the screws to cut through the femoral neck. Clearly, the anatomical molding of the plate did not fit with the topographic anatomy of the proximal femur (AO/OTA 32A) (**Fig 3.4-7**).

Case 3

This case contains more than one mistake. The periprosthetic fracture is clearly Vancouver B2 with a mobile stem, not B1. The less invasive stabilization system-distal femoral plate designed to fit the distal femur was applied to the lateral side. Although this plate has been used in periprosthetic hip and knee fractures, there is no indication in the current case for such an application as shown in **Fig 3.4-8**.

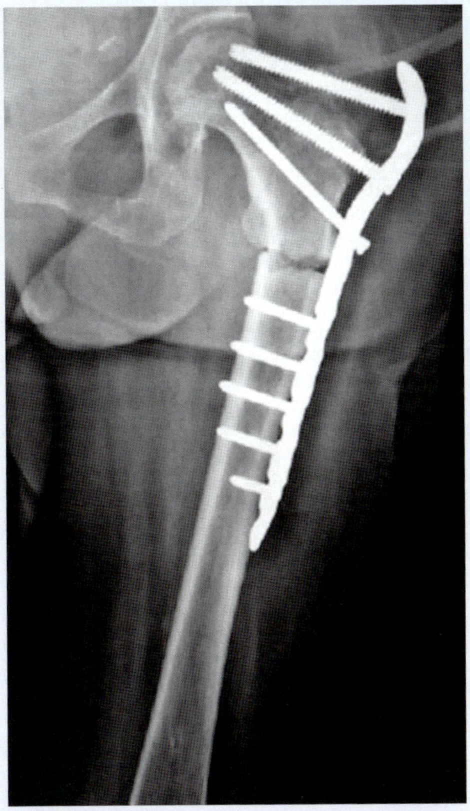

Fig 3.4-7 A large anatomical plate for the proximal femur used in a small femur results in the plate being partly detached from the femur and the screws cutting through the femoral neck.

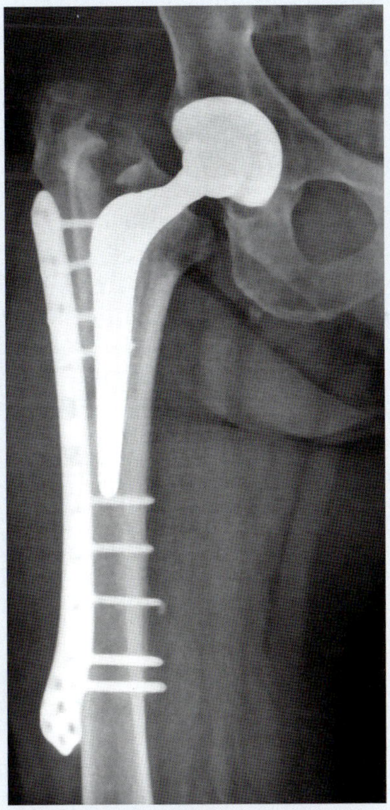

Fig 3.4-8 X-ray showing a less invasive stabilization system-distal femoral plate that was placed on the lateral side instead of the distal femur for which it was designed, leading to a failure.

Analysis of failure and reflection

When molded anatomical plates are used, surgeons must always keep in mind the anatomical variants of each individual and that trying to adapt the bone to the plate or reduce the bone to fit the plate without making small modifications can lead to failure. It is always necessary to keep in mind that modifying a plate with threaded holes can deform it and affect the angular stability of the plate with the locking screw.

The locking plate technique achieves stable fracture fixation without the need for compression of the plate to the bone surface. From a biomechanical point of view, a perfect fit between plate undersurface and bone is not required. However, basic mechanics of fixed-angle locking plates dictate that load transfer is most optimal when the plate–screw interface is closest to the near cortex.

Clinically, an anatomically well-fitting plate can greatly facilitate the process of reduction in terms of axial and rotational alignment of the main fragments. A nonfitting plate may protrude and therefore cause soft-tissue impingement/irritations **[Schmutz et al, 2008]**.

Key points to remember

- When using anatomical implants, surgeons must keep in mind that there exist significant differences in bone morphology, bone size and shape, which depend on such factors as the patient's age, gender, race, ethnic origin, and region.
- From the biomechanical point of view, a perfect fitting of the plate to the bone is not necessary if the plate is used as an internal fixator with angular stability criteria.
- The protrusion caused by a poor fit of the plate to the bone can cause soft-tissue impingement and/or irritation, especially in subcutaneous areas.
- The experience of the surgeon is important when determining the degree of molding required for the optimal fit of the plate. Molding the plate should be avoided at the level of the threaded holes, whether fixed-angle or variable-angle holes, because the molding can deform the thread.
- In periarticular threaded holes, the surgeons should always ensure that the locking screws are placed parallel to the articular surface.

References and suggested reading

Gustilo RB, Mendoza RM, Williams DN. Problems in the management of type III (severe) open fractures: a new classification of type III open fractures. *J Trauma.* 1984 Aug;24(8):742–746.

Heim U. Operationstaktik [Operative technique]. In: Heim U, Gächter A, eds. *The Pilon Tibial Fracture. Classification, Surgical Techniques, Results.* Berlin Heidelberg: Springer-Verlag; 1991:141–143.

Perren SM. Evolution and rationale of locked internal fixator technology. Introductory remarks. *Injury.* 2001 Sep;32 Suppl 2:B3–9.

Rüedi TP. Pilon-tibial-Frakturen: What's new? [Pilon tibial fractures: What's new?]. In: Heim U, Gächter A, eds. *The Pilon Tibial Fracture. Classification, Surgical Techniques, Results.* Berlin Heidelberg: Springer-Verlag; 1991:209–215.

Schmutz B, Wullschleger ME, Kim H, et al. Fit assessment of anatomic plates for the distal medial tibia. *J Orthop Trauma.* 2008 Apr;22(4):258–263.

Wagner M. General principles for the clinical use of the LCP. *Injury.* 2003 Nov;34 Suppl 2:B31–42.

White T, Folkens P. *The Human Bone Manual.* Burlington: Elsevier Academic Press; 2005.

3.5 Designs and techniques of intramedullary nailing

Suthorn Bavonratanavech, Joan Girós Torres, Josep Muñoz Vives, Roberto Rivero Sosa, Pol M Rommens, J Miquel Sales Pérez, Miquel Videla Cés

An evening in which everyone agrees, is a lost evening.

Albert Einstein

Intramedullary (IM) nailing of long bone shaft fractures is generally accepted as a standard treatment. The limits of nailing are related to the fracture location in the shaft and the fracture pattern. In polytrauma patients, early total care (ETC) with definitive stabilization with nails should not be performed in case of:

- Patients with severe head or chest trauma
- Hemorrhagic shock
- Patients with a high Injury Severity Score (ISS)

A challenge for nailing can also be the shape of the diaphysis as it occurs in the humerus, where the medullary cavity is cylindrical in the proximal third, elliptical in the middle third and nonexistent in the distal third where the margins are triangular and filled with compact bone. The triangular shape is particularly important as it can make fitting the nail more difficult (**Fig 3.5-1**).

The first-generation nails had an almost straight shape with hardly any curvature, so the use of the conventional Küntscher nail was restricted to relatively simple transverse and short oblique midshaft fractures.

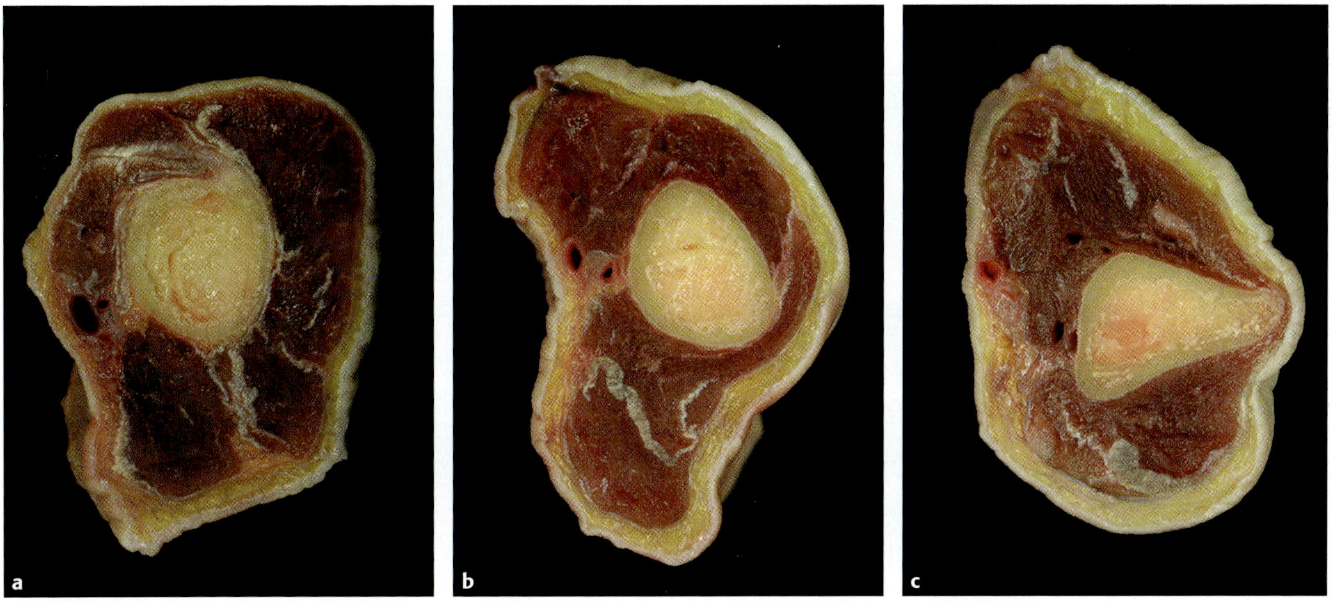

Fig 3.5-1a–c The morphology transition of the medullary canal of the humerus. The cylindrical medullary canal in the proximal third of the humeral shaft (**a**). The shape is elliptical in the middle third (**b**), and almost without canal in the distal third (**c**) where it is filled with compact bone, sometimes making it impossible to drill enough to insert a nail.

In the last decades of the 20th century, the need to address different fracture patterns, including open fractures, led to a great development in the design of a variety of IM nails. Surgeons started debating the need for reaming or not reaming the medullary cavity.

Reaming the medullary cavity increases the area of contact between the IM nail and bone. This is indicated in fractures which are more complex or more proximal or distal in the shaft. Reaming also improves the mechanical properties of the bone-implant interface by allowing the use of implants with larger diameters. However, the reaming process itself has some inherent biological disadvantages, especially when performed excessively. These include a considerable rise in IM pressure and temperature causing bone necrosis [Krettek, 2007].

For unreamed IM nails, there is an obvious need for a small diameter, solid IM nail that should be locked. If the insertion site is not optimally chosen, or the shape and radius of the IM canal diverge from those of the IM nail's geometry, a proper fit may be a problem.

Regardless of the type and shape of the IM nail, controlling length, alignment, axis, and rotation of the limb is essential. In any multifragmentary fractures the length of the limb can only be assessed radiographically after distal locking. Poor axial alignment is more frequent in marginal fractures in the shaft, either proximal or distal, especially in those cases where a narrow nail has been used.

Insertion techniques and preparation of the entry point

Selecting the correct entry point is crucial in IM nailing. A wrong choice of the nail insertion point can be the cause of axial and rotational misalignments.

During the nailing process, the axis and the rotation of the bone must be checked. There are several tricks to check the correct alignment in the lower limb; one of the most useful tricks for checking alignment in the coronal plane is the cable technique where the knee is fully extended and the patella must face anterior (**Fig 3.5-2**). A technical tip to assess the correct femoral rotation is the evaluation of the shape of the lesser trochanter for comparison with the contralateral

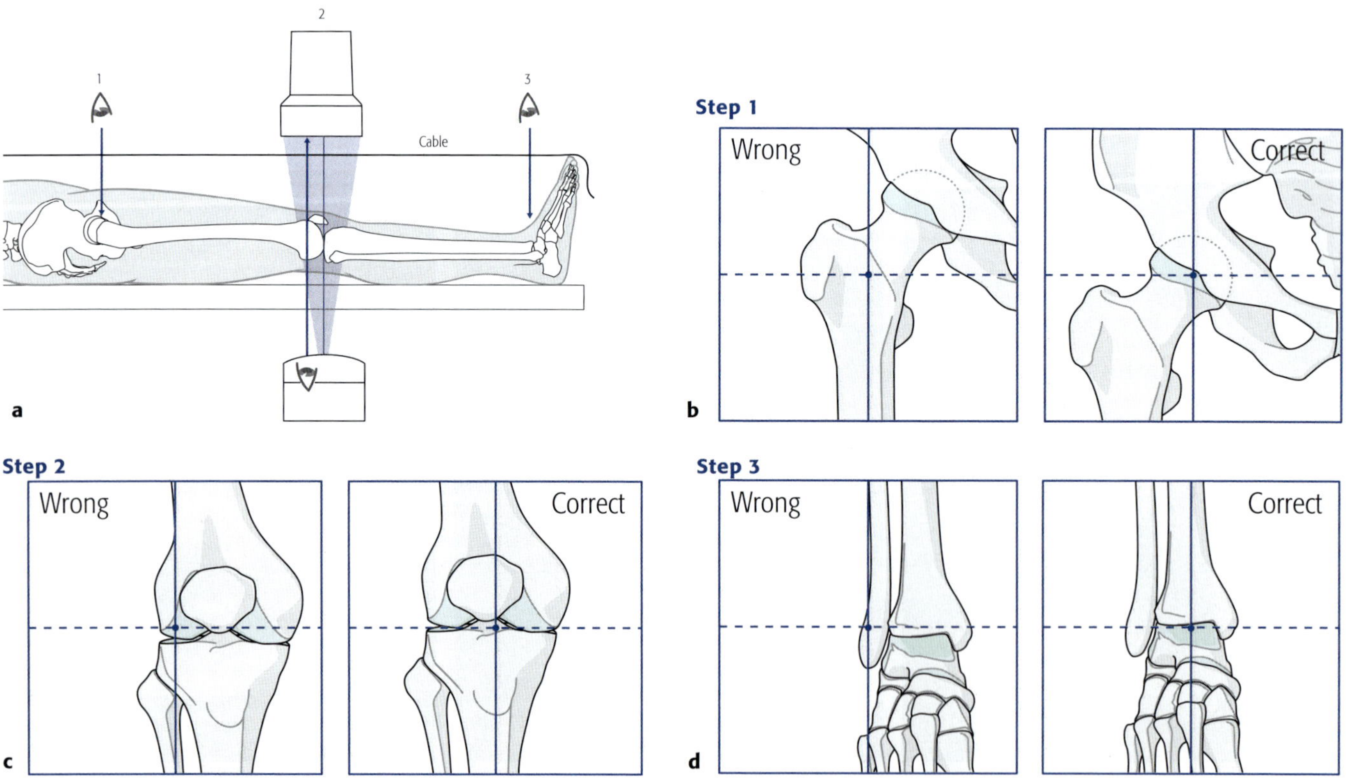

Fig 3.5-2a–d Cable technique for checking alignment in the coronal plane. The knee is fully extended and the patella must face anterior [Hessmann, 2017].

side. After distal locking with the patella facing anterior, the proximal fragment is rotated until the shape of the lesser trochanter matches the stored view of the intact side (**Fig 3.5-3**) [Hessmann, 2017].

Before starting surgery, the surgeon should plan how to achieve fracture reduction. It is also imperative to reduce the fracture before nailing, because IM nails alone can never achieve fracture reduction by themselves. Surgeons must not believe that the implant can improve the reduction of a fracture that has not been properly reduced.

Limited open techniques can greatly facilitate the reduction of closed fractures but raise concern about infection through exposure of the fracture site. The infection rate for open versus closed reductions is higher but not statistically significant [Tang et al, 2006].

Stab incision techniques have been developed for the femur and the tibia. In both bones, care must be taken to place the incisions in line with the axis of the medullary cavity and not too close to the chosen entry point on the bone [Hessmann, 2017].

The choice of the entry point is mainly based on the nail geometry, its angulation, and proximal and distal curvature. The use of an antegrade or retrograde technique determines the choice of entry points for the femur, as the choice of suprapatellar or infrapatellar technique does for tibial nailing.

Consensus seems to exist on the choice of the antegrade entry point in the humerus. When using the most recent straight nail designs, surgeons avoid the lateral approach and also avoid the transtendinous insertion of the rotator cuff. They are strongly advised to select a more medial entry

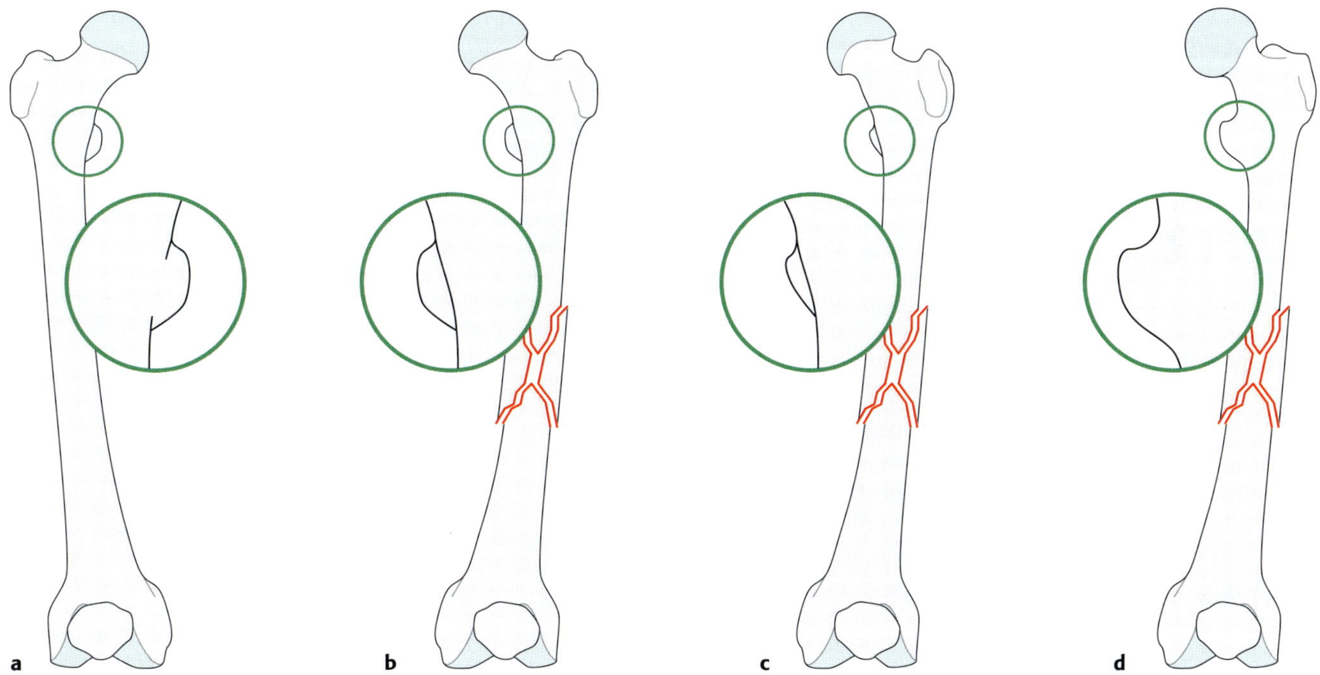

Fig 3.5-3a–d Intraoperative x-ray assessment of rotation. The shape of the lesser trochanter is compared with the contralateral side [Hessmann, 2017].

- **a** Before positioning the patient, the shape of the lesser trochanter should look like the one of the intact opposite side (with patella facing anterior).
- **b** After distal locking with the patella facing anterior, the proximal fragment is rotated until the shape of the lesser trochanter matches the stored view of the intact side.
- **c** With external malrotation, the lesser trochanter is smaller and partially hidden behind the proximal femoral shaft.
- **d** With internal malrotation, the lesser trochanter appears enlarged.

through the supraspinatus muscle mass, reaming the entry hole in the more proximal cartilage of the humeral head. Retrograde nailing of the humerus is a much more demanding technique with a high risk of causing supracondylar humeral fractures; increasingly, this technique is used less often, also because of a lack of appropriate implants and/or necessary instrumentation.

Almost all nails, whether reamed or unreamed, are locked. While locking is advisable in reamed IM nailing, it is mandatory in unreamed nailing procedures because the nails are thinner.

The locked IM nailing technique uses nails with holes for its fixation with screws inside the bone. The localization of the nail holes used for the distal locking turns out to be usually quite difficult. The distal fixation procedure is in fact performed manually through a centering framework connected to a C-arm that requires very long operating times, and consequently, long exposure to ionizing radiation for the surgical team and the patient [Ingrassia et al, 2011].

Proximal locking is performed through the guide attached to the insertion handle. Distally, at least two (femoral) or three (tibial) interlocking screws are recommended for the following reasons:

- As there is no tight fit between the interlocking screws and the IM nail, toggling may occur. This can lead to instability and malalignment, especially in the coronal plane. The insertion of two (femoral) or three (tibial) distal interlocking screws, which are usually not quite parallel, reduces the toggling.
- Breakage of an interlocking screw occurs because of the implant material, design, strength (due to diameter, eg, 5.0 mm locking screw is stronger than a 3.5 mm locking screw), surface finish, the load applied, and the number of cycles. With small-diameter nails (in unreamed systems), the interlocking screws are of a smaller core diameter, which results more frequently in screw breakage by fatigue [Eberle et al, 2010].

Poller screws

Intramedullary nailing of fractures in the metaphysis is associated with a higher rate of malalignment. A strong muscle pull and a wide medullary canal can lead to postfixation instability, even with locking. Placing screws adjacent to the IM nail has been proposed as a possible solution to prevent lateral or medial translation in both the tibia and the femur. These screws ("Poller screws") decrease the width of the metaphyseal medullary canal, forcing the IM nail to the center of the medullary cavity, and also increasing the mechanical stiffness of the bone-implant construct. Poller screws can be used for correcting alignment, stabilization, and manipulation. The screw is placed perpendicular to the direction in which the implant might displace. In oblique metaphyseal fractures of the distal tibia or femur, the Poller screw may be helpful for stabilization, as shear forces are transformed into compression forces.

The Poller screw may help to prevent displacement in situations where a previously misplaced IM nail tends to slip into the old nail path. It can also be used in situations where the entry point for antegrade IM nailing (eg, in the tibia) was originally poorly chosen, forcing the proximal bone fragment into malalignment: the IM nail must be removed temporarily and the Poller screw placed to block the incorrect path, while the IM nail is reinserted (**Fig 3.5-4**) [Krettek, 2007].

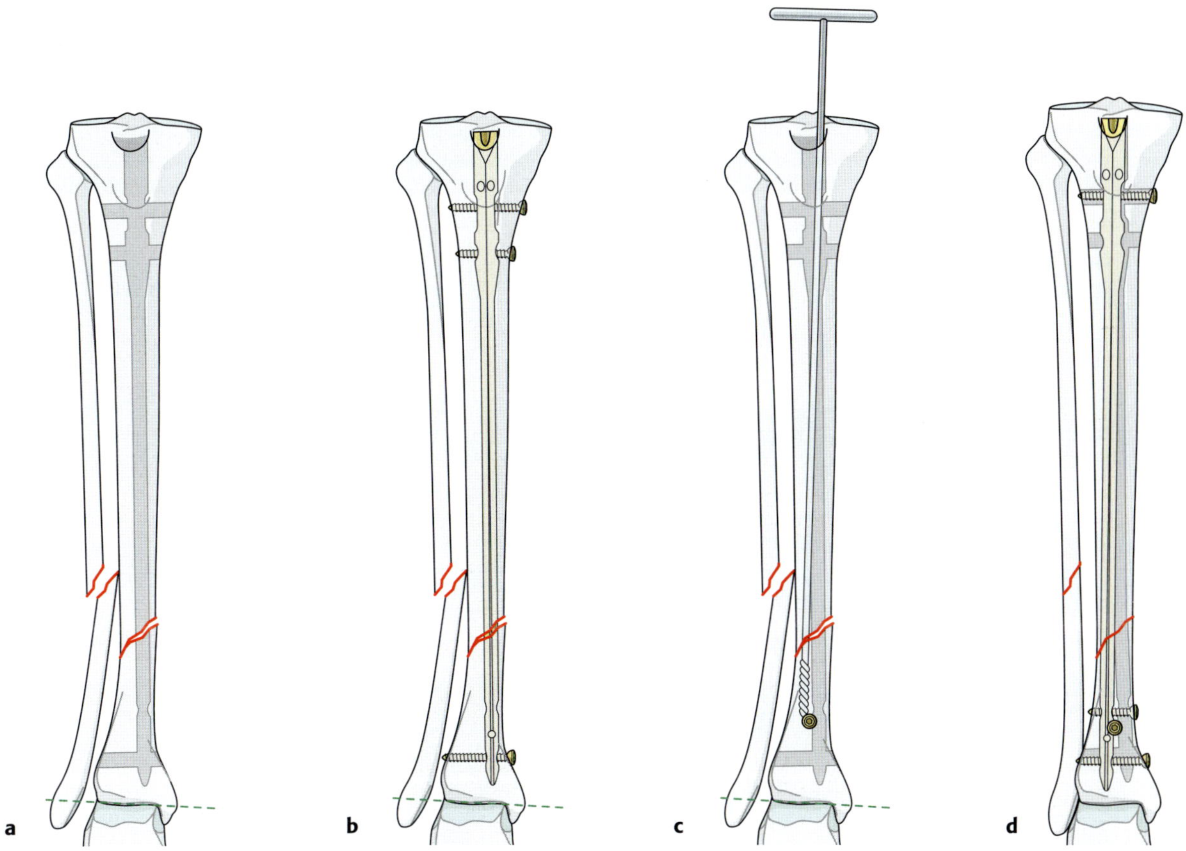

Fig 3.5-4a–d Poller screws **[Hessmann, 2017]**.

- **a** Schematic drawing of a clinical case: the fracture healed with valgus malalignment. After nail removal, a refracture occurred.
- **b** Since the original nail path is sclerotic, the new intramedullary (IM) nail follows the preexisting path with the same malalignment.
- **c** This problem can be solved by using a Poller screw as a reduction tool: the Poller screw is placed in the old IM nail path to block it, while a new path is prepared with a hand reamer.
- **d** Once the new nail path has been prepared, the new IM nail is inserted and locked, while the Poller screw remains in place.

CASE 1

Case description

An 87-year-old man presented with a closed fracture of the right intertrochanteric hip after falling on the floor (AO/OTA 31A3) (**Fig 3.5-5**). He was treated with a proximal femoral nail antirotation (PFNA). There was a slight valgus reduction causing a gap in the calcar area (**Fig 3.5-6**). The malposition of an implant is usually an indirect sign of malreduction. In this case, the nail tip was higher than the tip of the greater trochanter while the blade was on the lower half of the femoral neck. The fracture gap caused instability and eventually implant failure 1 month postoperatively (**Fig 3.5-7**). Implant removal and medialization of the distal fragment (shaft fragment) were performed to achieve better biomechanical stability. A 130° angled blade plate was used to fix the fracture (**Fig 3.5-6**). The initial preoperative salvage plan (**Fig 3.5-8**) was made before the 2-stage corrective surgery: first, the PFNA was removed (**Fig 3.5-9**) and second, the reduction and internal fixation with the 130° blade plate was performed (**Fig 3.5-10**). The medialization of the distal fragment was performed to achieve medial support for the fracture and a 130° angled blade plate was used to fix the fracture (**Fig 3.5-10**).

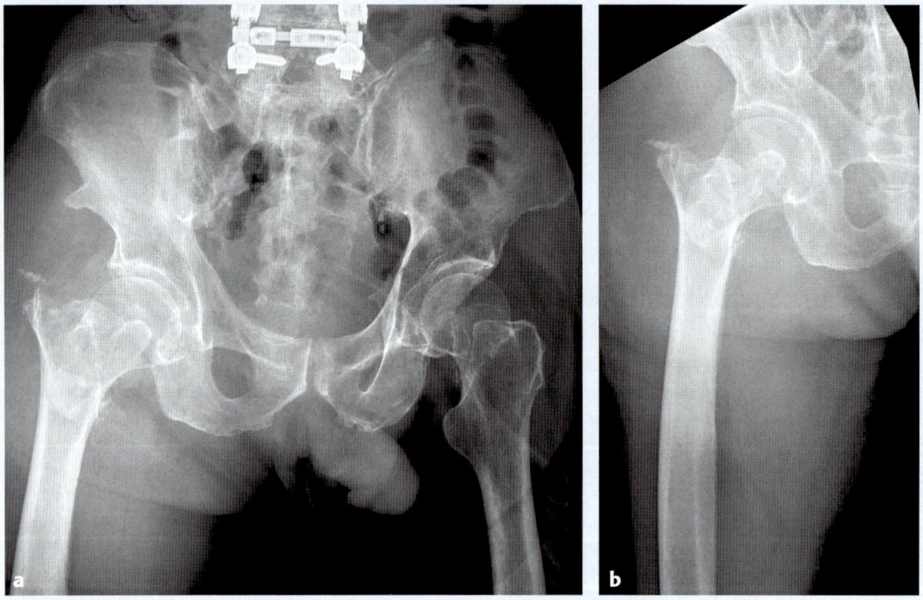

Fig 3.5-5a–b Preoperative x-rays showing a closed intertrochanteric fracture of the right hip.

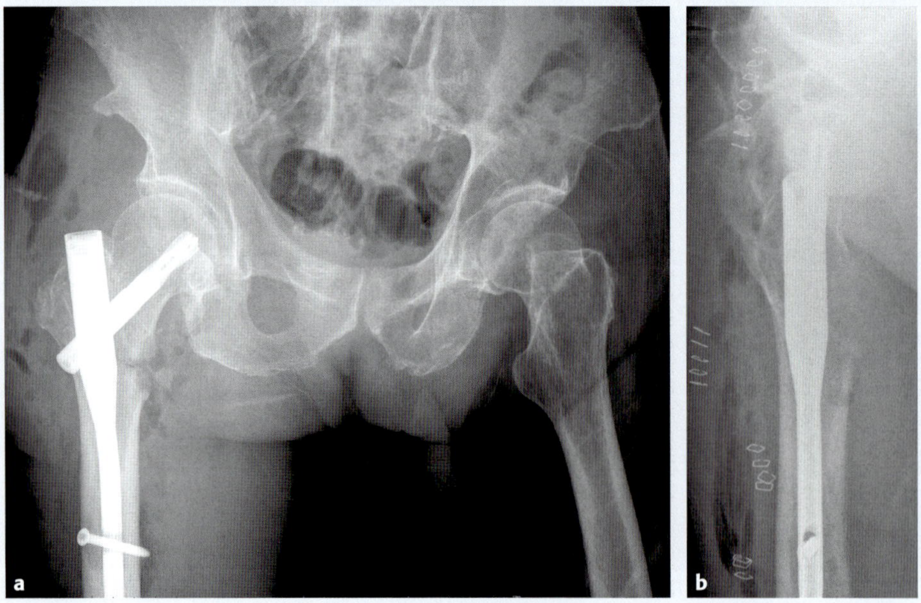

Fig 3.5-6a–d Postoperative x-rays.
a–b X-rays showing a slight valgus reduction that caused a gap in the calcar area resulting in instability.

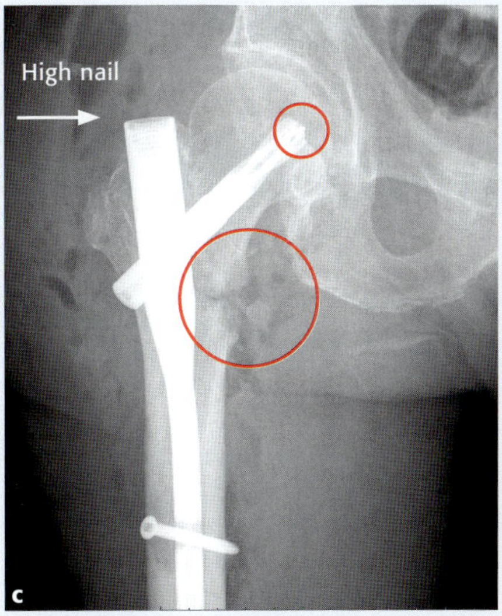

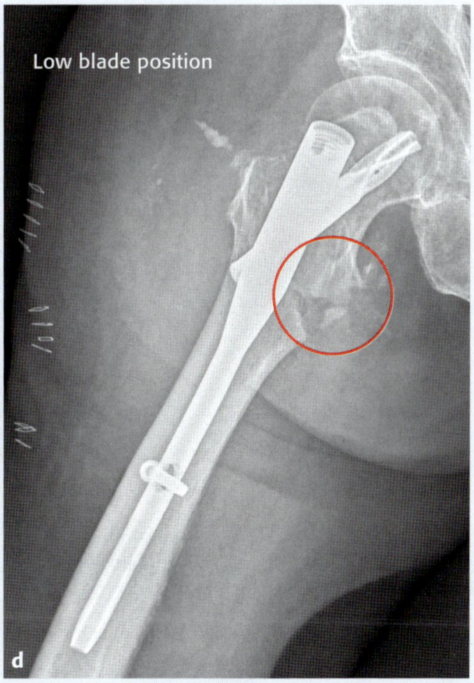

Fig 3.5-6a–d (cont) Postoperative x-rays.
c–d The implant malposition is an indirect sign of malreduction. In this case, the nail tip was higher than the tip of the greater trochanter (**c**) while the blade was on the posterior half of the femoral neck (**d**).

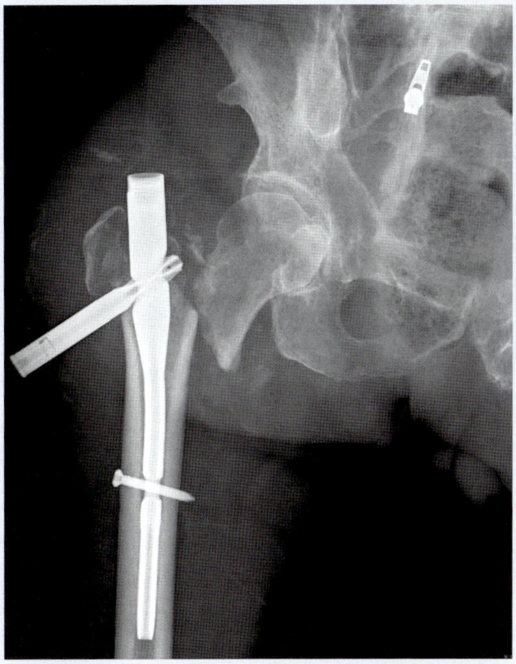

Fig 3.5-7 X-ray showing the failed implant: instability caused the proximal femoral nail antirotation blade to toggle inside the osteoporotic femoral head.

Analysis of failure and reflection

A slight valgus reduction caused a gap in the calcar area, which resulted in instability since there was no medial support. Implant malposition is an indirect sign of malreduction. In this case, the nail's tip was higher than the tip of the greater trochanter while the blade was on the posterior part of the femoral neck (**Fig 3.5-6c–d**). Instability from lack of medial support caused the PFNA blade to toggle inside the osteoporotic femoral head and eventually led to implant failure.

A careful and thorough analysis of the quality of reduction before inserting the implant can prevent devastating complications. It is important to remember that the nail used in a proximal femoral fracture cannot provide fracture reduction and to always check the fracture reduction during the operation.

Final outcome

The fracture healed uneventfully 6 months after the rescue surgery (**Fig 3.5-11**).

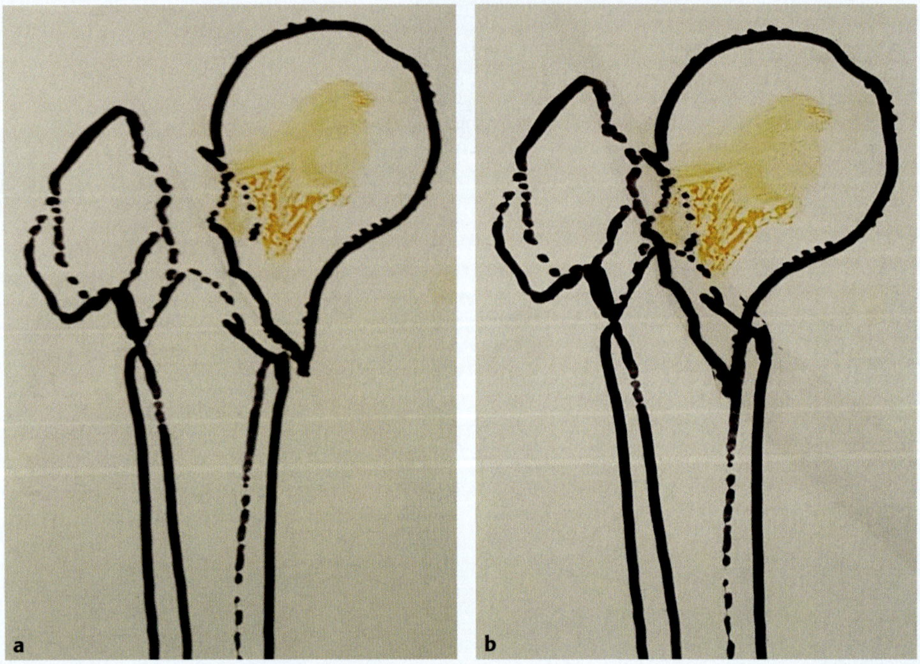

Fig 3.5-8a–b Preoperative plan to salvage the failed first surgery: medialization of the distal fragment to achieve medial support for the fracture.

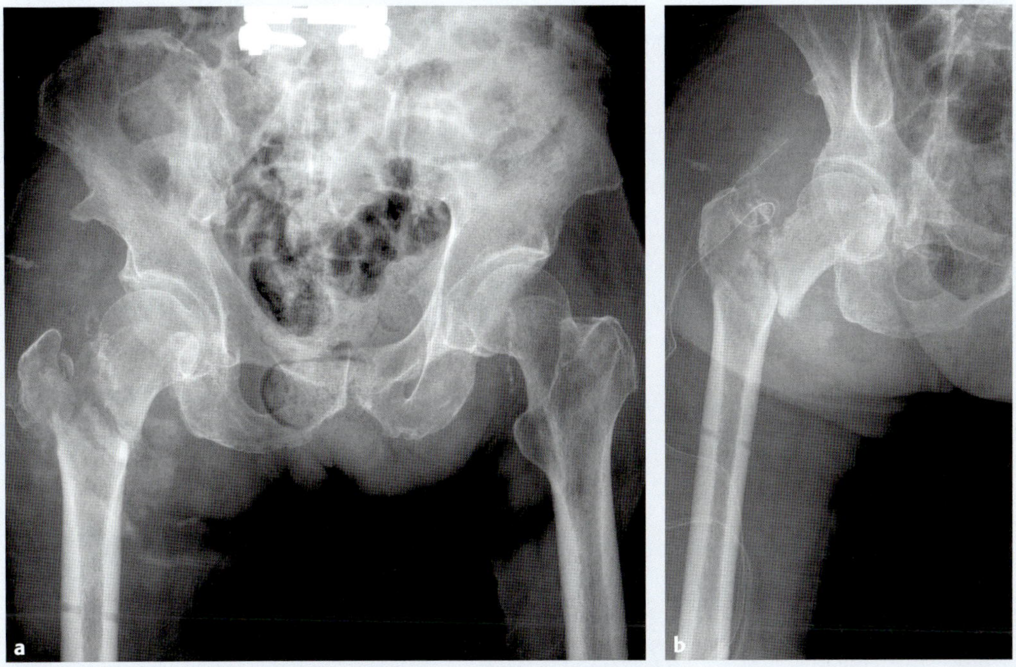

Fig 3.5-9a–b Removal of the proximal femoral nail antirotation (PFNA) revealed more information before the corrective surgery, ie, that toggling of the PFNA blade inside the osteoporotic femoral head had created a hole around the blade and emptied the femoral head and neck of bone, eventually leading to implant failure. The AP (**a**) and axial (**b**) x-rays after the PFNA removal shows the greater trochanter as one large separate piece.

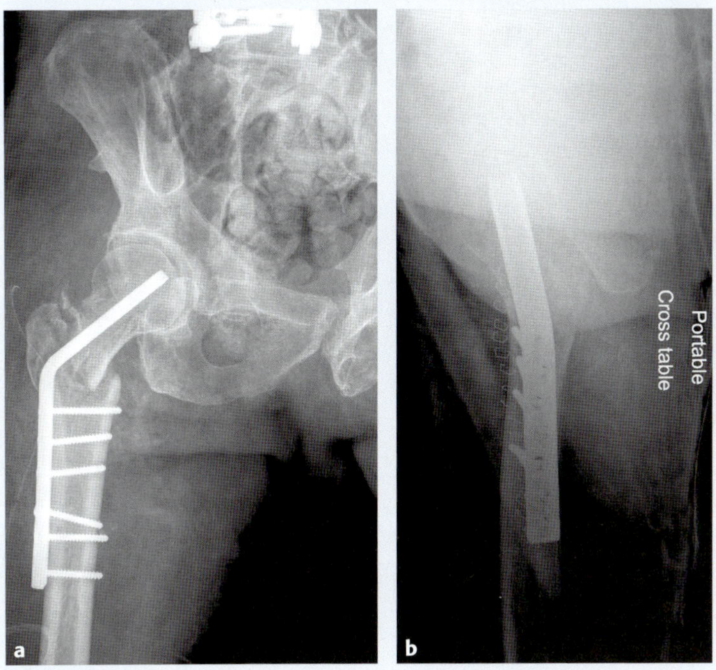

Fig 3.5-10a–b Rescue surgery using an angled blade plate. AP view (**a**) and axial view (**b**) of the final fixation with a 130° angled blade plate.

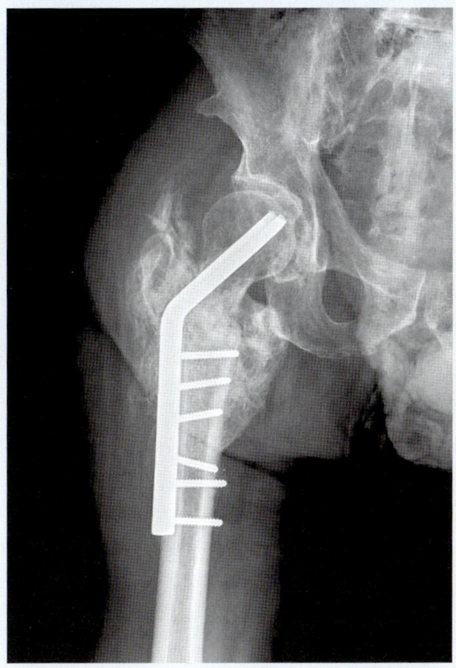

Fig 3.5-11 Six-month postoperative x-ray showing the healed fracture.

CASE 2

Case description

A 65-year-old woman fell from standing height sustaining a spiral humeral shaft fracture of the left arm (AO/OTA 12A1) (**Fig 3.5-12**). The patient had no comorbidities. Since nailing shaft fractures is considered the gold standard, the surgeon planned to use an expert humeral nail. The patient complained of elbow pain just after the surgery and the elbow range of motion was limited, both in flexion and extension. She also complained of shoulder pain and a significant disability. A distal periimplant fracture at the tip of the nail was not diagnosed until 2 months later (**Fig 3.5-13**). Proximally, the entry point of the nail seemed to be slightly lateral and the spiral blade was not completely impacted (**Fig 3.5-14**). For definitive treatment, the nail was removed, the proximal end of the medullary cavity overreamed, and both fractures fixed by minimally invasive plate osteosynthesis technique with a long and twisted PHILOS plate used as a helical plate (**Fig 3.5-15**).

In the immediate postoperative period, an assisted mobilization protocol of the elbow and shoulder was established, achieving a functional mobility in both joints at the 4-month follow-up control (**Fig 3.5-16**).

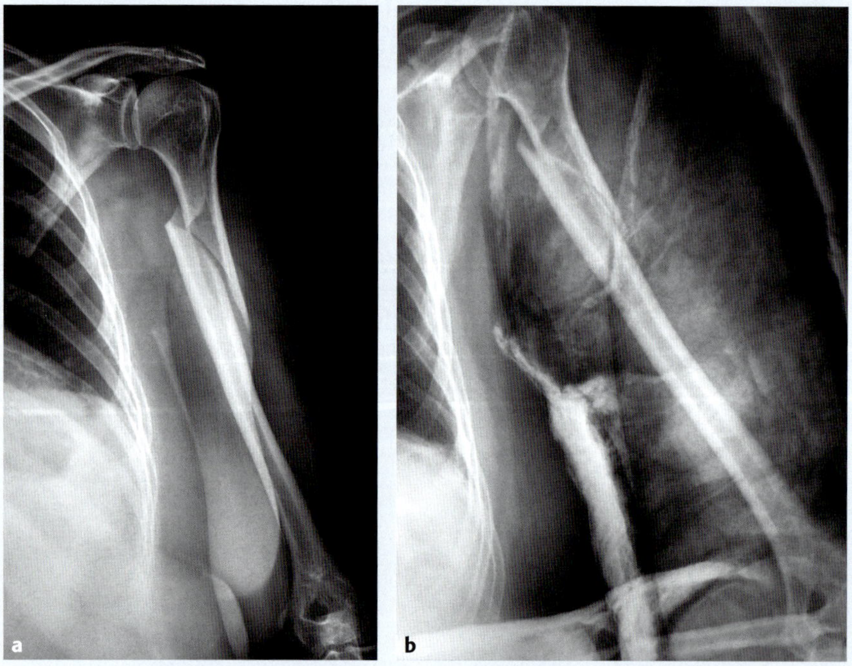

Fig 3.5-12a–b AP (**a**) and oblique (**b**) x-rays of a proximal spiral shaft fracture of the left humerus.

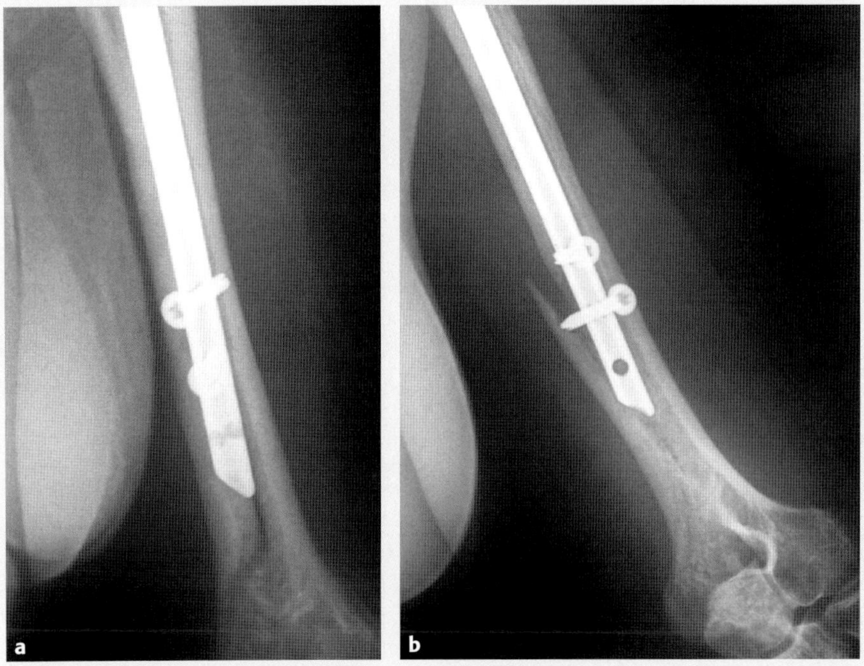

Fig 3.5-13a–b Detail of the distal third of the humerus, where the periimplant fracture can be clearly seen.

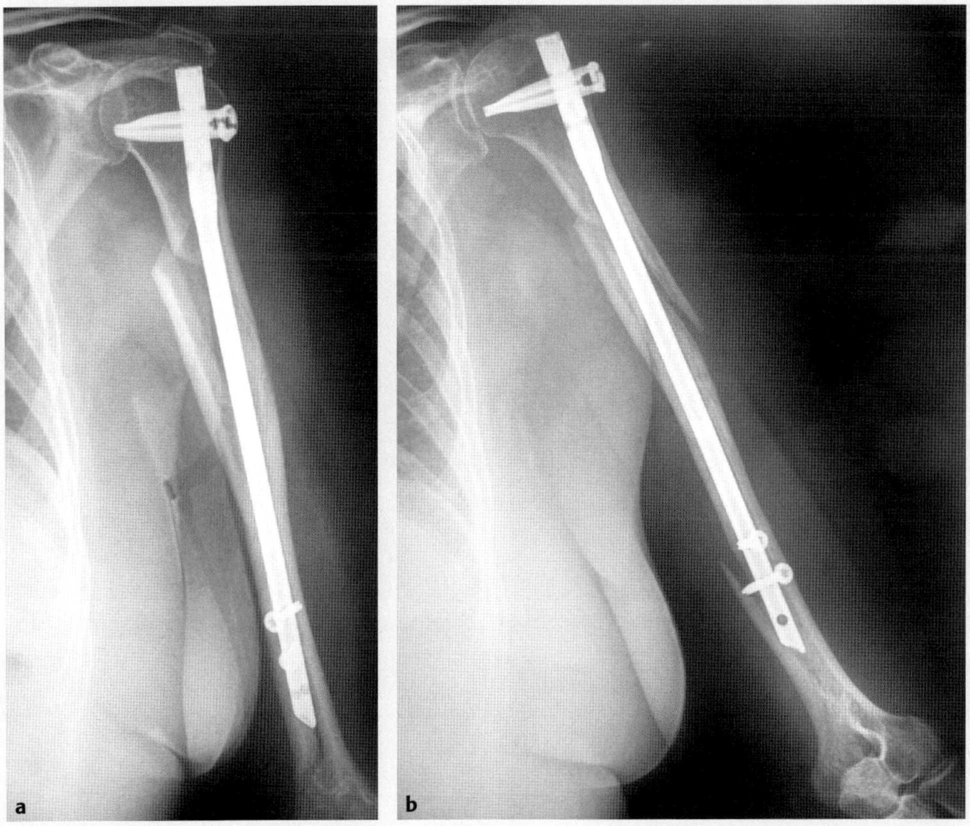

Fig 3.5-14a–b Two-month postoperative x-rays: a distal periimplant fracture at the tip of the nail is visible in the external rotation view (**b**).

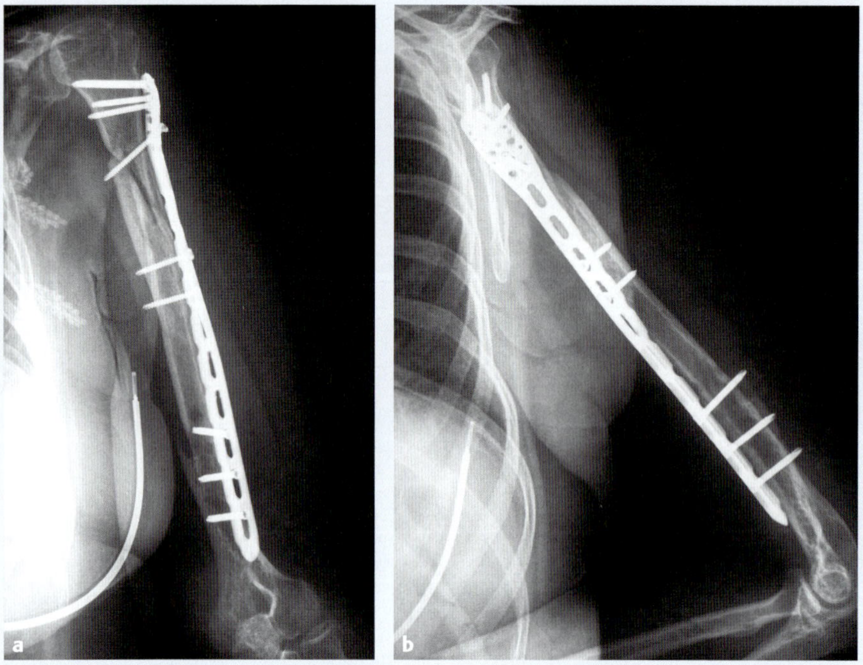

Fig 3.5-15a–b Four-month follow-up control x-rays of the revision surgery: the final fixation was done by minimally invasive plate osteosynthesis technique with a long and twisted PHILOS plate that was used as a helical plate.

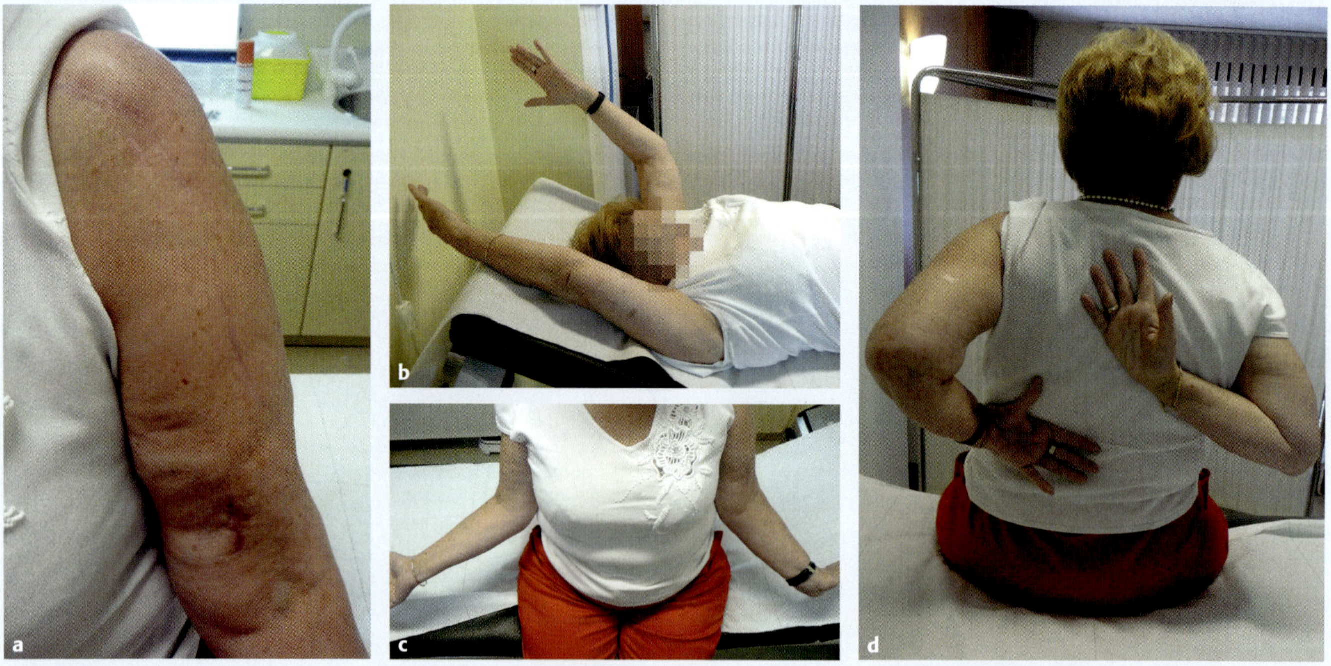

Fig 3.5-16a–d Patient at the 4-month clinical follow-up control.

Analysis of failure and reflection

Surgeons must know the topographic anatomy. The shape of the humeral shaft can be a challenge for nailing, as the geometry of the humeral shaft cavity changes from cylindrical in the proximal third to elliptical in the middle third and is nonexistent in the distal third, where the margins of the humerus are triangular and filled with compact bone (**Fig 3.5-17**).

Surgeons also need to carefully reflect on what could and should have been done differently. If the insertion site is not optimally chosen, or the shape and radius of the intramedullary canal diverge from those of the intramedullary nail geometry, a proper fit may be a problem.

Final outcome

The patient achieved full functional mobility of elbow and shoulder 4 months after surgery and assisted mobilization (**Fig 3.5-16** and **Fig 3.5-17**).

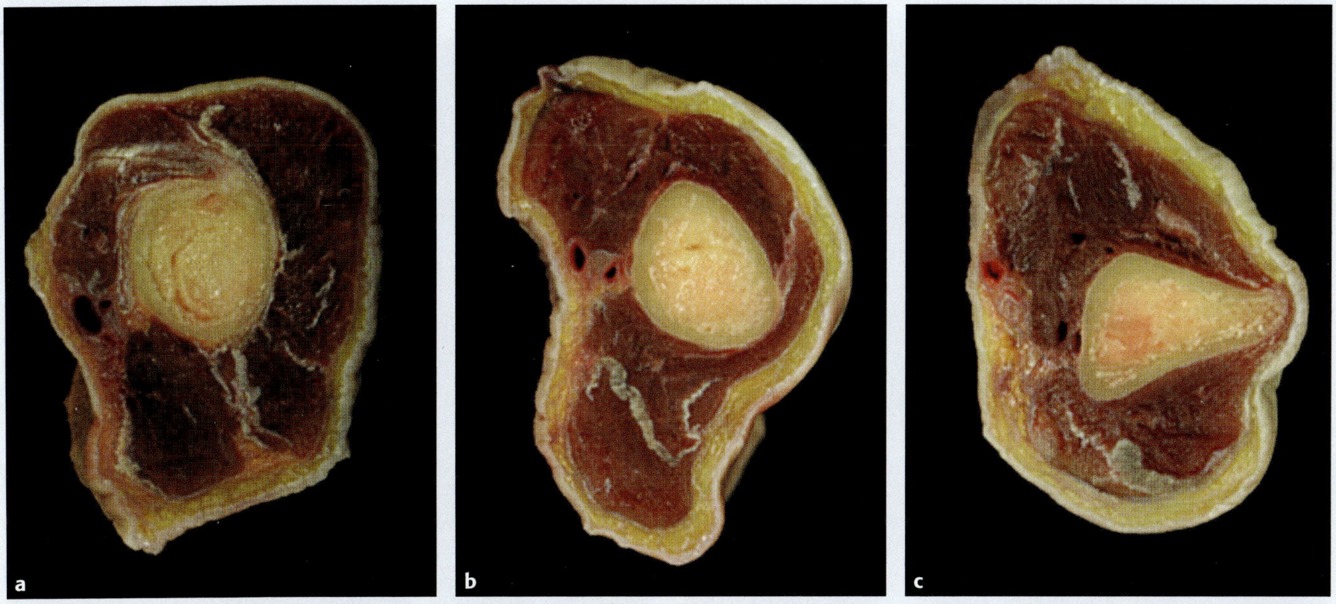

Fig 3.5-17a–c The morphology transition of the medullary canal of the humerus: a cylindrical channel can be seen in the proximal third of the humeral shaft (**a**), while the shape is elliptical in the middle third (**b**), and almost without canal in the distal third (**c**) and full of compact bone, through which it is sometimes impossible to insert a nail.

CASE 3

Case description

A 55-year-old obese patient (BMI > 30) lost his footing while getting on a bus, which resulted in immediate intense pain in the left lower leg and inability to walk. X-rays of the lower leg in AP and lateral views revealed a nondisplaced oblique fracture in the upper third of the tibial shaft (AO/OTA 42A2) (**Fig 3.5-18**). The fracture was treated with intramedullary nailing and the postoperative x-rays revealed an antecurvatum (apex anterior deformity) at the fracture site (**Fig 3.5-19**). The postoperative result was accepted and early rehabilitation initiated, but a nonunion developed. Three additional surgeries were performed before achieving bone healing (ie, first, dynamization; second, nail removal and plate osteosynthesis with cancellous bone grafting; third, second bone grafting), resulting in a 20° varus deformity and 3 cm shortening of the leg (**Fig 3.5-20**).

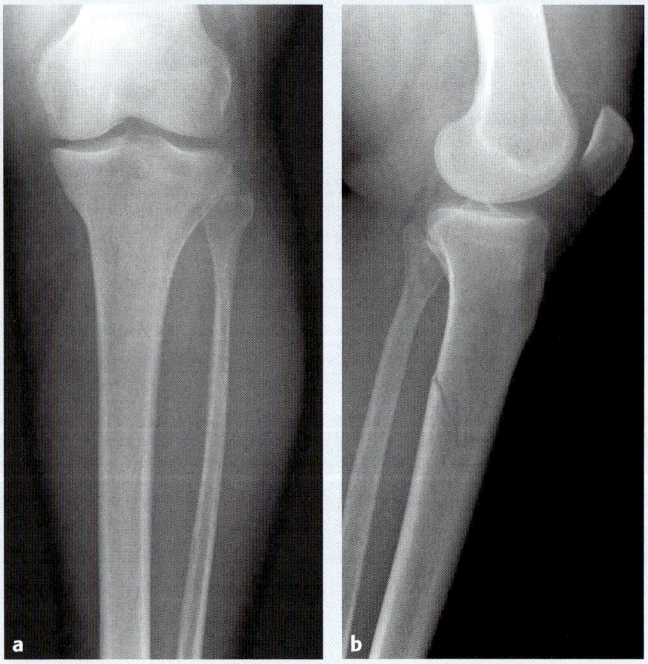

Fig 3.5-18a–b Preoperative x-rays of a nondisplaced oblique tibial shaft fracture.

- **a** AP x-ray of the left knee joint and lower leg reveals a cortical split at the lateral cortex in the proximal third of the shaft. Two slightly oblique fracture lines can be detected near this cortical break. There is no displacement of the fracture fragments.
- **b** Lateral view of the knee joint and left lower leg. The nondisplaced fracture can be seen more clearly in this view than in the AP x-ray.

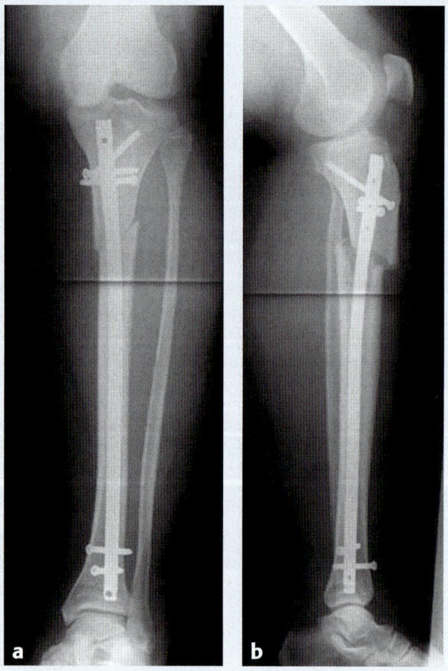

Fig 3.5-19a–b Immediate postoperative x-rays of the fracture.

- **a** Postoperative AP x-ray of the entire left lower leg. The fracture has been stabilized with a cannulated intramedullary nail. The proximal fragment is fixed with three interlocking screws, the distal fragment with two. Although alignment seems correct, there is a slight displacement of the proximal fragment towards medial.
- **b** Postoperative lateral x-ray of the entire left lower leg. The displacement of the proximal fragment in the sagittal plane is more severe now than before the surgery when it was barely perceptible. There is a translation of the proximal fragment towards anterior, together with a slight antecurvatum. The main fragments are not firmly connected but are statically interlocked.

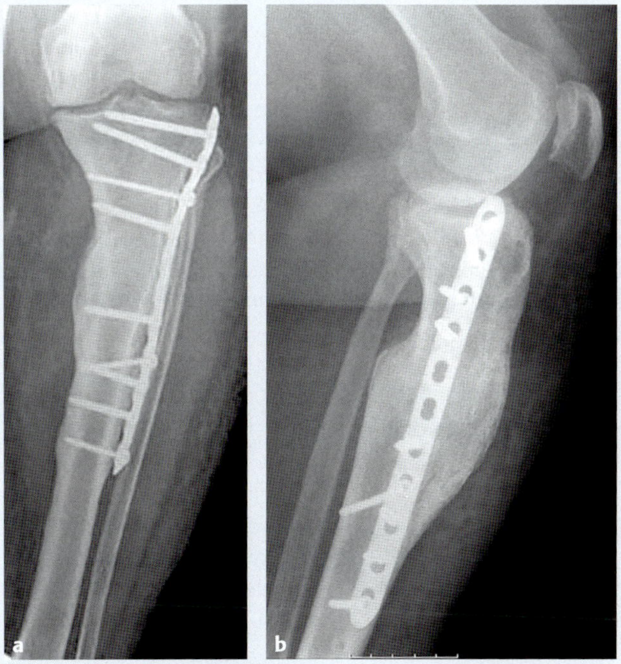

Fig 3.5-20a–b X-rays taken 8 years after the accident.
a AP view showing that the nail has been removed and lateral plate osteosynthesis with cancellous bone grafting performed.
b Lateral x-ray of the knee joint and left lower leg.

Analysis of failure and reflection

The surgical team decided to perform intramedullary nailing to stabilize this fracture. During the nailing procedure, the nondisplaced fracture became displaced and malaligned. Postoperatively, there was almost no contact between the bone fragments. Both fragments were statically interlocked with several screws. Diastasis and malalignment in a highly stable environment led to nonunion. Displacement of the proximal fragment towards anterior and antecurvatum is a typical problem in nailing of proximal tibial fractures. Displacement occurs when the straight nail enters into the medullary canal of the tibia through an eccentric entry portal. When the tip of the nail hits the posterior cortex and glides along this cortex towards distal, a bending force is created on the proximal fragment which leads to displacement (**Fig 3.5-21**). This complication can be avoided by several techniques:

- Flexing the knee joint over 110° prevents conflict between the patella and the pathway for nail insertion.
- Provisionally fixing the fracture with a pointed reduction forceps.
- Fixing the fracture with a lag screw which is inserted outside the medullary canal.
- Inserting a Poller screw from medial to lateral in the proximal fragment anterior to its posterior cortex.
- Performing a suprapatellar nailing with the knee joint in slight flexion.

Final outcome

As was to be expected, the fracture developed into a nonunion. The patient complained of continuous and disabling pain while walking with partial weight bearing. In an attempt to accelerate bone healing, the nail was dynamized by removing both distal screws. Because the fibula was intact, shortening of the tibia with closure of the fracture gap did not occur. After 8 months, the nail was removed and a lateral plate osteosynthesis with a nonangular stable plate and cancellous bone grafting was performed. Due to delayed bone healing, a third reoperation with a second cancellous bone grafting was necessary. Healing eventually occurred after more than 30 months. **Fig 3.5-20** shows x-rays of the left lower leg 8 years after the accident. There was a varus malunion of 20° due to a varus malalignment and leg shortening of 3 cm. The patient refused further surgical interventions.

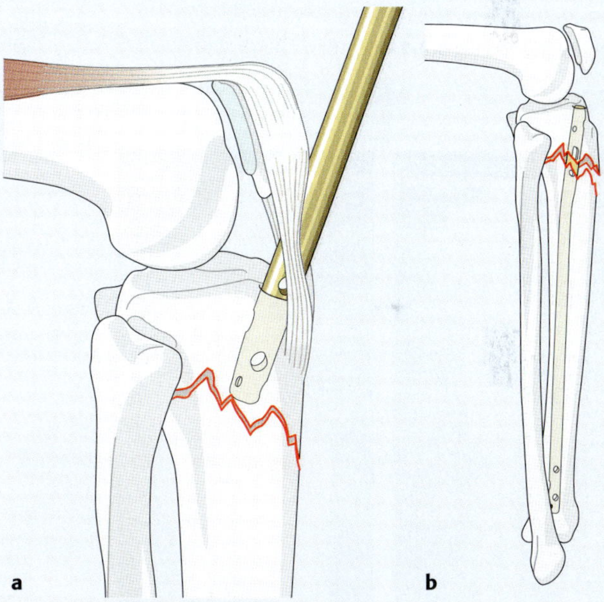

Fig 3.5-21a–b A bending force on the proximal fragment leading to displacement (illustrations adapted from Rommens et al [2015]).
a A straight nail is inserted through an entry portal which is not in line with the axis of the endomedullary canal for stabilizing an oblique nondisplaced proximal metaphyseal tibial fracture.
b Displacement of the proximal fragment towards anterior and in antecurvatum occurs during nail insertion. When the nail tip hits the posterior cortex and glides down along this cortex, a bending force is put on the proximal fragment leading to antecurvatum (apex anterior deformity).

CASE 4

Case description

A 44-year-old man with no significant medical history suffered a sports accident with a twisting injury to his right leg. He presented with a Gustilo type I simple, spiral fracture of the medial-distal third of the tibial diaphysis with an associated proximal fibular fracture (AO/OTA 42A1; Gustilo type I) (**Fig 3.5-22**).

Antibiotic treatment was started and an intervention with proximal and distal reamed and locked intramedullary (IM) nailing was performed 4 days later (**Fig 3.5-23**). The patient was discharged on the third day after surgery with permission to walk with partial weight bearing using crutches. At the outpatient follow-ups, the patient reported pain in the anteromedial compartment of the knee and patellar ligament with pseudo locking upon flexion. At an outpatient check-up 6 months postfracture (**Fig 3.5-24**), the pain persisted at the level of the fracture site and breakage of the distal screws of the nail was detected. The patient also complained of pain upon knee flexion. At subsequent check-ups, consolidation of the fracture and protrusion of the proximal end of the nail under the skin were observed; thus, removal of the nail was proposed 13 months after the intervention (**Fig 3.5-25**).

In the surgical intervention to remove the osteosynthesis material, the proximal screws were completely removed and the distal screws only partially, with the fragments of the screw stems remaining broken in the nail holes. Nail extraction was attempted using intense and continued tapping with the nail extractor and the mallet, which turned out to be futile as the distal fragments of the screw stems were impacted at the level of the fracture callus (**Fig 3.5-26**). The nail was distally impacted and the intervention carried out without successfully extracting the nail (**Fig 3.5-27**). The patient reported persistent knee pain and limitations in performing normal activities of daily living.

One month after the first intervention, another well-planned surgery to extract the osteosynthesis material was performed. The patient was placed in supine decubitus position leaving the limb free. The leg was positioned to permit rotation on a support. A posterointernal surgical approach was made at the level of the distal locking screws for the extraction of the residual fragments through windows made in the tibial cortex (**Fig 3.5-28**). Once the distal fragments of the locking screws were removed, the nail was extracted using the nail extraction tools (**Fig 3.5-29**).

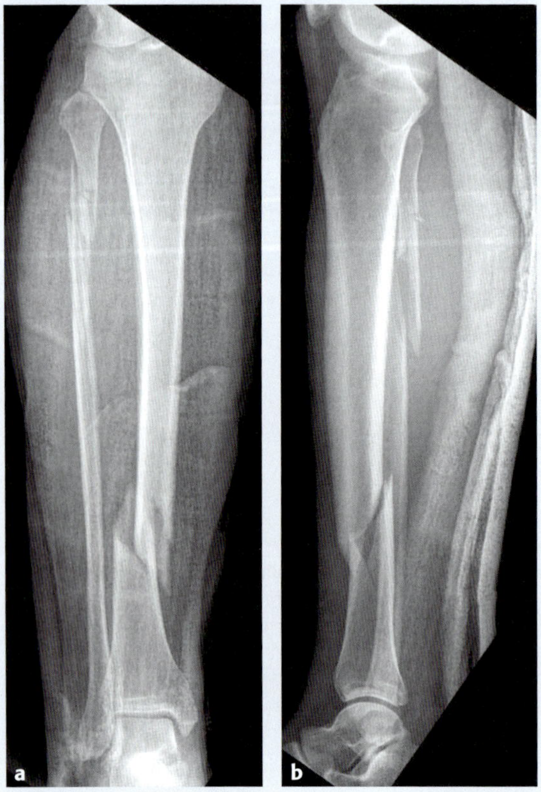

Fig 3.5-22a–b AP (**a**) and lateral (**b**) x-rays of the distal diaphyseal tibial fracture.

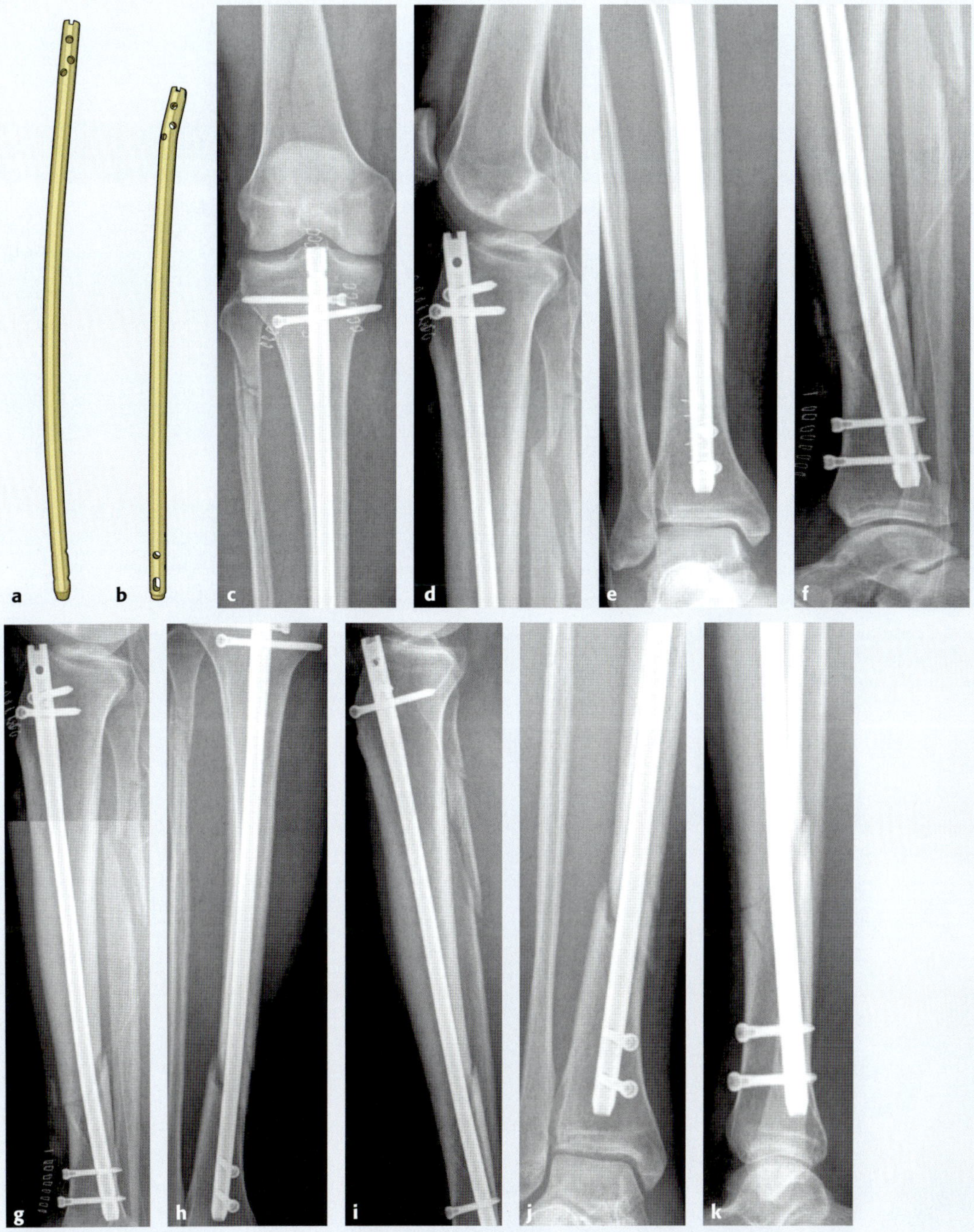

Fig 3.5-23a–k X-rays of the fracture after reamed and locked intramedullary (IM) nailing.

a–b Antegrade IM nail for the femur (**a**) and IM nail for the tibia (**b**). The design and radius of curvature are different, adapted to the shape of each bone.

c–f Immediate postoperative x-rays of the tibial fracture nailing.

g In the lateral view, the design of the nail without the typical proximal curvature of tibial nails can be seen. The uniform curvature of the femoral nail takes its distal part to the rearmost part of the distal tibia which could displace the fracture even further.

h–k Control x-rays 2 months after the intervention.

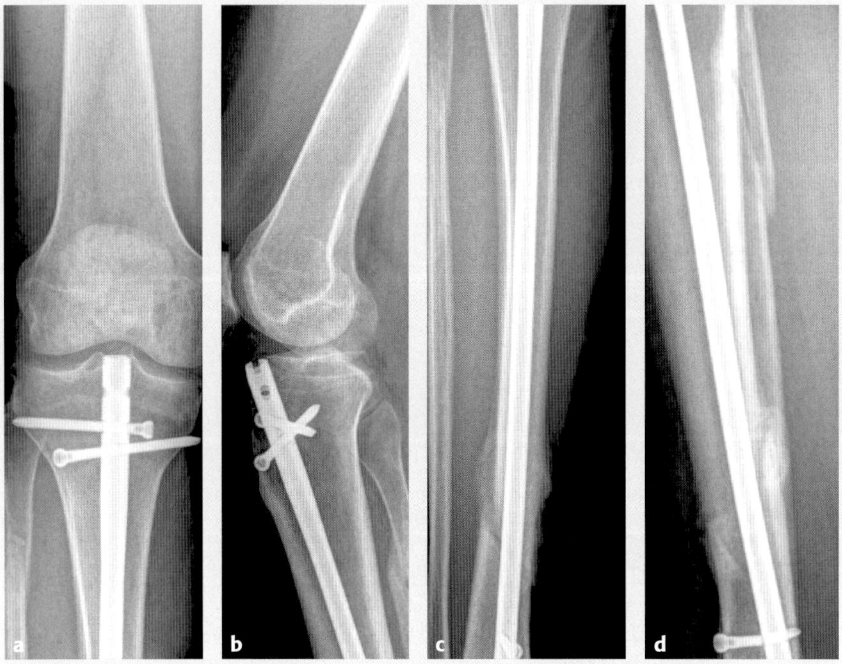

Fig 3.5-24a–d Control x-rays at 6 months after surgery (**a–d**). Breakage of the distal locking bolt (**d**) leads to the collapse and close contact of the main fracture fragments (**c–d**), which facilitates fracture consolidation and the healing process.

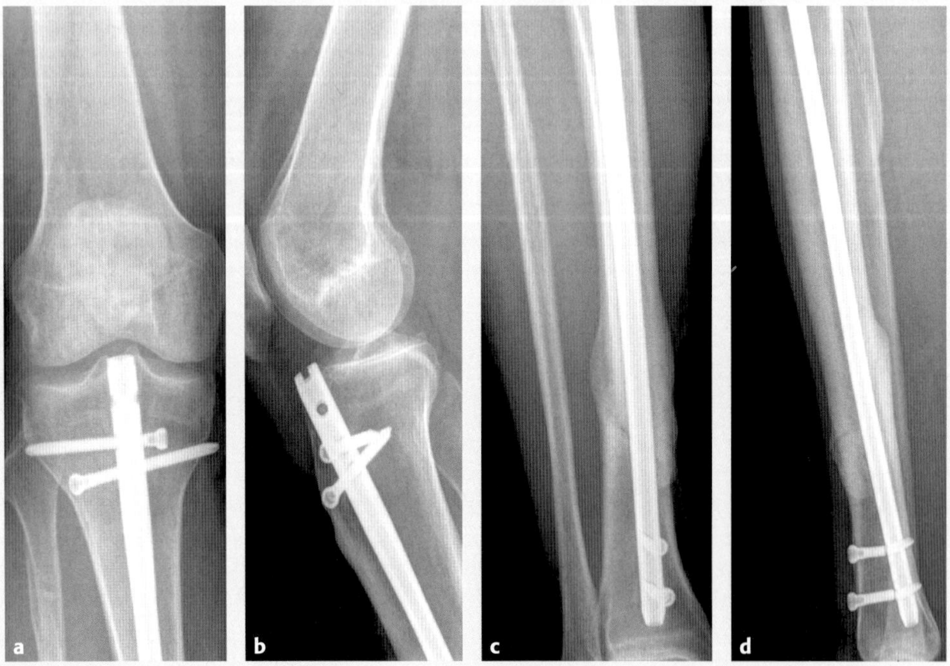

Fig 3.5-25a–d Control x-rays taken 13 months after the intervention (**a–d**). The breakage of the distal screws and the consolidation of the fracture can be seen (**c–d**). The proximal end of the nail protrudes under the skin, causing pain and inflammation in the patellar ligament.

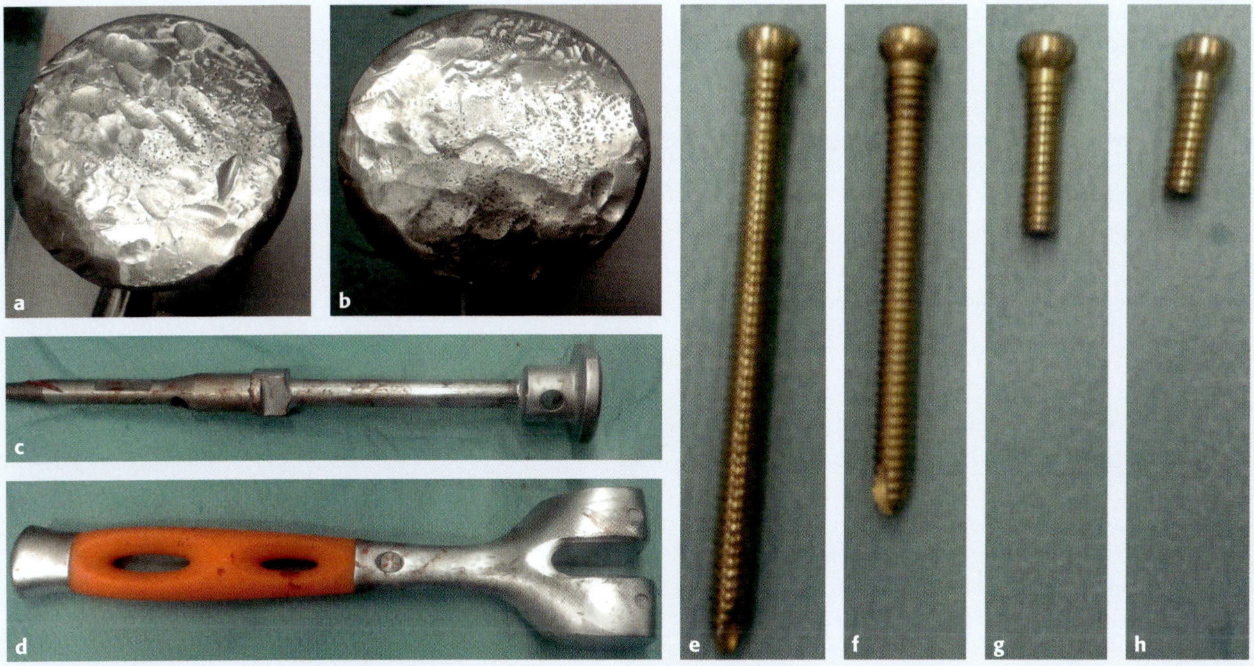

Fig 3.5-26a–h Tools used to extract the nail (**a–d**) and the extracted screws (**e–h**).
a–b Note the dents in the hammer produced by the intensity of the force used.
c Nail extractor.
d Slotted hammer.
e–f Locking screws.
g–h Broken locking screws.

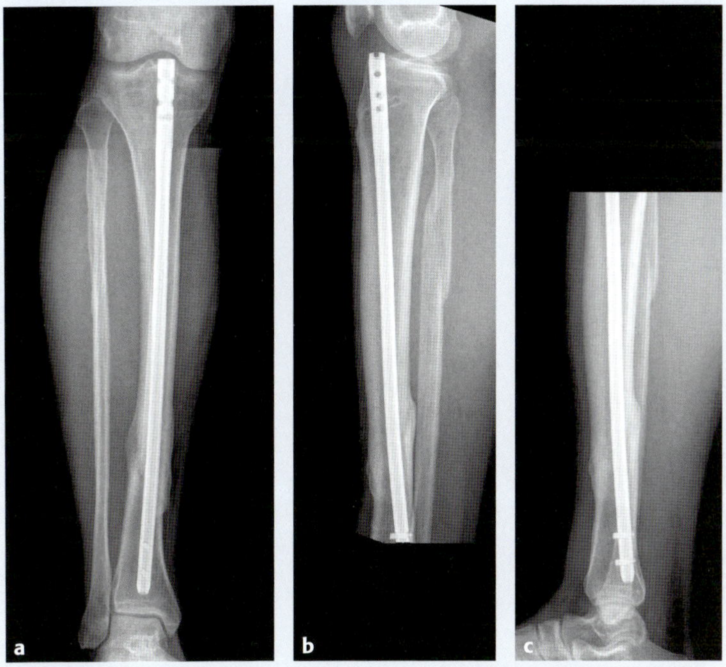

Fig 3.5-27a–c Control x-rays taken in the immediate postoperative period after attempting to extract the intramedullary nail. Note the remnant fragments inside the distal holes of the nail (**b–c**).

Analysis of failure and reflection

A fracture that can be treated by anatomical reduction through careful anatomical access across the soft tissues needs to be done under general conditions of asepsis. By placing the broad fractured surfaces of the collapsed main fragments in contact with each other and compressing them with a lag screw, absolute stability can be obtained and protected by a contoured and prestressed protection plate screwed to the main proximal and distal fragments. The lag screw can be placed through one of the holes in the plate or outside the plate. If perfect reduction and stability are achieved, this leads to consolidation by first intention without a radiographically visible callus.

These shaft fractures can also be treated with a locked IM nail, at least in the distal region where the tibia is wider and the screw does not exercise sufficient hold. Especially the latest generation IM nails allow an approach to the most proximal and distal ends of the diaphysis. Before performing distal fixation with locks, special attention must always be paid to avoiding varus or valgus deformation at the level of the ankle joint, which otherwise would result in bone misalignment.

Nailing allows the patient to walk with weight bearing soon after surgery, but it is also a demanding technique that may become complicated both during nail placement and extraction (when required) as occurred in the present case. First, the wrong nail was used. The intention in this case was to use an IM knee nail indicated for retrograde femoral and antegrade techniques, but the selected nail was for femoral diaphyseal fractures. Unlike the femoral nail, which has a homogeneous curvature that adapts well to the femur, the tibial nail does not have this characteristic and therefore the femoral nail does not easily adapt to the tibia. The biomechanical task is therefore different, and proximal protrusion of the tibial nail may be more likely because of its shape. The position of the distal locking screws is also different from those usually used with a tibial nail. In addition, the implant was not carefully checked when it was unwrapped and before it was inserted; it may have already been damaged as a result of incorrect storage prior to surgery.

The retrograde extraction of a nail with screw fragments trapped in its locking holes may mean that these become impacted into the narrower zone of the fracture site or an IM plug (if it exists). To extract the screw fragments, it may be necessary to open a small window of bone so that under image intensifier control the fragment(s) can be pushed from inside the nail hole or from the opposite cortex to detach from the nail. Using force to extract an impacted nail may cause greater complications, ie, it may become completely stuck causing new fractures, and cause injuries to the soft tissues.

Final outcome

Fortunately, in this case it was decided not to extract the nail by force, which may have led to serious complications.

At the 1-year follow-up visit, the patient presented good postoperative clinical and x-ray evolution, was pain free, and had regained full function (**Fig 3.5-30**).

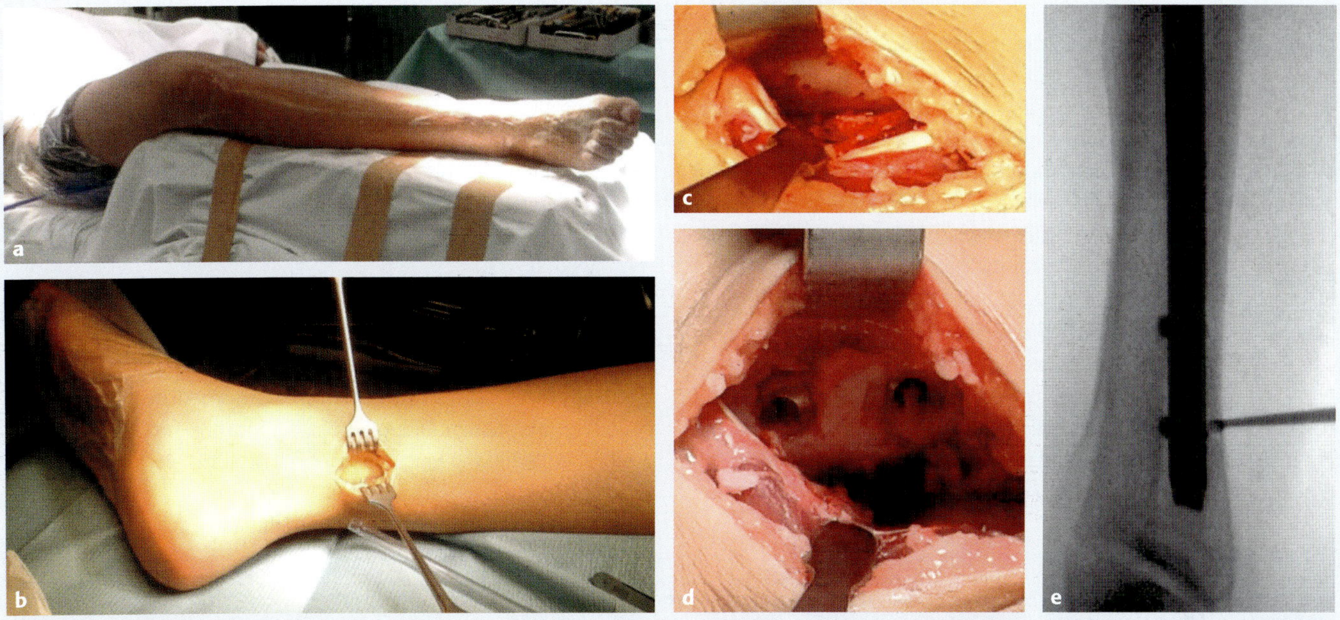

Fig 3.5-28a–e The patient is placed in the supine decubitus position for the reintervention surgery to remove the osteosynthesis material (**a–b**). A lengthwise medial incision is made at the level of the distal tibia and dissection is made layer by layer at the level of the distal screws (**c–d**). Windows are made in the tibial cortex to achieve extraction of the residual locking fragments (**e**).

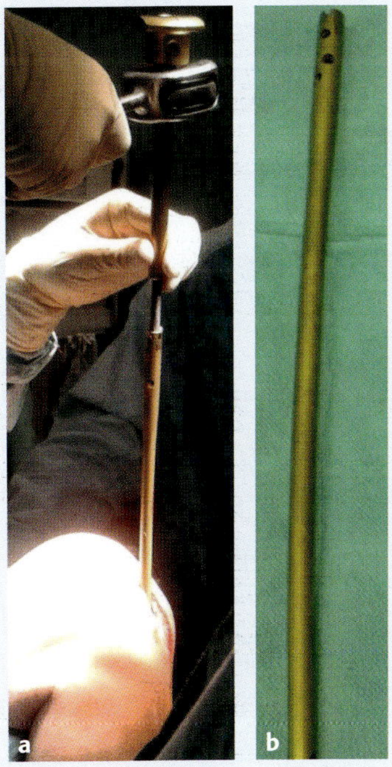

Fig 3.5-29a–b Clinical image shows the extraction of the intramedullary nail done in the usual way and without complications (**a**). Clinical image of the femoral nail extracted from the tibia (**b**).

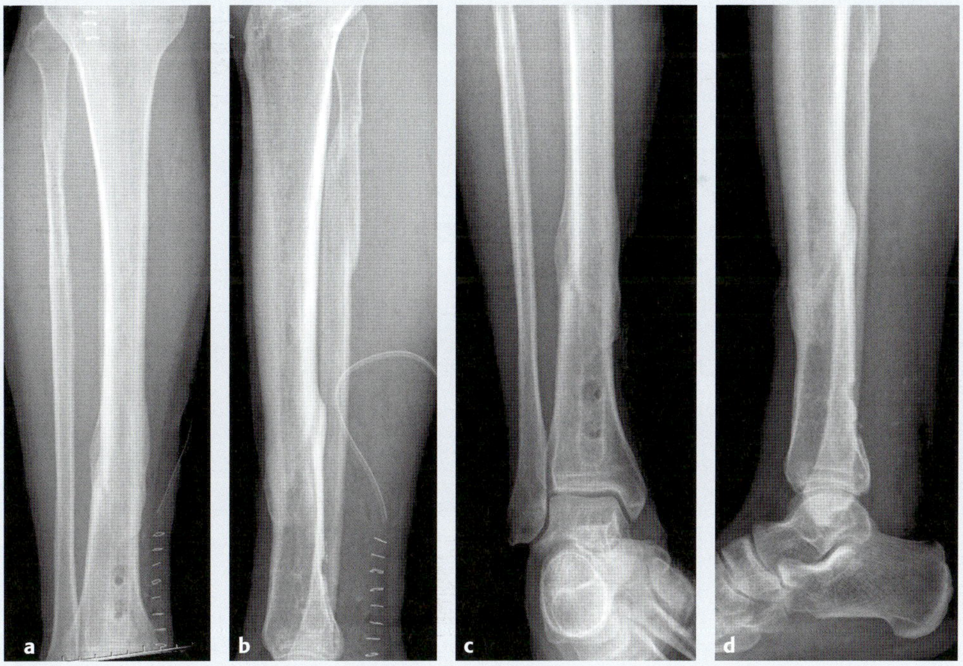

Fig 3.5-30a–d Postoperative (**a–b**) and 1-year follow-up (**c–d**) x-rays.
a–b Postoperative control x-rays in AP (**a**) and lateral (**b**) views.
c–d Control x-rays 1 year after removal of the material in AP (**a**) and lateral (**b**) views.

CASE 5

Case description

A 17-year-old boy had a motorbike accident sustaining a multifragmentary (fragmentary segmental) left femoral fracture (AO/OTA 32C3). Upon arrival at the emergency department, the airway, breathing, circulation, disability, exposure/examination (ABCDE following advanced trauma life support) was fine, but the patient presented with multiple contusions and a fractured left femur (**Fig 3.5-31**). A transosseous traction was applied before taking the patient to the operating room for the first surgery.

Surgery was planned with a helical-shaped lateral femoral nail (LFN), which was a new device in the armamentarium in 2013. The lateral entry into the trochanteric region appears to have facilitated the surgery. Choosing the right entry point can sometimes be difficult, but is essential as the helical design of the LFN can alter the result of the reduction if the entry point is not correct.

In the immediate postoperative period, the patient showed external malrotation of the left leg of more than 30° (**Fig 3.5-32**). The computed tomographic scan revealed an extra external rotation of 36° of the femoral fracture center (**Fig 3.5-33**). The comminution of the trochanteric lateral cortex may have caused a malorientation and an entry point that was too anterior, which could have been the starting point for failure (**Fig 3.5-34**).

Nail removal, correction of the rotational deformity, and renailing were performed. The correct entry point was chosen and a new LFN improved the alignment and the assessment of rotation, achieving symmetry of the lower extremities. In the immediate postoperative period, an assisted mobilization protocol for the hip and knee was established, achieving functional mobility in both joints at the 4-month follow-up control.

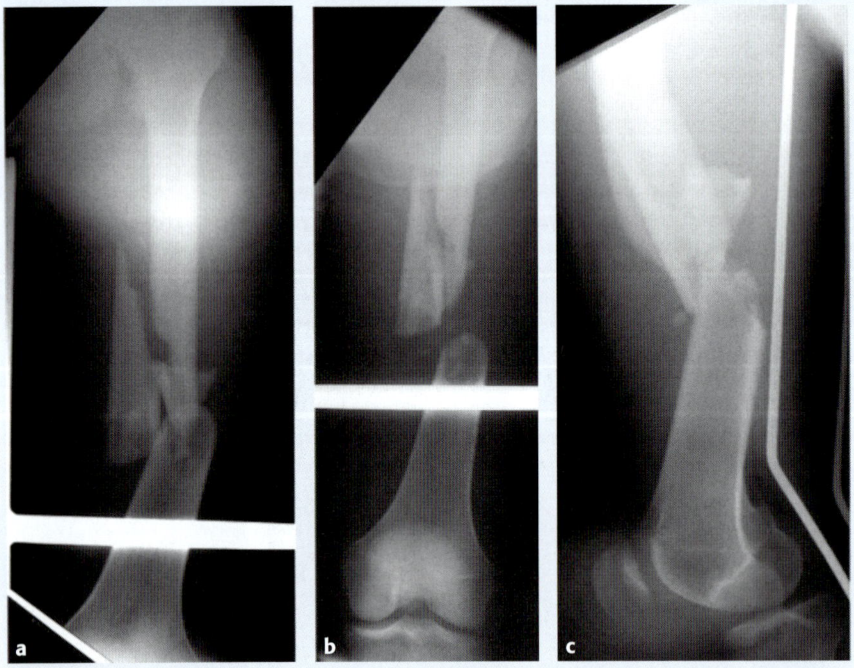

Fig 3.5-31a–c AP (**a**) and posterior (**b–c**) x-rays showing a multifragmentary fracture of the left femur.

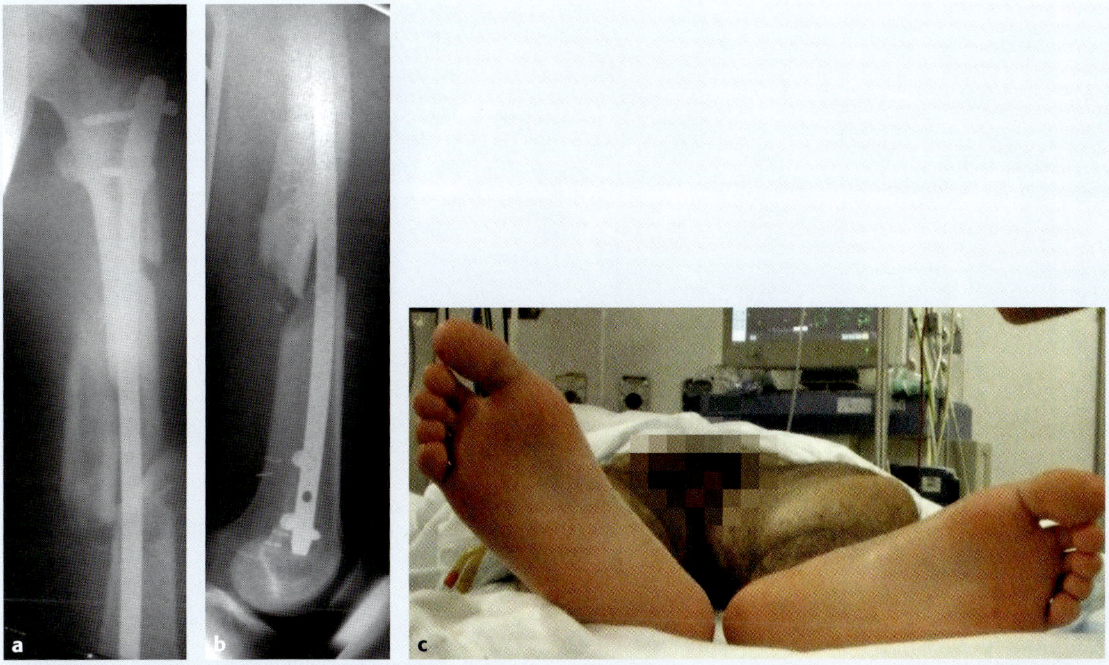

Fig 3.5-32a–c Immediate postoperative x-rays (**a–b**) and clinical photograph (**c**) of the externally malrotated left lower limb.

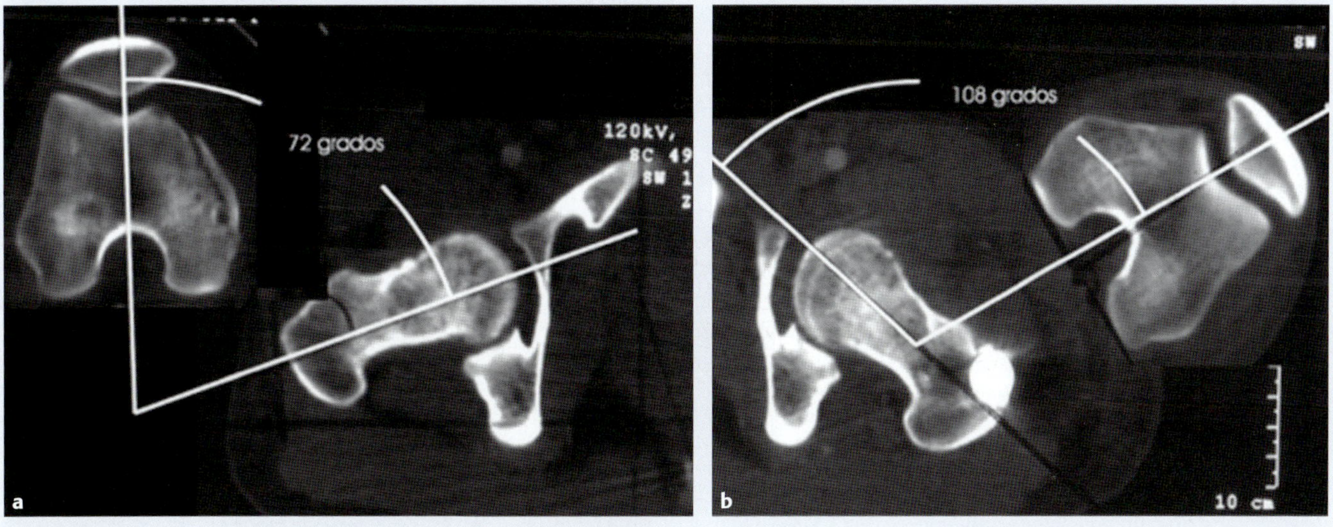

Fig 3.5-33a–b Immediate postoperative computed tomographic scans that show an external malrotated femoral reduction of approximately 36°.

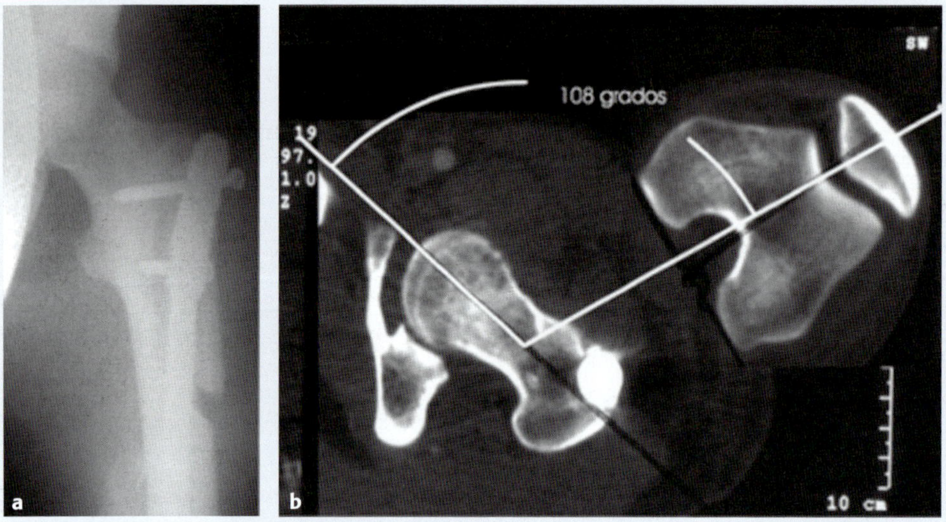

Fig 3.5-34a–b The comminution of the lateral cortex caused an incorrect orientation of the leg and an entry point too anterior.

Analysis of failure and reflection

Selection of the correct entry point in the lateral trochanteric cortex of the proximal fragment and a central position of the intramedullary (IM) nail in the distal fragment are the most important points to avoid malalignment and malrotation.

The development of new IM nails designed for different indications has greatly expanded the spectrum of IM nailing in terms of fracture pattern, fracture location, and concomitant injuries. Each new device has its own technique and its own specific set of tools.

The entry point can be different for each nail and/or brand, and they may also have their own technical tricks. It is mandatory to check the technical guide before using a new device for the first time. Using a new specific device in simple cases first may help the surgeon to improve her or his learning curve. But we must have patience and perhaps have lower expectations during the learning period.

Final outcome

The fracture healed properly after the second surgery with no changes in length, axis, and rotation of the femur and leg (**Fig 3.5-35**). Normal function and activity were recovered within 4 months after the second surgery (**Fig 3.5-36**). The hardware was removed 1 year after the second surgery (**Fig 3.5-37**) and the function of the left lower limb was restored completely, enabling the patient to carry out his sports activities.

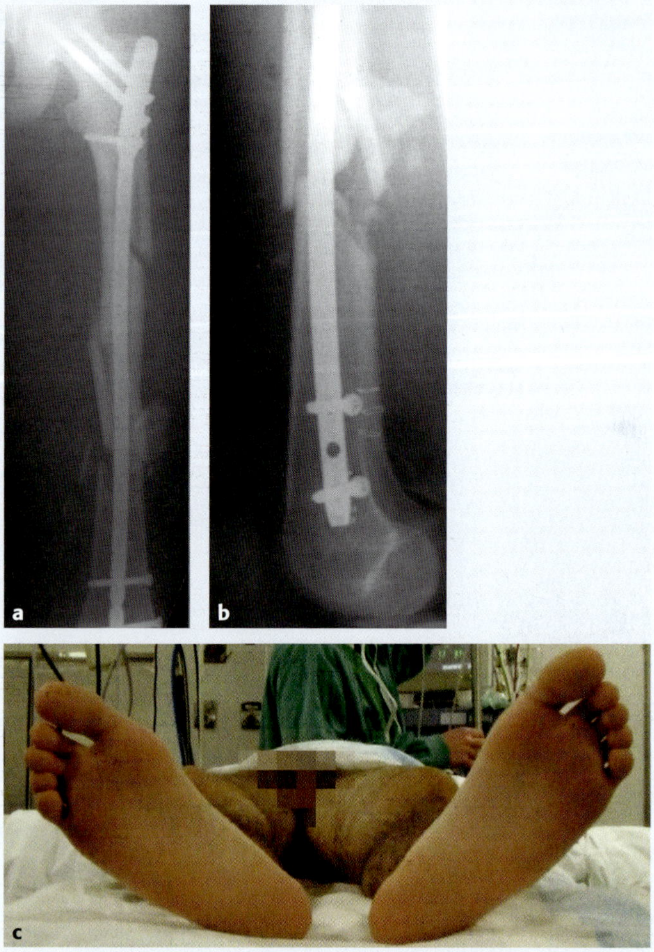

Fig 3.5-35a–c Postoperative x-rays (**a–b**) and clinical photograph (**c**) of the left lower limb after the second surgery where symmetry and rotation were achieved.

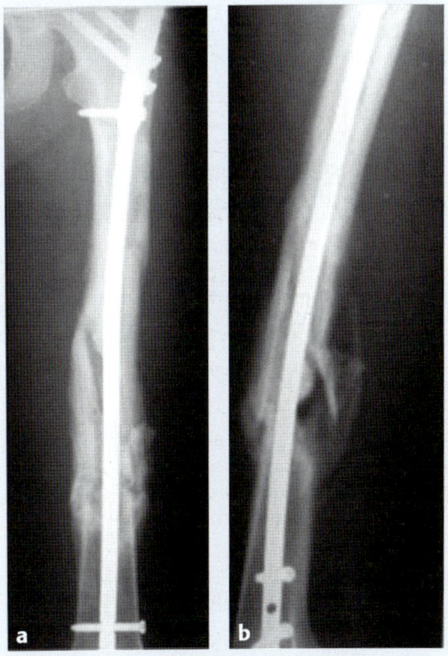

Fig 3.5-36a–b Four-month control x-rays after the second surgery.

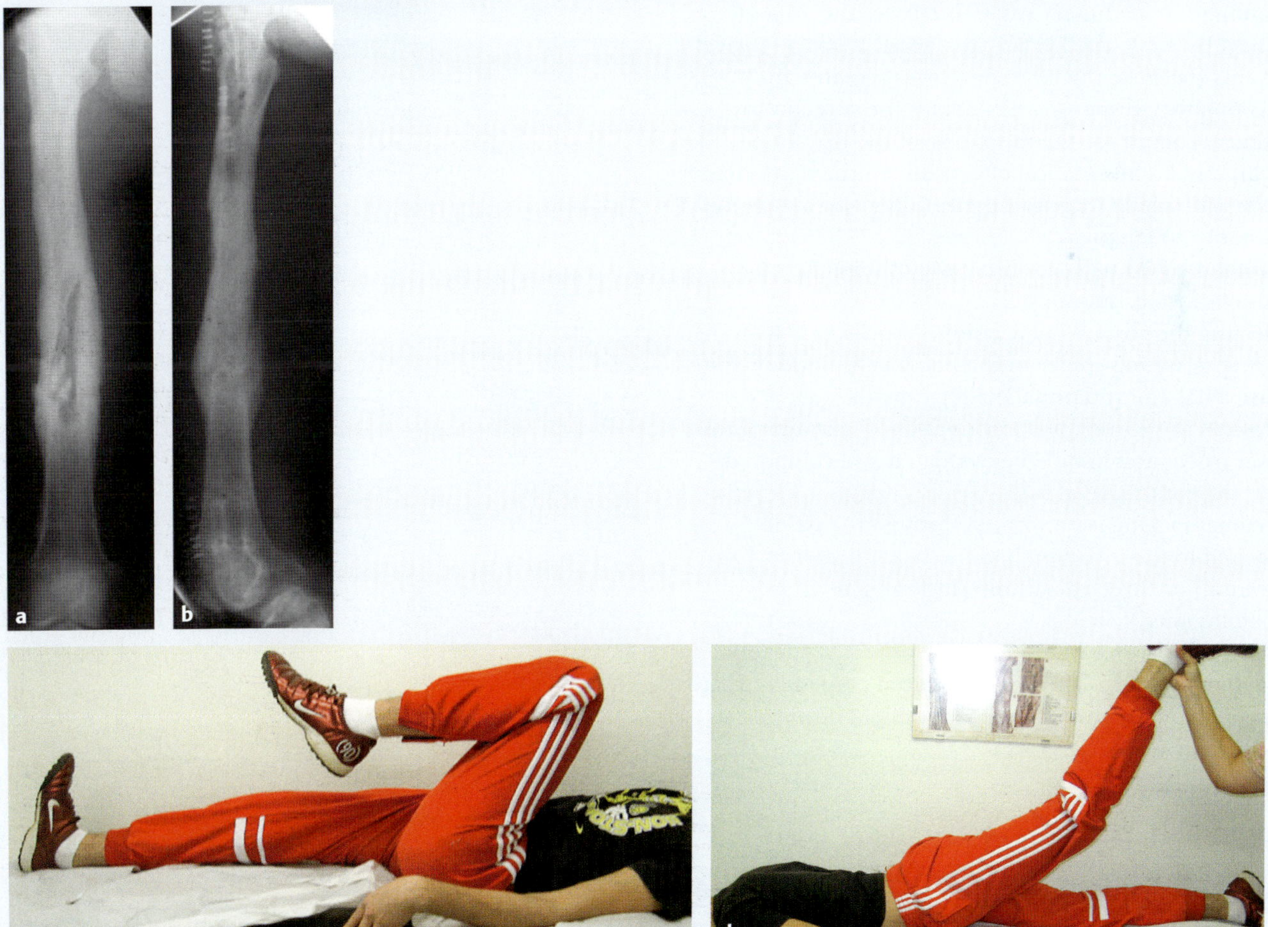

Fig 3.5-37a–d Control x-rays after the nail removal (**a–b**). Clinical photographs of the hip function after removing the nail (**c–d**).

Key points to remember

- Before starting surgery, the surgeon should plan how to obtain fracture reduction. Reducing a fracture before nailing is imperative, because simply inserting an intramedullary nail will never achieve fracture reduction.
- The limits of nailing are related to the fracture location in the shaft and the fracture pattern. In polytrauma patients with severe head or chest trauma, hemorrhagic shock, or a high ISS, ETC with definitive stabilization with nails should not be performed.
- The shape of the medullary canal in the humerus varies from the proximal third to the distal end; the medullary cavity is cylindrical in the proximal third, elliptical in the middle third, and nonexistent in the distal third, where the margins of the humerus are triangular and filled with compact bone.
- Retrograde nailing of the humerus is a much more demanding technique with a high risk of causing supracondylar humeral fractures.
- Reaming the medullary cavity increases the area of contact between the IM nail and bone. It has biological benefits (because the reaming process creates an inflammatory response and enables the surgeon to obtain autograft for the inner side of the diaphyseal canal) and biomechanical effects due to the tightening of the nail which increases the bending and rotational resistance to fatigue.
- If unreamed IM nails are used, they should be small-diameter, solid, and locked.
- Selecting the correct entry point is crucial in IM nailing. A wrong choice of the nail insertion point can cause axial and rotational malalignments.
- To assess the correct femoral rotation, the shape of the lesser trochanter should be evaluated and compared with the contralateral side.
- Proximal locking is performed through the guide attached to the insertion handle. Distally, at least two (femoral) or three (tibial) interlocking screws are recommended.
- Poller screws can be used for alignment, stabilization, and manipulation. The screw is placed perpendicular to the direction in which the implant might displace.

References and suggested reading

Eberle S, Bauer C, Gerber C, et al. The stability of a hip fracture determines the fatigue of an intramedullary nail. *Proc Inst Mech Eng H.* 2010;224(4):577–584.

Hessmann MH. Intramedullary nailing. In: Buckley RE, Moran CG, Apivatthakakul T, eds. *AO Principles of Fracture Management.* 3rd ed. Stuttgart New York: Thieme; 2017:217–240.

Ingrassia T, Mancuso A, Ricotta V. Design of a new tibial intramedullary nail. Paper presented at: Proceedings of the IMProVe 2011. *International conference on Innovative Methods in Product Design;* June 15–17, 2011; Venice.

Krettek C. Intramedullary nailing. In: Rüedi TP, Buckley RE, Moran CG, eds. *Principles of Fracture Management.* 2nd ed. Stuttgart New York: Thieme; 2007:257–284.

Rommens PM, Hessmann MH. Proximal Tibia. In: Rommens PM, Hessmann MH, eds. *Intramedullary Nailing: A Comprehensive Guide.* London: Springer; 2015:331–346.

Tang P, Gates C, Hawes J, et al. Does open reduction increase the chance of infection during intramedullary nailing of closed tibial shaft fractures? *J Orthop Trauma.* 2006 May;20(5):317–322.

3.6 Failures due to guided targeting and implant assembly

Arancha Capel Agúndez, Joan Girós Torres, Roberto Rivero Sosa, J Miquel Sales Pérez, Miquel Videla Cés

Reason does not guide, but our actions decide.
Tim Pethick

Locked implants, especially locking plates, represent a major advancement in fracture care due to the improvement in construct stability [Fernández et al, 2019; Tejwani et al, 2011].

The aiming devices allow percutaneous insertion of screws with less impact on biology. It is assumed that fixed angle locking screws stay locked when inserted correctly under guidance. Locked fixed angle screw implants with angular stability have been developed to improve the pullout strength. These plates provide more secure fixation, especially in weak or osteoporotic bone. The construct loses strength when the locking head thread is not firmly screwed into the threaded plate hole, provoking screw loosening both from the plate and bone. This could affect the quality of the fracture reduction and lead to failure [Clavert et al, 2010].

Many implants, especially intramedullary (IM) nails, need to be inserted into the bone using a guide wire aiming device to which they should be firmly and correctly connected (**Fig 3.6-1a–b**). These guiding devices must be carefully manipulated. Strong pressure on or hammering in the weak zones of the insertion handle should be avoided, as this can deform the aiming device and affect the guided insertion of the screws or blades. If necessary, the hammering connector can be placed on the insertion handle and light hammer blows can be used on the connector to help insert the nail.

In the case of trochanteric nails, the guide wire aiming device also helps surgeons to properly position and insert the screws into the femoral head and neck area. With the short trochanteric nails, the insertion of the distal locking bolts is guided, either statically or dynamically, using the same aiming device used as insertion handle. Deformation in the handle or insufficient tightening of this device could lead to a failure between the bolt and the shaft of the nail [Pardiwala et al, 2001]. Surgeons should ensure that the connection between the trochanteric IM nail and the insertion handle is tight. From time to time during surgery it may be necessary to retighten it to avoid deviations when inserting the screw through the aiming arm.

When using guided implants (nails or plates), there is a learning curve for fracture reduction and implant insertion, as with any device or technique. When percutaneous techniques are used, fracture reduction can be more challenging than with traditional open surgical procedures. Choosing an assembled and tightened construction is not justification for improper reduction of the fracture.

An implant should always be inserted in an already reduced fracture, but we cannot expect that the implant itself can improve a poor reduction.

It is recommended to carefully check that all components are correctly placed and properly tightened. It is also necessary to clarify that the result correlates with the surgeon's preoperative planning: that the location of the implants inside the bone is correct and that the intraoperative C-arm controls do not show any bone deformation. Visualizing a supposed good fracture reduction and a correct implant placement in only one radiographical plane is insufficient; it is mandatory to check that a good result is achieved in all views before wound closure.

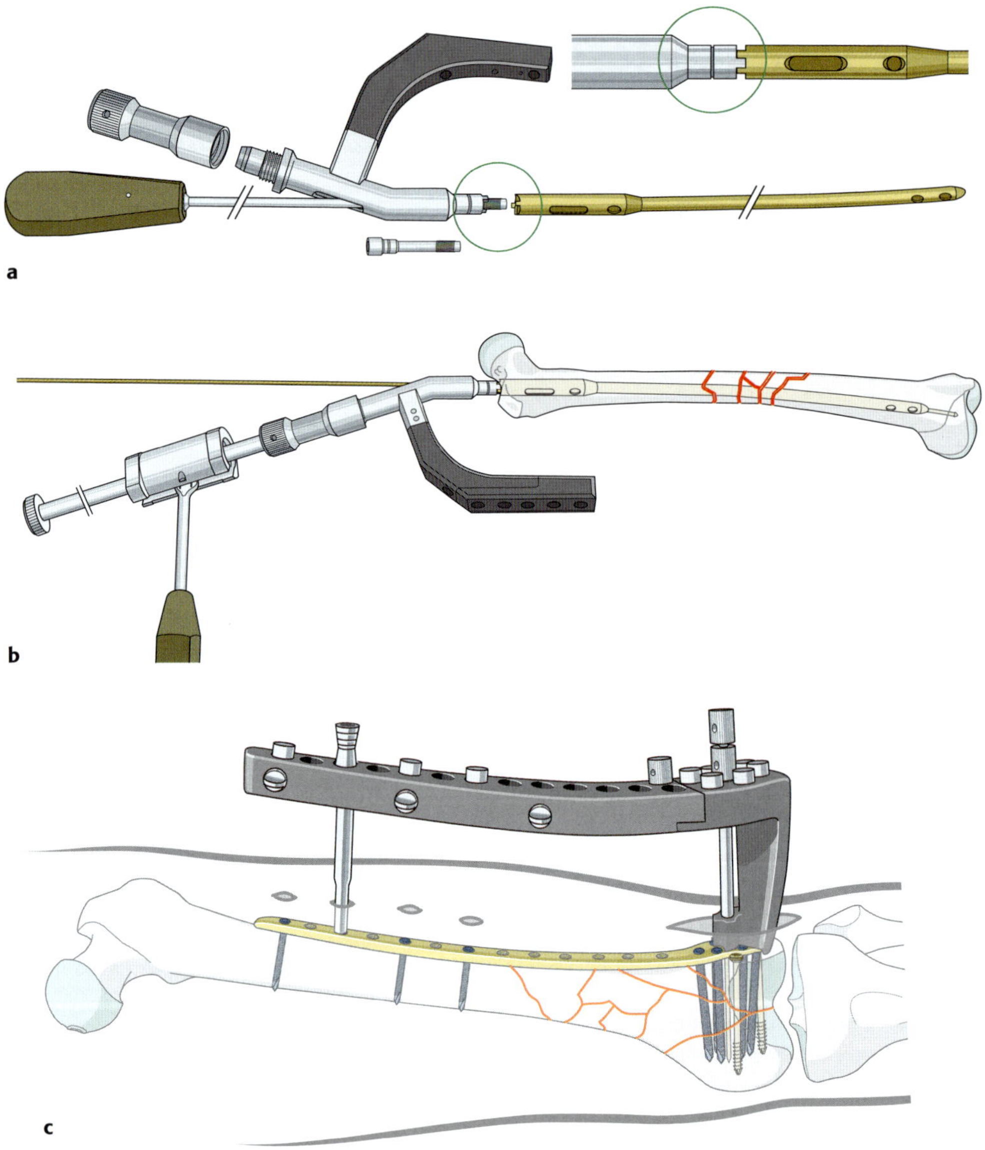

Fig 3.6-1a–c Assembly of implant and guide wire aiming device.

Case description

An 85-year-old woman fell from standing height while walking down the street. Her airway, breathing, and circulation (according to the ABC of advanced trauma life support) were satisfactory; however, she suffered from hypertension. She sustained a right supracondylar fracture (AO/OTA 33A3) (**Fig 3.6-2**). A minimally invasive plate osteosynthesis (MIPO) with a long splinting less invasive stabilization system-distal femur (LISS DF) was planned.

Surgery was performed with the patient in a supine position, the knee was free and with a moderate flexion. Three windows were made for the surgical approach. The plate was pushed with the insertion guide and was slipped submuscularly from distal to proximal. The collinear clamp was used to temporarily attach the plate onto the bone. Finally, the locked distal screws were screwed with the screwdriver attached to the power tool. They were not manually tightened with the torque-limiting screwdriver as is recommended, because the surgeon thought that cold fusion would not occur with steel.

In the postoperative control x-rays, the fracture showed a correct axis but with a medial displacement of the joint fragment. The most distal screws were parallel to the joint surface. Distally, the location of the LISS DF plate seems to be fixed too anterior in the epiphysis (**Fig 3.6-3**). In the immediate postoperative period, the affected limb remained unloaded with active mobilization of the hip and knee.

The patient was discharged from hospital and transferred to a nursing home 5 days after surgery. The 6-week control x-rays showed a loss of reduction with mobilization and migration of the distal locking screws with loss of distal anchorage (**Fig 3.6-4**).

The open salvage surgery consisted in the removal of the LISS DF plate, decortication of the fracture ends, cancellous autograft, and a new internal fixation with lag screws of the articular fragments and a long dynamic condylar screw (DCS) plate (**Fig 3.6-5**).

In the postoperative period, the affected limb remained unloaded for 6 more weeks with a protocol of active and assisted mobilization of the hip and knee. She was allowed to walk with a walker in week 7. The x-ray follow-up control at 3 months showed evidence of callus at the level of the fracture site without screw loosening (**Fig 3.6-6**).

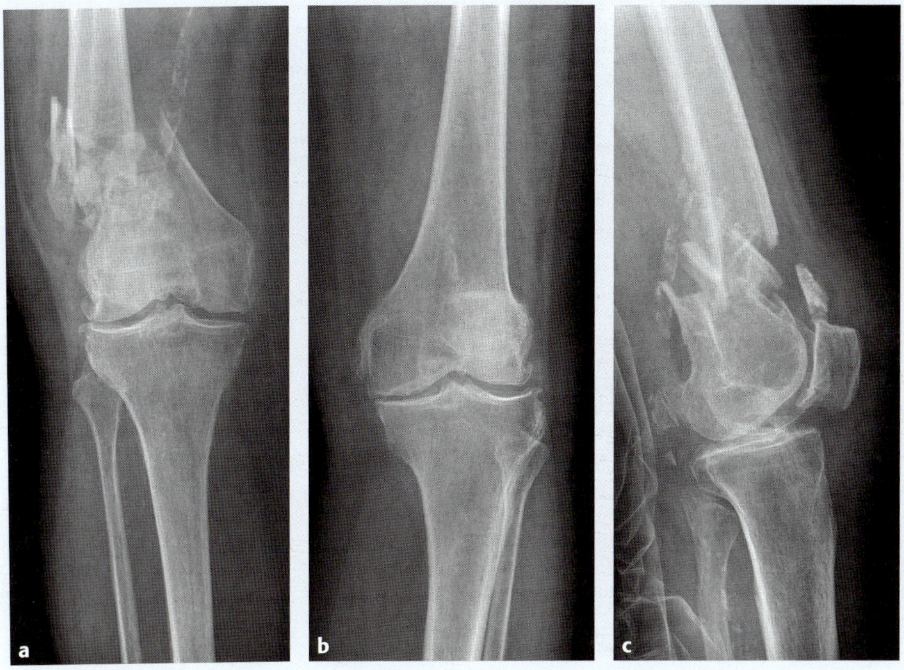

Fig 3.6-2a–c X-rays showing a supracondylar right femoral fracture.

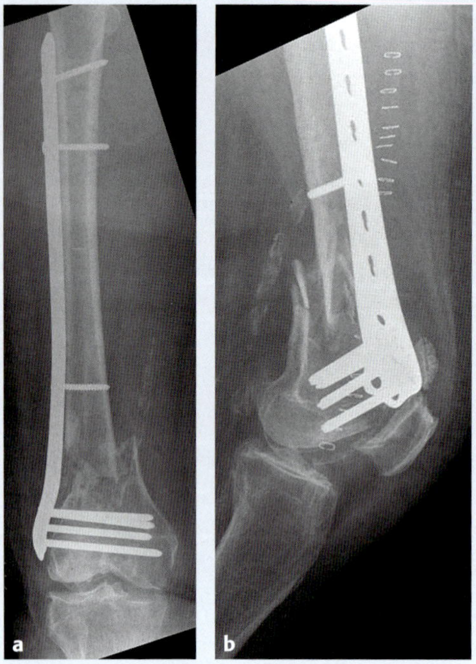

Fig 3.6-3a–b Postoperative x-rays showing a correct axis but with a medial displacement of the joint fragment. The most distal screws were parallel to the joint surface. Note that distally, the location of the less invasive stabilization system-distal femoral plate seems to be fixed too anterior in the epiphysis.

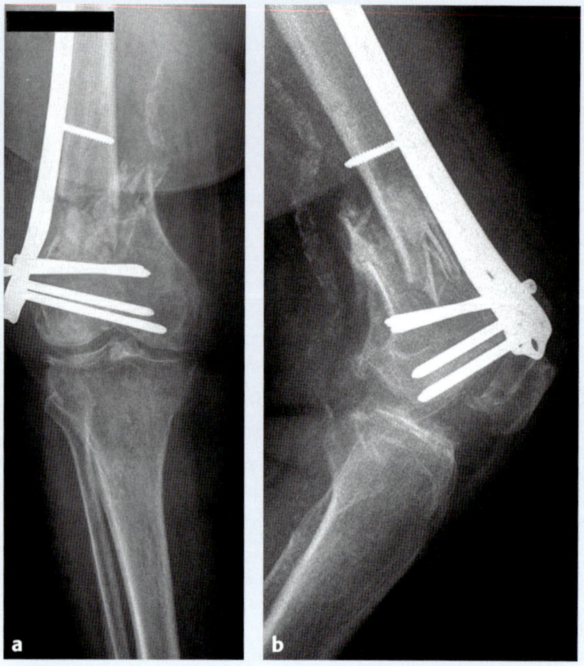

Fig 3.6-4a–b The 6-week control x-rays show a loss of reduction with mobilization and migration of the distal locking screws with loss of distal anchorage.

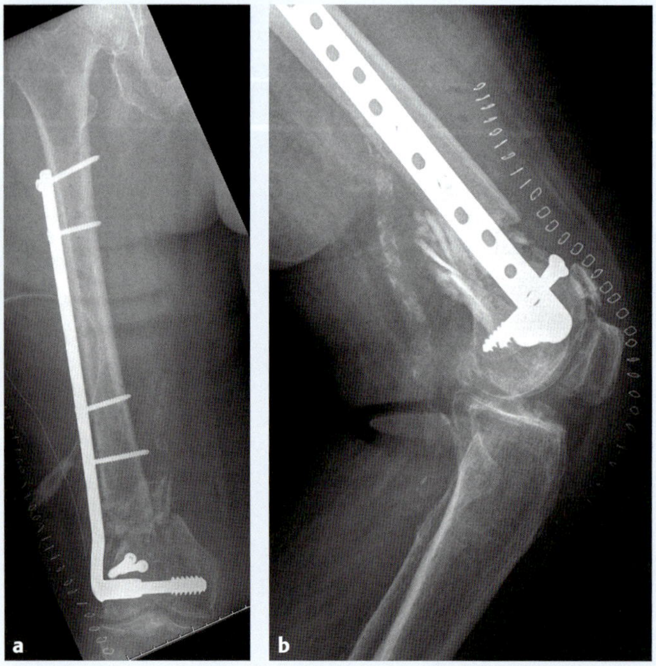

Fig 3.6-5a–b X-rays of the salvage operation showing removal of the less invasive stabilization system-distal femoral plate, decortication of the fracture ends, cancellous autograft, and a new internal fixation with lag screws of the articular fragments and a long dynamic condylar screw plate.

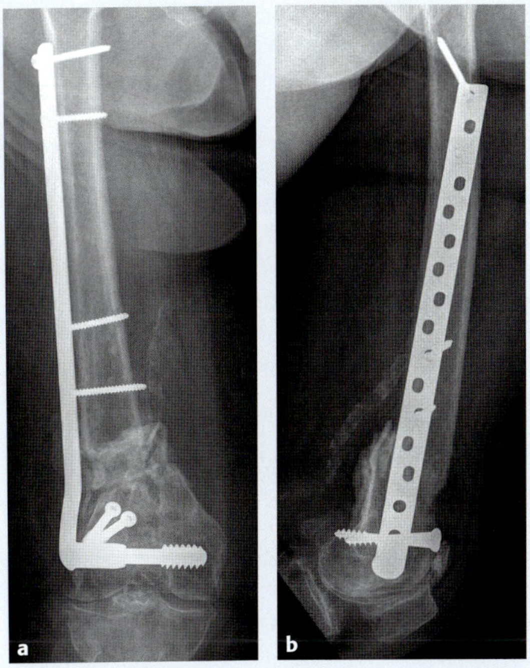

Fig 3.6-6a–b Control x-rays at the 3-month follow-up show evidence of callus at the level of the fracture site without screw loosening.

Analysis of failure and reflection

Although the alignment of the fracture after the first surgery was acceptable, the medial displacement of the joint segment caused the reduction to be suboptimal. Prior to the insertion of the guided implant, the surgeon should have checked that the drill sleeves match the guided aiming device and the threaded holes of the plate. This should be verified with the C-arm to obtain accurate and true AP and lateral views of the knee, which is mandatory before starting the surgery.

The correct way to insert the locking screw using a power tool is to fit a torque limiter to the power tool and insert the screwdriver shaft into the torque limiter. Insert the locking screw into the plate hole through the drill sleeve for LISS DF insertion guide. To insert the screw, start the power tool slowly, increase the speed and then reduce it again before the screw is fully tightened. Tighten the screw manually with the torque-limiting screwdriver. The optimum torque is reached after one click **[Egol et al, 2004]**.

It is advisable to perform the three-dimensional (AP and lateral or axial views) control before the end of the surgery and try to correct any visible problems. The location of the LISS DF plate in the most anterior third of the distal femur can cause protrusion and irritation at the level of the iliotibial band, so it is important to maintain the plate flat up against the cortex to ensure an optimal fit against the bone.

The elderly are physically unable to walk with partial weight bearing; therefore, when they walk they put the full weight on the leg. When there is not enough fracture callus, the implant has to bear the full weight, which can lead to metal implant fatigue and failure. No weight bearing for several weeks causes severe sarcopenia with inability to walk, which decreases these patients' quality of life.

The key to success is related to the surgeon's compliance with the principles of internal fixation and ability to accurately follow the steps of the technique. It can be helpful to make a checklist of the different mechanical steps required, especially when insertion handles should be used.

Final outcome

The fracture healed and the patient recovered the ability to walk with a walker. She is almost pain free and recovered sufficient functionality to return home, but she lost quality of life for the first 6 months after the fracture.

CASE 2

Case description

An 83-year-old woman fell from standing height at the home she shared with one of her daughters. Her airway, breathing, and circulation were satisfactory (according to the ABC of advanced trauma life support). She had comorbidities of hypertension, hearing loss, and chronic anemia. The patient sustained a right pertrochanteric fracture (AO/OTA 31A1) (**Fig 3.6-7**).

A trochanteric proximal femoral nail antirotation (PFNA) was planned (130°, 170 mm long, 10 mm diameter with static locking screw). The surgical team did not check the connections between nail and insertion handle and the surgeon tried to place a 130° PFNA with the aiming device for 125° PFNA . Once they realized the mistake, the nail was removed and the correct 130° aiming device was attached. However, the operating room personal and the surgeon did not tighten the connections between nail and insertion handle, which remained unlocked and incorrectly aligned. This resulted in the surgeon being unaware that the locking screw was placed outside the locking hole. Unusually, the tip of the nail is supported on the medial wall and the locking screw seems to be inserted into the nail through the distal locking hole in the intraoperative C-arm view (one plane), but it was a misleading image (similar to a false negative or a false positive), which may have led the surgeon to make the mistake (**Fig 3.6-8**). The postoperative control x-rays in AP and axial views showed a loss of fracture reduction and that the locking screw was not inserted through the locking hole of the nail. Instead it was located proximal and posterior in the proximal femoral shaft. Importantly, the leg showed a shortening and an external rotation deformity, and the patient was unable to stand or even sit without hip pain (**Fig 3.6-9**).

Due to operating room availability and in order to reverse the effect of enoxaparin, the rescue surgery was performed 2 days after the first internal fixation. For many anesthetists in many countries, coagulation monitoring is essential to perform surgery. In the rescue surgery a fracture occurred in the lateral cortex of the most proximal third of the femoral shaft, so a cerclage wire was used before nailing.

Reoperation was performed under C-arm control. Tips and tricks were necessary to help the reduction. The hook helped to close the reduction of the femoral neck and the cerclage wire was used to fix the lateral wall fracture that could not be seen in the first fracture (**Fig 3.6-10**).

The planned surgical steps were: first to remove the implant with the patient placed on a radiolucent surgical table and second, on a traction table, to achieve rereduction and renailing with cement augmentation. A 125° PFNA (240 mm long, 10 mm diameter) with dynamic locking screw was chosen and correctly used with the appropriate aiming device. The surgical team checked that the sleeves matched the guided insertion handle of the nail. During the replacement of the nail, a fracture occurred in the lateral cortex of the most proximal third of the femoral shaft, so a cerclage wire was used to reduce this fracture before nailing (**Fig 3.6-10** and **Fig 3.6-11**). Cement augmentation was used to fill the neck and head defect of the femur.

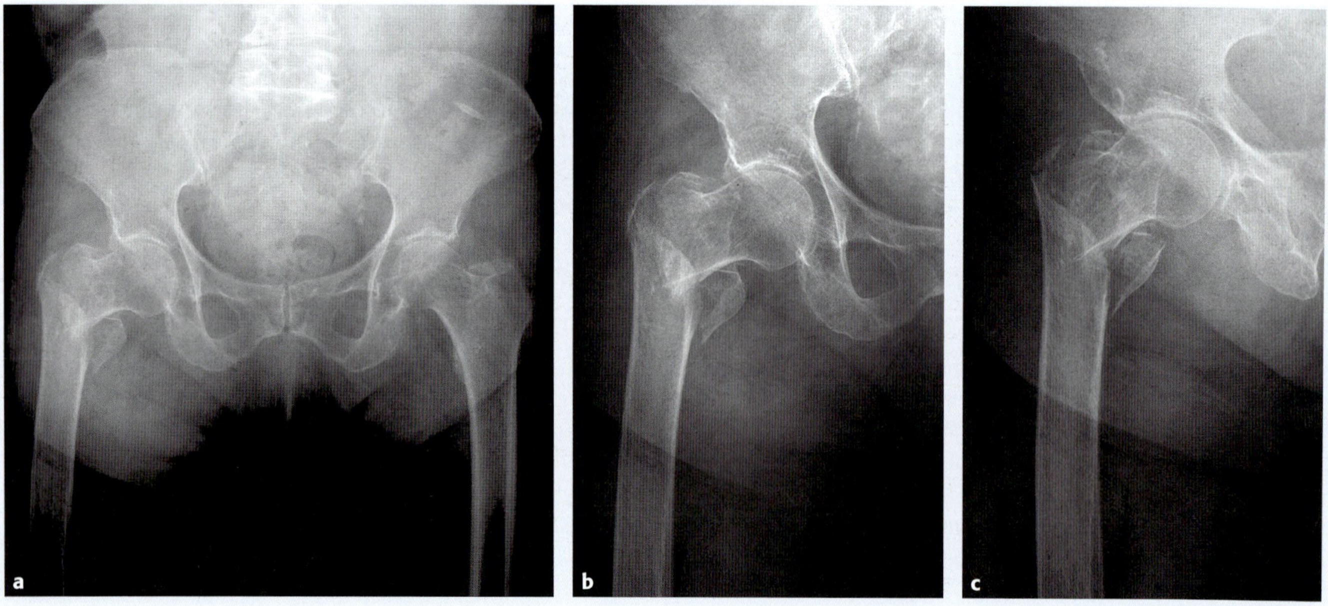

Fig 3.6-7a–c X-rays showing a pertrochanteric right femoral fracture (**a–b**) and axial view of the pelvis (**c**).

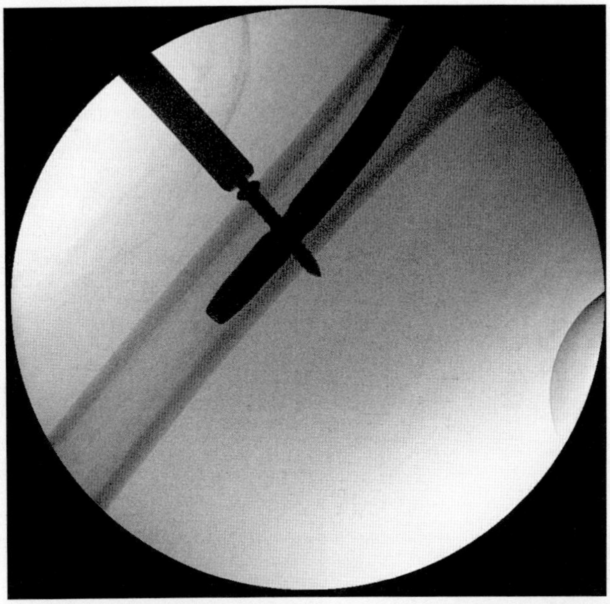

Fig 3.6-8 C-arm view from the first surgery: Unusually, the tip of the nail is supported on the medial wall and the locking screw seems to be linked to the nail through the distal locking hole, but this is a "false" image, which may have led the surgeon to make the mistake.

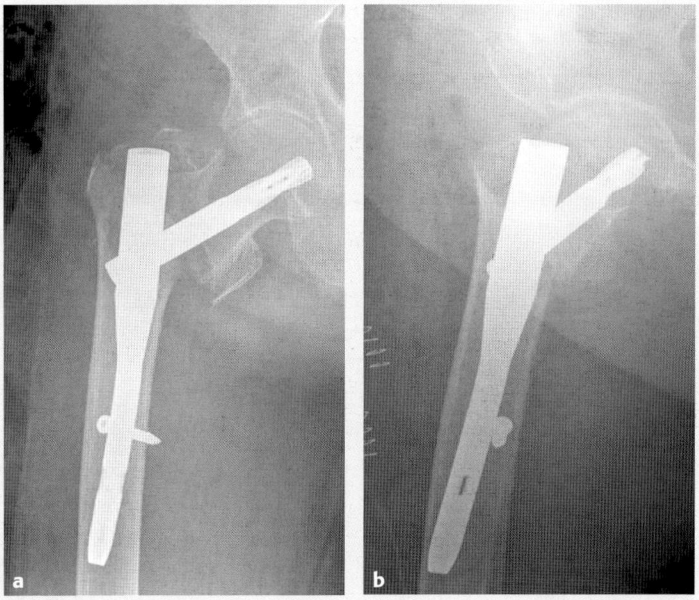

Fig 3.6-9a–b Postoperative x-rays showing loss of reduction. The locking screw was outside the locking hole of the nail, it was located proximal and posterior in the proximal femoral shaft. The leg showed a shortening and an external rotation deformity.

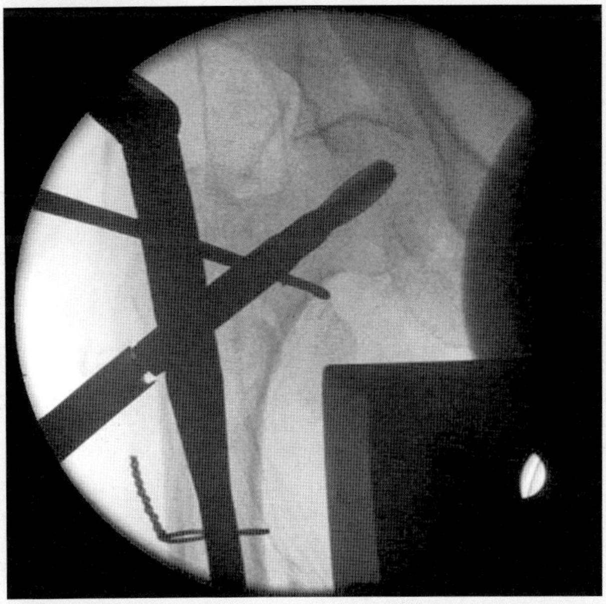

Fig 3.6-10 C-arm view of the reoperation. The hook helped to close the reduction of the femoral neck and the cerclage wire was used to fix the lateral wall fracture, which was not visible in the first fracture.

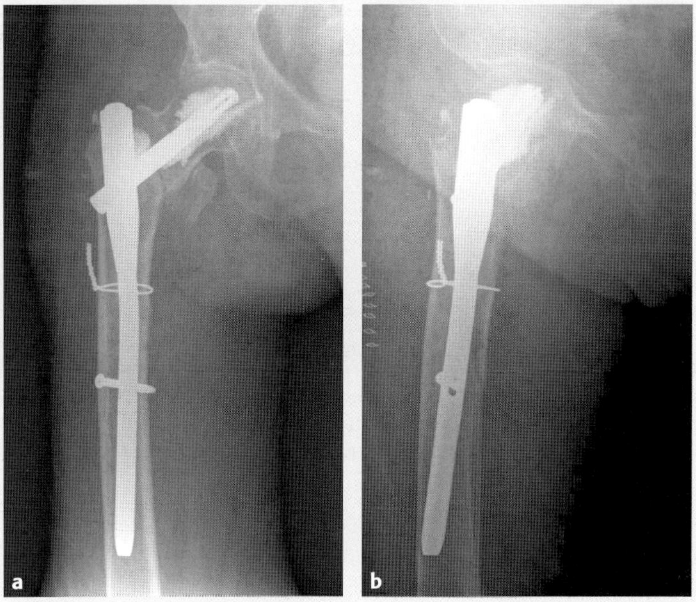

Fig 3.6-11a–b X-rays of the rescue surgery. Removal of the previous implant and renailing with polymethylmethacrylate cement augmentation of the femoral head was planned. A cerclage wire was used before nailing to hold the new fracture.

Analysis of failure and reflection

The reduction of the fracture was considered suboptimal and the locking screw not inserted through the nail. This caused a malreduction with an unstable situation, probably due to an incorrect assembly of the nail to the insertion handle. The mistake in choosing the incorrect aiming device is not uncommon. To avoid this error, a checklist must be made and followed to verify that the implant chosen in the planning corresponds to the correct insertion handle.

It is mandatory to check the connections between nail and insertion handle. Before insertion of the guided implant, it must be checked that the drill sleeves match the guided aiming device and the holes of the nail. Before starting surgery, the surgeon must use the C-arm to check for true AP and lateral views.

In the small and medium trochanteric nails, the insertion of the locking screw is guided using the correct aiming device connected to the insertion handle. The decision between static or dynamic distal locking lies in the morphology and primary stability of the fracture. It is advisable to perform the three-dimensional control x-rays (in AP and lateral or axial views) before the end of the surgery and try to correct the possible problems.

Final outcome

The fracture healed and the patient recovered the ability to walk with crutches. She recovered sufficient functionality, but she lost some quality of life in the first year after the fracture (**Fig 3.6-12**).

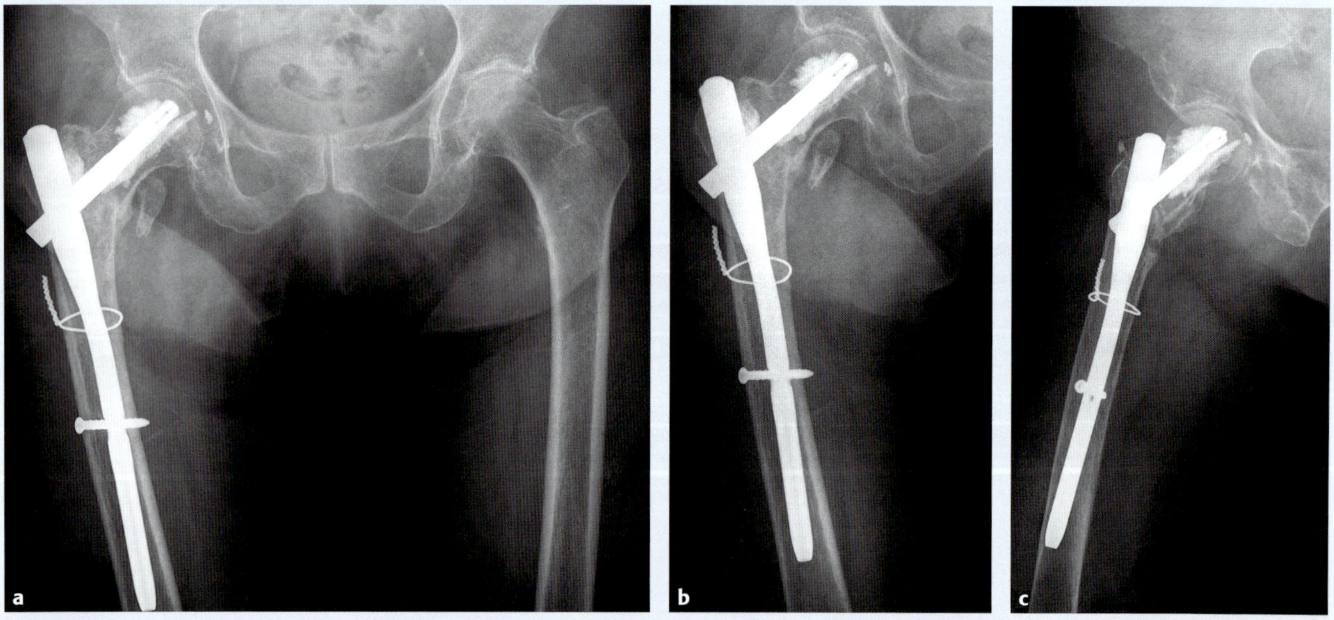

Fig 3.6-12a–c Six-month follow-up control x-rays. Both the AP (**b**) and axial (**c**) views show a correct consolidation of the fracture, for both the subtrochanteric lateral cortex and pertrochanteric fractures. The view of the pelvis (**a**) shows no shortening of the right leg. The proximal femoral nail antirotation spiral blade remains in place without loosening, migration or interface between the cement and the bone, or between the cement and the implant.

Case description

A 46-year-old man sustained an unstable subtrochanteric fracture of the right femur after a fall from a 2 m high staircase (AO/OTA 31A3) (**Fig 3.6-13**). The patient, who was 174 cm tall and weighed 105 kg, suffered from obesity, but otherwise had no comorbidities. He was initially treated with trochanteric nails. After 4 months the patient complained about pain in the left hip so hip prosthesis was performed subsequently.

Unstable proximal femoral fractures are best treated with trochanteric intramedullary (IM) nails, because they give better mechanical support than extramedullary implants. In low and extended subtrochanteric fractures the use of long trochanteric nails is indicated.

Trochanteric IM nailing was chosen as surgical treatment with long proximal femoral nails. Mechanically, they provide better support to the bending forces on the medial side of the subtrochanteric area.

The postoperative x-rays obtained at 1 week (**Fig 3.6-14**) and at 1 month (**Fig 3.6-15**) show a proper evolution of the healing process.

At the 4-month follow-up, the patient complained about pain in the trochanteric region of the left hip. Owing to gluteal insufficiency he walked with a Trendelenburg limp and needed a cane for support.

The hip had full range of motion, but the patient suffered from pain and muscular atrophy in his thigh (**Fig 3.6-16**).

The 4-month postoperative axial view of the proximal femur (**Fig 3.6-15e–f**) showed that the femoral neck screw was located posteriorly and outside the proximal end of the nail and that the proximal hole in the nail was empty. Both findings indicated that the femoral neck screw and the hip pin were misplaced and not connected to the nail.

Review of the postoperative x-rays taken 1 week after surgery (**Fig 3.6-17a–b**) showed a deficiency of implant assembly:

- Proximal screw placement was not parallel in the AP view (**Fig 3.6-15a** and **Fig 3.6-17a**).
- Screws were located outside the nail holes, which is evident in the axial view (**Fig 3.6-15b** and **Fig 3.6-17b**).

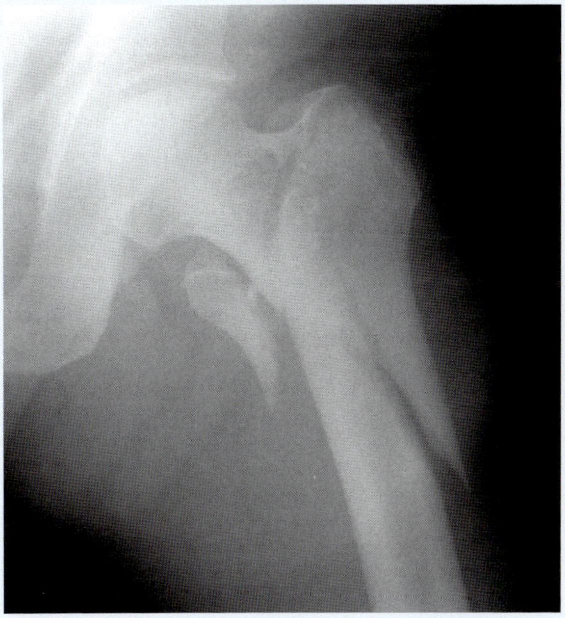

Fig 3.6-13 Preoperative x-ray shows a subtrochanteric fracture of the left femur.

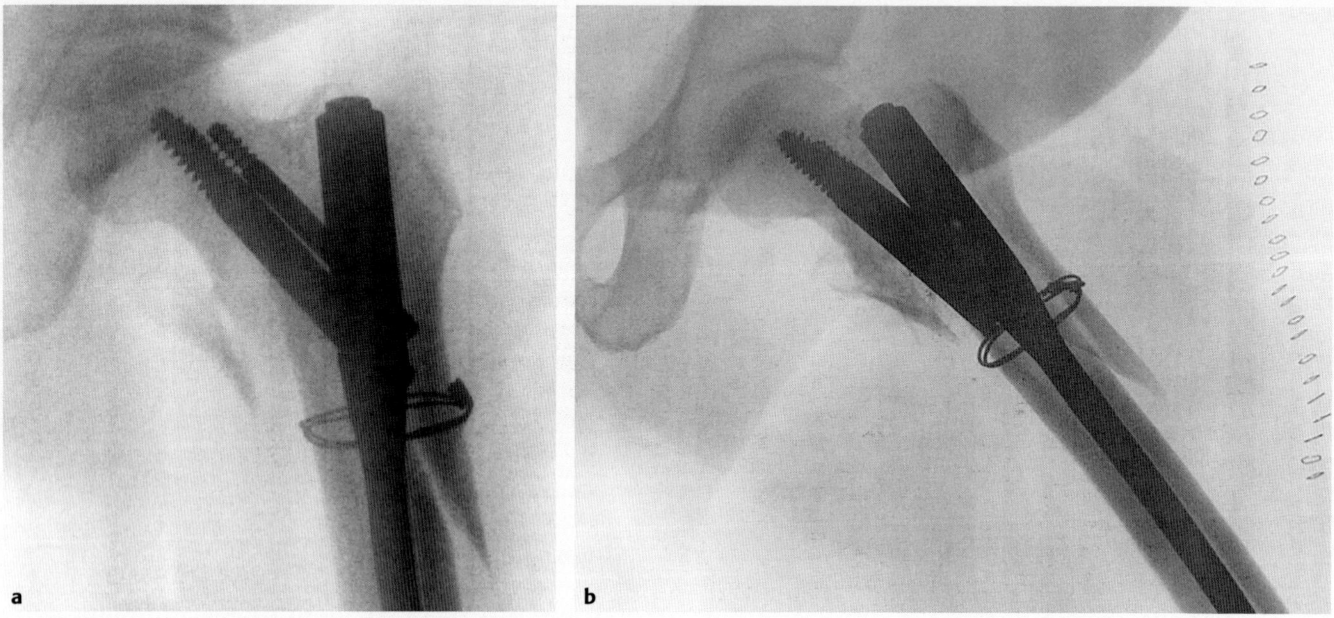

Fig 3.6-14a–b Postoperative x-rays at 1 week.

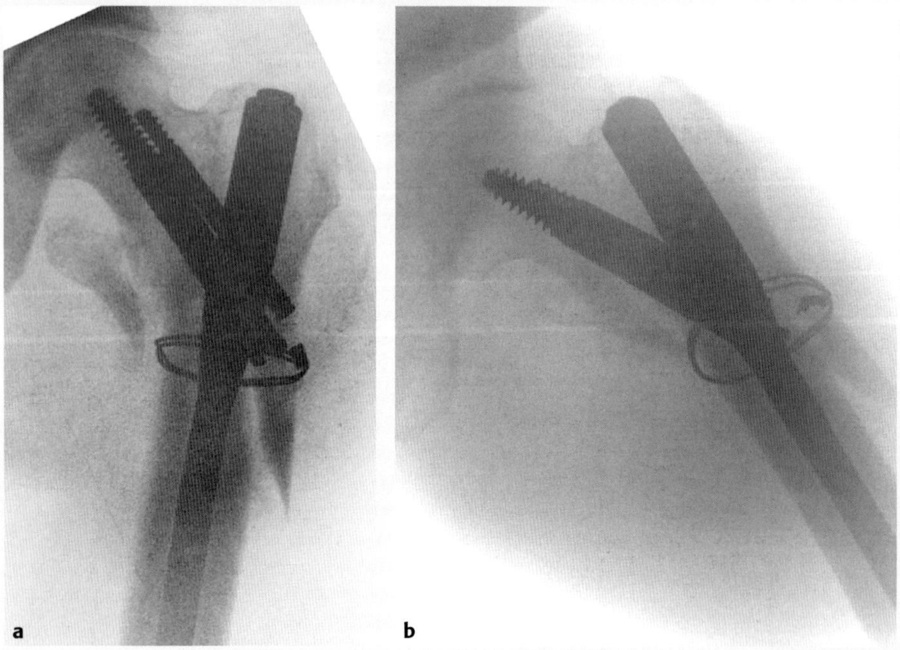

Fig 3.6-15a–b X-rays taken at the 1-month postoperative follow-up.

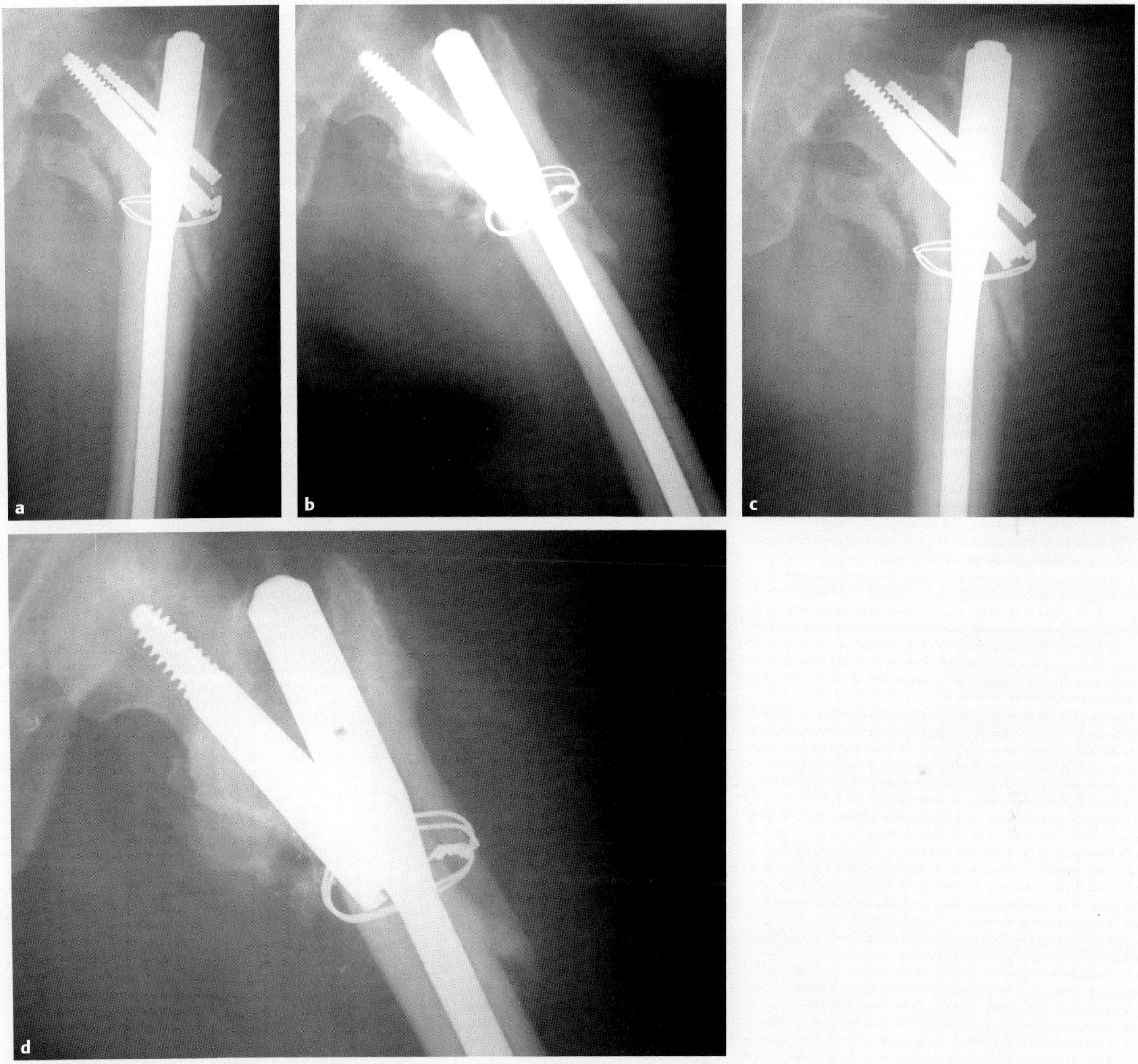

Fig 3.6-16a–f X-rays taken at the 4-month postoperative follow-up (axial view).

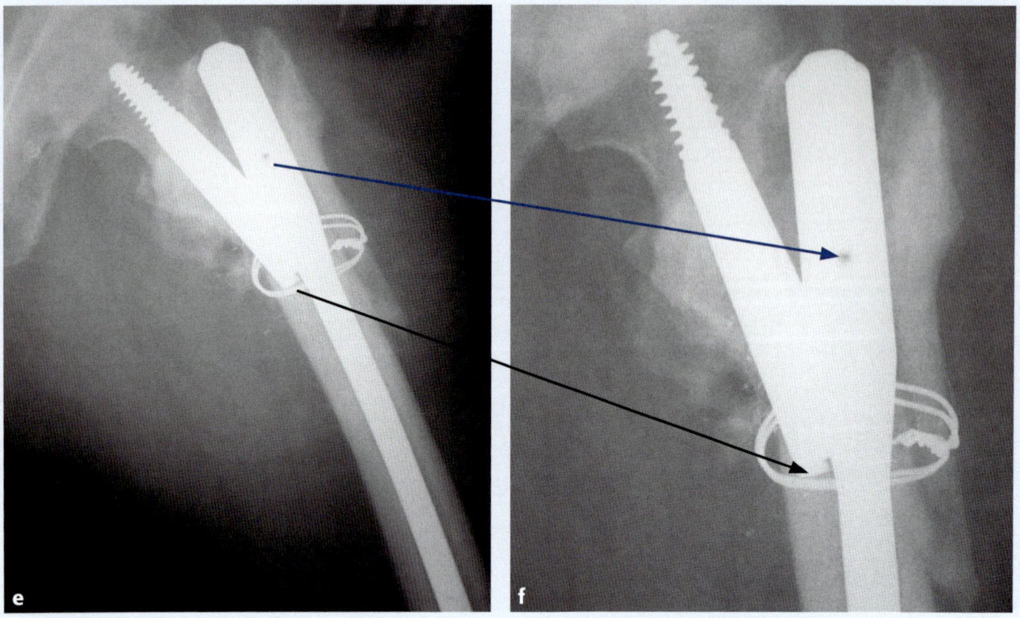

Fig 3.6-16a–f (cont) X-rays taken at the 4-month postoperative follow-up (axial view). Enlargement (**e–f**): the black arrow shows the location of the screw on the outside of the nail; the blue arrow indicates that the proximal hole is empty.

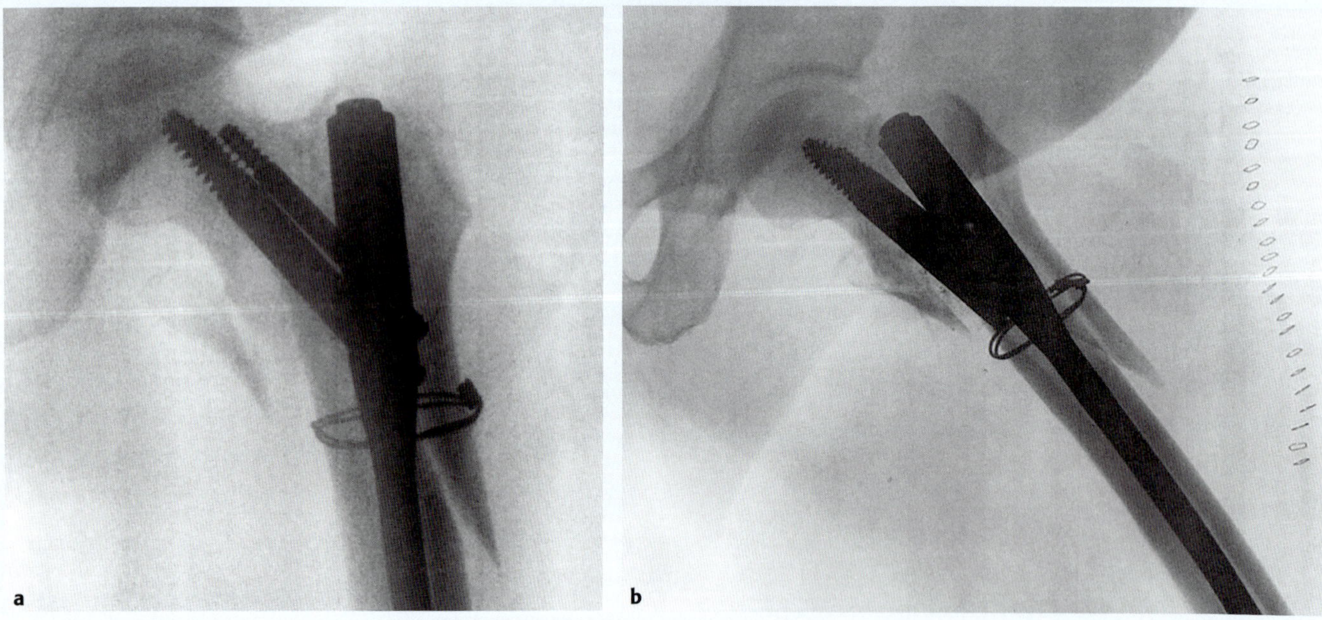

Fig 3.6-17a–b Review of x-rays taken 1 week postoperatively.

Analysis of failure and reflection

Postoperative limb mobilization was hampered by a large leg edema. Deep vein thrombosis was suspected, but analytical and ultrasound tests ruled this out.

The patient was suffering from groin pain during the immediate postoperative period and was therefore noncompliant with the prescribed weight-bearing target load and exercises during postoperative recovery.

In this case, the failures were due to:

- Improperly guided targeting and implant assembly.
- A poor follow-up leading to a misreading and misunderstanding of the x-ray images.

The failures could be attributed to either a learning curve failure or an error related to lack of knowledge about the surgical technique by the surgeon, assistants (including staff that handle the C-arm), or the operating room personnel. The operating room personnel should always check the aiming device insertion handle, ie, check not only how tight it is, but also the guided targeting of the wires and drills. It is also mandatory to achieve good x-ray views, but the main responsibility for the final result lies with the surgeon. A surgery cannot be finished before checking the final reduction and the correct positioning of the implant in the bone.

To correct the failure and improve the patient's situation during surgery, the surgeon should have taken the following measures:

- Checked the connections between nail and insertion handle.
- Checked the guide wire aiming device for the correct orientation of drill sleeves and screws.
- Verified the reduction and fixation with good C-arm images in AP and lateral views, as is also mandatory before starting the surgery.

The surgeon found and analyzed the following failures after finishing surgery:

- Technical problems in assembling the nail with the instruments for insertion.
- Lack of three-dimensional checking before ending surgery.
- Poor clinical and x-ray evaluation in the follow-up.

Final outcome

Total hip replacement was subsequently done as the last revision.

CASE 4

Case description

A 78-year-old woman fell from standing height in the street. Her airway, breathing, and circulation (according to the ABC of advanced trauma life support) were satisfactory, but she suffered from the comorbid condition of hypothyroidism. She sustained a right subtrochanteric fracture (AO/OTA 32B2) (**Fig 3.6-18**).

A long trochanteric nail was planned (long proximal femoral nail antirotation [PFNA]). The surgical team did not check the connections between nail and insertion handle. The postoperative AP control x-ray view showed the fracture was nicely reduced with a well-placed implant (**Fig 3.6-19a**). However, the patient complained of hip pain and was not able to stand or walk. The postoperative axial x-ray view showed the PFNA spiral blade outside the proximal nail hole (**Fig 3.6-19b**).

Rescue surgery was performed 1 week after the first internal fixation (**Fig 3.6-20**). The planned surgical steps were first to remove the hardware, then rereduce and renail after checking that the sleeves matched the guided insertion handle of the nail.

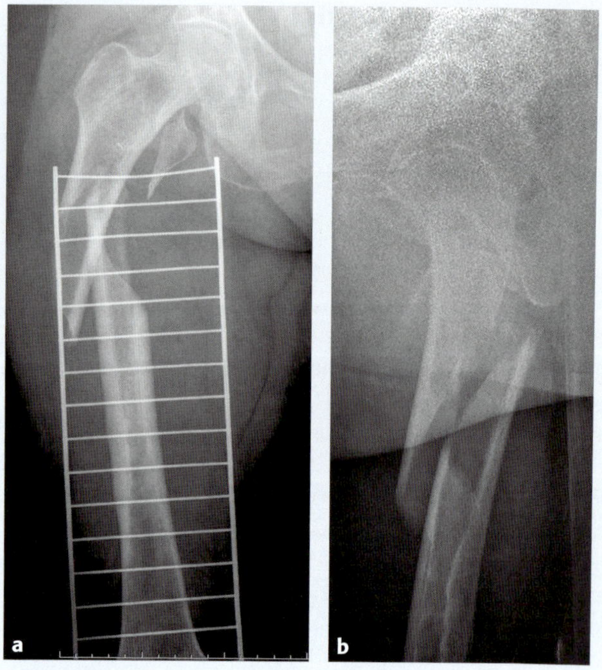

Fig 3.6-18a–b X-ray showing a subtrochanteric right femoral fracture due to a ground-level fall.

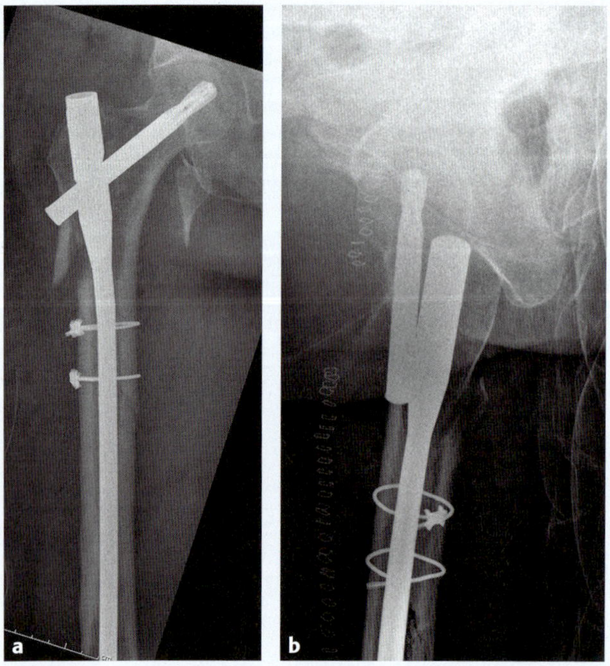

Fig 3.6-19a–b Postoperative x-rays. A nice reduction and a well-placed implant visible in the AP view (**a**). The axial view shows the spiral blade placed anterior in the femoral neck, not linked to the proximal femoral nail antirotation (**b**).

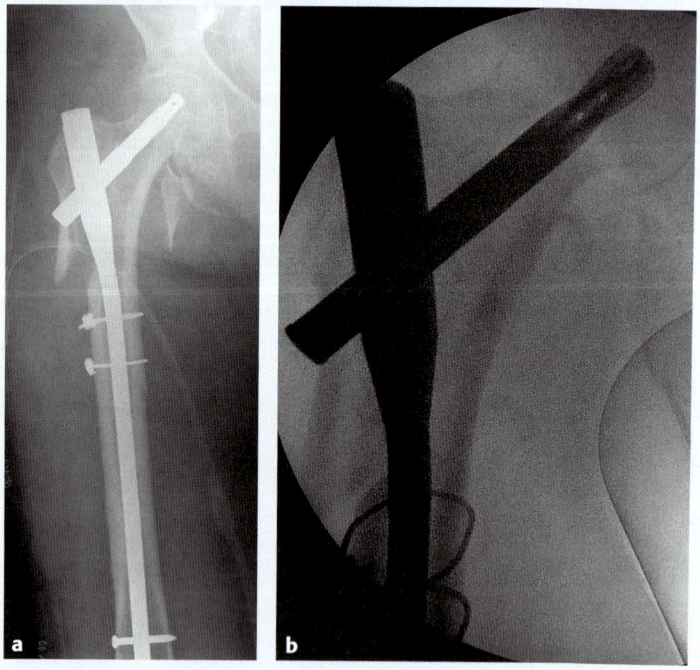

Fig 3.6-20a–b X-rays of the rescue surgery. Removal of the previous implant and renailing after checking that the sleeves matched the guided insertion handle of the nail (**a**). The C-arm oblique view shows the spiral blade is linked to the proximal end of the nail (**b**).

Analysis of failure and reflection

The PFNA spiral blade was placed outside the proximal nail hole, probably due to an incorrect assembly of the nail to its insertion handle. It is mandatory to check the connections between nail and insertion handle before insertion of the nail. Before insertion of the guided implant, it should be checked that the drill sleeves match the guided aiming device and the holes of the nail.

The C-arm must be used to obtain true AP and lateral views, which is mandatory before starting surgery. Distal locking of a long nail is a difficult surgical step. Although some guided devices exist, most of the time the distal locking screws in long PFNA are inserted by free-hand technique, so true lateral views are needed for the distal screw locking insertion. It is advisable to perform the three-dimensional control x-rays (in AP and lateral or axial views) before the end of the surgery and try to correct the possible problems.

Final outcome

The fracture healed and the patient was able to walk with crutches. She is pain free and she has recovered sufficient functionality but lost quality of life in the first year after the fracture (**Fig 3.6-21**).

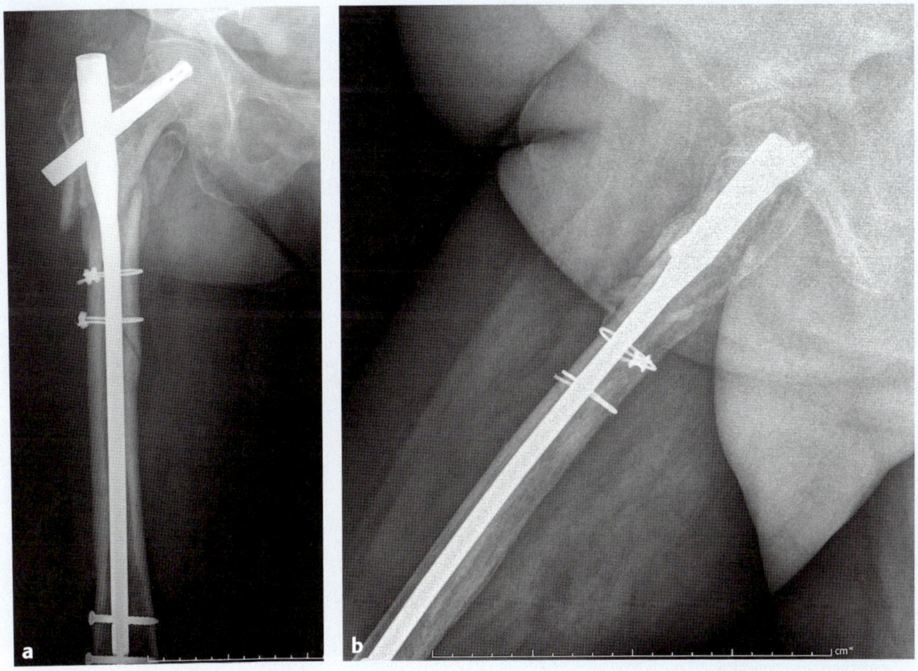

Fig 3.6-21a–b One-year follow-up control x-rays. Both the AP (**a**) and axial (**b**) views show a correct consolidation of the fracture. There are no signs of periimplant lysis or mobilization. The spiral blade remains connected to the proximal end of the proximal femoral nail antirotation.

CASE 5

Case description

An 86-year-old woman fell from standing height. Her airway, breathing, and circulation (according to the ABC of advanced trauma life support) were satisfactory. She had comorbidities of hypertension, type 1 diabetes mellitus, heart failure, and renal failure. She sustained a right multifragmentary intertrochanteric fracture (AO/OTA 31A3) (**Fig 3.6-22**).

A long trochanteric nail was planned (long proximal femoral nail antirotation [PFNA]). The surgical team did not check the connections between nail and insertion handle. In the postoperative control x-rays, the fracture showed a loss of reduction with a light varus malreduction (**Fig 3.6-23**). Due to hip pain, the patient was unable to stand or walk. The computed tomographic (CT) scan showed the PFNA spiral blade outside the proximal nail hole (**Fig 3.6-24**).

The rescue surgery was performed 1 day after the first internal fixation (**Fig 3.6-25**). The planned surgical steps were first to remove the hardware, then rereduce and renail after checking that the sleeves matched the guided insertion handle of the nail.

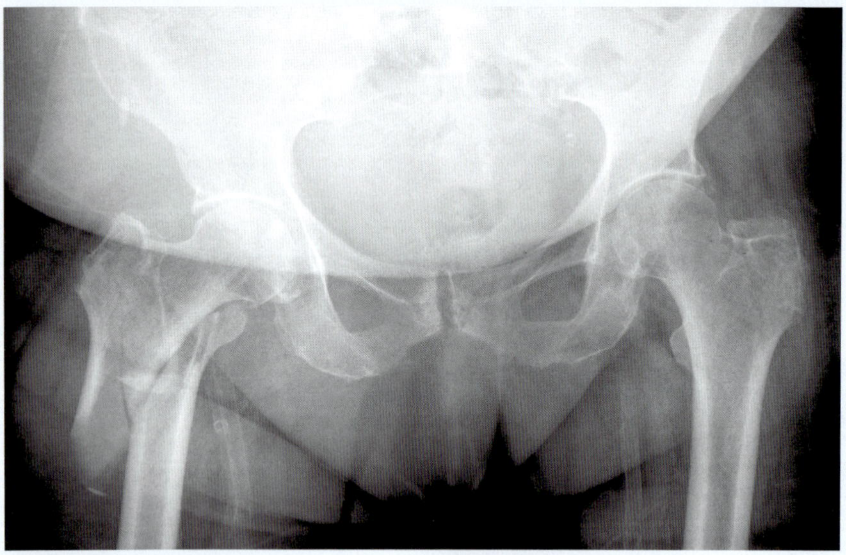

Fig 3.6-22 An intertrochanteric right femoral fracture due to a ground-level fall.

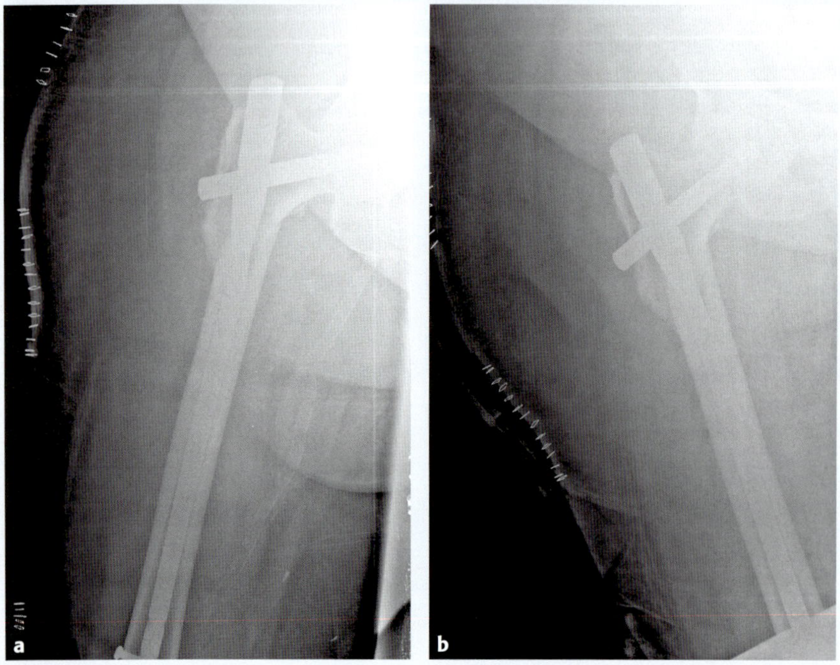

Fig 3.6-23a–b Postoperative x-rays showing a malreduction of the trochanteric fracture with a light varus malreduction in the AP (**a**) and oblique (**b**) views.

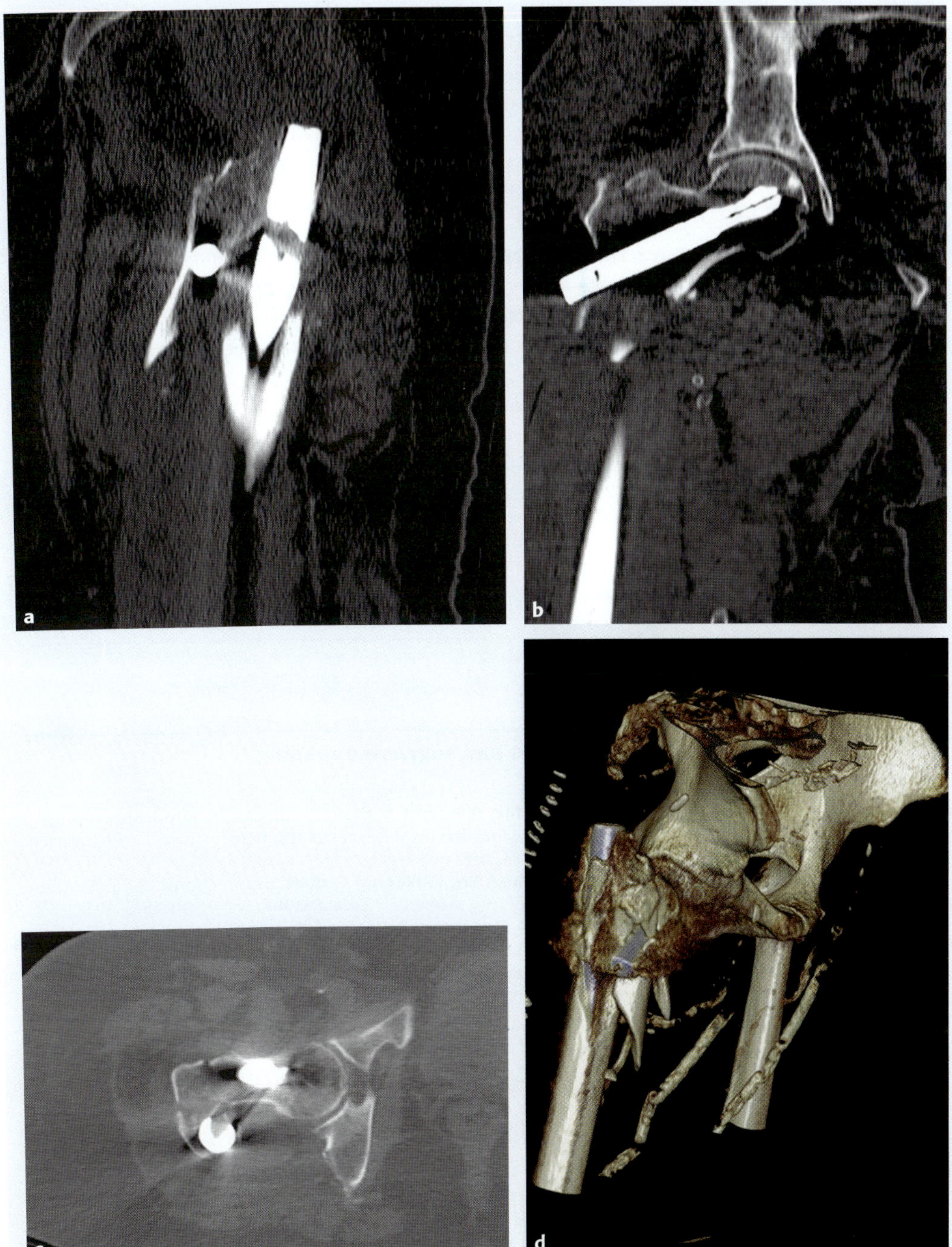

Fig 3.6-24a–d Two-dimensional and three-dimensional computed tomographic (CT) scans of the implant.

a–c Two-dimensional CT scans of the sagittal (**a**), frontal (**b**), and coronal (**c**) views showing that the implant (spiral blade) extending through the neck into the head is not linked to the trochanteric nail.

d Three-dimensional CT scan showing the nail in the posterior corner of the greater trochanter and the spiral blade extending into the head in anterior aspect of the femoral neck.

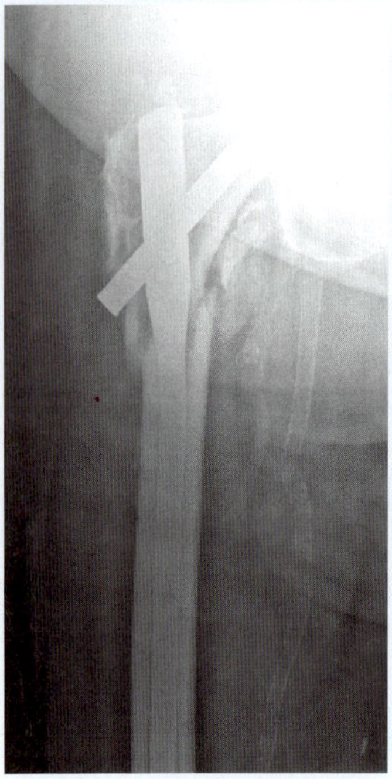

Fig 3.6-25 Rescue surgery: removal of a previous implant, rereduction, and renailing after checking that the sleeves matched the guided insertion handle of the nail. The valgus angulation was restored and the spiral blade is linked to the proximal end of the nail.

Analysis of failure and reflection

The PFNA spiral blade was placed outside the nail's proximal hole, probably due to an incorrect assembly of the nail to the insertion handle. It is mandatory to check the connections between nail and insertion handle. Before insertion of the guided implant, it should be checked that the drill sleeves match the guided aiming device and the holes of the nail.

The C-arm must be used to obtain true AP and lateral views, which is mandatory before starting the surgery. It is advisable to perform the three-dimensional control x-rays (in AP and lateral or axial views) before the end of the surgery and try to correct the possible problems.

Final outcome

The patient died 6 weeks after the rescue surgery due to problems related to her fragility and numerous comorbidities.

Key points to remember

- Strong pressure on or hammering in the weak zones of the insertion handle should be avoided, as this may deform the aiming device and affect the guided insertion of the screws or blades.
- Before inserting the nail, it is mandatory for the surgeon to check that the drill sleeves match the aiming device and the holes of the nail.
- After the insertion of the nail either with oscillating movements or hammering, the connection mechanism between the nail and the aiming device must be retightened.
- Before closing the surgical incisions, the surgeon must ensure with correct C-arm views that all the connections between the modular components of the nail are perfectly interconnected and in a correct position.
- When a percutaneous minimally invasive plate osteosynthesis technique has been performed and an aiming device for screws used, it is mandatory for the surgeon to test the perfect connection between the aiming device, the sleeve, and the threaded hole of the plate.

References and suggested reading

Clavert P, Adam P, Bevort A, et al. Pitfalls and complications with locking plate for proximal humerus fracture. *J Shoulder Elbow Surg.* 2010 Jun;19(4):489–494.

Egol KA, Kubiak EN, Fulkerson E, et al. Biomechanics of locked plates and screws. *J Orthop Trauma.* 2004 Sep;18(8):488–493.

Fernández A, Regazzoni P, Perren SM. Does locking last in metaphyseal screws with guided or free-hand insertion? £2019 Feb. *ICUC One-Page Paper.* Available at: www.icuc.net/multimedia/#papers. Accessed May 2019.

Pardiwala D, Prabhu V, Dudhniwala G, et al. The AO distal locking aiming device: an evaluation of efficacy and learning curve. *Injury.* 2001 Nov;32(9):713–718.

Tejwani NC, Guerado E. Improving fixation of the osteoporotic fracture: the role of locked plating. *J Orthop Trauma.* 2011 Jun;25 Suppl 2:S56–60.

Section 4
Surgical team

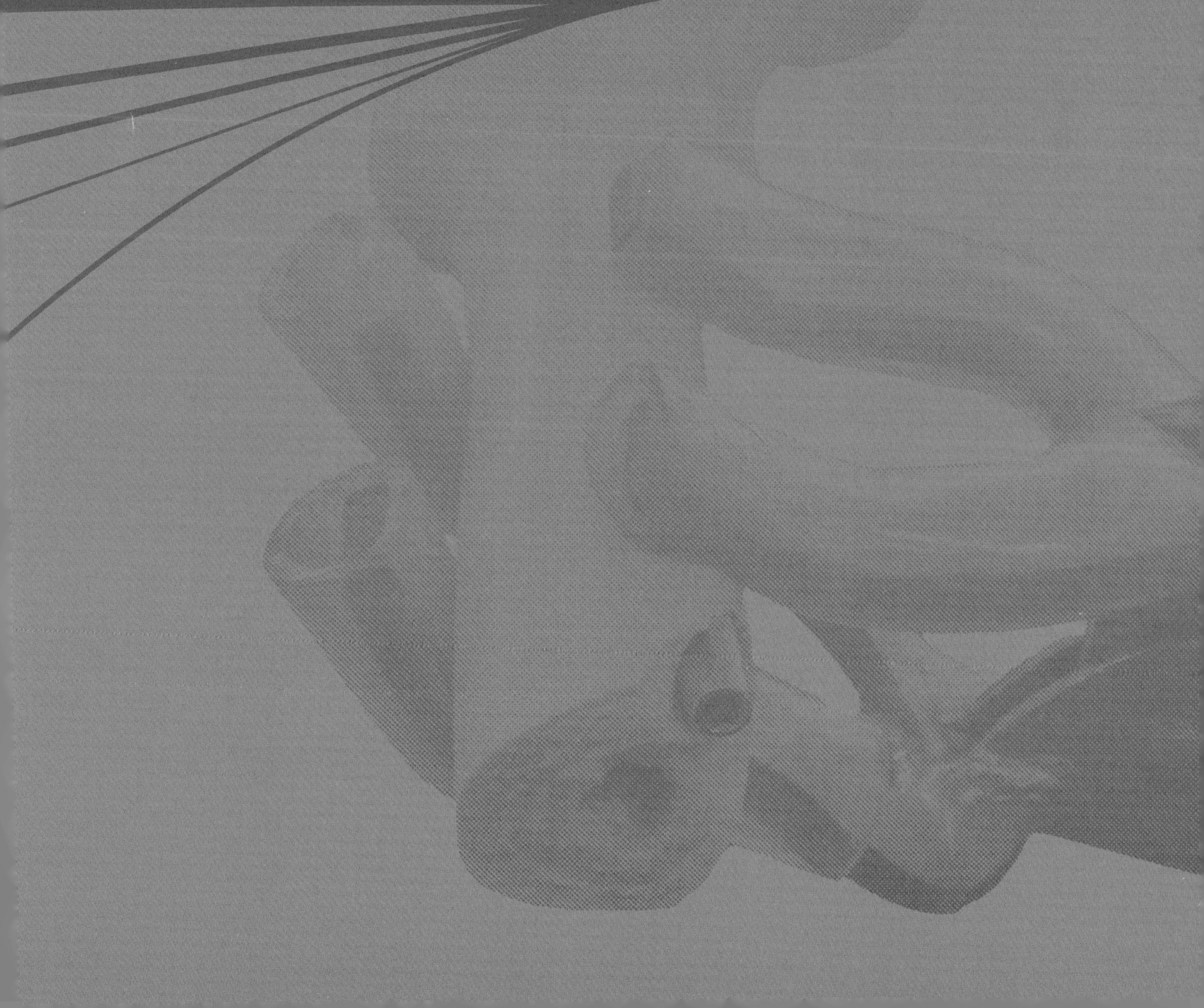

Section 4
Surgical team

4.1 Determining factors for failures relating to the surgical team

J Miquel Sales Pérez
Joan Girós Torres, Roberto Rivero Sosa, Miquel Videla Cés

Decisions are more important than incisions.

Neil Sinart

The procedure for assessing the patient's clinical situation, fracture characteristics, and ensuring the availability of all the technical requirements to carry out the surgical treatment is complex but well known and is the primary function of the entire surgical team. Although on occasion some factors are undervalued or overlooked, each factor that influences the treatment is important for the good outcome hoped for by both the patient and surgical team. The team, led by the surgeon, must be aware of each factor and stage of the process to be able to plan the treatment in a rational way.

The determining factors in planning the fracture treatment can be divided into three groups: the patient, the fracture, and the technical conditions required for its treatment. All these factors influence the results expected over the course of the procedure (**Table 4.1-1**).

While writing this book, the reason(s) for which a treatment may fail have been considered. For educational purposes, the cases have been grouped into different categories. However, the reason for failure never exists in isolation. In each case presented, there are various factors determining the result that have not been taken into account before or during the treatment.

In each surgical team and in each injured patient there is a convergence of needs and responsibilities that are sometimes not covered, not necessarily due to negligence or carelessness. The pressures on emergency department services and the coordination that should exist is not always dealt with in the most desirable way. In some cases this regrettably leads to failures that otherwise could have been avoided. The main goal of the surgical team is always that their patients receive the best possible treatment and completely recover.

In this chapter we emphasize various factors related to the surgical team:

- The importance of *treatment planning,* essential for proper execution of the method.
- We also mention the need to possess sufficient *anatomical knowledge* to tackle fractures using internal fixation Modern osteosynthesis tries, on occasion, to tackle major difficulties associated with the severity of the injury (combined fractures, high-energy accidents, marked osteoporosis, etc). These are sometimes impossible to resolve completely, and despite advocating for method simplicity, they are more demanding and require in-depth knowledge of new surgical approaches and anatomically preshaped implants.
- The rigorous technique required for osteosynthesis always goes hand in hand with the need to respect *asepsis protocols* to avoid a much-dreaded infection, which of all possible complications is the one most feared by the surgeon.
- The *experience of the surgical team* is fundamental for performing the osteosynthesis method. The long learning curve requires tenacity and the assimilation of all the concepts necessary for its practice. Understanding specific technical details in the cases presented here may help surgeons in this long learning process.
- Finally, cases are presented in which it is sometimes difficult to single out one predominant failure; many exist in combination which increases their consequences. Difficult cases nearly always present an *accumulation of failures* occurring after one initial failure, in a cascade effect. Understanding what has happened with these patients will help us to avoid similar failures in future cases.

Category	Factors
Patient	• General condition of patient and prior medical conditions (eg, obesity, rheumatic disorders, neurological disorders, chronic medications, polytrauma). An adequate multidisciplinary evaluation may be necessary. • Functional demand: prior ambulatory capacity and daily needs • Motivation and expectations of the patient • Bone quality, osteoporosis, etc • Condition of the soft tissues • Neurovascular status of the limb • Patient's social support
Fracture	• Localization, morphology, and classification • Displacement of the fracture • Stage of treatment (pre-, intra-, or postoperative) • Local conditions of bone and soft tissues (eg, infection, areas of osteolysis) • Existence of prior deformities • Preexisting implant: - Osteosynthesis or arthroplasty - Study the whole bone - Prior surgeries - Selection of the appropriate implant • State of prior arthroplasty if one exists: - Stability or looseness of the components - Ligament stability - Know the type and size of the components • Stability of the prior implant if one exists: - Prior stability - Type and size of the implant - Improve constructions between implants • Relationship with previous implant and distance between implants • Local biological and biomechanical aspects • Bone remnants and need for graft if bone defects exist • Achieve adequate stability (ie, mobility and union) • Prevention of future complications • Timing of surgery
Technical conditions	• Adequate diagnostic and intraoperative imaging studies (eg, computed tomographic radiology) • Experience of the surgeon (ie, technical knowledge of reduction techniques, internal fixation, and revision arthroplasties) • Adequate and individualized preoperative planning • Choice of implant • Availability and knowledge of adequate instruments and implants • Patient care conditions for preoperative preparation of patient and postoperative care (eg, hospitalization units, rehabilitation, and support) • Adequate facilities (ie, pre-, intra-, and postoperative) • Postoperative planning (rehabilitation, etc) and prevention of new fractures (stress zones, etc) • Adequate social conditions (ie, patient's environment, care, and assistance) • Alternative planning where necessary

Table 4.1-1 Determining factors in planning for the treatment of fractures.

Key points to remember

- Evaluating the patient and her or his fracture and ensuring the technical needs are met is the responsibility of the entire surgical team.
- All factors that can influence treatment of the patient must be evaluated.
- All aspects of how a treatment may fail should also be considered.

References and suggested reading

Agnoletti V, Buccioli M, Padovani E, et al. Operating room data management: improving efficiency and safety in a surgical block. *BMC Surg.* 2013 Mar 11;13:7.

Antoniadis S, Passauer-Baierl S, Baschnegger H, et al. Identification and interference of intraoperative distractions and interruptions in operating rooms. *J Surg Res.* 2014 May 1;188(1): 21–29.

Aveling EL, Stone J, Sundt T, et al. Factors Influencing Team Behaviors in Surgery: A Qualitative Study to Inform Teamwork Interventions. *Ann Thorac Surg.* 2018 Jul;106(1):115–120.

Bhattacharyya T, Vrahas MS, Morrison SM, et al. The value of the dedicated orthopaedic trauma operating room. *J Trauma.* 2006 Jun;60(6):1336–1340; discussion 1340–1331.

Bogner MS. *Human Error in Medicine.* Hillsdale, NJ: Lawrence Erlbaum; 1994.

Elder GM, Harvey EJ, Vaidya R, et al. The effectiveness of orthopaedic trauma theatres in decreasing morbidity and mortality: a study of 701 displaced subcapital hip fractures in two trauma centres. *Injury.* 2005 Sep;36(9):1060–1066.

Halverson AL, Casey JT, Andersson J, et al. Communication failure in the operating room. *Surgery.* 2011 Mar;149(3):305–310.

Leach LS, Myrtle RC, Weaver FA. Surgical teams: role perspectives and role dynamics in the operating room. *Health Serv Manage Res.* 2011 May;24(2):81–90.

Min W, Wolinsky PR. The dedicated orthopedic trauma operating room. *J Trauma.* 2011 Aug;71(2):513–515.

Stone JL, Aveling EL, Frean M, et al. Effective Leadership of Surgical Teams: A Mixed Methods Study of Surgeon Behaviors and Functions. *Ann Thorac Surg.* 2017 Aug;104(2):530–537.

Suliman A, Klaber RE, Warren OJ. Exploiting opportunities for leadership development of surgeons within the operating theatre. *Int J Surg.* 2013;11(1):6–11.

Walker IA, Reshamwalla S, Wilson IH. Surgical safety checklists: do they improve outcomes? *Br J Anaesth.* 2012 Jul;109(1):47–54.

4.2 Insufficient preparatory planning, including alternatives

Matej Cimerman, Joan Girós Torres, Anze Kristan, Roberto Rivero Sosa, Pol M Rommens, J Miquel Sales Pérez, Miquel Videla Cés

If you fail to plan, you are planning to fail.
Benjamin Franklin

Advances in investigative techniques, metallurgy, and surgical techniques, coupled with the development of biological concepts (eg, minimal biological aggression) and mechanics (eg, optimal stability) have enabled an even higher standard (ie, better results achieved due to increased knowledge) of osteosynthesis in the treatment of fractures and the correction of bone defects by means of osteotomy. Since the founding of the AO in the 1950s, one of the main goals has been and continues to be an educative model; teaching concepts to improve internal fixation methods with increased likelihood of success and less improvisation. Improvisation is a poor companion to osteosynthesis that results in bad and on occasion catastrophic results. For treatment to be effective, teaching is essential; it plays a fundamental role in the acquisition of basic concepts for the indication and judicious implementation of method.

The AO teaching places particular emphasis on preoperative planning. While "art" (ie, use of correct implant size, right number and size of screws, and correct distribution in the bone, etc) may play some part in osteosynthesis procedures, such procedures are technically demanding, even when faced with simple fractures. Planning will avoid the need for improvisation in both pre- and postoperative processes.

When young surgeons with limited experience indicate the placement of a specific implant for the treatment of a determined fracture based solely on the observation of similar and previously treated cases, then this represents a deterioration of the philosophy of osteosynthesis. The indication that "we're going to insert a pin or a plate" in a fracture is made without being fully aware of precisely what the implant will do, and without the intellectual process of having previously rationalized the treatment based on principals of osteosynthesis. An implant is only a means to meet determined functions for the treatment of a fracture, rather than an end in itself. The surgeon must look at the type of stability that is required and which implant will best serve that specific function. To base our knowledge of osteosynthesis solely on a reading of the specific part of the *AO Principles of Fracture Management* [Rüedi et al, 2007], ie, the part that deals directly with the treatment of different fractures, while skipping the first, more general part, which explains the different injuries and the biological and mechanical reasoning for the treatment, represents a deterioration in terms of training. Moreover, attempting an osteosynthesis without prior planning, due to the lack of knowledge and understanding about these basic concepts, is an even greater folly.

Professor Maurice E Müller always used to repeat the phrase "the theatre is where you go to operate, not to think". Thinking about what is required to treat a patient, ie, preoperative planning, comes before the operative treatment begins. Planning must occur before the patient is brought into the operating room. It allows the surgeon to carry out an in-depth analysis of the fracture, along with the patient needs and care that must be met for that treatment to be successfully carried out.

Critical review of results following analysis of the documentation of cases being treated through internal fixation identifies lack of preoperative planning as the most influential on results.

The main goal in the treatment of fractures is the application of the basic principles of stability with the minimum possible alteration of vascularization. The technique is demanding and sophisticated and it is unacceptable that we should solely base performance on the surgeon's skill or surgical resources. Planning requires a mental effort in terms of anticipation, which will pay off by paving the way for the application of the surgical technique, while also simplifying communication with the rest of the team and ensuring that the work will be done much more effectively. It is recommended for all procedures.

Preoperative planning is essential to fully understand the fracture, recognize its outlines and the forces that caused the injury, define the tactics to be applied to counteract those injuries, and achieve the reduction via direct and indirect techniques.

Preoperative planning needs to define the segment affected by the fracture. In cases of fracture of the humeral, femoral, or tibial diaphysis, the shaft of the limb will have to be restored, avoiding angulations on frontal and sagittal planes, while in the horizontal plane it is necessary to ensure correct rotational alignment. The shortening or lengthening of lower limbs must be avoided in view of the required levels of weight bearing. Anatomical reduction is not critical and is not the goal, particularly if there is devascularization of the anatomy around the fracture. The same principals have to be followed in the metaphyseal region, although bone grafts will have to be inserted if there are areas of bone loss due to impaction of the cancellous bone. In the joint area anatomical reduction is required, with the articular surface requiring an adequate replacement of displaced bone fragments to ensure the congruency of the articular surface.

During preoperative planning we need to determine the mechanical stability that needs to be applied to the fracture, depending on type and location, as well as the instruments and implants required to adapt to the fractured bone. During preoperative planning, surgical tactics and the execution of the different maneuvers must be anticipated and annotated, which will also allow the surgeon to anticipate other possible needs in advance, establishing variations of the technique or an alternative treatment plan. This will allow the surgeon to deal with such contingencies or incidents during the operation.

Working out why the injuries occurred, the treatment is needed, and how to apply it will turn the process into an intellectual rather than a merely manual exercise and will also favor the successful achievement of the goals. Mere observation cannot replace a good knowledge of surgery or a good understanding of cause and effect of fracture treatment. Improvisation must be avoided, insofar as this is frequently the root cause of subsequent problems. Understanding the difficulties in advance also helps to reduce intervention times by minimizing exposure and associated devascularization in the area of the fracture and by decreasing the likelihood of complications associated with prolonged exposure times.

Preoperative planning allows the surgeon to evaluate in advance whether all the necessary information about the fracture has been revealed, or whether additional complementary imaging studies are needed and, in this way, limiting the possibility that unexpected difficulties could arise during the operation. The same planning process will also anticipate aspects such as the positioning of the patient on the operating table, adequate surgical access, and postoperative recuperation phases (eg, weight bearing and mobility).

While different forms of planning exist (eg, manually tracing with transparent paper and marker, preoperative planning computer software programs), the goal of this book is not to describe them, rather it is recommended that the reader consult the existing body of published literature on preoperative planning.

Case description

An 89-year-old woman with significant comorbidities due to a history of high blood pressure, cardiac arrhythmia due to atrial fibrillation, ischemic cerebrovascular accident (stroke) (ie, ischemic brain injury), total arthroplasty of the left knee, and left ischemia of both lower limbs with femoral and popliteal stent in the left lower limb, fell at home. She presented with pain and functional impairment in both knees with deformity in the right knee where a supracondylar femoral fracture was detected radiographically. It was an irregular, extraarticular, multifragmentary, metaphyseal fracture of the distal femur (AO/OTA 33A3) (**Fig 4.2-1**).

The patient had advanced osteoporosis. Due to comorbidities of high surgical risk, she underwent tibial skeletal traction for stabilization of her medical problems during hospital admission before undergoing surgical intervention. A computed tomographic scan was performed to rule out articular involvement (**Fig 4.2-2**).

Closed reduction and osteosynthesis were performed using a retrograde long intramedullary locking nail to initiate early mobilization of the patient. A transpatellar approach was chosen, and during the nailing procedure, it was discovered that the patient had previously undergone ipsilateral total hip arthroplasty. The decision was taken to change the indication and use a short 150 mm intramedullary nail. Before completing the surgical procedure, articular protrusion of the nail preventing mobilization of the knee was detected; therefore, the bolts were removed and the nail was introduced further. During perforation of the new holes for the proximal locking, a longitudinal fracture occurred through the holes made in the cortex due to bone weakness. Cerclage wires were applied to bring the fragments closer to the intramedullary nail, external immobilization was used with a groin-to-toe plaster cast, and no weight bearing was prescribed for the limb (**Fig 4.2-3**).

One month after the intervention a new fracture site was detected at the proximal end of the nail (**Fig 4.2-4**).

A new surgical intervention was performed 1 month after the first one to remove the intramedullary nail and cerclage wires. The reduction of the fracture was achieved by using a lateral approach and performing osteosynthesis with a long less invasive stabilization system plate with bicortical and monocortical locking screws and cerclages with steel cable. The osteosynthesis with a long plate protected the area between the implants and also avoided possible new fractures (**Fig 4.2-5**).

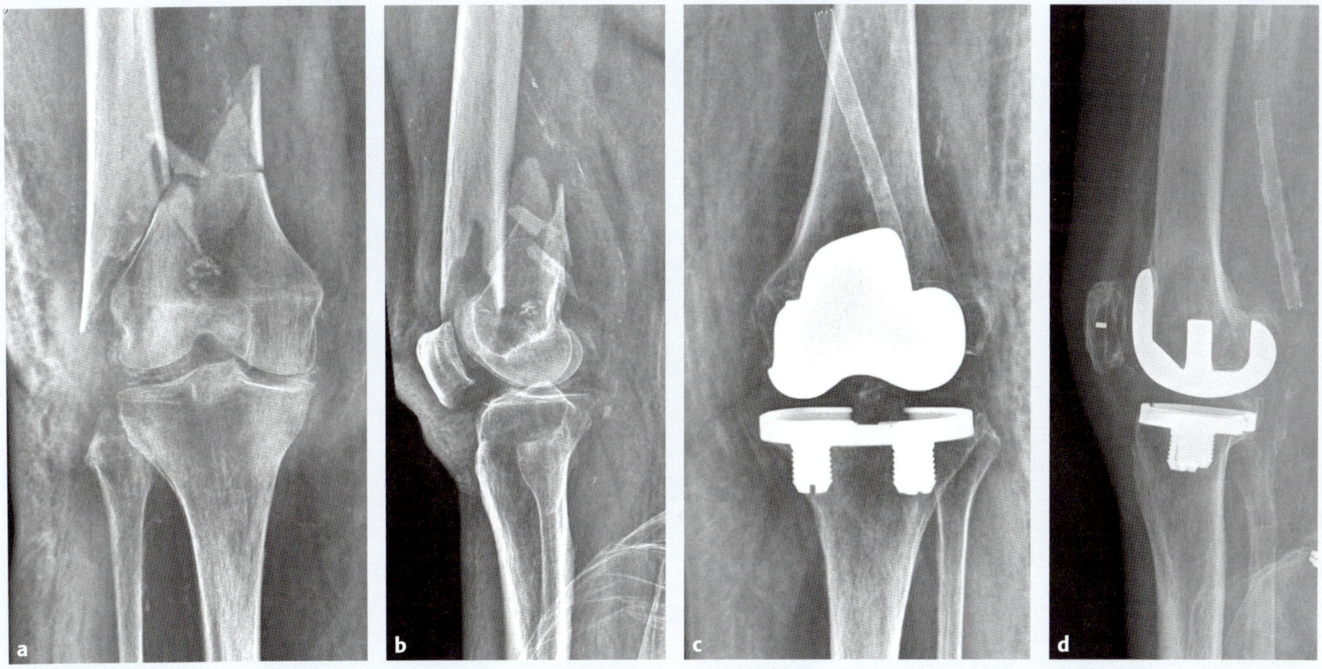

Fig 4.2-1a–d X-rays of the right knee fracture (**a–b**) and left knee with a total knee arthroplasty and vascular bypass (**c–d**).

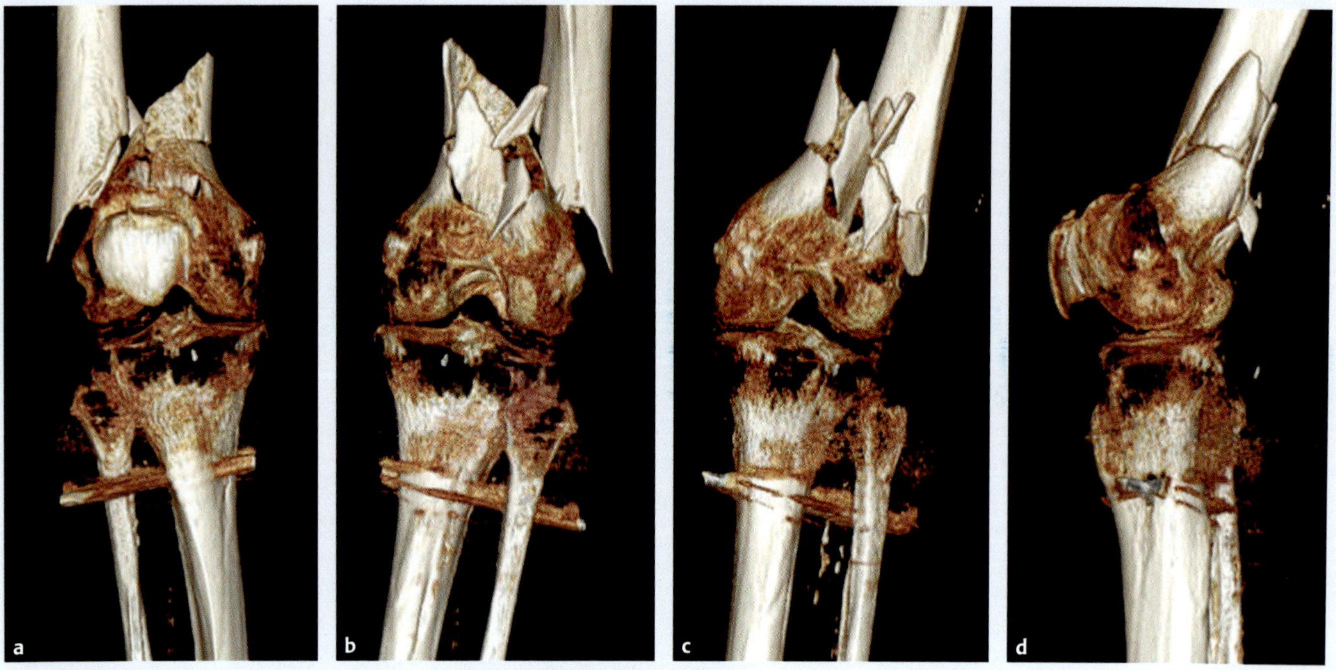

Fig 4.2-2a–d Reconstruction of the fracture using 3D computed tomography.

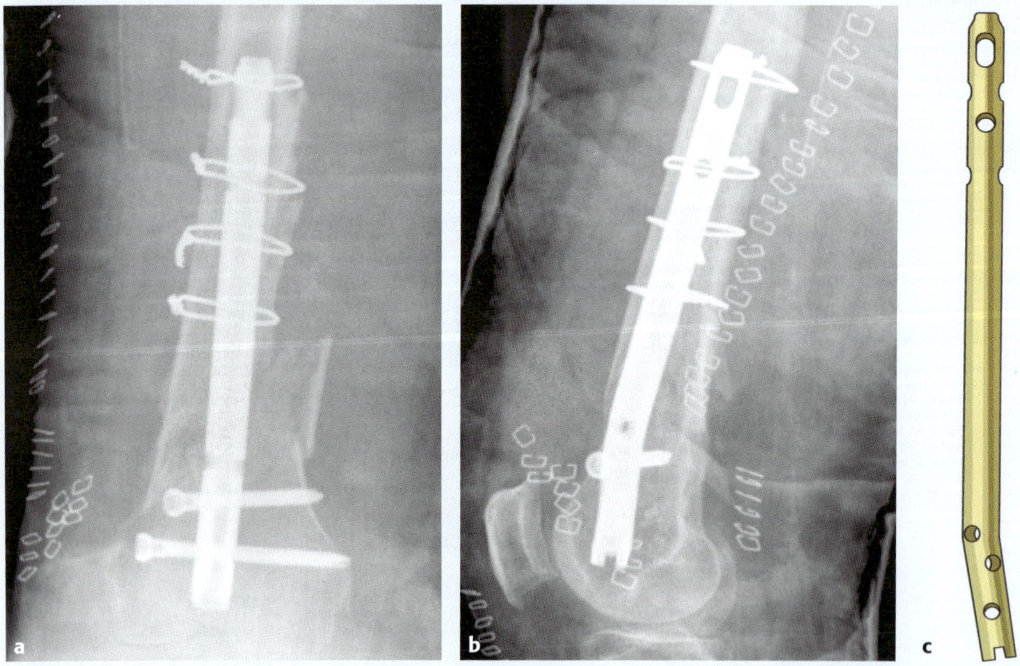

Fig 4.2-3a–g Postoperative control x-rays showing the intramedullary nail and longitudinal fracture produced between the proximal locking holes.
a–b Immediate postoperative x-rays of retrograde short nail in AP (**a**) and lateral (**b**) views.
c Retrograde short femoral intramedullary nail.

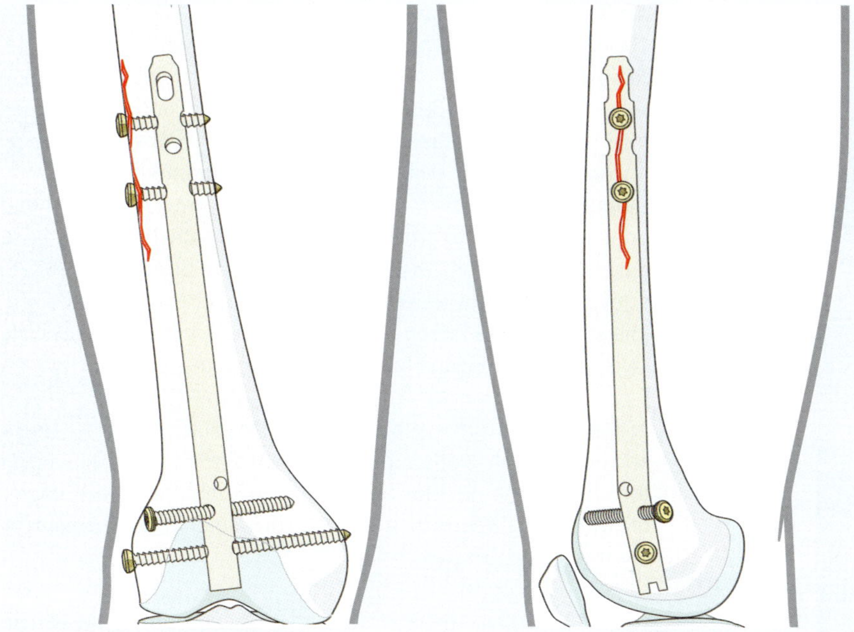

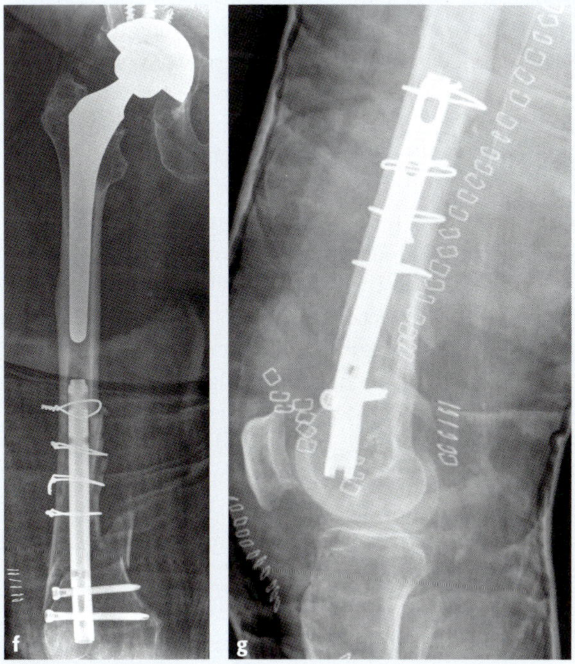

Fig 4.2-3a–g (cont) Postoperative control x-rays showing the intramedullary nail and longitudinal fracture produced between the proximal locking holes.

d–e Outline of the breakage of the femoral cortex through the holes made in the proximal locking of the nail.

f–g Immediate postoperative AP (**f**) and lateral (**g**) x-rays of the short retrograde nail in the femur.

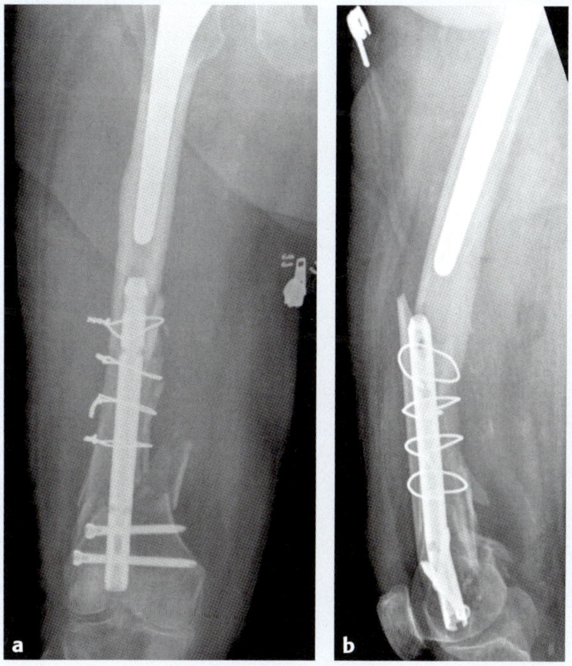

Fig 4.2-4a–b
Postoperative evolution x-ray at 1 month showing the fracture and displacement of the site.

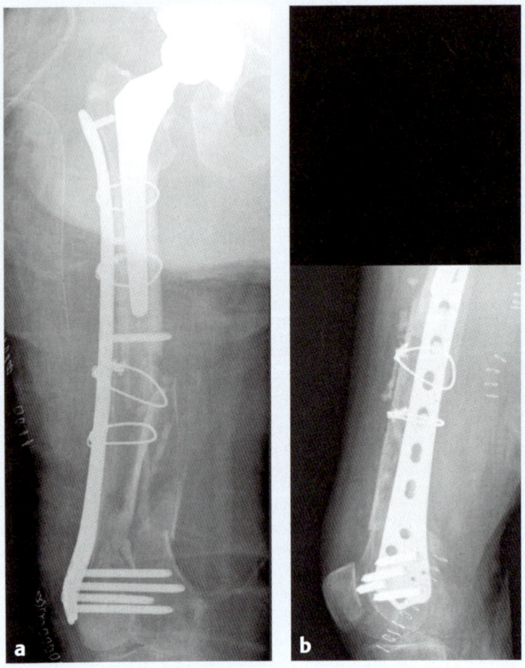

Fig 4.2-5a–b Control x-rays of the reintervention with AP (**a**) and lateral (**b**) views of plate.

Analysis of failure and reflection

The aim for a fracture with metaphyseal comminution that is difficult to treat should not be to reduce the numerous intermediate fragments. By applying adequate traction, with the knee in flexion, the fragments can be reassembled approximately in the metaphyseal region. The implant, which can be locked intramedullary or extramedullary, manages to bridge the area to provide stability that enhances the healing process while respecting the bone alignment, length, and rotation. The entry points in the bone made for the screws are points of lesser resistance and concentration of tensions. The stresses on a locked nail increase because the nail acts like a lever, concentrating the tensions at the proximal end.

In this case, the osteosynthesis was insufficient to permit movement and bear weight. Furthermore, it left the intermediate area between the stem of the hip prosthesis and the distal femoral nail unprotected, leaving a zone of stress that could lead to new fractures in the future.

Currently, special emphasis is placed on the increasing rate of fractures around prior implants because of either osteosynthesis of previous fractures in the same bone (ie, periimplant fractures) or prosthesis for joint replacement in hip and knee alike (ie, periprosthetic fractures). The surge of these types of fractures due to increased life expectancy among patients who have previously undergone surgery indicates that we cannot always rely on prior planning of a surgery with implants but have to consider other factors and the patient's history. That is to say, in planning the treatment of a fracture, we must always think about the possibility of a relationship with an osteosynthesis or arthroplasty previously implanted in the same bone. Individualized treatments must take into account the recent fracture that we have to treat and its relationship with the previously implanted material, the protection of the remaining bone, the survival of an arthroplasty, etc. In these increasingly common cases, patients receive individualized treatments depending on their needs and prior implants that aim to treat the recent fracture, preserving the bone protection of the previous implant, and/or the survival of the joint prosthesis already implanted. The planning of the osteosynthesis assembly must consider the type, dimension, arrangement, stability, and combination of implants. Performing technically difficult surgery requires knowledge of biological and biomechanical concepts and the ability to carefully perform complex internal fixations and revision arthroplasty techniques. The role of minimally invasive surgery (ie, opening only what is necessary) is also important in these cases to avoid aggressive approaches.

In this patient, displacement occurred during flexion leading to the collapse of the fracture. The insufficient medical history and physical examination of the patient, the incomplete x-ray series, and nonexistent preoperative planning are notable. When recording a patient's medical history, additionally it is vital to note overall activities of daily living and living circumstances and to know if previous interventions have been made in the fractured bone that may require surgery, and to inspect old scars, if any.

The intermediate solution after the cortical breakage was insufficient. This possibility should have been considered beforehand in case any unforeseen incidents occurred during nailing, as this would have allowed the surgeons to have other implants and strategies for the definitive treatment at their disposal.

The prolonged period of time that elapsed between the complication and the definitive treatment was excessively extended in this case, especially considering that this was an elderly patient who should be mobilized as soon as possible to avoid general complications.

Final outcome

Partial weight bearing was recommended for 3 months. The patient started to ambulate using a walker and an articular balance of the limb from 0° to 90° was achieved, along with later pain-free ambulation (**Fig 4.2-6**).

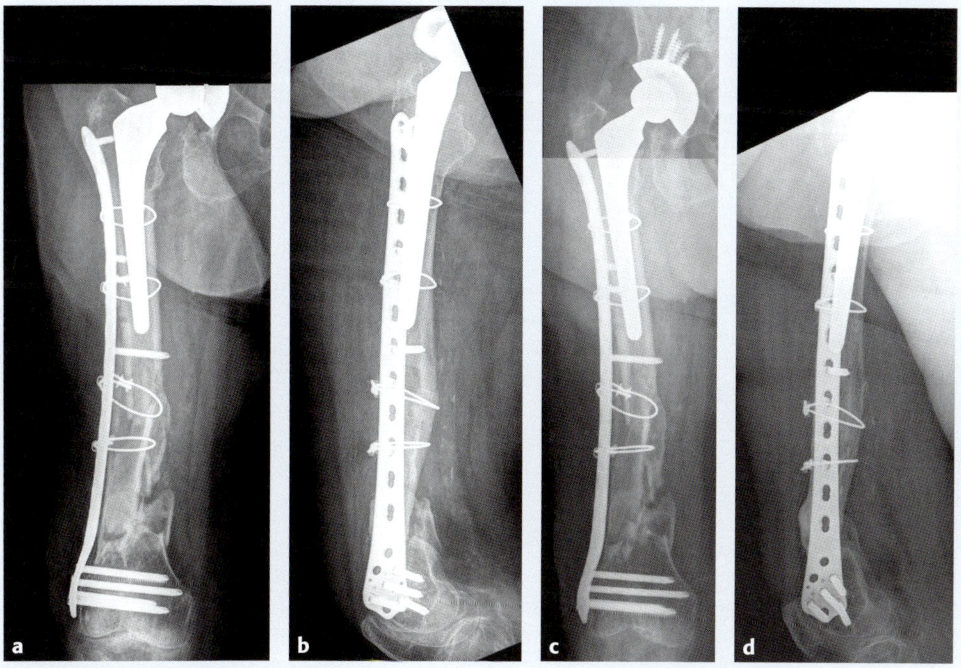

Fig 4.2-6a–d Postoperative control x-rays 6 and 8 months after surgery, respectively.
a–b X-rays at 6 months in AP (**a**) and lateral (**b**) views.
c–d X-rays in AP (**c**) and lateral (**d**) views 1.5 years following the reintervention.

CASE 2

Case description

A 49-year-old woman suffered a high-energy trauma after a sporting injury that affected her left arm. She presented with intense pain and inflammation of the soft tissues but without wounds or neuromuscular damage. X-rays revealed a proximal multifragmentary fracture of the diaphysis in the left humerus (AO/OTA 12C3) with severe displacement of several fracture fragments. The surgical team decided to implant an intramedullary nail to stabilize the fractures. The nail did not achieve adequate stability between the fracture fragments. The bone fragments with sharp edges were not reduced either and they continued to perforate the surrounding soft tissues. The postoperative x-rays showed incorrect alignment between the fragments of the humeral head and the diaphysis due to an incorrect entry portal (**Fig 4.2-7**).

Due to the pain and major functional limitation, it was decided to extract the nail and perform an osteosynthesis with a long angular stability plate (ie, long PHILOS plate), which would stabilize the fracture site from the humeral head to the distal humerus. The displaced fragments were reduced and fixed with traction screws while they remained joined to the soft tissues (**Fig 4.2-8**).

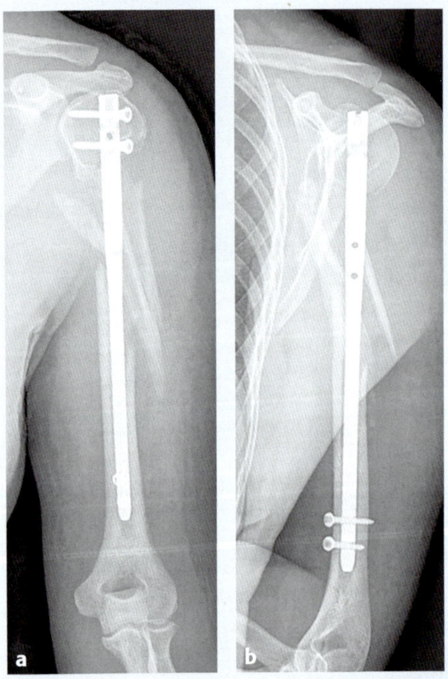

Fig 4.2-7a–b Postoperative x-rays taken after intramedullary nailing of the multifragmentary proximal fracture of the humeral diaphysis. A large space exists at the fracture site and there is no contact between the humeral head and the fragments of the proximal half of the humeral diaphysis. There are at least three long wedge fragments, which previously constituted the medullary canal of the proximal humerus. Due to their displacement, there is no longer any medullary canal in this area. There is a poor alignment of the humeral head and the major displacement of the wedge fragments is clearly visible.

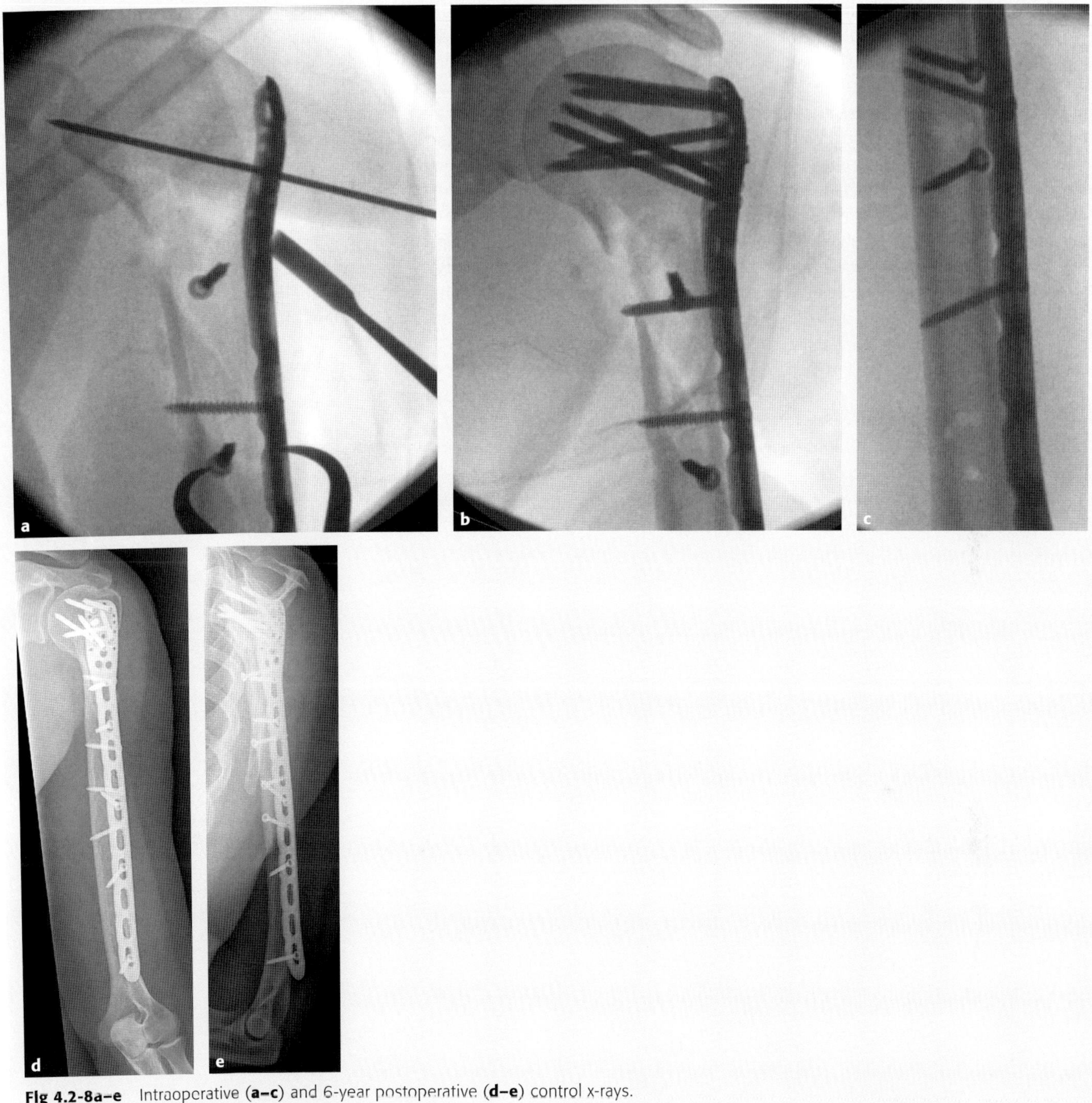

Fig 4.2-8a–e Intraoperative (**a–c**) and 6-year postoperative (**d–e**) control x-rays.

a–c Intraoperative x-rays with image intensifier of the left humeral head and the diaphysis of the proximal humerus during the reconstruction procedure. The wedge fragments were carefully released, reduced, and fixed with traction screws. The humeral head is turned to reposition it. The plate is adapted to the humerus, pressed against it with a small periosteal elevator, and provisionally fixed with reduction forceps. An intraoperative image of the left humeral head and proximal humerus was taken after plate fixation. The humeral head is fixed with seven angular stability screws to obtain the greatest possible stability. This is necessary due to the bone defect in the medial metaphysis and to the longer healing time. Intraoperative view of the left distal humerus shows the anatomical reduction of the fracture, the fixation with traction screws, and the perfect adaptation of the plate along the lateral cortex of the humeral diaphysis.

d–e X-ray in AP and lateral views of the humerus 6 years after the osteosynthesis with screwed plate showing complete healing with remodeling of the humerus.

Analysis of failure and reflection

This patient sustained a complex multifragmentary fracture of the proximal humeral diaphysis. There were various thin, long, and sharp wedge-shaped fragments that were severely displaced. We can identify at least three of these fragments, which were situated between the humeral head and the humeral diaphysis. In this area, the medullary canal has disappeared and the diaphysis, formed by cortical bone, has burst. Intramedullary nailing is not an adequate way to stabilize these types of fractures. The benefits of nailing are overestimated. When fragments are unreduced, the fracture will never heal, nor will healing occur with any other type of osteosynthesis. Furthermore, there was a lack of stability in the overall ensemble. The extensive fracture zone was bridged with a nail and only two screws in the proximal fragment. Since these two screws provided not enough cortical purchase but were found in the porous bone of the humeral head, they did not provide enough stability to counteract the axial, flexion, and rotational forces that the osteosynthesis must bear during healing. The loosening of the screws and/or a cutting phenomenon could occur. Stability in the distal fragment is enough when using two screws for cortical locking and the nail is well situated in the medullary canal.

There was also a lack of reduction of the humeral head fragment. The nail entry point was incorrect, ie, too lateral for this straight nail, and there was a significantly poor rotatory alignment of the humeral head (**Fig 4.2-9**). This will cause an important limitation of shoulder function. Stability and healing after nailing would only have been possible after careful reduction and fixation of the fracture fragments displaced around the nail with the help of cerclage wires or sutures.

Since the open reduction of the fracture fragments was inevitable and replacing the nail would have led to a second entry point through the humeral head cartilage, the preferred option was an osteosynthesis with an open reduction and utilization of the plate as a rescue procedure.

Final outcome

Six years following the reintervention, the patient has full function of her left upper limb. A slight limitation of abduction and elevation exists, but she has no pain and has good muscular strength. The patient does not want the osteosynthesis material to be removed.

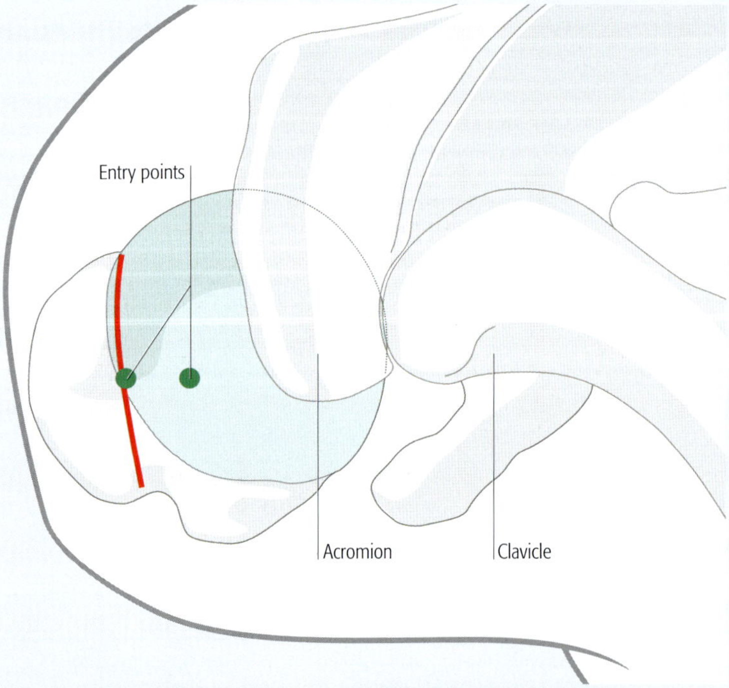

Fig 4.2-9 The correct entry point depends on the design of the nail. In straight nails, the entry point must be more medial, on the top of the humeral head. In curved nails, the entry point can be more lateral, but damaging the insertion of the rotator cuff at the greater tubercle should be avoided.

Case description

A 49-year-old woman fell from a height of 2 m and sustained a Gustilo type II fracture of her right leg [Gustilo et al, 1984]. The initial x-rays showed a tibial pilon fracture (AO/OTA 43C3) (**Fig 4.2-10**).

An intervention was undertaken on the same day using the wound on the medial side as an approach to the tibia. The fibula was also stabilized (**Fig 4.2-11**).

The postoperative x-ray showed that the articular fracture of the tibia was not anatomically reduced. Computed tomographic (CT) scans were performed (**Fig 4.2-12**) which clearly showed unreduced fragments of the distal tibia.

Reintervention was indicated. The decision was taken to treat the fracture with open reduction and a new osteosynthesis, which was performed once the soft tissues were in a suitable condition (**Fig 4.2-13**).

The patient underwent surgical reintervention 17 days after the initial operation. From the first operation there was a lateral wound that was a little more posterior and a straight medial wound. The wounds evolved well and healed. The plan was to remove the plate from the medial side, carry out anatomical reduction of the tibiotalar joint and stable fixation using compression screws and an anterolateral tibial distal plate. The surgeons decided to use one large incision and several punctiform incisions. The main incision was a straight anterior incision mobilizing the soft tissues to approach the medial and lateral parts of the distal tibia.

After removing the tibial plate, the surgeons performed the anatomical reduction of the articulation and fixed it with screws, then they joined the joint fragment to the metaphysis using a locking compression plate for the anterolateral distal tibia. Finally, they applied a compression plate on the medial side (**Fig 4.2-13**).

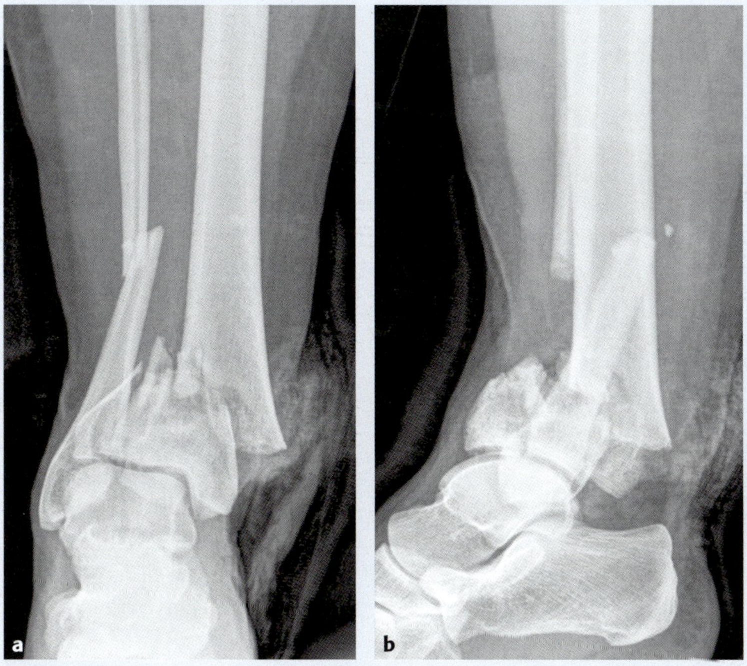

Fig 4.2-10a–b Preoperative AP (**a**) and lateral (**b**) x-rays.

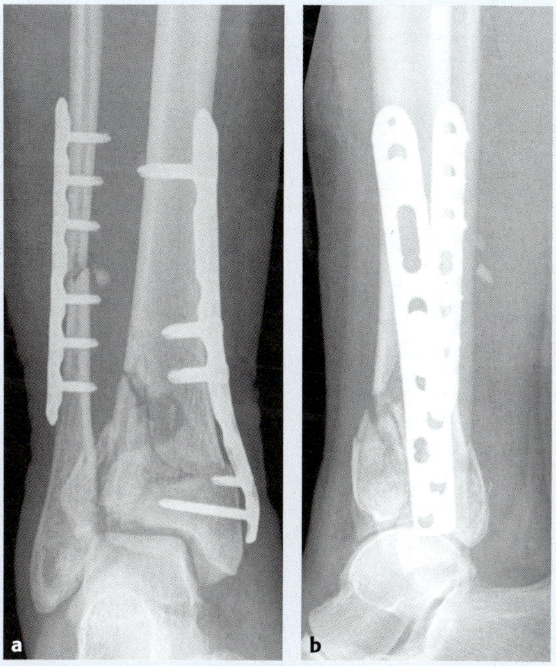

Fig 4.2-11a–b AP (**a**) and lateral (**b**) x-rays taken 2 days postoperatively.

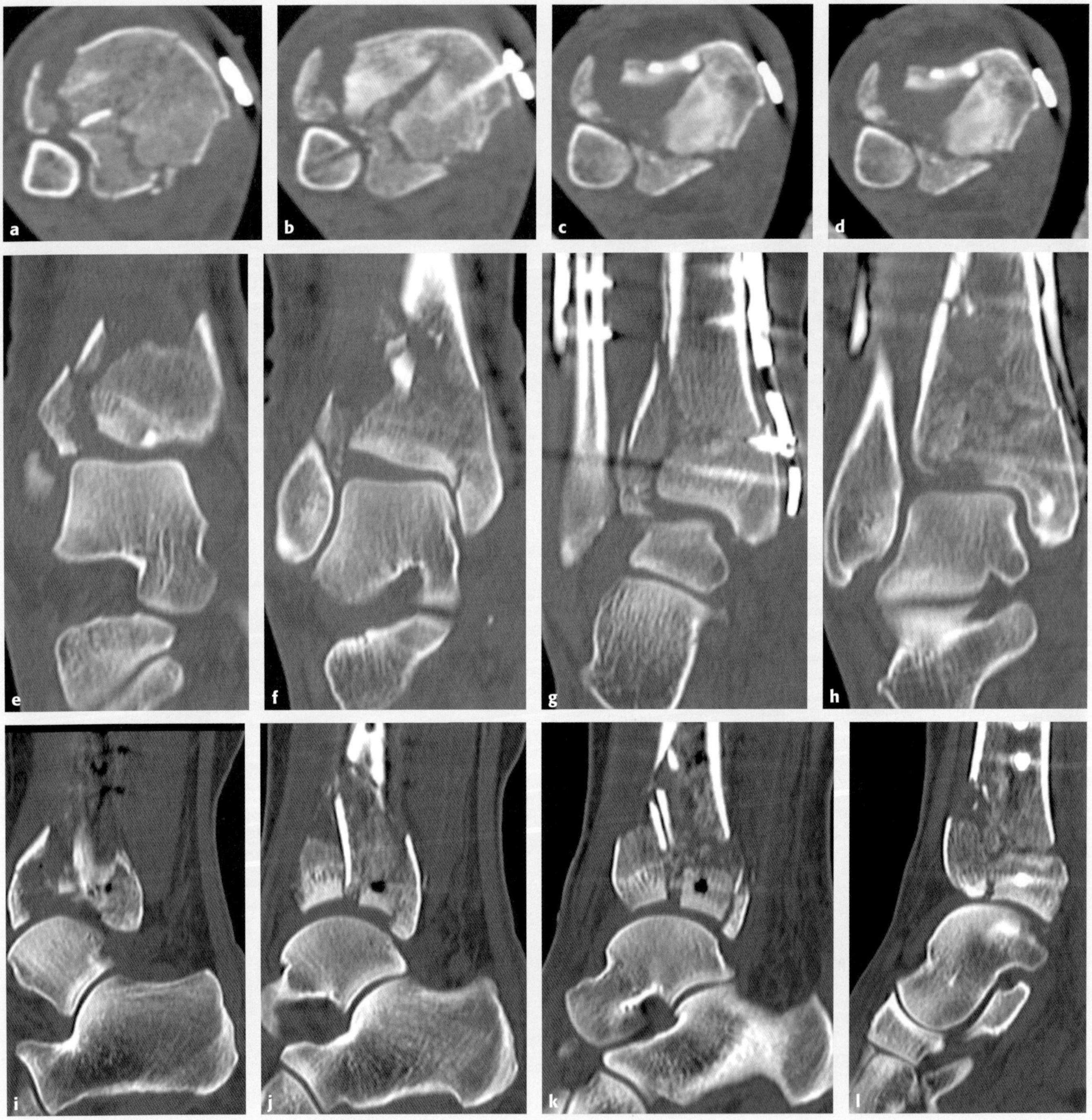

Fig 4.2-12a–o Postoperative computed tomographic scans showing the lack of reduction of the tibiotalar joint with screws in nonreduced bone fragments.
a–d Axial view.
e–h Coronal view.
i–l Sagittal view.

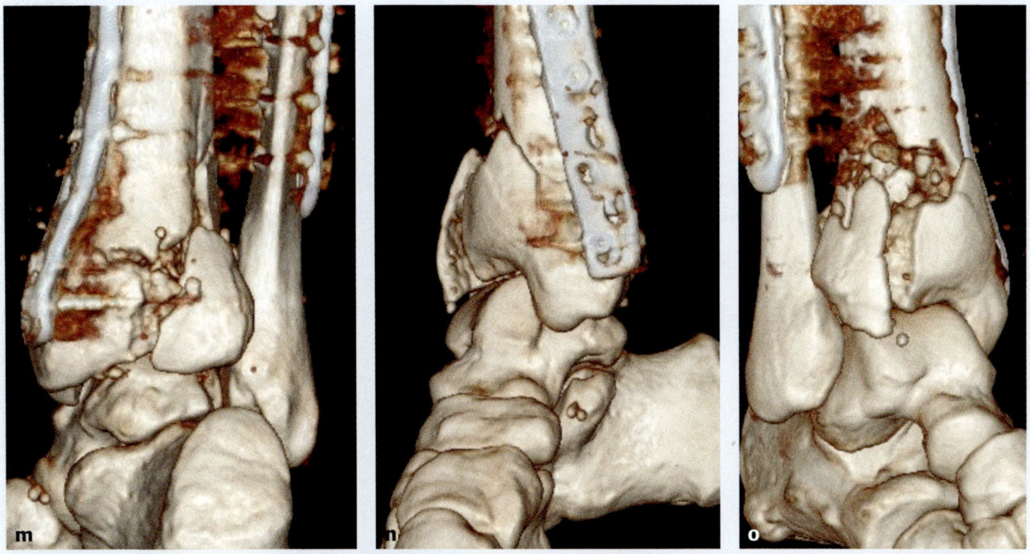

Fig 4.2-12a–o (cont) Postoperative computed tomographic scans showing the lack of reduction of the tibiotalar joint with screws in nonreduced bone fragments.
m–o Three-dimensional reconstruction.

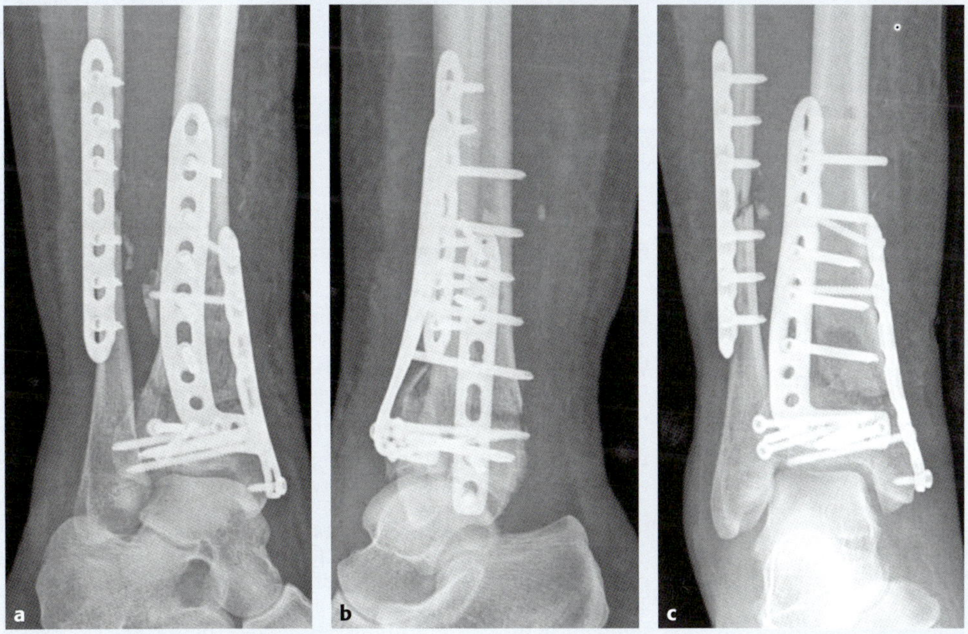

Fig 4.2-13a–c Immediate postoperative x-rays following the second intervention.

Analysis of failure and reflection

Open comminuted fractures of the tibial pilon should be treated in two phases. In this case, the main surgeon knew that it was a two-phase procedure and planned it accordingly. The objective of the first operation was, according to the surgeon's notes, to obtain length, rotation, and axis of the fibula without reducing the joint. The plan was that the articular part of the fracture would be treated at a later stage. During the procedure, the surgeon changed the plan and tried to complete the open reduction and internal fixation of the tibial pilon. She or he decided on a very risky tactic and used the medial wound as the approach. The reduction of the intraarticular tibial fragments was deficient.

The correct procedure would have been debridement of the wound and external fixation of the ankle joint. Given that the fibular fracture was simple, it would be an option (but not necessary) to carry out open reduction and internal fixation of the fibula. The wound was closed, but if this had not been possible, negative-pressure wound therapy (NPWT) (eg, vacuum-assisted wound closure [VAC]) could have been applied. After the initial treatment, a CT scan should have been performed and the definitive treatment planned.

This case shows that the adequate procedural sequence, including planning, is extremely important. Intraarticular fractures must be anatomically reduced and fixed. Changing the plan during the operation without a very good reason usually leads to a bad result.

Final outcome

The postoperative course was uneventful. The patient was discharged from hospital 9 days after the reintervention. The last outpatient examination took place 1 year after the operation. At that time, the patient was able to walk more than 5 km and the ankle had normal mobility (**Fig 4.2-14**).

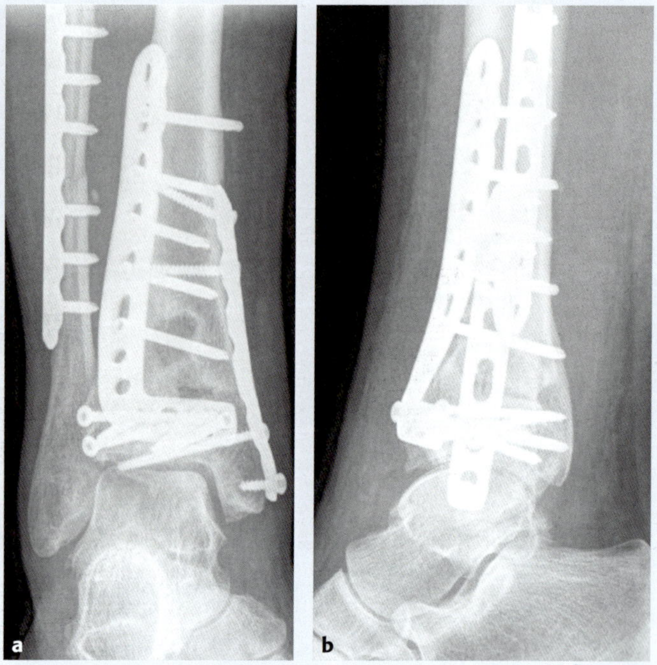

Fig 4.2-14a–b Postoperative x-rays at 1 year.

Key points to remember

- Teaching is essential and emphasizing preoperative planning is important.
- Careful preoperative planning must be performed for the proper execution of the osteosynthesis.
- Lack of preoperative planning is one of the greater influences on the results. Improvisation leads to bad results and an incorrect or insufficient preoperative plan can cause avoidable complications.
- Planning covers the pre-, intra- and postoperative periods.
- Different solutions with the use of different implants must always comply with the established principles.
- The injury must be fully understood to plan the treatment properly.

References and suggested reading

Buckley RE, Moran CG, Apivatthakakul T. *AO Principles of Fracture Management.* 3rd ed. Stuttgart New York: Thieme; 2017.
Gustilo RB, Mendoza RM, Williams DN. Problems in the management of type III (severe) open fractures: a new classification of type III open fractures. *J Trauma.* 1984 Aug;24(8):742–746.
Hak DJ, Rose J, Stahel PF. Preoperative planning in orthopedic trauma: benefits and contemporary uses. *Orthopedics.* 2010 Aug;33(8):581–584.
Hankemeier S, Gosling T, Richter M, et al. Computer-assisted analysis of lower limb geometry: higher intraobserver reliability compared to conventional method. *Comput Aided Surg.* 2006 Mar;11(2):81–86.
Holdsworth BJ. Planning in fracture surgery. In: Bunker TD, Colton CL, Webb JK, eds. *Frontiers in Fracture Surgery.* London: Martin Dunitz; 1989:1–15.
Mast J, Jakob R, Ganz R. *Planning and Reduction Technique in Fracture Surgery.* Berlin Heidelberg: Springer-Verlag; 1989.
Mast JW. Preoperative planning in the surgical correction of tibial nonunions and malunions. *Clin Orthop Relat Res.* 1983 Sep(178):26–30.
Porteous M, Bäuerle S. *Techniques and Principles for the Operating Room.* Stuttgart New York: Thieme; 2010.
Rüedi TP, Buckley RE, Moran CG. *AO Principles of Fracture Management.* 2nd ed. Stuttgart, New York: Thieme Verlag; 2007.
Rüedi TP, Murphy WM. *AO Principles of Fracture Management.* 1st ed. Stuttgart New York: Thieme; 2000.
Suero EM, Hufner T, Stubig T, et al. Use of a virtual 3D software for planning of tibial plateau fracture reconstruction. *Injury.* 2010 Jun;41(6):589–591.

4.3 Lack of anatomical knowledge

Joan Girós Torres, Roberto Rivero Sosa, J Miquel Sales Pérez, Juan Carlos Serfaty Soler, Miquel Videla Cés

All things acquire importance when we realize that they exist.

André Gide

To perform a surgical intervention on the musculoskeletal system, it is necessary to know not only the surgical approach but also the topographic anatomy of the region. Anatomical knowledge cannot be substituted by any other ability or with enthusiasm. Knowledge of bone anatomy and respect for the soft tissues is essential for the healing of fractures.

Traditionally, the approach to fractures was carried out through safe, generally large anatomical routes for exposure of the fractured region, respecting the neurovascular structures and splitting the soft tissues in a limited way to guarantee the manipulation of fragments. Both structures are essential for fracture healing and for normal limb function without sequelae. With study and better knowledge of the anatomy, internervous plane approaches have been developed to avoid damaging structures that would otherwise lead to often definitive functional deficits. Knowledge of the vascular tree that nourishes and drains the anatomy must be respected as one of the principles for osteosynthesis. Knowing the anatomy of the different bones, their stabilizing elements during mobilization, and their interrelations with other anatomical structures is fundamental for the surgeon to be able to reduce and stabilize the fracture and achieve functional recovery.

Today, due especially to the need for treatment of multifragmentary fractures, new approaches to certain anatomical regions have been described that enable them to be reduced and stabilized, often with implants designed specifically for the bone anatomy and the mechanical conditioning factors of the injury. When the implants are preshaped or have to be molded for application to a specific region of the bone, it is necessary to know the anatomical form of that bone. If the original form of the bone to be treated is not accurately known, including its cortical diaphyseal areas, metaphyseal porous bone areas, and articular areas with cartilaginous covering, then it is impossible to adapt the osteosynthesis to the bone in an adequate arrangement, let alone attempt to reconstruct its anatomy. No bone is straight and uniform, which has anatomical and biomechanical implications. The arrangement and adaptation of implants requires exact knowledge of the bone anatomy (ie, rotation, inclination, angulation of bone axes, etc).

Advances in biological and mechanical knowledge have favored minimally invasive interventions to preserve the biological process of the fracture site hematoma and respect the soft tissues of the limb (ie, biological fixation) preserving bone vascularization during surgery. During execution of the technique, the bone is partially accessed through small windows, without a view of the entire bone, with the aim of minimizing the damage to soft tissues during surgery. For this reason, it is necessary to be familiar with the location and three-dimensional (3D) arrangement of the anatomical structures and points of reference, thus conserving soft-tissue insertions and only exposing those areas necessary for insertion of the implants and carrying out those reduction maneuvers necessary. The limited field of vision requires the use of intraoperative imaging techniques. This involves advanced knowledge of the topographical anatomy of the region and bone surfaces, with detailed knowledge of the anatomy being even more necessary than when it is performed by direct visualization, given the possibility of causing hidden damage. An additional influencing factor during implant insertion is the surgeon's intellectual capacity for 3D construction.

Performing osteosynthesis requires a long learning process and deep knowledge of the anatomy, and this occupies a large percentage of surgeons' training. Under expert supervision, this training is carried out with practical exercises using plastic models and anatomical specimens to achieve perfect knowledge of the needs and difficulties in plate application, with painstaking planning of surgical approaches (**Fig 4.3-1**).

Lack of anatomical knowledge leads to failures during application of the osteosynthesis method which, as described, requires demanding knowledge and techniques.

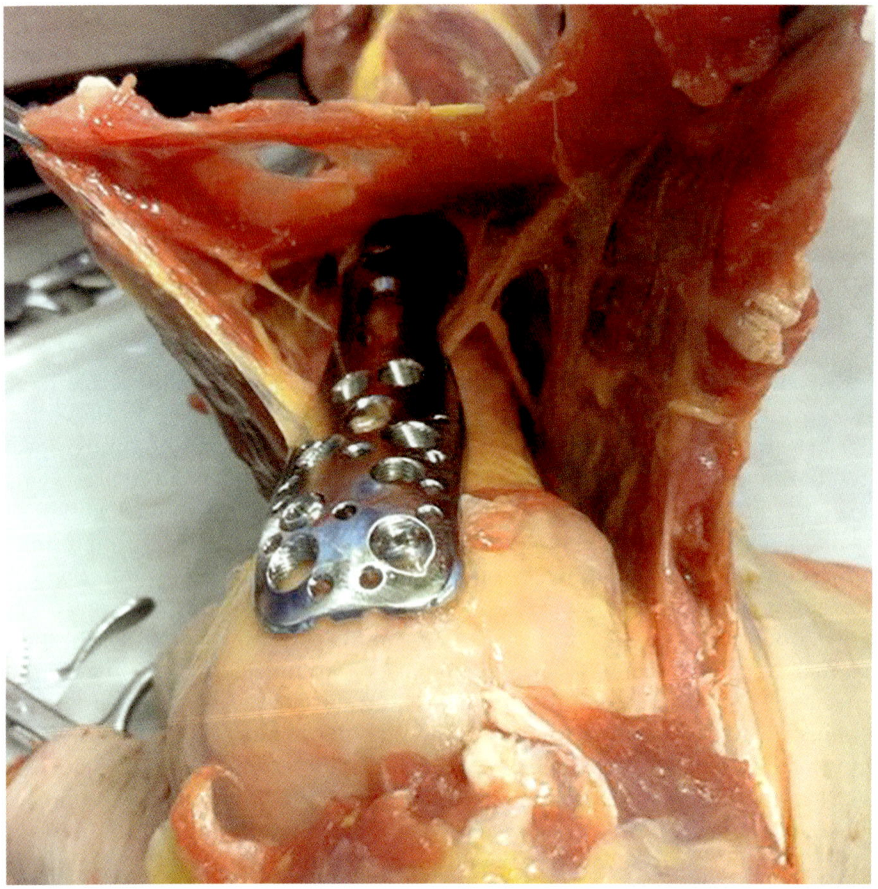

Fig 4.3-1 Anatomical specimen exercise for percutaneous placing of a PHILOS plate on the proximal humerus. After placing the plate, the anatomical window is opened to visualize the correct placement and the relationship with the neighboring anatomical structures. In this case it was clear that the circumflex nerve was injured during plate placement. Learning in practical workshops aims to avoid similar situations during clinical practice.

Case description

A 33-year-old man presented with a right ankle fracture (AO/OTA 44C2,4F2) after a motorbike accident (**Fig 4.3-2**).

Surgical intervention was required. Open reduction and osteosynthesis was performed using a one-third tubular plate for the fibula and two 4.0 mm cancellous screws for the internal malleolus. Posterior malleolar reduction was done with one posteroanterior 4.0 mm cancellous screw and the placement of one intertibiofibular screw. In the postoperative control x-rays there was evidence of 4 mm diastasis in the posterior malleolar fracture site, confirmed with a computed tomographic (CT) scan (**Fig 4.3-3**).

A reintervention was performed to remove the intertibiofibular and posteroanterior screws. Through a posterolateral approach the posterior malleolus was stabilized with two cancellous screws reoriented in line with the fracture pattern. Finally, the intertibiofibular screw was repositioned (**Fig 4.3-4**).

The patient was not allowed to bear weight during the postoperative period. When the intertibiofibular screw was removed in the seventh week, he started progressive partial weight bearing. During the rehabilitation period the patient was diagnosed with complex regional pain syndrome, receiving the recommended medical and rehabilitation treatment to deal with this complication.

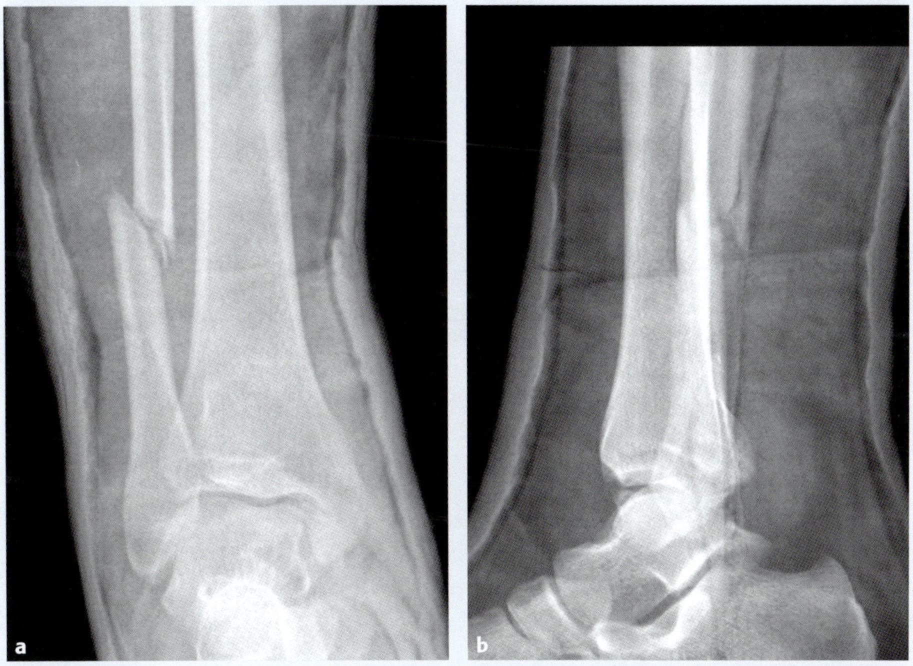

Fig 4.3-2a–b Preoperative x-rays showing the fracture of the right ankle in AP (**a**) and lateral (**b**) views.

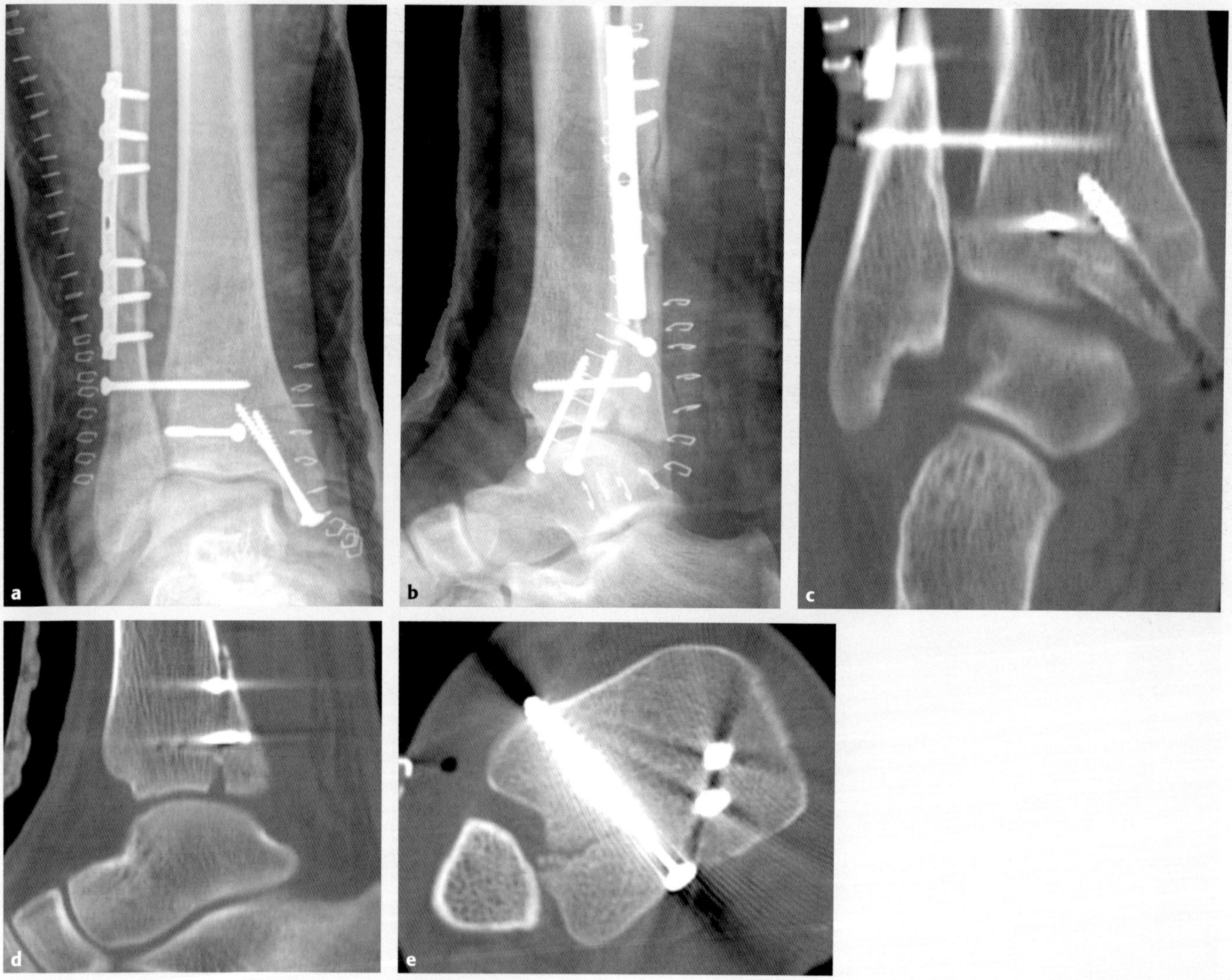

Fig 4.3-3a–e Postoperative x-ray and computed tomographic (CT) scan.

a–b Immediate postoperative x-ray. AP (**a**) and lateral (**b**) views showing diastasis of the posterior malleolus.

c–e Incorrect joint reduction. Postoperative CT scan in AP view showing joint incongruence (subsidence) on the articular surface of the tibia (**c**); CT scan showing diastasis of the posterior malleolus in lateral view (**d**); CT scan in coronal view (**e**) showing the failure in the orientation of the posteroanterior screw.

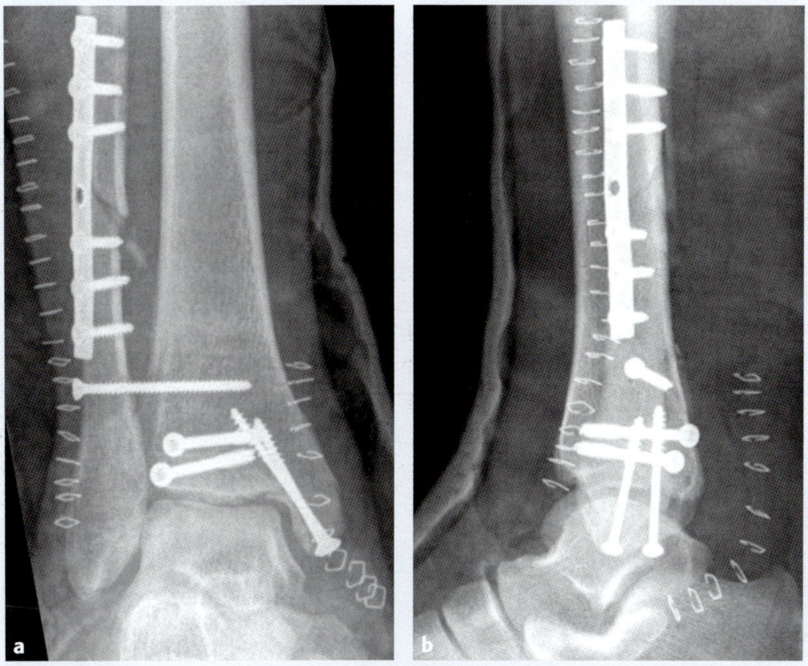

Fig 4.3-4a–b Immediate postoperative x-rays of the reintervention in AP (**a**) and lateral (**b**) views showing the anatomical reduction of the posterior malleolus.

Analysis of failure and reflection

This case failed because the surgeons knew neither how to correctly interpret the posterior malleolus fracture pattern nor how to perform the osteosynthesis without three-dimensional criteria. It would have been extremely useful to have a CT scan or more x-rays (ie, x-rays of internal/external rotation) before the surgical intervention to accurately plan the osteosynthesis. It is imperative that surgeons know all the fracture patterns to be able to perform adequate preoperative planning, geared towards resolving the injury in a single surgical intervention and avoid complications.

Final outcome

Eight months after the injury, fracture consolidation could be observed. The clinical outcome was with limited flexion and extension (ie, plantar flexion 20°, dorsal flexion 20°) (**Fig 4.3-5**).

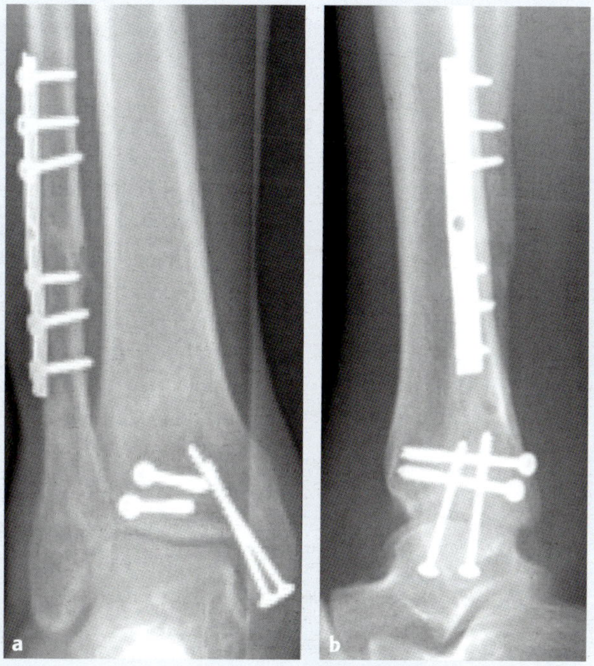

Fig 4.3-5a–b Control x-rays at 8 months after reintervention showing fracture union in AP (**a**) and lateral (**b**) views.

CASE 2

Case description

A 45-year-old woman had a motorbike accident, sustaining a sprain of the left foot with a Lisfranc fracture dislocation (AO/OTA 80D5) (**Fig 4.3-6**).

In the emergency department an attempt was made to reduce and fix the fracture dislocation with K-wires. Lack of knowledge of the pathological anatomy of the Lisfranc injury and inflammation of the foot made immobilization with a plaster cast necessary without having achieved reduction (**Fig 4.3-7**).

Forty-eight hours later, the inflammation was under control, so a reintervention was carried out opting for open reduction and internal fixation to achieve congruity in the Lisfranc joint. To resolve the dislocation, 4.5 mm cannulated screws were used (**Fig 4.3-8**).

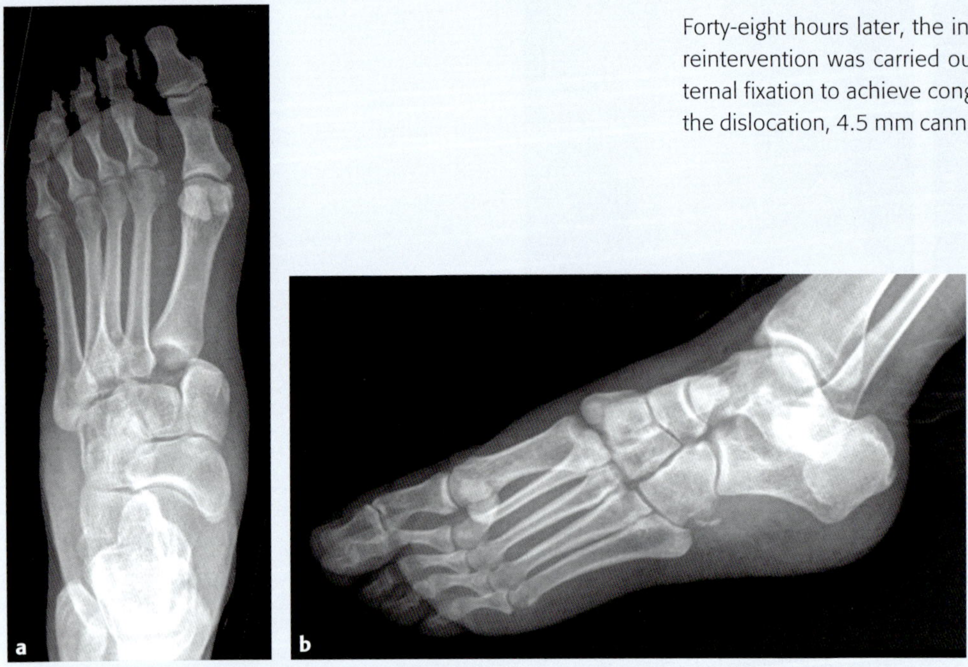

Fig 4.3-6a–b Preoperative x-rays of the Lisfranc fracture dislocation.

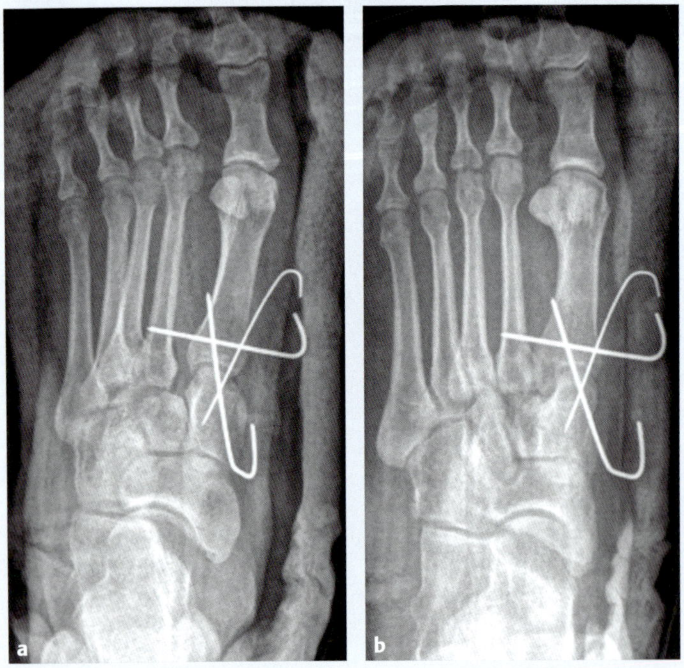

Fig 4.3-7a–b Immediate postoperative AP (**a**) and oblique (**b**) x-rays showing the lack of reduction of the Lisfranc fracture dislocation.

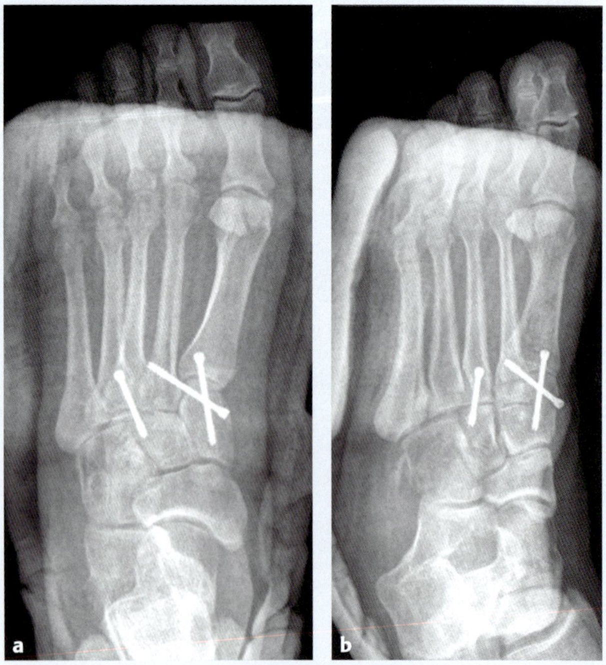

Fig 4.3-8a–b Immediate postoperative AP (**a**) and oblique (**b**) x-rays of the reduction and osteosynthesis achieved.

Analysis of failure and reflection

Despite having a good diagnosis with only emergency department x-rays, it is recommended that a CT scan is performed to acquire a good knowledge of the fracture anatomy and obtain a three-dimensional orientation, necessary for treating all fractures that feature articular involvement.

Surgeons must understand the fracture anatomy, classify it with the images available, and select the adequate surgical technique to approach, reduce, and repair the Lisfranc injury. Emergency treatment does not mean it can be done without sufficient knowledge, otherwise surgeons must seek the advice of an expert.

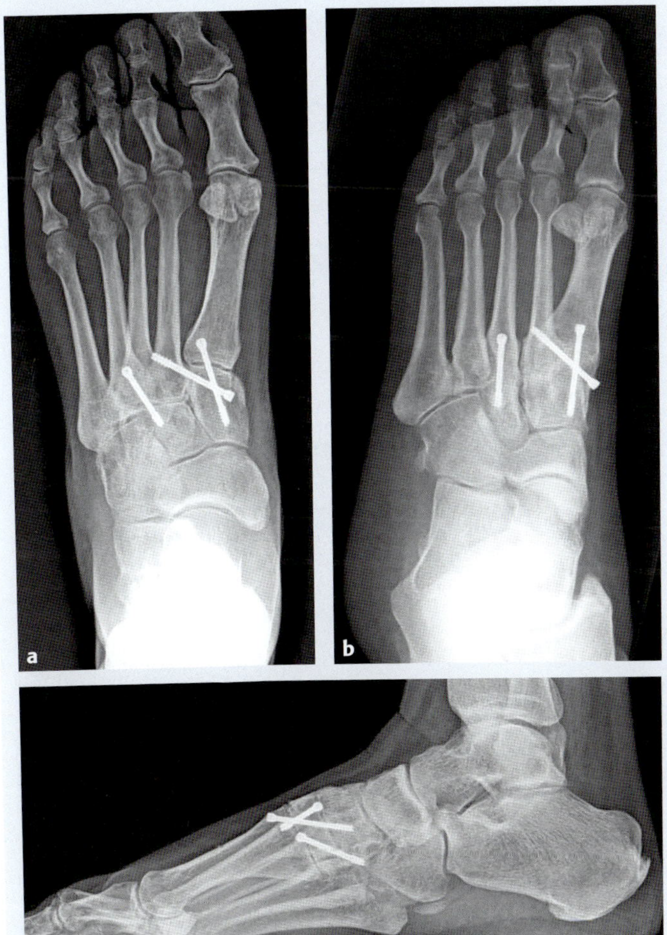

Fig 4.3-9a–c X-rays showing the final result after reduction of the Lisfranc fracture dislocation.

Final outcome

Immobilization was maintained with a plaster cast for 3 weeks and the patient was not allowed to bear weight for 6 weeks after surgery. She commenced rehabilitation sessions and was able to resume working at 14 weeks (**Fig 4.3-9**).

CASE 3

Case description

A 42-year-old man sustained a left diaphyseal clavicular fracture with comminution of the fracture site after a motorbike accident (AO/OTA 15.2C) (**Fig 4.3-10**).

He underwent surgical intervention. Open reduction and stabilization with an anatomically preshaped superior plate was performed (**Fig 4.3-11**). The fracture was immobilized with a Gilchrist bandage and rehabilitation started 3 weeks after the fracture. At the post-operative control 2 weeks after the intervention, the patient reported pain and functional impairment, which was confirmed by the control x-ray that showed failure of the osteosynthesis (**Fig 4.3-12**).

At 6 weeks, the control x-ray showed that the fracture had been displaced and the osteosynthesis had become completely unanchored (**Fig 4.3-13**). In the computed tomographic scan, a lack of fixation of the plate in the main proximal fragment was observed (**Fig 4.3-14**).

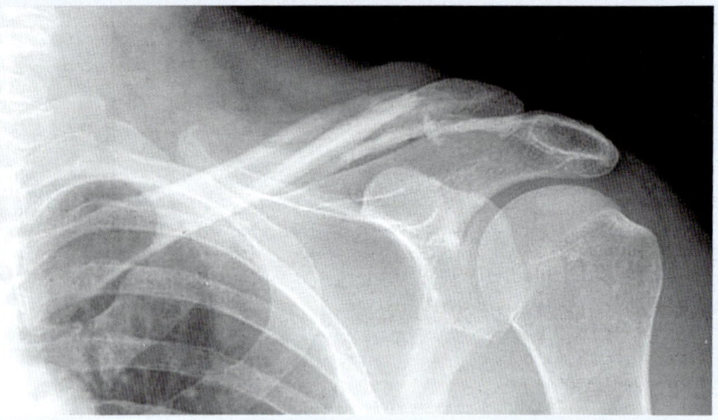

Fig 4.3-10 Preoperative x-ray of the fracture.

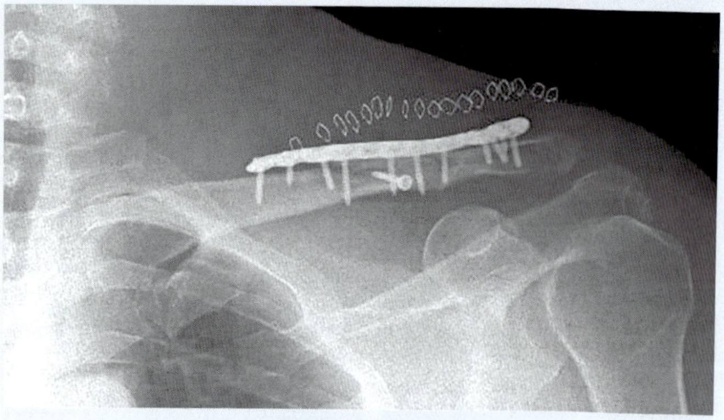

Fig 4.3-11 Immediate postoperative control x-ray.

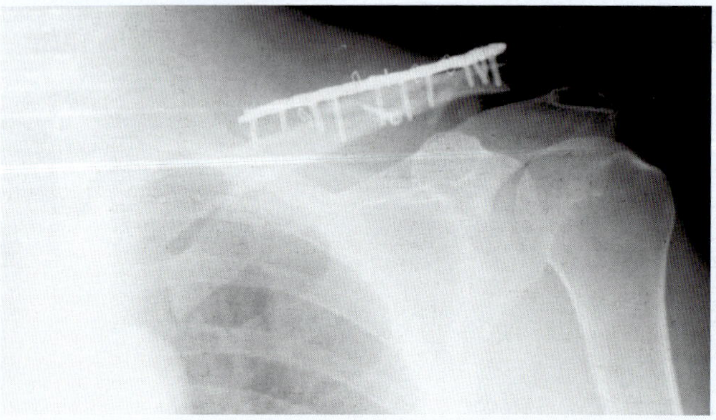

Fig 4.3-12 X-ray at 2 weeks showing failure of the osteosynthesis.

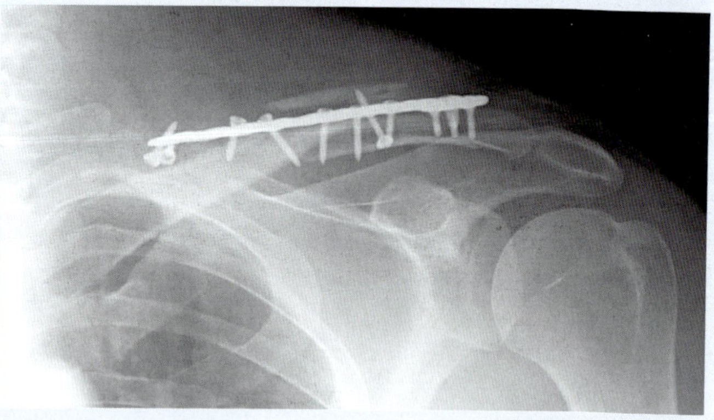

Fig 4.3-13 X-ray taken at 6 weeks showing the dislodged osteosynthesis implant.

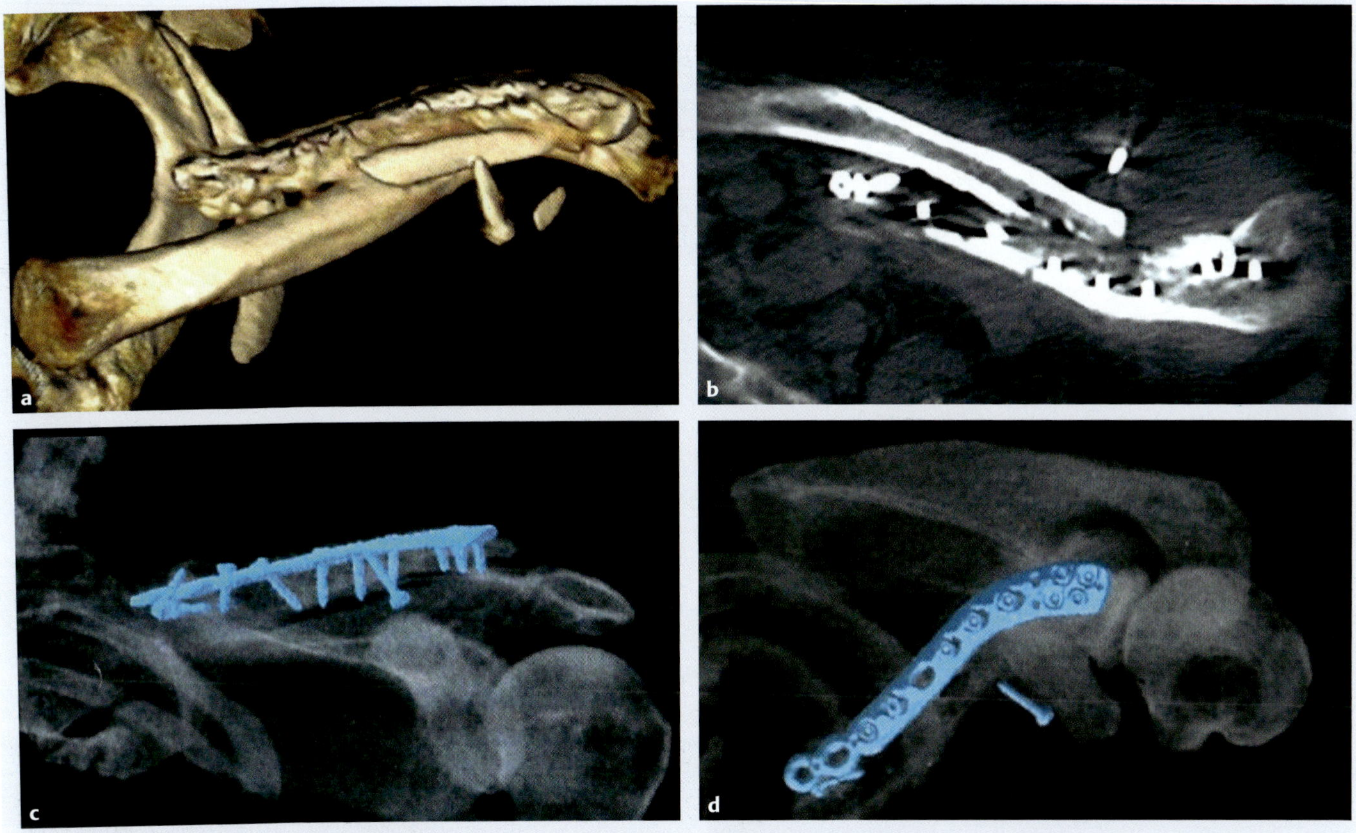

Fig 4.3-14a–d A 3D computed tomographic scan reconstruction of the osteosynthesis failure.

Analysis of failure and reflection

Preshaped clavicular plates today present different configurations depending on the superior or anterior position in which their application is planned. Furthermore, laterality (ie, whether plates are intended for the right or the left side) is also a configuration to bear in mind (**Fig 4.3-15**).

In the opinion of many surgeons, perfect adaptation of these plates to the clavicle is difficult to achieve and depends on the anatomy and size of the bone, the type of fracture, and its location; sometimes the application is also complicated.

This case shows how perfect open reduction has not been achieved despite the extensive exposure of the fracture site. The fixation of the screws in the proximal fragment was insufficient and can be attributed to a lack of anatomical knowledge, which was the principal error.

Final outcome

A new intervention was necessary to remove the osteosynthesis material and achieve a stabilized anatomical reduction with a new anatomically preshaped plate (**Fig 4.3-16**).

Fixation of the proximal area was achieved by osteosynthesis with plate anchorage in the cortices of both main fragments. At the last control 1 year following the reintervention, the clavicle showed a restored anatomy with fracture union and clinically, the patient presented no sequelae (**Fig 4.3-17**).

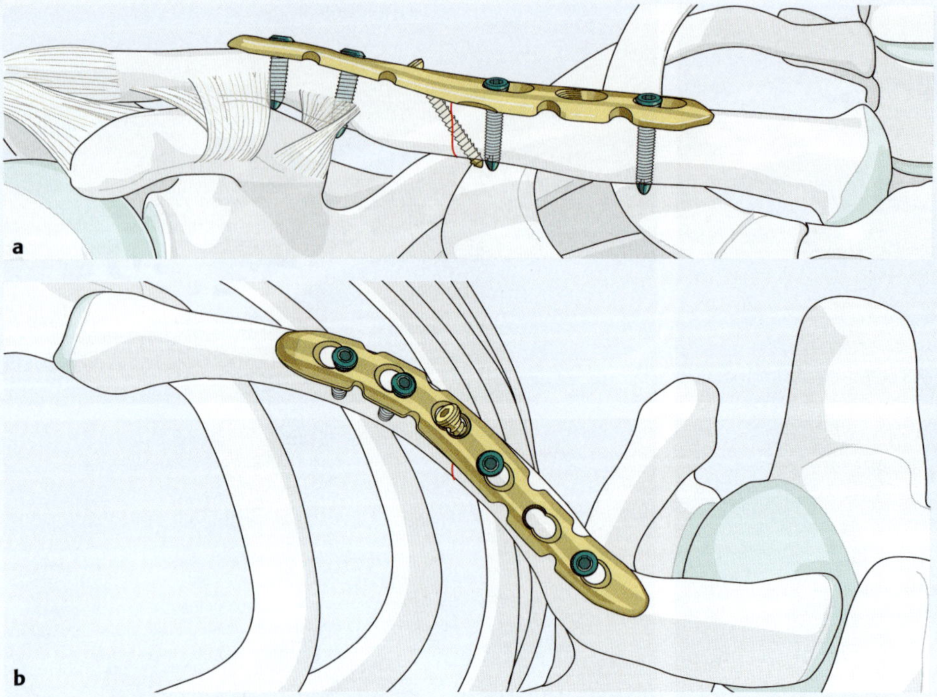

Fig 4.3-15a–b Preshaped clavicular plates. Although the plates can be molded and formed into their final shape with a hand press, they will adapt to fit the anatomical form of the clavicle, which varies depending on position and laterality.

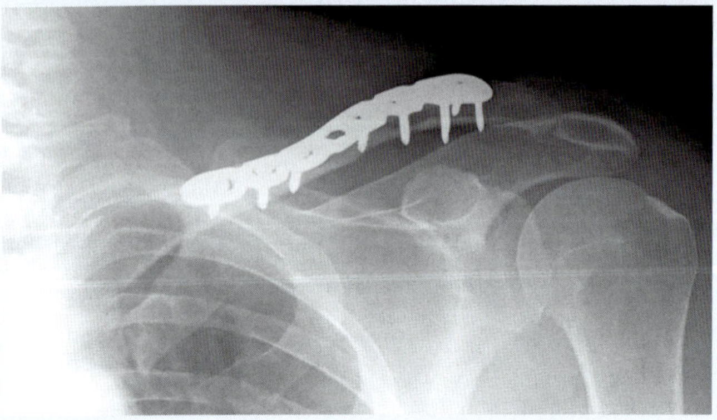

Fig 4.3-16 Postoperative control x-ray following reintervention.

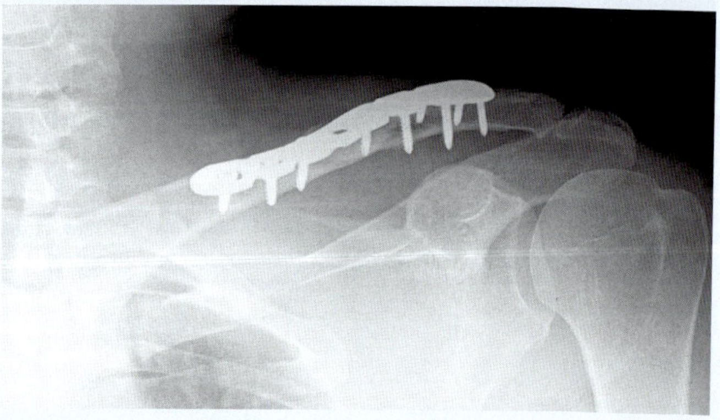

Fig 4.3-17 X-ray taken 1 year after the reintervention.

Key points to remember

- Knowledge of bone anatomy and its relationship with other anatomical structures as well as respect for soft tissues are essential for fracture healing.
- The arrangement and adaptation of the implants requires precise knowledge of both the topographical anatomy of the region and of the bone surfaces.
- The surgeon's skills to render and ability to interpret 3D reconstruction are important.
- Osteosynthesis requires a deep knowledge of the anatomy, and ability and experience to perform the demanding techniques.
- Urgent treatment does not mean performing surgery without sufficient anatomical knowledge.

References and suggested reading

Hoppenfeld S, deBoer P, Buckley R. *Surgical Exposures in Orthopedics: the Anatomic Approach.* Philadelphia: Lippincott Williams & Wilkins; 2016.

Miller MD, Chhabra AB, Hurwitz SR, et al. *Orthopaedic Surgical Approaches.* Philadelphia: Saunders Elsevier; 2008.

Rüedi TP, von Hochstetter AHC, Schlumpf R. *Surgical Approaches for Internal Fixation.* Berlin Heidelberg: Springer-Verlag; 1984.

Sales JM, Videla M, Forcada P, et al. *Atlas de Osteosíntesis. Fracturas de los huesos largos. Vias de acceso quirúrgico.* 2nd ed. Barcelona: Elsevier Masson; 2009.

4.4 Insufficient asepsis protocols

Matej Cimerman, Joan Girós Torres, Roberto Rivero Sosa, J Miquel Sales Pérez, Bostjan Sluga, Miquel Videla Cés

It is hard to believe how difficult it is to consider inevitable things that have already happened.

Stendhal

The presence of infection stands out above all other complications in the practice of osteosynthesis. The presence of vascular and soft-tissue alterations in addition to the trauma and greater susceptibility of the bone tissue to infection by bacterial contamination may result in serious sequelae, lengthening the hospital stay, and considerably increasing the financial and social costs for invalidity. Infection is the worst complication that can occur in the surgical treatment of a fracture. For the patient it is catastrophic and means almost certain sequelae and consequences. The presence of infection in the postoperative period of patients affected by fracture means the method of fixation has failed. Occasionally, even less aggressive infections cause nonunion and increased suffering for the patient.

Treatment of infection in a fracture that has been operated on is difficult to resolve and has an uncertain prognosis. This often leads to several interventions with repeated debridements, resection of bone areas and soft tissues, extraction of the osteosynthesis material to eliminate the layer of biofilm formed by microbial aggregates that cover the implants and prevent antibiotics from working, the placing of spacers with antibiotics, and reoperations for rescue once the infection has subsided. Sometimes this long path does not lead to healing and leaves permanent sequelae that require repeated antibiotic treatments and in extreme cases amputation. The best treatment for infection is prevention. The statement "it is preferable to suffer a closed pseudarthrosis than a perfect osteosynthesis that is infected" reflects the importance of this complication.

The main risk factors usually occur during the perioperative period; therefore, the prevention measures are concentrated in this period. Less frequently, infection may arise through postoperative contamination by the patient through the blood or skin or following new surgeries in the area.

Risk factors that may influence the appearance of infections may be related to the patient (eg, cutaneous flora, carrier of resistant germs, underlying diseases, preexisting infection, polytrauma) and/or factors related to the treatment environment (eg, operating room rules, air and water quality, surgical team hygiene, hand washing, adequate intravenous antibiotic prophylaxis, preparation of the patient and of the material). Awareness of these risk factors is paramount to detecting them and acting to diminish the risk of infection. The adherence to valid protocols in patient preparation, the correct actions in the operating room and during the hospital stay are fundamental measures that must be respected to avoid increase in infection rates. Noncompliance with the regulations and protocols increases the likelihood of infection in the postoperative period.

Contamination may cause infection depending on its level, the virulence of the germs, and the patient's resistance. Contamination can be reduced with prevention, hygiene, and antibiotic prophylaxis. During the preoperative period it is important to detect those factors that may facilitate contamination and subsequent infection, whether localized or due to preexisting diseases (eg, diabetes, corticoid therapy, obesity, smoking, chronic immunosuppressive medication, malnutrition, hematological diseases, liver diseases). Opportune measures must be taken to reduce risks of contamination in the perioperative period (eg, preoperative hygiene and proper skin preparation).

The operating room, as an environment for the definitive treatment of fractures, must fulfil certain established conditions, including the circulation of clean and used materials, design and set-up of the operating room, cleaning, air and ventilation control, water control, movement of hospital personnel and patient, temperature and humidity control, and treatment of the instruments.

The surgical team and personnel in the operating room must be well disciplined and follow the protocols that exist to limit factors that may facilitate infection. For example, it is necessary to follow rigorous asepsis protocol to reduce the possibility of infection and its consequences during surgery. The importance of the correct preparation of instrument tables, care in the donning of gowns and gloves of the entire surgical team, the preparation of the operating area in a convenient way is widely known. Despite this, the authors occasionally see that basic operating room rules are relaxed, such as access and circulation of personnel, and that distances to the surgical area (ie, instrument tables, etc) are not respected. Asepsis conditions must be maximized because if not, an infection can lead to the total failure of the operative procedure and to permanent sequelae. While the percentages of infection in orthopedic surgery and traumatology are low, the effects are catastrophic for patients, for the healthcare team, and for the social economy (eg, enterprises, organizations, and insurance providers). Contamination occurs via direct contact with surgical instruments and the contaminated hands of the surgical team where particles loaded with environmental germs are deposited. Prolonged surgical exposure brings with it increased risk of contamination by such germs. The correct cutaneous preparation of the patient especially in the operating room is crucial to avoid the colonization of tissues by germs that under normal conditions do not cross the cutaneous barrier.

A surgical technique that does not respect the soft tissues and the vascularization of the bone fragments is also a factor that increases the risk of infection and its consequences. The surgical technique and perioperative care of the soft tissues is fundamental for respecting the tissues and not increasing necrosis and devascularization, which are breeding grounds for the germs that cause infection.

Open fractures are an exception to the low percentages of infection in planned surgery and the surgery of fractures without traumatic exposure of soft tissues (closed fracture fixation). Following treatment protocols with physical asepsis measures and antibiotic treatments reduces the incidence of infection and expands the indications to perform definitive emergency surgery. In cases of open fractures, the situation becomes complicated depending on the size of the wounds and the attrition of the soft tissues, requiring exhaustive debridement and cleaning, early stabilization of the fracture, and correct coverage of the soft tissues and closure of the wound, if possible. The collection of samples after debridement and wound cleaning during surgery can help subsequent evaluation of the decontamination obtained and guide surgeons regarding the different pathogenic agents that exist and their response to treatment with different antibiotics. Antibiotic treatment following hospital protocols should begin as soon as possible.

In polytrauma patients, the situation becomes more difficult because of the other associated injuries (eg, vascular, visceral) and additional invasive procedures for resuscitation or stabilization. This, together with the body's response mechanisms to trauma and preexisting diseases (eg, diabetes, urinary infections), increases the seriousness of these patients' situations and the possibility of infection. These polytrauma patients should be treated emergently for damage control when it is not possible to carry out definitive treatment, stabilizing fractures with external fixation. The initial treatment must be performed to reduce the likelihood of infectious complications: debriding hematomas and devascularized tissues and stabilizing the bone injury that would otherwise increase the edema and likelihood of infection. The possibility of occult lesions must also be considered in the first examinations which may later worsen the prognosis.

Case description

A 60-year-old man without prior relevant medical conditions fell on his left foot from a 2 m high wall and sustained a Gustilo type II fracture of the distal tibia and fibula (AO/OTA 43C2,4F2B) (**Fig 4.4-1**).

The patient was first treated in the emergency department of a local hospital while he was on holiday. The wound was cleaned, debrided, and the fracture aligned and immobilized with a plaster cast. After 48 hours he was transferred to another hospital where the wound was again debrided on the medial surface of the ankle and the first external fixator was applied (**Fig 4.4-2**). No attempt was made to reduce the fibular fracture, which resulted in worsening of the distal tibial fracture alignment. The valgus deformity caused further damage to the skin wound at the fracture level (**Fig 4.4-3**). A protocol of empirical treatment with antibiotics was initiated.

Three weeks later the patient underwent surgical revision. Internal fixation was performed on the fibula, which allowed the tibial fracture to be aligned and the pressure on the wound area to be reduced (**Fig 4.4-4**).

At 4 months, the patient presented with a fistula. Secretion cultures were negative, but bone scintigraphy showed septic pseudarthrosis (**Fig 4.4-5**).

It was planned to treat the septic pseudarthrosis with a resection of the infected area and restoration of the bone defect using an induced membrane technique (Masquelet technique) **[Giannoudis et al, 2016]**. During the first stage of the Masquelet technique, a fistulectomy was performed. The 4 cm resection of the tibia at the level of the infected pseudarthrosis area was filled with a gentamicin- and vancomycin-loaded polymethylmethacrylate (PMMA) spacer (**Fig 4.4-6a**). The cutaneous defect was covered with a reverse sural flap and the external fixator was put back in place (**Fig 4.4-6b–e**).

After 10 weeks, the sural flap had become integrated, which allowed the second stage of the Masquelet technique to be performed: removal of the antibiotic spacer, curettage of the ends of the bone defect, and filling with autogenous graft obtained from the iliac crest and an osteoinductive bone graft substance and mesenchymal cell aspirate (**Fig 4.4-7a**). The osteosynthesis was performed using a medial locking compression plate for the distal tibia (**Fig 4.4-7b**).

Nonweight bearing with active mobilization of the ankle and foot was implemented, with progressive partial weight bearing from the fourth month. At 12 months, the patient was walking without crutches and from 18 months resumed snowshoeing.

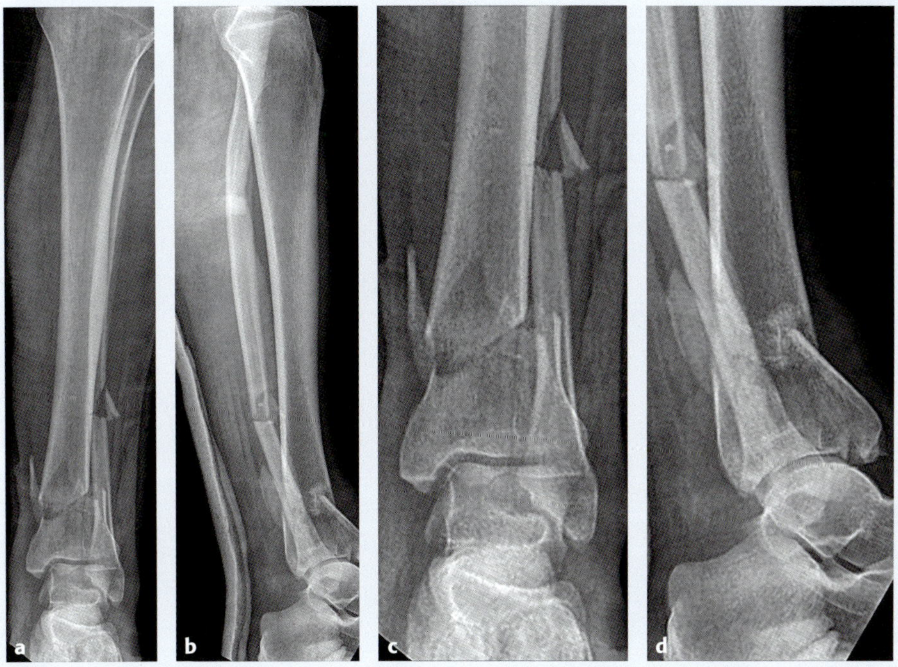

Fig 4.4-1a–d Preoperative x-rays.
a–b AP (**a**) and lateral (**b**) views of the Gustilo type II fracture of the distal tibia and fibula.
c–d X-rays of the ankle in AP (**c**) and lateral (**d**) views of the Gustilo type II fracture of the distal tibia and fibula.

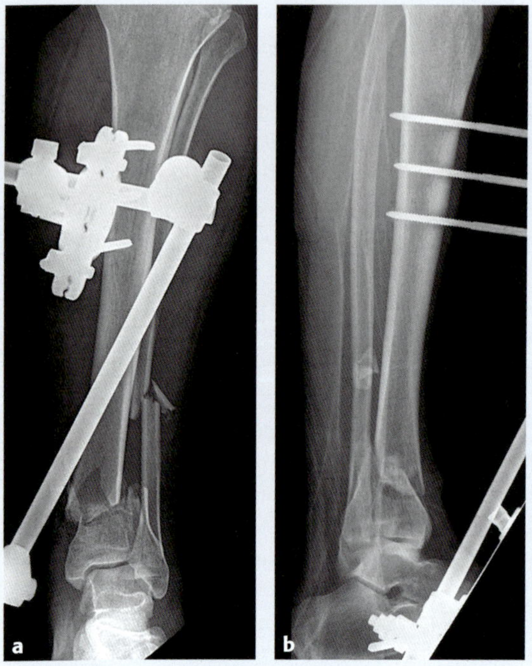

Fig 4.4-2a–b Postoperative x-rays of the first surgery that involved debridement and application of the external fixator, showing an incorrect reduction of the distal tibial fracture that caused a valgus deformity. In this first surgery the fibula was not fixed.

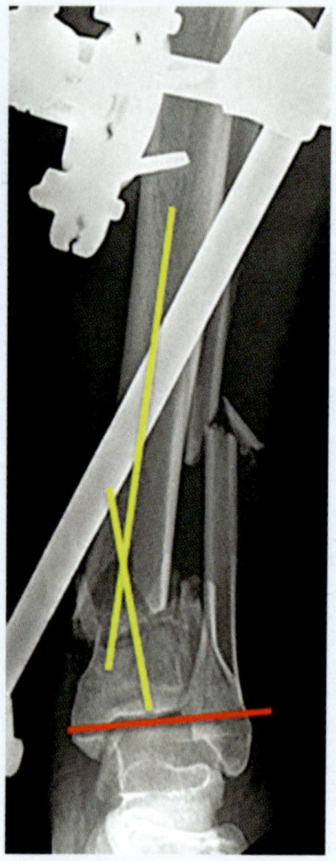

Fig 4.4-3 Detail of the poor valgus alignment of the distal tibia, which led to an increase in tension and pressure sore on the medial side of the wound.

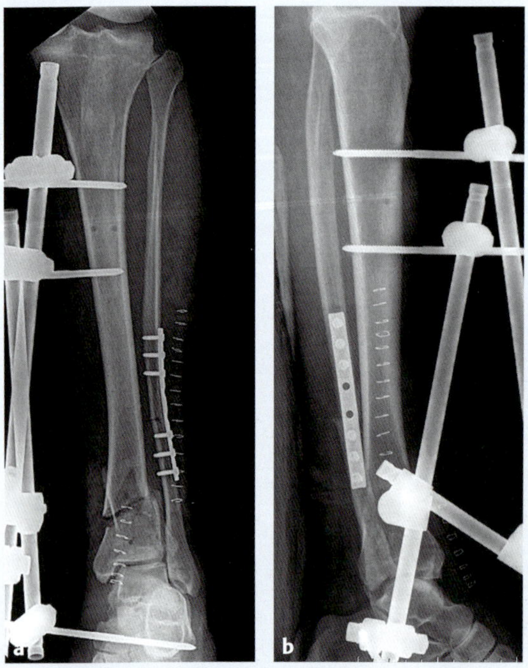

Fig 4.4-4a–b A second surgical intervention with a new debridement of the medial wound was performed along with osteosynthesis of the fibula, which was essential for aligning the tibial fracture.

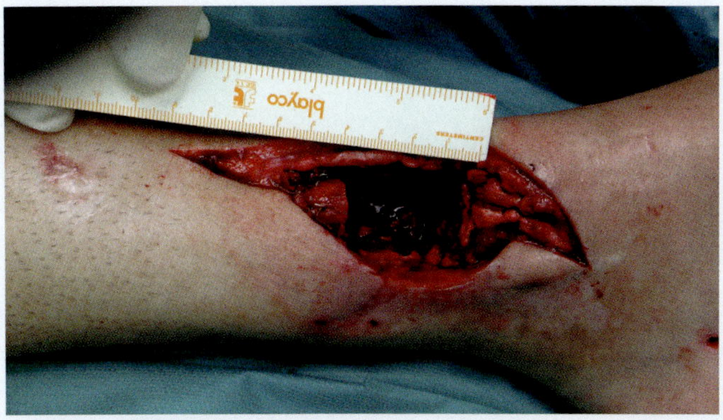

Fig 4.4-5 Major bone and coverage defect following the fistulectomy and the resection of the infected pseudarthrosis site in the first-stage Masquelet technique.

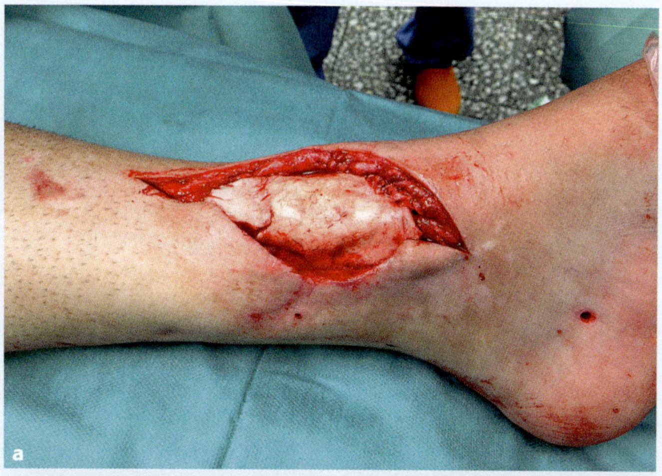

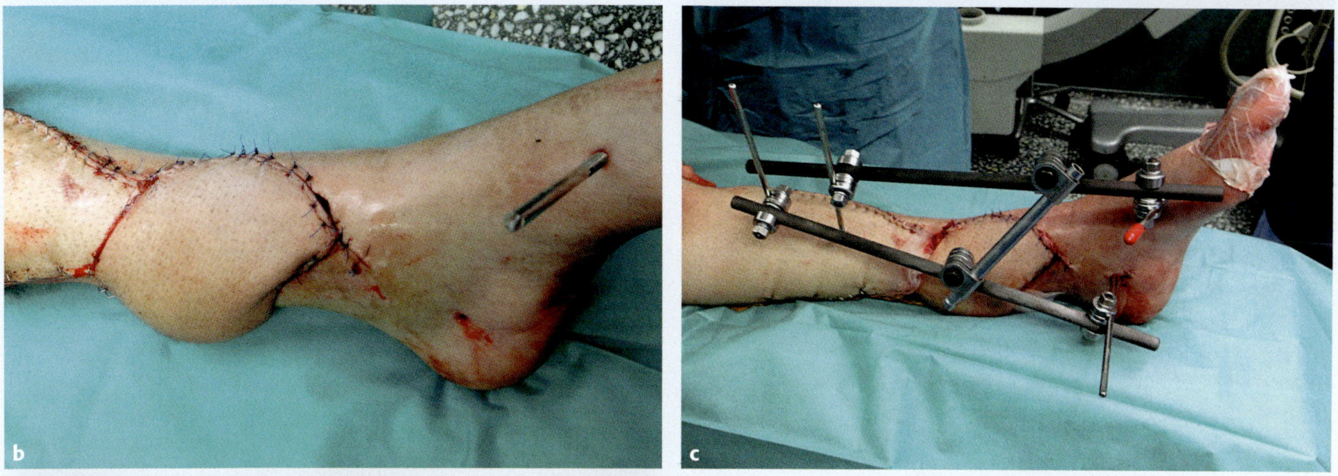

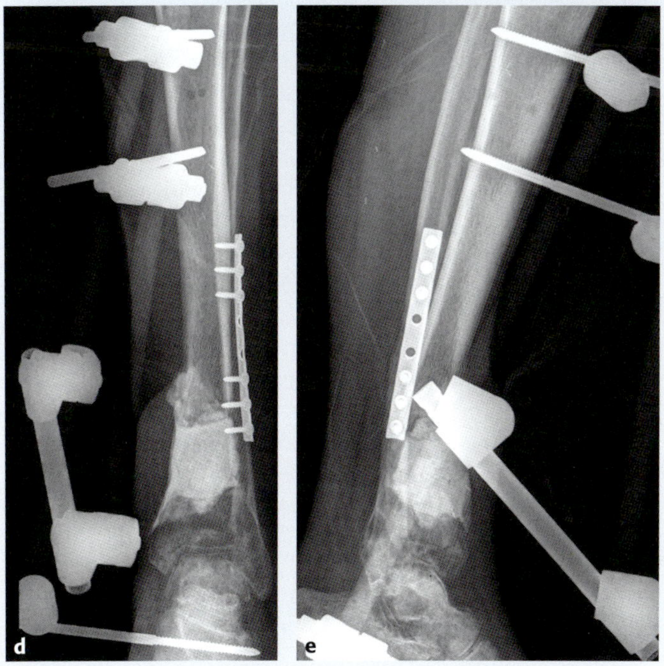

Fig 4.4-6a–e Clinical photographs and x-rays of the surgical procedure.

- **a** Filling the resection defect with a gentamicin and vancomycin-loaded polymethylmethacrylate spacer.
- **b** Appearance of the reverse sural flap that was used as coverage of the bone defect and antibiotic spacer.
- **c** Repositioning of the external fixator as the final step of the first-stage Masquelet technique.
- **d–e** X-rays 9 weeks into the first Masquelet stage showing the stability of the spacer, the tolerance of the fixator, and the tolerance of the fixator given the absence of lysis on the anchorage of the pins.

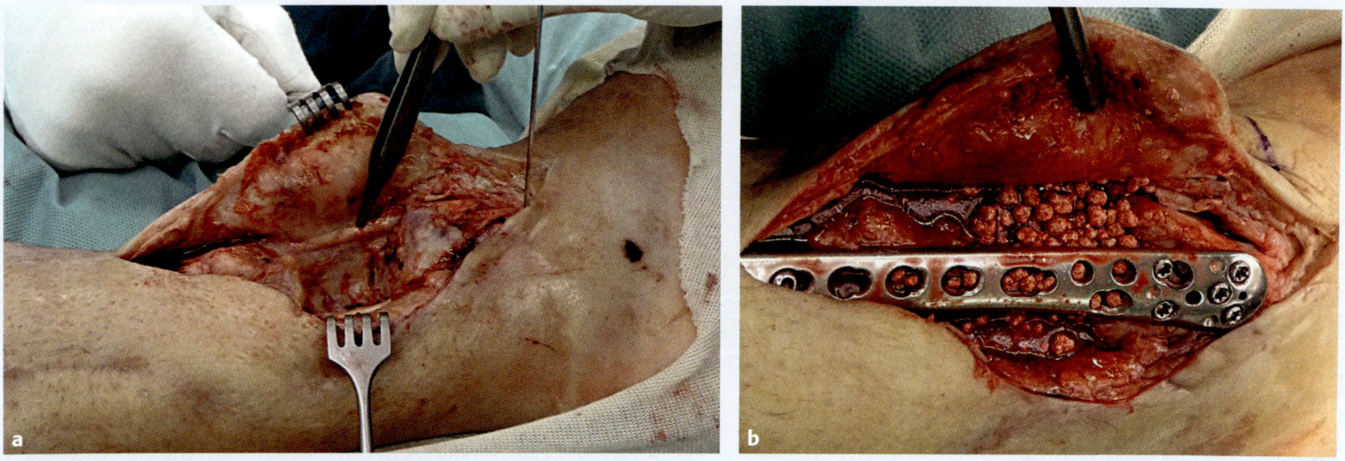

Fig 4.4-7a–b Second-stage of the Masquelet technique.
a The synovial pseudarthrosis after the removal of the antibiotic spacer.
b The cavity filled with autogenous graft and osteoinductive and osteoconductive granules. A medial locking compression plate was used for the distal tibia before closure of the fasciocutaneous flap.

Analysis of failure and reflection

The cleaning of the open fracture wound and immobilization with a plaster cast seems to be neither a state-of-the-art nor an adequate treatment for the soft tissues, although in this case the fracture alignment was satisfactory.

Treating an open fracture does not mean just applying an external fixator. It is necessary to align and reduce the fracture in the best way possible. At the surgical check-up carried out 48 hours after the accident, priority was given to the application of the external fixator. The fracture showed poor reduction with a valgus deviation, revealing a much worse result than with the plaster cast.

In a Gustilo type II fracture [Gustilo et al, 1984], if the state of the soft tissues, the swelling, and edema allow, there is the possibility of performing a definitive fracture treatment, above all in articular fractures where the restitution of the articular surface is essential.

After the first phase of controlling the soft tissues, definitive treatment of the intraarticular tibial pilon fracture should have been considered. In the consecutive stages of treatment of tibial pilon fractures, it is recommended in the first stage to perform synthesis of the fibula to avoid shortening. Once the soft tissues permit safe surgical access, the medial component of the fracture is reconstructed in a second surgical stage (**Fig 4.4-8**) [Sirkin et al, 2004].

Compromised soft tissues and an infection with fistula are some of the most serious and challenging complications in the treatment of distal tibial fractures. The deficient management of the soft tissues increases the risk of problems and of wound dehiscence and osteomyelitis.

It seems that delays in decision making, both at the time of the emergency and at the follow-up visit, were responsible for the subsequent treatment involving four surgical interventions over more than 3 years.

When treating infected pseudarthrosis, surgeons may consider the possibility of performing a bone transport, autogenous grafting with vascularized fibula, and the Masquelet technique of induced membrane. The decision to use the induced membrane technique was made to try to shorten the external fixation period, as this allowed for an osteosynthesis with a correct fasciocutaneous coverage following the second surgical stage of the Masquelet technique (**Fig 4.4-9**).

Final outcome

The bone infection healed and the fracture united, leading to a good axis of the leg. The functionality of the ankle was restored and the patient regained his preinjury level of walking 1 year after the rescue surgery and returned to his sports activities 3 years after the primary injury (**Fig 4.4-10**).

The moderate residual functional deficit in the range of motion of the ankle is due to the union in hyperextension of the distal metaphysis of the tibia. However, this has not had any consequences in terms of pain or clinical deformity, except for the aesthetic deficit in the donor area and in the recipient site of the reverse sural fasciocutaneous flap.

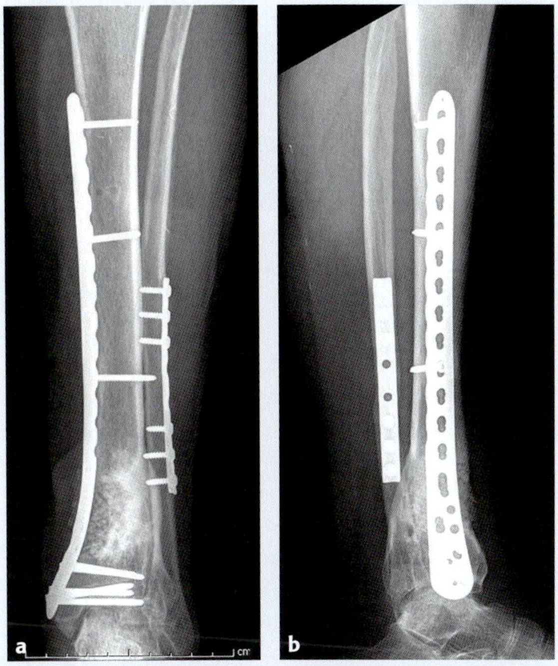

Fig 4.4-8a–b X-rays at 2.5 years after the second-stage Masquelet technique showing the union of the bone defect.

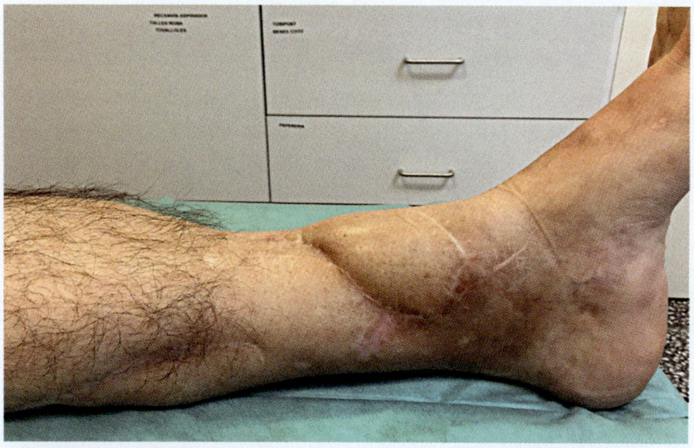

Fig 4.4-9 Appearance of the reverse sural fasciocutaneous flap at 2.5 years after the second stage of the Masquelet technique.

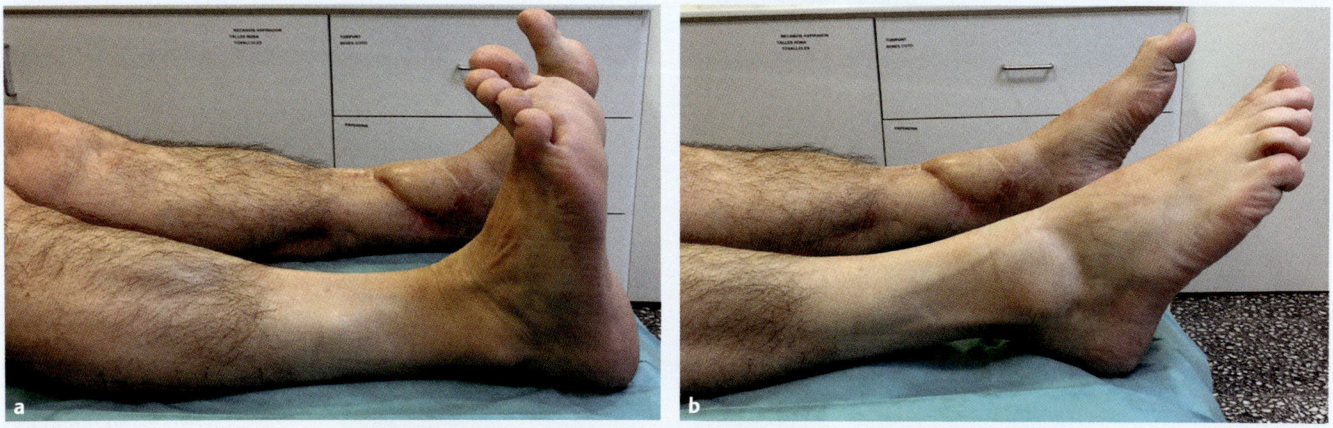

Fig 4.4-10a–b The patient shows a satisfactory range of motion and function of the left ankle at 2.5 years after the second stage of the Masquelet technique (3 years after the primary injury).

CASE 2

Case description

An 84-year-old woman with a history of penicillin allergy, insulin-dependent diabetes, high blood pressure, obesity, and hemiparesis secondary to stroke with significant functional limitation tripped and fell at home (low-energy trauma). She presented with the inability to walk as well as shortening and marked external rotation of the lower right limb. The x-rays taken in the emergency department showed a pertrochanteric fracture (AO/OTA 31A2) (**Fig 4.4-11**).

A reduction was planned with internal fixation with a plate and a sliding screw (ie, dynamic hip screw [DHS]). The surgery was performed 72 hours after hospitalization. The postoperative control x-rays showed a correct reduction of the fracture, with the head and neck screw located in a center-center position on the femoral neck with a tip-apex distance at the femoral head close to the limit of 2.5 cm (**Fig 4.4-12**).

Two weeks after surgery, the patient had another fall and presented with a dehiscence of the surgical wound with serosanguineous secretion. Cultures were taken with abundant colonies of *Citrobacter koseri, Streptococcus agalactiae, Escherichia coli,* and *Proteus mirabilis* and isolated. Antibiotic therapy began in accordance with the antibiogram and three surgical cleanings were performed without removing the implant. In the control x-rays taken at 6 weeks, a medial displacement of the diaphysis was evident, without evidence of lysis around the implant (**Fig 4.4-13**).

Although her surgical wound evolved towards scar formation, her C-reactive protein levels remained high, and at 3 months she presented with an implant cut-out in the femoral head of probable septic etiology (**Fig 4.4-14a–b**). At that point it was decided to remove the osteosynthesis material, carry out surgical cleaning and insert gentamicin beads as a spacer (**Fig 4.4-14c**).

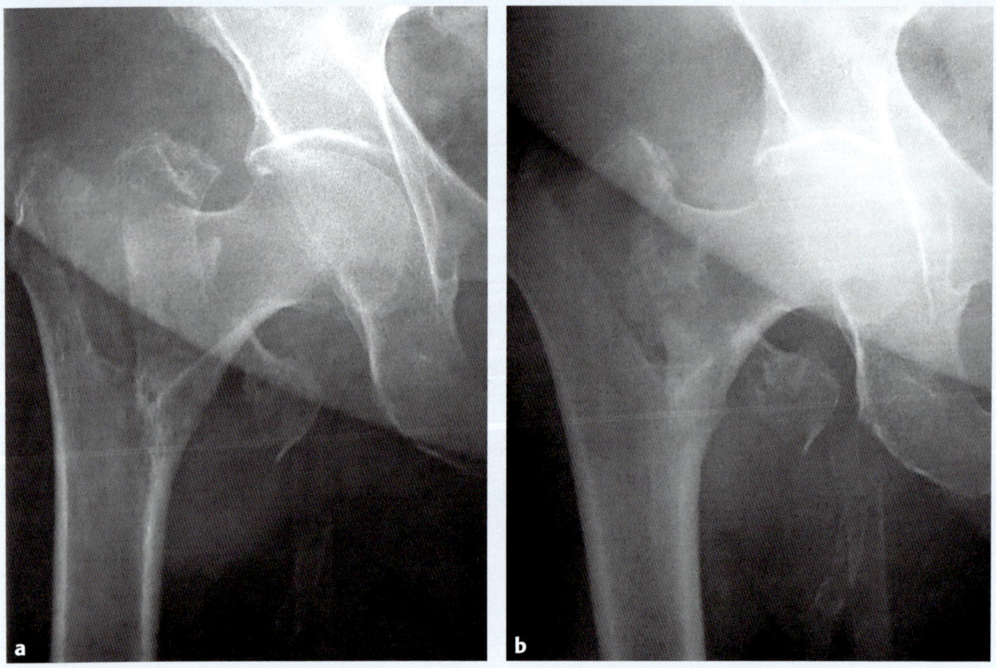

Fig 4.4-11a–b Preoperative x-rays of the extraarticular multifragmentary pertrochanteric fracture. The lesser trochanter fragment is small and the greater trochanter appears to be intact.

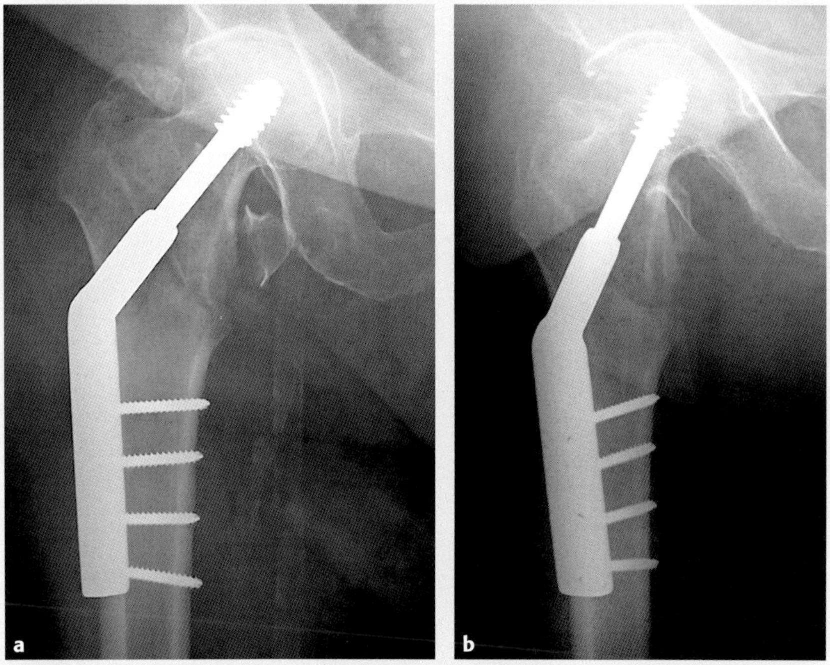

Fig 4.4-12a–b Postoperative x-rays. The fracture remains reduced, with the head and neck screw centered in the neck region of the femoral head and with a tip-apex distance at the femoral head of approximately 2.5 cm.

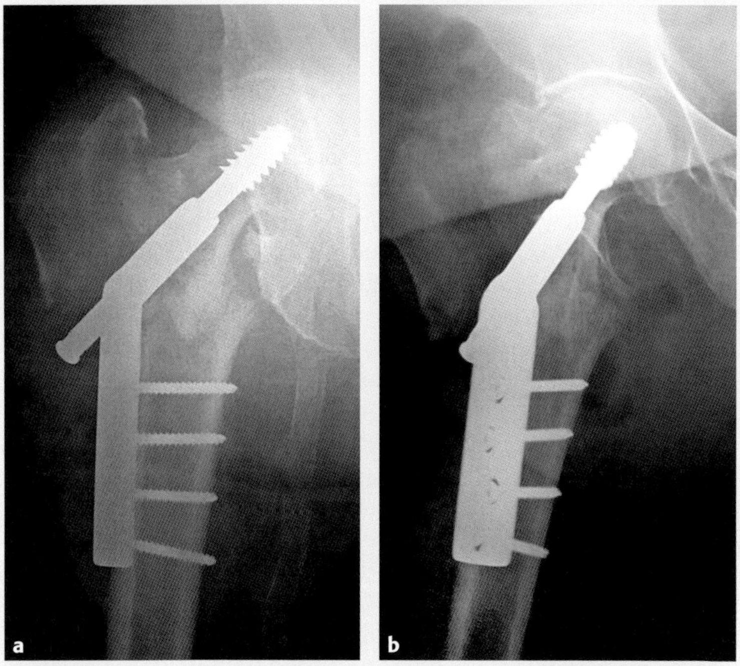

Fig 4.4-13a–b X-rays at 6 weeks showing a major dynamization of the sliding screw with medial displacement of the femoral axis and a displaced fracture of the greater trochanter. No lysis is observed around the implant nor loss of anchorage of the screws.

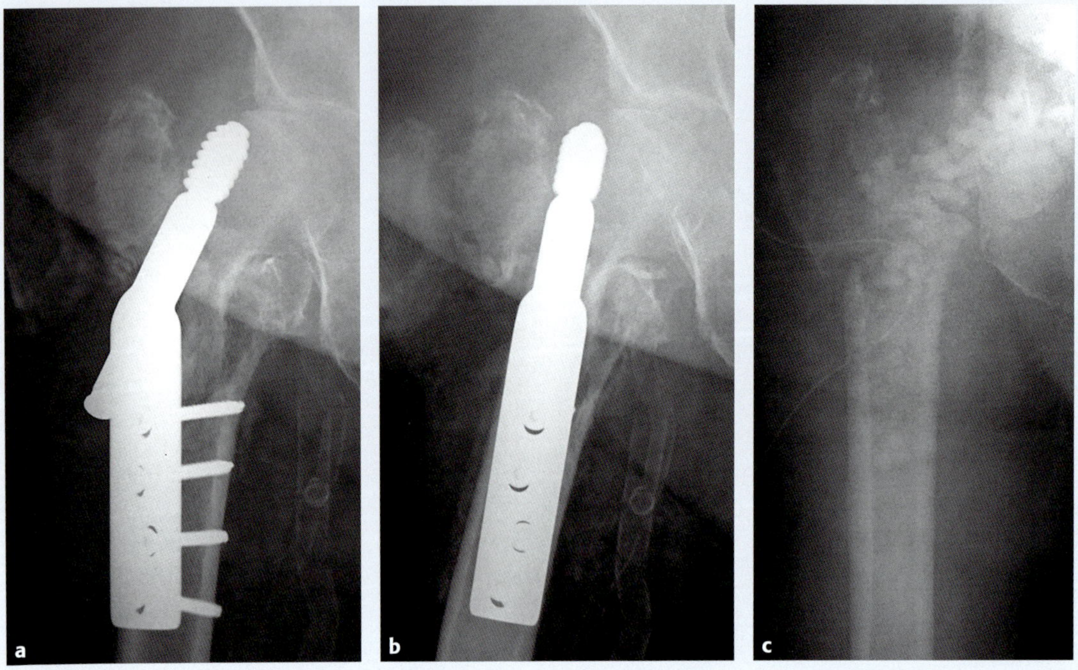

Fig 4.4-14a–c X-rays of the implant cut-out and after the extraction of osteosynthesis material.
a–b X-rays showing the cut-out in the femoral head at 3 months postfracture.
c Extraction of the osteosynthesis material (ie, dynamic hip screw) and insertion of gentamicin beads as an antibiotic spacer.

Analysis of failure and reflection

Although different studies do not show significant differences between DHS plates and trochanteric nails in the treatment of pertrochanteric fractures, the current trend is to use extramedullary implants in stable trochanteric fractures (AO/OTA 31A1) and trochanteric intramedullary nails in unstable fractures (AO/OTA 31A2,31A3).

In this case, the surgeon considered the fracture as stable and chose to use a plate with a sliding screw (ie, DHS), which achieved a good fracture reduction with the implant in the correct position, highlighting only a tip-apex distance at the limit.

The dehiscence of the wound after a simple fall only 15 days after the surgery might have been indicative of a problem, probably of a septic nature. "Wait and see" should not be our attitude. Surgical debridement and cleaning must be performed at the first signs of suspected infection, and the attitude toward treatment must be more demanding and aggressive in fragile patients with major comorbidities.

The medial displacement observed at the first control visits generally does not affect the process of fracture union, although functional compensation is lost due to the effect of tension in the gluteal muscles, which causes a Trendelenburg gait but not dissymmetry. The medial displacement is usually due to weakening of the lateral cortex of the greater trochanter during the perforation of the head screw, aggravated by the patient's fall in the immediate postoperative period. The surgeon must also evaluate a probable osteolysis around the implant resulting from the septic process. In the context of instability, it makes no sense to perform surgical cleaning without removing the osteosynthesis material, as the biofilm is thus never eliminated, limiting the response to antibiotics.

Final outcome

The different surgeries to which the patient was subjected weakened and worsened her fragility even further. Her kidney function deteriorated and she died due to multiorgan failure 3.5 months after the fracture.

Case description

A 77-year-old man, a former tobacco-user who receives no family support and suffers from arterial hypertension, chronic obstructive pulmonary disorder, and atrial flutter, sustained a fracture of the right ankle following a fall on a public road. The patient was transferred from another care center with a bivalve plaster cast for immobilization.

In the emergency department x-rays were taken showing a bimalleolar fracture dislocation of the right ankle (AO/OTA 44C2) (**Fig 4.4-15**).

Manual reduction was performed followed by immobilization with a below-the-knee plaster cast (**Fig 4.4-16**). One day after revision of the skin condition, trophic changes were detected due to previously undiagnosed possible chronic vascular insufficiency.

A surgical intervention was planned, performing open reduction and osteosynthesis with a traction screw in the fibula, a one-third tubular plate with protection effect, and an intertibiofibular screw to stabilize the syndesmosis. The tibial malleolus was reduced and stabilized with two traction screws. The postoperative control x-rays were considered to be correct (**Fig 4.4-17**).

The patient was discharged 2 weeks after the intervention, as he was free of fever and pain and there was minimum serous secretion from the wound. One month after surgery he was readmitted due to dehiscence of the lateral wound and ulceration on the medial wound with purulent drainage in the fibular area. Antibiotic treatment was started and the osteosynthesis material removed (**Fig 4.4-18**).

In the cultures from samples obtained during the intervention, it was possible to isolate *Enterobacter cloacae* that are resistant to first-generation cephalosporins, ampicillin, and amoxicillin/clavulanic acid. Due to persistent purulent secretion, a new surgical debridement was performed 48 hours later, resulting in bone and tendon exposure in the anterior face of the ankle. Five days after the second debridement, negative-pressure wound therapy (NPWT) (eg, vacuum-assisted wound closure [VAC]) began. During the hospital stay the patient presented with thoracic pain and was diagnosed with acute myocardial infarction. Evaluation of the wounds was requested by the plastic surgery department and treatment continued without obtaining any satisfactory results. With exposed and devitalized bone on the back of the ankle region, amputation of the limb was necessary (**Fig 4.4-19**). The indication was endorsed after evaluation by a vascular surgeon due to the patient's chronic vascular disorder and the affected limb was subsequently amputated in the supracondylar region of the femur.

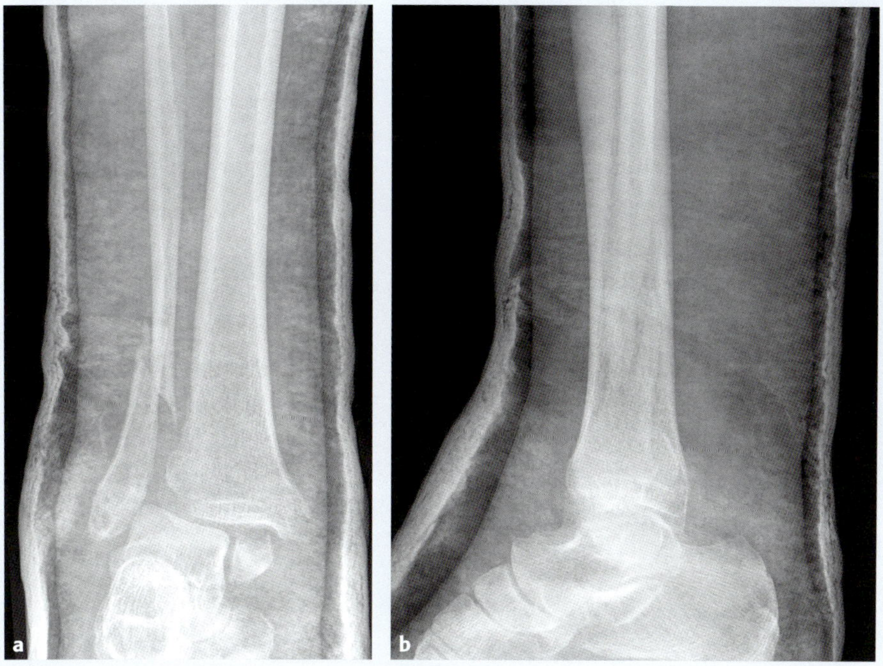

Fig 4.4-15a–b Control x-rays in AP (**a**) and lateral (**b**) views taken at admission of the patient, showing a bimalleolar fracture dislocation of the right ankle.

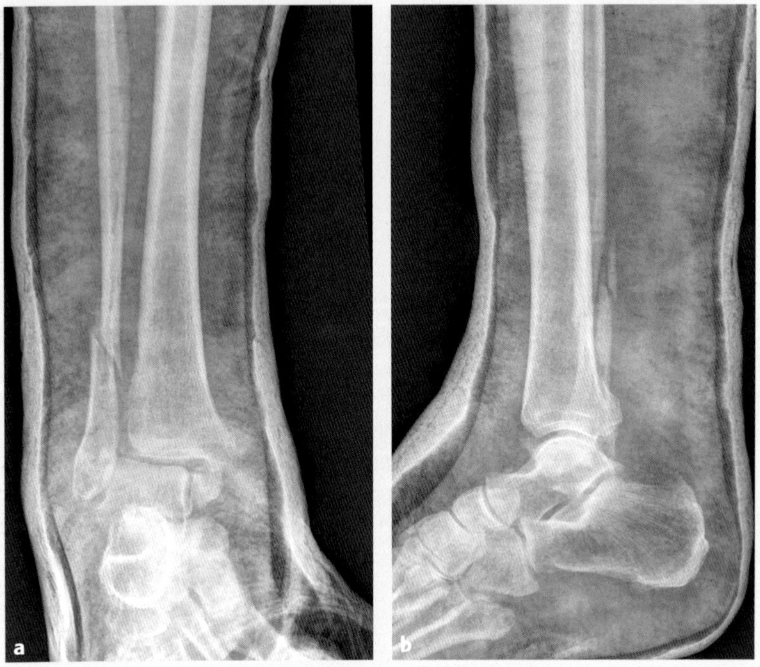

Fig 4.4-16a–b AP (**a**) and lateral (**b**) control x-rays after closed reduction and immobilization with a below-the-knee plaster cast.

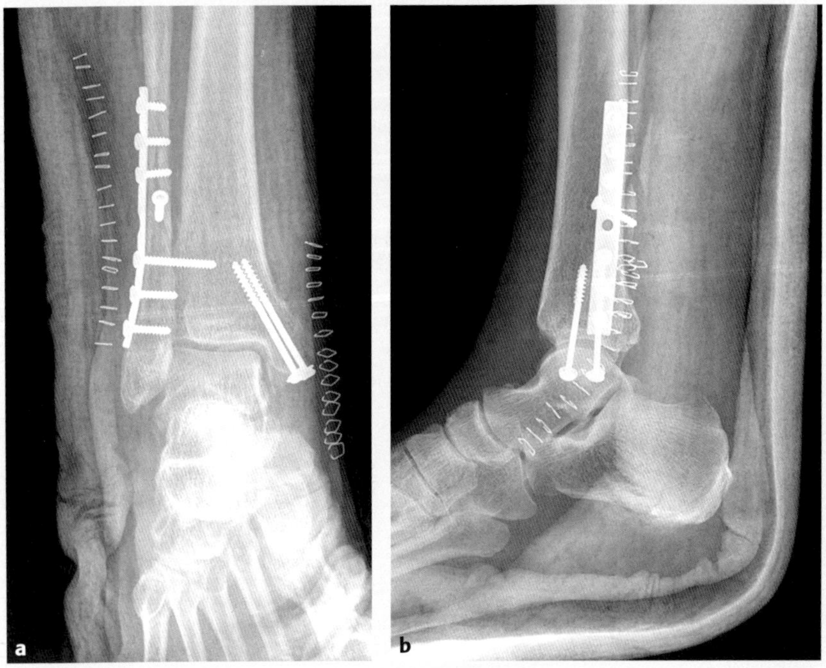

Fig 4.4-17a–b AP (**a**) and lateral (**b**) x-rays taken in the immediate postoperative period.

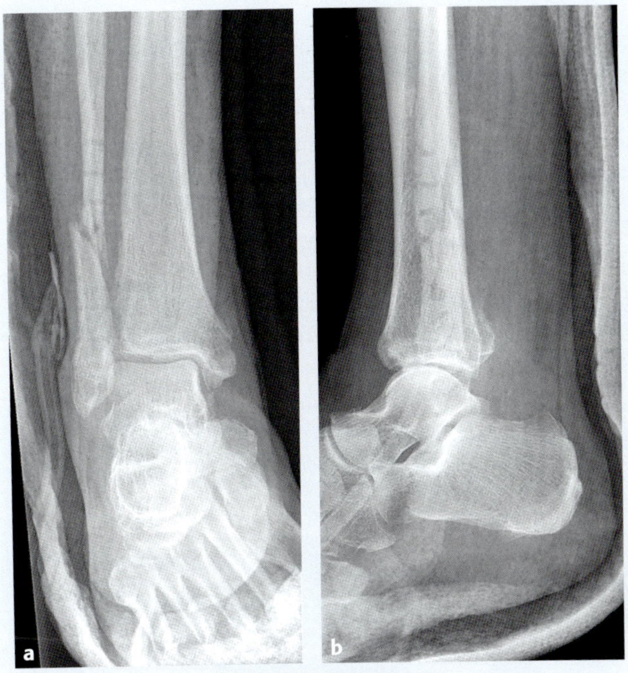

Fig 4.4-18a–b X-rays in AP (**a**) and lateral (**b**) views following removal of the osteosynthesis material.

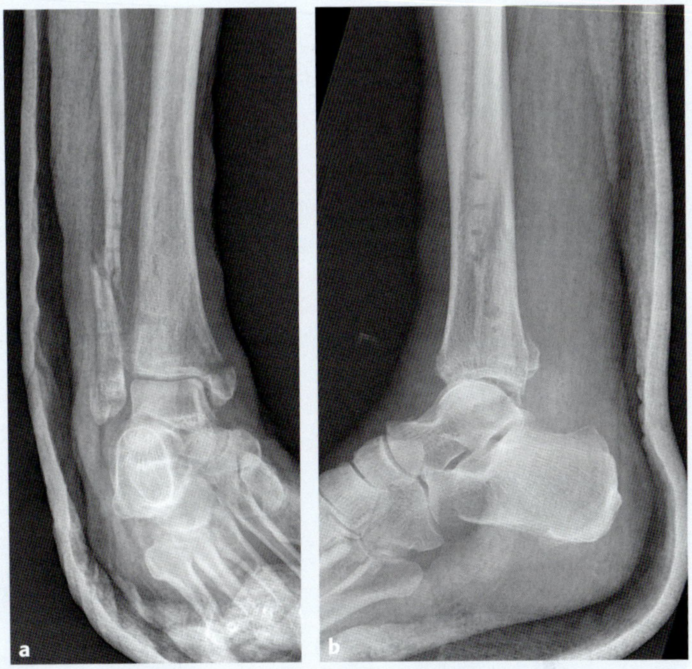

Fig 4.4-19a–b X-rays 3 months after removal of the osteosynthesis material in AP (**a**) and lateral (**b**) views.

Analysis of failure and reflection

Just like in many other cases in this book, the failure in this case is also multifactorial. For educational purposes, though, we single out one factor where possible. There is almost always a combination of causes that lead to poor evolution and a bad final result. Immediate reduction and immobilization are important to avoid the displacement or movement of the fracture fragments. If, for some reason, the patient needs to be transferred or the intervention is deferred, the articulation and the fracture must be reduced and immobilized in the best anatomical position possible with a slightly padded, rigid bandage. Otherwise, the surrounding soft tissues continue to swell, further compromising them and thus increasing the risk of possible complications. It is unjustifiable to place an immobilization plaster cast on an articular fracture dislocation without reducing it.

If the vascular system of the patient's limb had been studied before the first surgical intervention, the indication and timing of surgery may have been different.

The importance of postoperative care and follow-ups have been underestimated. In this case, serous secretion from the surgical wounds evolved initially towards frank suppuration, dehiscence, and ulceration of the wounds. All wounds must be correctly evaluated. In patients that present with slow and difficult wound healing or with a history of complications, strict control needs to be exercised. Given the poor evolution of the wounds, the removal of the osteosynthesis material and aggressive cleaning of the wounds should have been done earlier.

Final outcome

Owing to the poor evolution of the soft tissues, which was due to wound dehiscence and infection, and despite repeated attempts to eradicate the infection through specific antibiotic treatment, debridements, negative-pressure wound therapy (NPWT) (eg, vacuum assisted closure [VAC]), and removal of the osteosynthesis material, the patient ultimately required supracondylar amputation of the affected limb.

CASE 4

Case description

A 13-year-old boy fell from a 1 m high concrete wall into a muddy field and sustained an open fracture of his left distal leg (AO/OTA 42A2,4F2A) (**Fig 4.4-20**).

The patient was admitted to the local hospital and he was operated on the first day under local anesthesia. Debridement was performed with revision and suturing of the wound. A plaster cast was applied to immobilize the leg. Surgery was done again the next morning, and a percutaneous reduction and osteosynthesis with a locking compression plate for the distal medial tibia was performed (**Fig 4.4-21**).

After 3 days a secretion started coming out from the wound, so the patient was treated with antibiotics for a week. There was no improvement, the wound edges dehisced, and the plate became exposed. The surgeon decided to remove the plate and screws and apply an external fixator (**Fig 4.4-22**).

After debridement the wound was treated using a negative-pressure wound dressing (NPWD). The dressing was then changed every 3 days under general anesthesia for 1 month. Because of pin-track infection, the external fixator was removed after 2 weeks and a plaster cast was applied again. There was no improvement after 12 NPWD changes and the patient was admitted to the author's hospital.

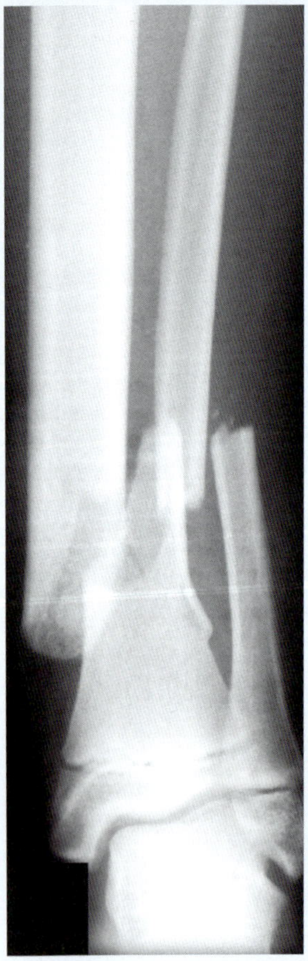

Fig 4.4-20 Preoperative AP x-ray of the distal leg fracture with two butterfly fragments in the tibial fracture.

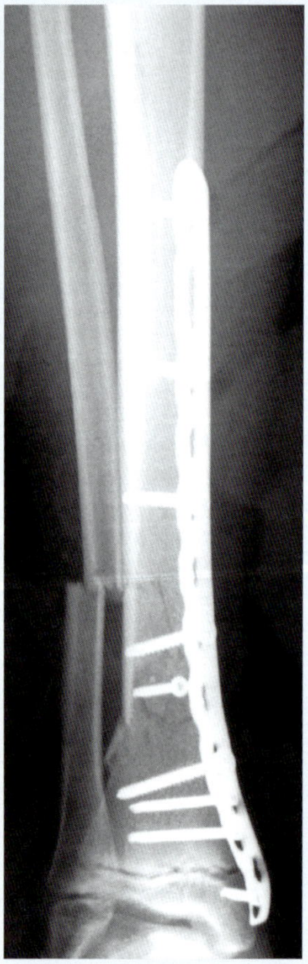

Fig 4.4-21 Postoperative AP x-ray showing the internal fixation performed the day after admission with an insufficient reduction.

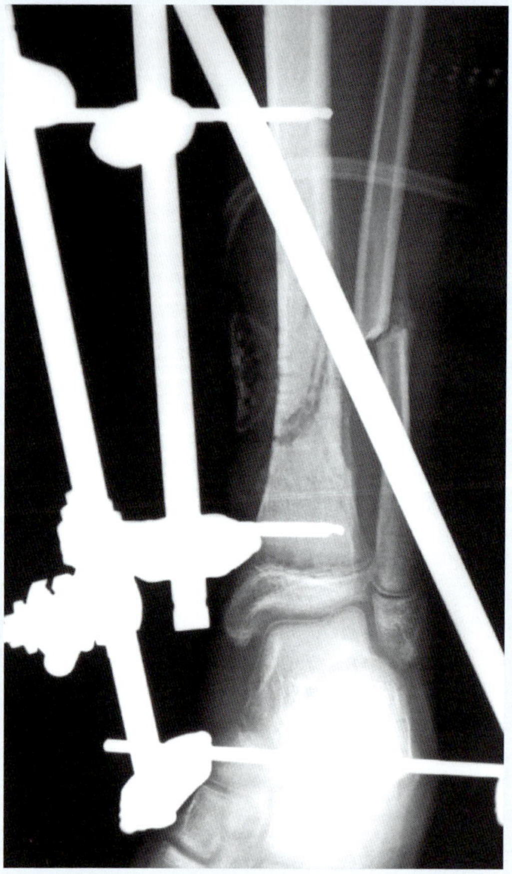

Fig 4.4-22 X-ray after the revision surgery and the application of an external fixator.

At admission to the author's hospital, the wound was about 10 x 8 cm and covered with granulation tissue and purulent exudation. The fracture part of the distal leg was unstable and painful. Treatment was started about 6 weeks after the injury:

First operation: Segmental resection of the affected necrotic bone was performed, followed by debridement of soft tissues (some foreign tissue particles were still present), therapy with septopal beads, and treatment with a hybrid external fixator (**Fig 4.4-23**).

A multibacterial infection was recognized (ie, *Enterococcus faecalis, Clostridium glycolicum*, and *Escherichia coli*). Appropriate antibiotic treatment was introduced thereafter.

Second operation: As soon as the wound was free of infection (**Fig 4.4-24a**), a serratus flap procedure was performed by a plastic surgeon 10 days after the first operation (**Fig 4.4-24b**).

Third operation: One month later, a proximal percutaneous corticotomy was performed and a bone transport with a unilateral fixator was started. The flap was already in place. The external fixator was used for the bone transport. The bone defect was 7 cm (**Fig 4.4-25**).

Fourth operation: Two months later bone grafting of the docking site was performed (**Fig 4.4-26** and **Fig 4.4-27**).

Fifth operation: The external fixator was removed 3.5 months later. One month after fixator removal the patient started full weight bearing (**Fig 4.4-28**).

Analysis of failure and reflection

The open fracture was treated inadequately from the very beginning:

1. The first debridement of the highly contaminated wound was performed under local anesthesia. It is impossible to do radical debridement in that manner. General anesthesia and radical debridement should have been performed.
2. The next morning minimally invasive osteosynthesis was done, obviously with no additional debridement and rinsing. The highly contaminated wound should have been thoroughly debrided and rinsed a second time before performing minimally invasive osteosynthesis.
3. With postoperative secretion from the wound and signs of infection, the continuation of antibiotic treatment with no operative revision of the wound was incorrect. The correct thing would have been to carry out an extended debridement of the surgical wound (as explained in 2).
4. Although debridement was not performed, operative revision with removal of implant or osteosynthesis material, tissue samples for microbiology, and application of an external fixator was the right approach.
5. No extensive debridement was performed but only antibiotics were relied upon. Extensive debridement and NPWT would have been the right way to treat the patient at that stage (ie, after the intervention with plaque and when the first signs of infection appeared), but a radical debridement is a cornerstone of success. If there is no improvement after 1–2 weeks, the surgeon should be very suspicious about ongoing infection and insufficient debridement.
6. The lack of reduction and instability caused poor evolution of the soft tissues around the fracture. Removing the external fixator from the unstable fracture with soft-tissue problems would not have helped. Plaster casting was not a solution in this case, as gypsum would not have achieved good stability and would not have allowed the surgeon to take adequate care of the soft tissues; instead, a new external fixator should have been applied.
7. The soft tissue was not taken care of properly and the bone was left without soft-tissue coverage. Since bone with no soft-tissue coverage will die, the aim of treatment should be to clean the wound and cover the bone. The involvement of a plastic surgeon is essential.

Initial treatment of the contaminated open simple distal tibial fracture was inappropriate. The patient should have been operated on admission under general anesthesia. Debridement and rinsing of the wound are very important, and treatment with antibiotics is essential, lasting for at least a few days, depending on the grade of the open fracture. Stability of the fracture enables soft tissue to heal. The fixation of a Gustilo type I and type II fracture could be internal or external. In highly contaminated wounds, external fixation (temporary or final) is safer because it provides stability for the fracture and allows the soft tissues to evolve towards healing.

Final outcome

Physiotherapy for the knee and ankle had already started during the bone transport phase, so the range of motion of both joints was perfect by the time of fixator removal. Two years later the patient was doing well, had no pain in the leg, and no problems in doing recreational sports (**Fig 4.4-29**).

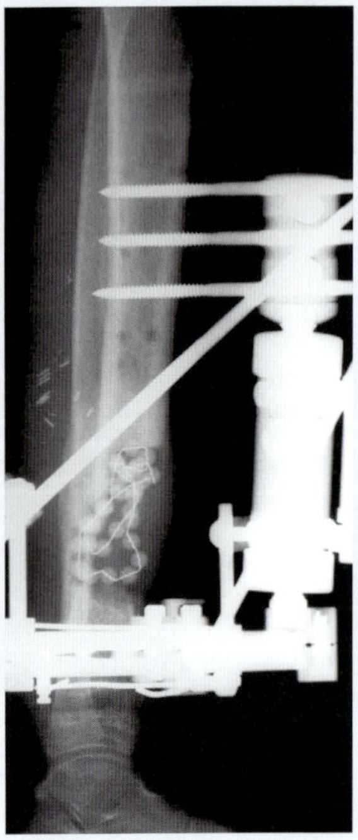

Fig 4.4-23 X-ray after segmental resection, septopal beads application, and hybrid external fixation.

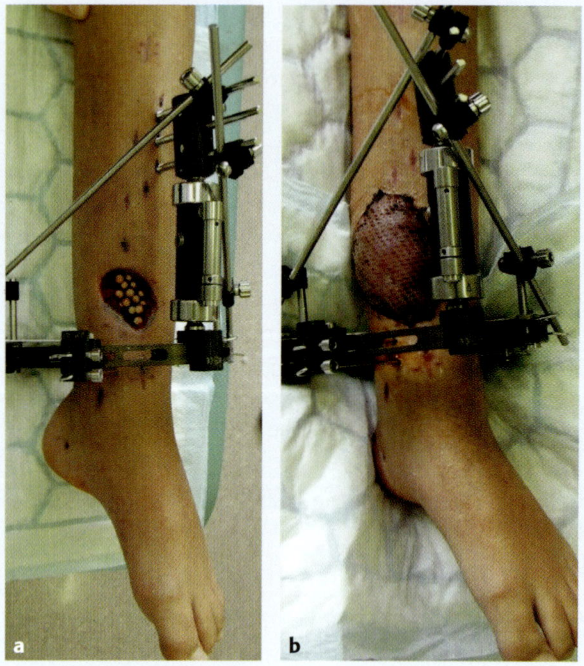

Fig 4.4-24a–b The leg before and after the flap with serratus muscle.

a Clinical appearance 10 days after radical debridement.

b Clinical appearance 1 week after coverage with a serratus muscle flap.

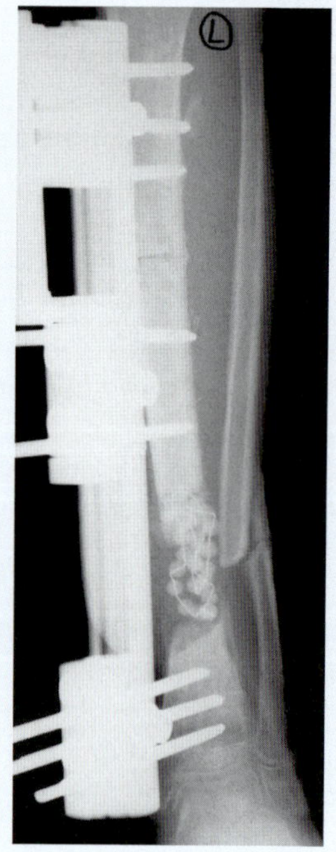

Fig 4.4-25 Postoperative x-ray after proximal corticotomy and unilateral bone transport with external fixator.

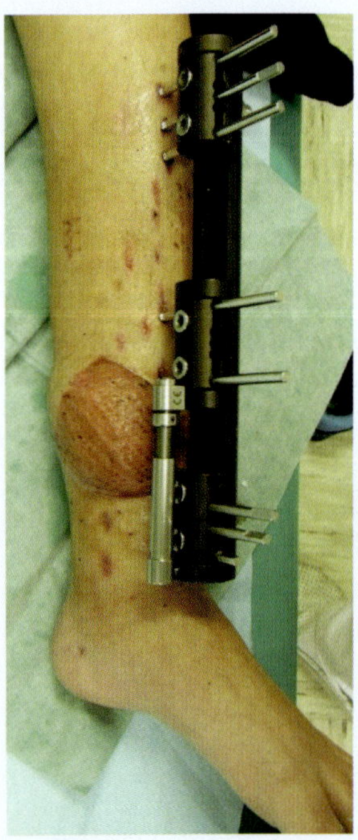

Fig 4.4-26 The docking site before bone grafting.

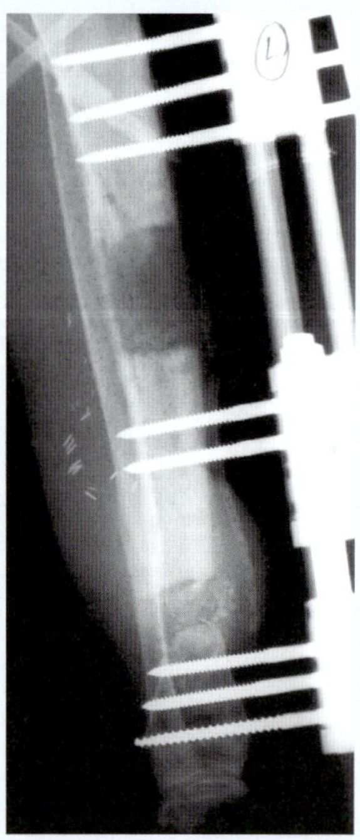

Fig 4.4-27 Postoperative x-ray just after bone grafting of the docking site.

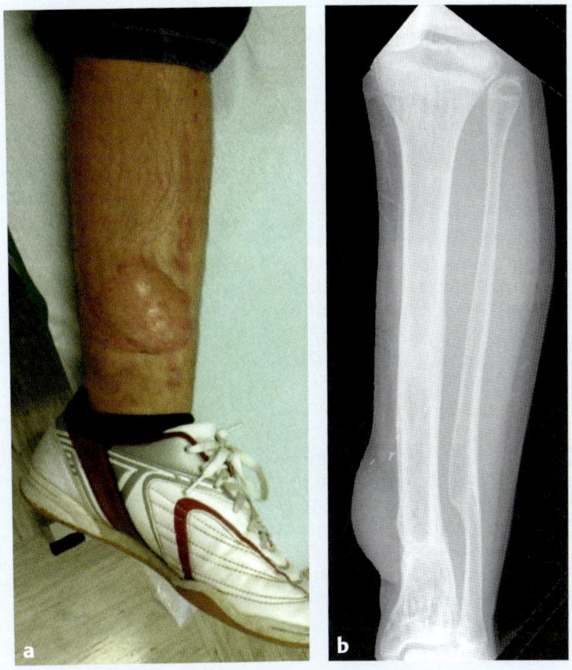

Fig 4.4-28a–b Bone transport and consolidation.
a Six months after fixator removal.
b X-ray 1 year after fixator removal.

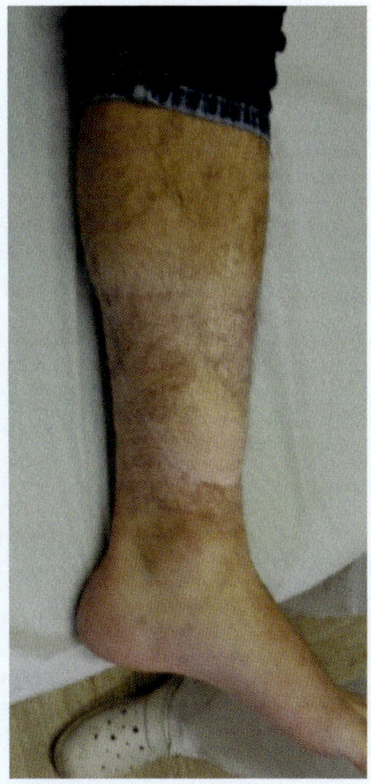

Fig 4.4-29 Two years after completion of treatment.

Key points to remember

- Infection is the worst complication that can occur in the surgical treatment of a fracture and means the method has failed.
- The best treatment for infection is prevention. A rigorous asepsis protocol must be followed to reduce the possibility of infection.
- Failure to comply with asepsis rules and protocols increases the rate of infection in the postoperative period. Aseptic conditions should be maximized.
- A surgical technique that does not respect the soft tissues and the vascularization of the bone fragments increases the risk of infection.
- Contamination can cause infection depending on the level of contamination, the virulence of the germs, and the resistance of the patient.

References and suggested reading

Borens O, Yusuf E, Trampuz A. Surgical Site Infections (SSIs): Risk factors and Prevention Strategies. Paper presented at: 14th EFORT Congress, European Federation of National Associations of Orthopaedics and Traumatology (EFORT); June 5–8, 2013; Istanbul.

Giannoudis PV, Harwood PJ, Tosounidis T, et al. Restoration of long bone defects treated with the induced membrane technique: protocol and outcomes. *Injury.* 2016 Dec;47 Suppl 6:S53–S61.

Gross T, Kaim AH, Regazzoni P, et al. Current concepts in posttraumatic osteomyelitis: a diagnostic challenge with new imaging options. *J Trauma.* 2002 Jun;52(6):1210–1219.

Gustilo RB, Mendoza RM, Williams DN. Problems in the management of type III (severe) open fractures: a new classification of type III open fractures. *J Trauma.* 1984 Aug;24(8):742–746.

Sirkin M, Sanders R, DiPasquale T, et al. A staged protocol for soft tissue management in the treatment of complex pilon fractures. *J Orthop Trauma.* 2004 Sep;18(8 Suppl):S32–38.

Trampuz A, Widmer AF. Infections associated with orthopedic implants. *Curr Opin Infect Dis.* 2006 Aug;19(4):349–356.

Trampuz A, Zimmerli W. Diagnosis and treatment of infections associated with fracture-fixation devices. *Injury.* 2006 May;37 Suppl 2:S59–66.

4.5 Proficiency and experience

Jordi Bertrán Padrós, Joan Girós Torres, Roberto Rivero Sosa, J Miquel Sales Pérez, Miquel Videla Cés

Victory has a thousand fathers but defeat is an orphan.

John F Kennedy

Before performing surgical treatment on a fracture, a fundamental requirement is the theoretical knowledge of the biological and mechanical conditioning factors necessary. However, this alone does not guarantee a good clinical result. Mastery of the surgical technique requires training and is acquired with practice. Practical learning is achieved by attending workshops to practice with plastic bones and on anatomical specimens, acquiring skills alongside surgeons with greater experience. These are obligatory requirements for achieving good results.

Learning to understand the importance of each kind of fracture, the essential technical needs for the correct use of instruments, the adequate application of implants, and the level of experience and skill of the surgeon all require time and dedication to achieve before the surgeon can adequately treat fractures. A self-critical attitude is also necessary when reviewing case follow-up documentation. The critical review of one's own results is essential, and helps to assimilate concepts, and recognize one's own technical capabilities. The x-ray results of the surgical treatment of a fracture show the technique used and whether this has been performed by someone with experience. Without self-evaluation, a surgeon can never know if the knowledge acquired has been sufficient and correctly applied. Repeatedly making errors because of inadequate evaluation of the results is, at the very least, dangerous.

During the learning period surgeons tend to commit a series of understandable small errors of little clinical significance until the necessary skills and feel for the surgery are acquired and refined. One needs time and experience, a sense of balance, a sense of the relationship between instruments and implants, and an understanding of the principles of osteosynthesis for its correct application. Depending on the number of fractures treated as well as their level of difficulty to repair and severity, which must be addressed progressively, the surgeon will gradually acquire experience in applying the theory and practice of fracture treatment.

The surgeon's experience encompasses the entire process during treatment. For example, in the preoperative period, it helps her or him to perform a correct evaluation of the fracture, to decide the best timing for the surgery, the necessary care that she or he must give to the soft tissues prior to surgery, the positioning of the patient, to know the functions of the implants, the planning of the treatment, the choice of implant, and the conditions for its placement (for example when an implant can contribute to the reduction of a fracture and at the same time stabilize it as in the case of a reamed nail). During the surgery itself, experience reveals knowledge of "tricks" in the use of instruments helping to reduce the fracture without periosteal stripping of the bone fragments, the biomechanically balanced placement of implants, the three-dimensional orientation positioning, etc. But the surgeon must also not forget to control the evolution of the fracture in the postoperative follow-up, to give the correct indications as to nonweight-bearing times, and adequate rehabilitation, etc. All this and more must be considered in the attempt to achieve the perfect osteosynthesis and, above all, to avoid any failure or combination of failures.

CASE 1

Case description

A 24-year-old man suffered a strained right ankle while playing football and presented with a suprasyndesmotic facture of the ankle (AO/OTA 44C3) (**Fig 4.5-1**).

An internal fixation was performed in the emergency department. The surgeon chose a minimally invasive plate osteosynthesis technique using screws to repair the medial malleolus and implanted a tibiofibular screw to keep the distal tibiofibular articulation closed, without direct repair of the anterior syndesmosis complex. In the immediate postoperative control x-rays a poor reduction of the syndesmosis was detected. It continued in diastasis, with the inter-tibiofibular screw oriented the wrong way without applying distal pressure on the tibia as it passed posterior to the bone (**Fig 4.5-2**).

Two days later the patient underwent another intervention with the intertibiofibular screw being placed in the correct direction after reduction of the syndesmosis space (**Fig 4.5-3**).

The intertibiofibular screw was removed at 8 weeks. Fortunately, the ankle joint showed good congruity without signs of dystrophy.

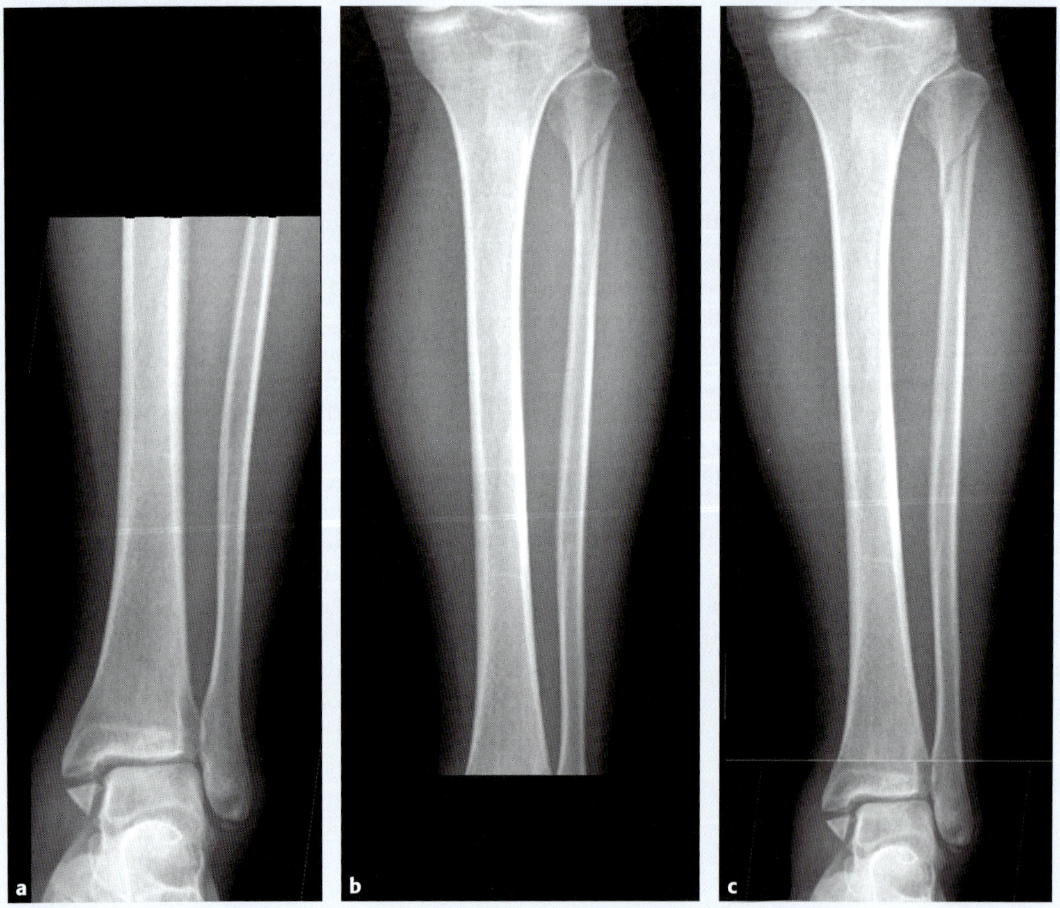

Fig 4.5-1a–c Preoperative x-rays showing a bimalleolar fracture with proximal subcapital fracture of the fibula.

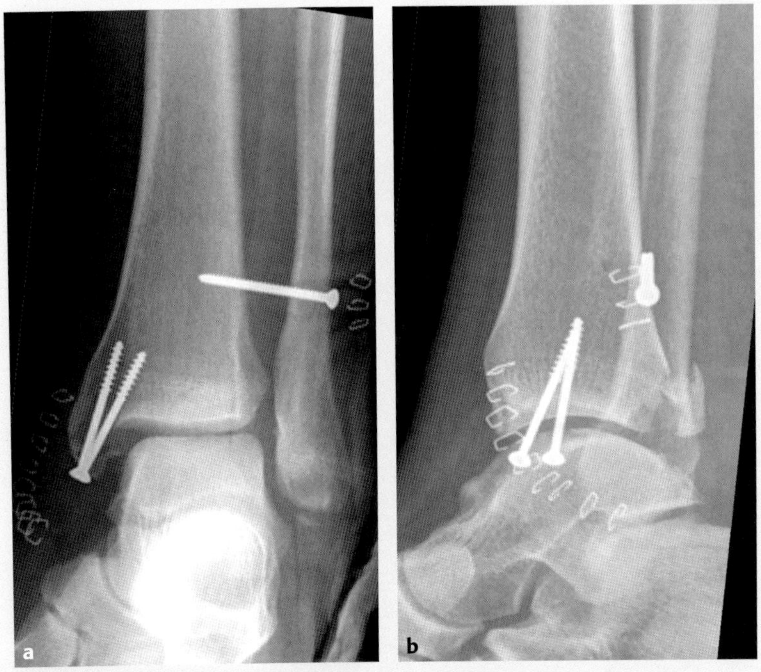

Fig 4.5-2a–b Control x-rays in the immediate postoperative period of the first surgery. The reduction of the syndesmosis was not achieved and the intertibiofibular screw was not oriented correctly, therefore, it did not grip the tibia.

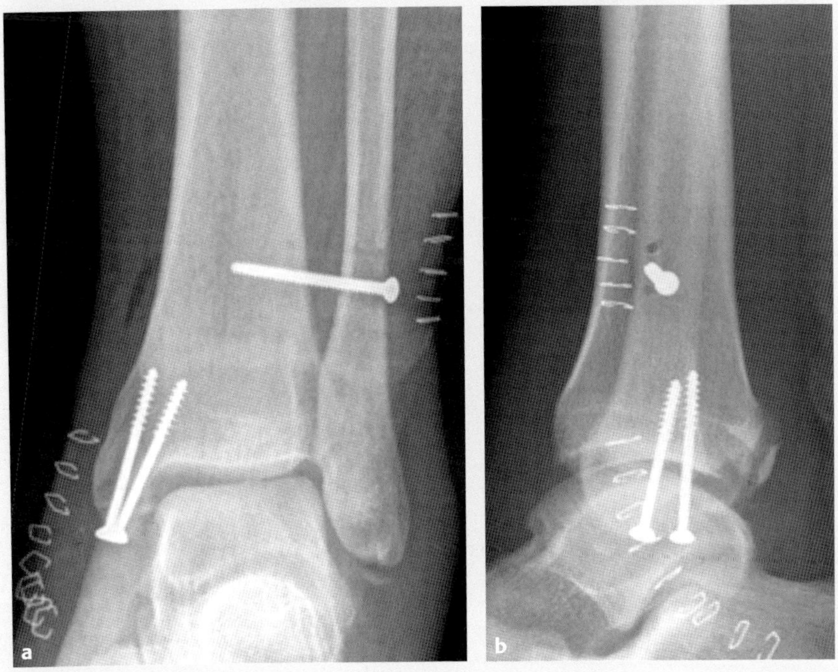

Fig 4.5-3a–b Control x-rays in the postoperative phase of the second surgery. The ankle joint has been reduced.

Analysis of failure and reflection

The surgeon must have a good x-ray study of the injury and evaluate the state of the soft tissues to choose the best approach for treating the fracture. If the status of the skin and the degree of inflammation do not allow for intervention, surgery must be postponed until there is a better chance of success.

In the sagittal plane, the fibula is located behind the tibia, therefore the direction of the screw must be posterior to anterior with an approximate angulation of 30°. This ensures that it can reach the tibia and perform its function as a positioning screw stabilizing the space between both bones, once it has been reduced to the adequate distance by manipulation while healing the syndesmosis (**Fig 4.5-4**). During screw placement the ankle must be at 90° of dorsal flexion to maintain the precise space as indicated in the *Manual of Internal Fixation* [**Willenegger et al, 1970**].

Final outcome

The immobilization was maintained with a plaster cast for 3 weeks to care for the soft tissues and nonweight bearing continued for 8 weeks until after the extraction of the tibiofibular screw.

The patient began sessions of rehabilitation and was able to return to activities of daily living at 16 weeks (**Fig 4.5-5**).

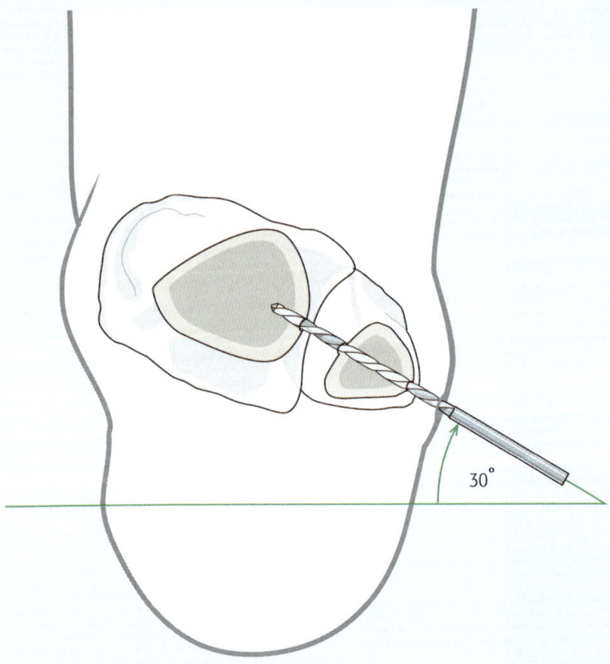

Fig 4.5-4 The direction that the intertibiofibular screw should follow in the sagittal plane when inserted.

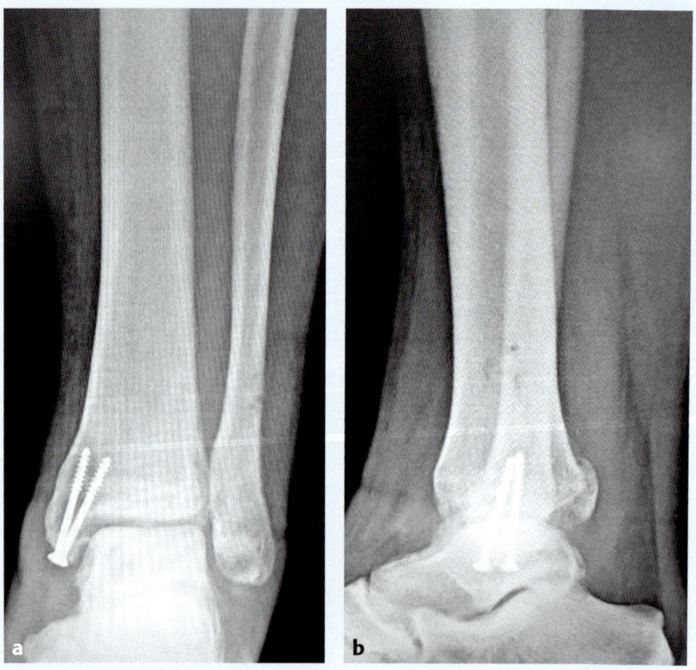

Fig 4.5-5a–b Control x-rays at 4 months after the second surgery. The ankle joint is reduced. The small posterior, extraarticular fragment does not cause any functional problems.

Case description

An 83-year-old woman suffered a casual fall, presenting a subcapital fracture of the right femur, impacted with slight valgus bowing (AO/OTA 31B1) (**Fig 4.5-6**).

It was treated with three 6.5 mm short threaded screws for cancellous bone (**Fig 4.5-7**). The concentration of stress in a small area of the lateral femoral cortex caused a fracture in the subtrochanteric region where the screws were inserted (AO/OTA 32A1) (**Fig 4.5-8**).

In a second intervention, the screws were removed and an intramedullary nail (eg, proximal femoral nail antirotation [PFNA]) was chosen to stabilize the fracture. The head and neck blade of the PFNA nail was placed in an excessively subchondral position (**Fig 4.5-9**).

Trochanteric nails are less dynamic than the sliding screw plate (dynamic hip screw [DHS]), therefore the subchondral position of the blade would lead to implant cut-out in the femoral head [**Flores et al, 2016**].

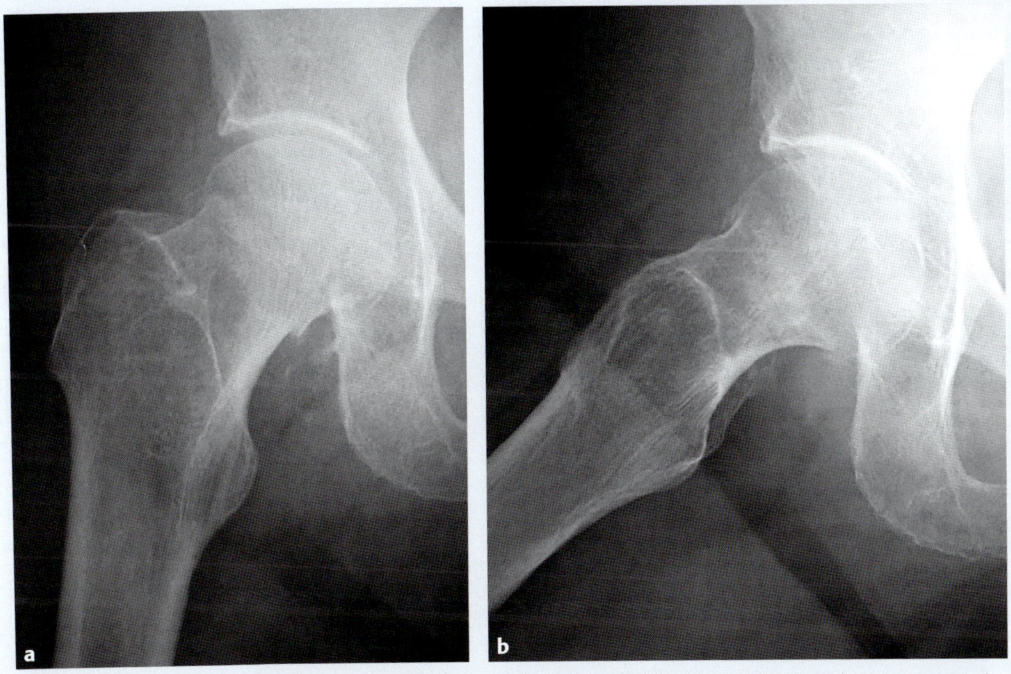

a b

Fig 4.5-6a–b X-rays in AP (**a**) and axial (**b**) views of the subcapital fracture of the right femur, impacted in slight valgus. There is no displacement in retroversion in the axial view.

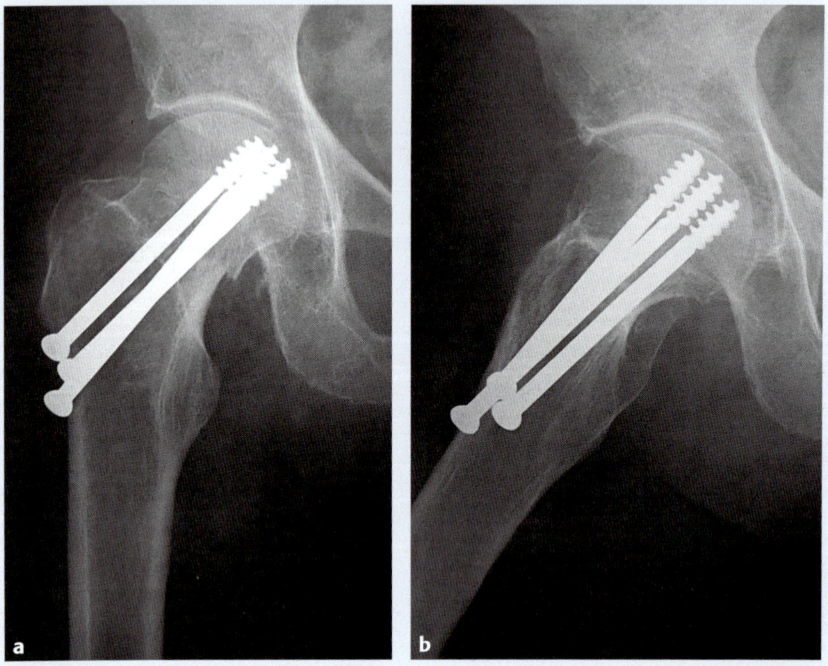

Fig 4.5-7a–b Immediate postoperative control x-rays of the fixation of the humeral head with three screws.

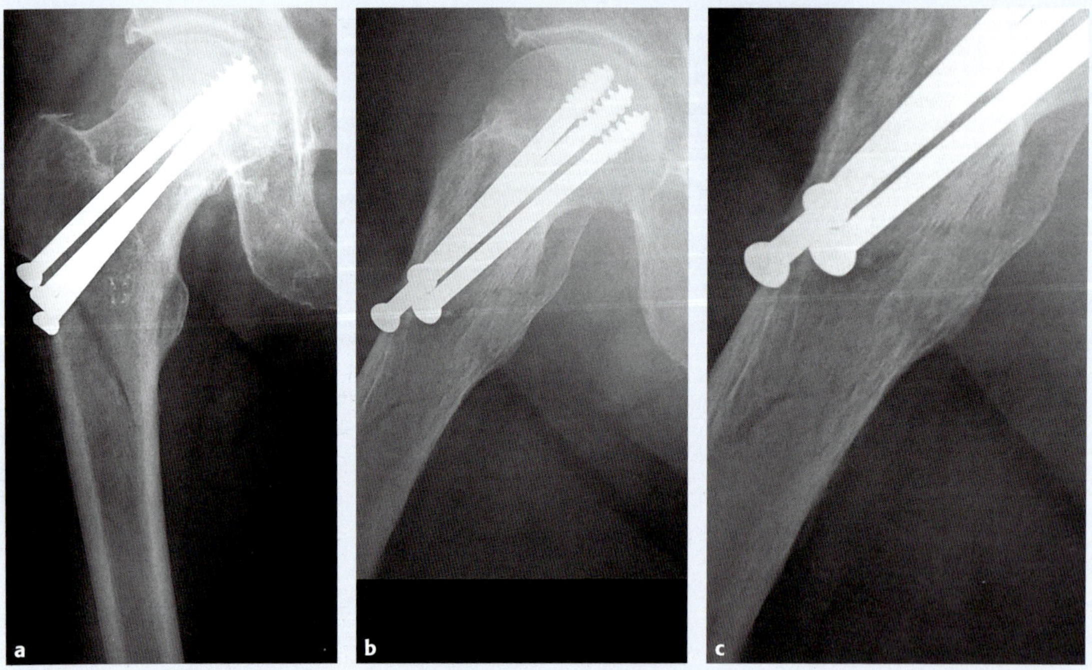

Fig 4.5-8a–c Subsequent control x-rays showing a fracture in the subtrochanteric zone of the femur, beginning at the external cortex of the femur in the holes made for the placement of screws.

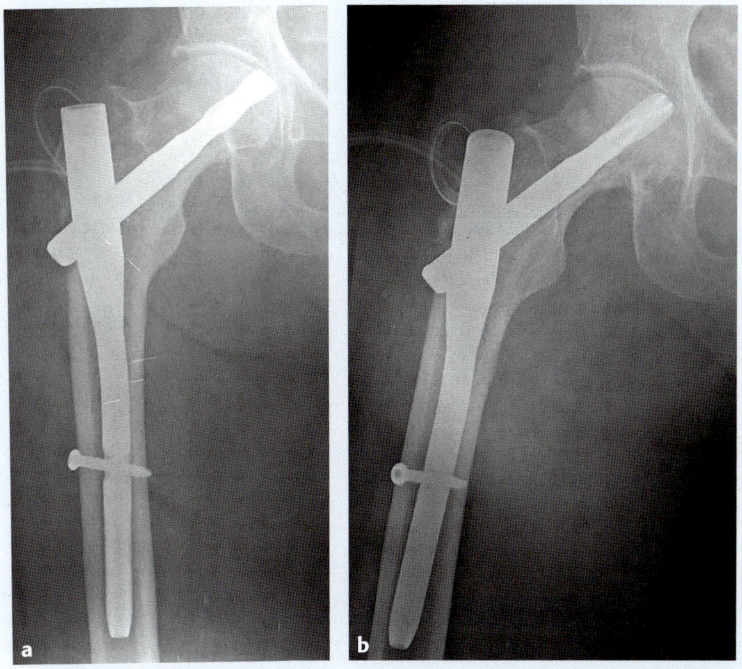

Fig 4.5-9a–b Postoperative control x-rays of the second intervention. The trochanteric nail presents an excessively subchondral position of the head and neck blade.

Analysis of failure and reflection

The tolerable limit for the insertion of screws in the treatment of subcapital fractures of the femur must not be distal to the level of the lesser trochanter.

The geometrical positioning of the screws in the treatment of subcapital fractures slightly displaced in valgus is important. The arrangement of the triangle of the distal base is mechanically more effective, but it debilitates the lateral cortex of the femur. It is important to avoid the concentration of stresses. The safety distance between the heads of the screws of 10–13 mm depending on the washers must be respected.

Placing a blade in the head and neck region of the femur seems to be the best option in this case, since the screws implanted in the first intervention reduced the amount of bone tissue that could hinder the placement of another screw even if of greater size. In cases with poor bone content, an augmentation system can also be used to give more density to the area so that the implant can better perform its weight-bearing function.

Final outcome

The patient did not present with implant cut-out and the fracture achieved union, with the patient able to walk once more.

CASE 3

Case description

An 82-year-old woman suffered a casual fall on a public thoroughfare, hitting her right arm. She presented with a spiral fracture with an intact wedge, in the proximal third of the humerus, and an associated radial paralysis (AO/OTA 12B2) (**Fig 4.5-10**).

The plan was an open reduction and internal fixation with a long PHILOS plate and revision of the radial nerve, enabling confirmation that it was bruised but intact. The postoperative control x-rays showed good alignment of the fracture, but the aiming device of the PHILOS plate was still joined to the plate because it had not been removed during the intervention (**Fig 4.5-11**).

The patient underwent reintervention 48 hours later to remove the aiming device (**Fig 4.5-12**).

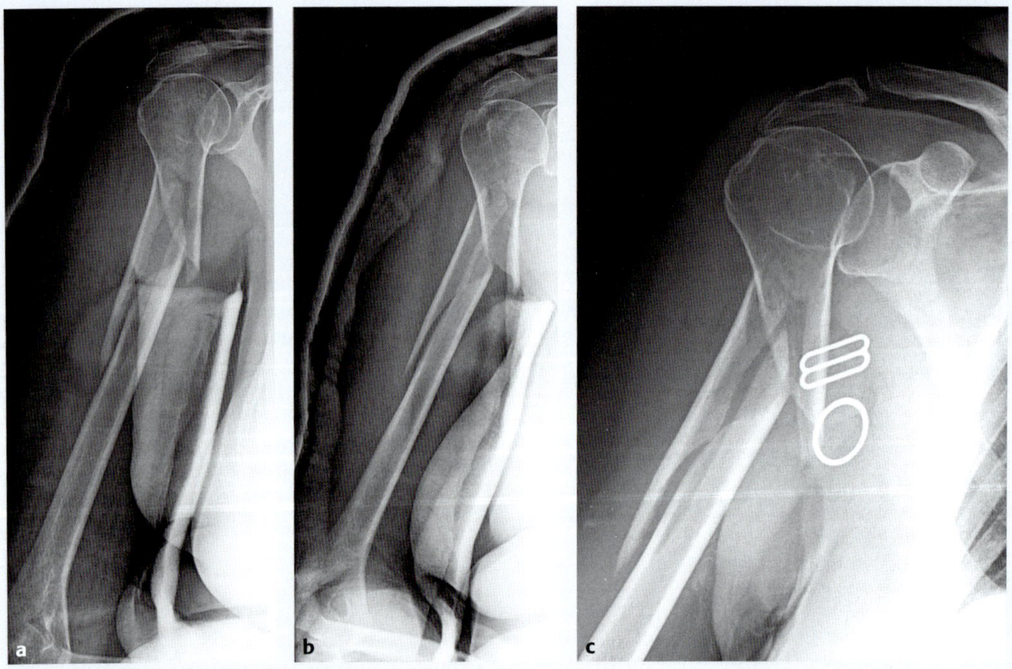

Fig 4.5-10a–c X-ray study of the fracture.
a–b Preoperative x-rays showing the proximal humeral diaphyseal fracture with a third fragment due to torsion.
c Detail of the proximal humeral fracture.

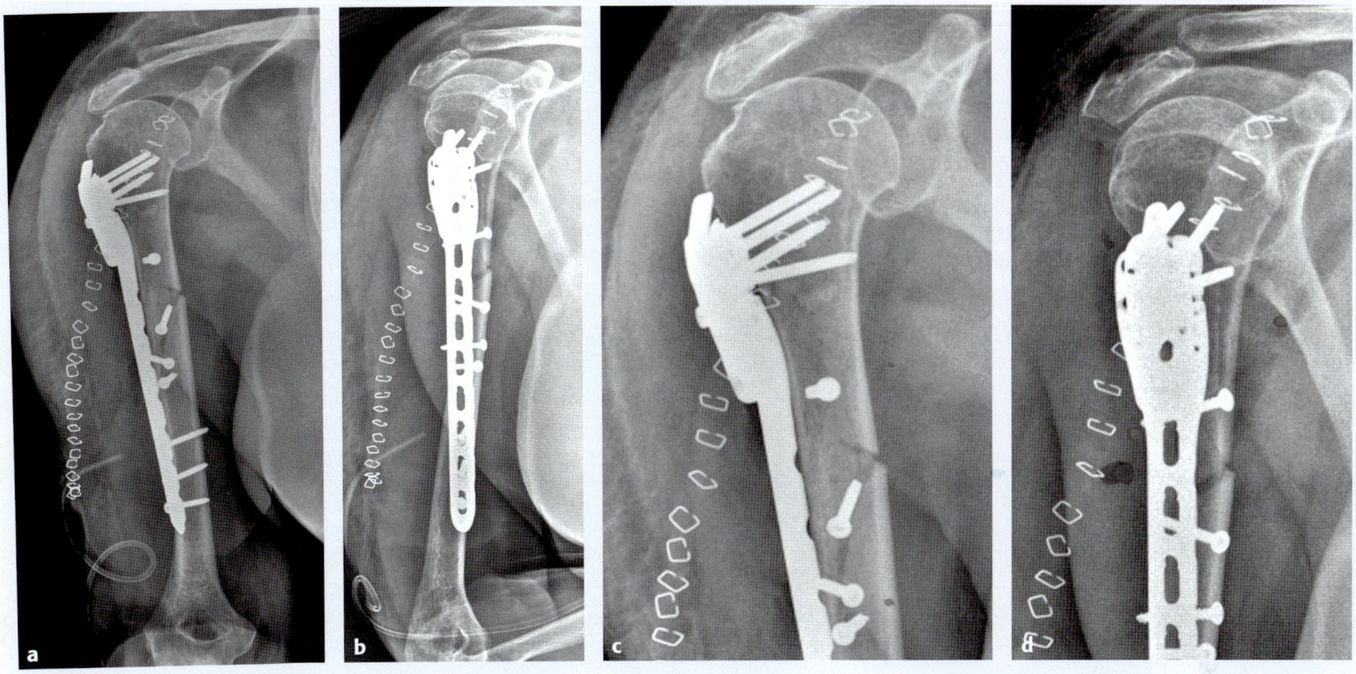

Fig 4.5-11a–d Postoperative control x-rays.

a–b Postoperative x-rays of the proximal humeral fracture. Good reduction of the fracture and stability was achieved with a PHILOS plate. The third intact fragment has achieved union with the traction screws. However, the aiming device of the PHILOS plate remains screwed to the plate and has not been removed.

c–d Postoperative x-rays of the PHILOS plate with the aiming device still in place.

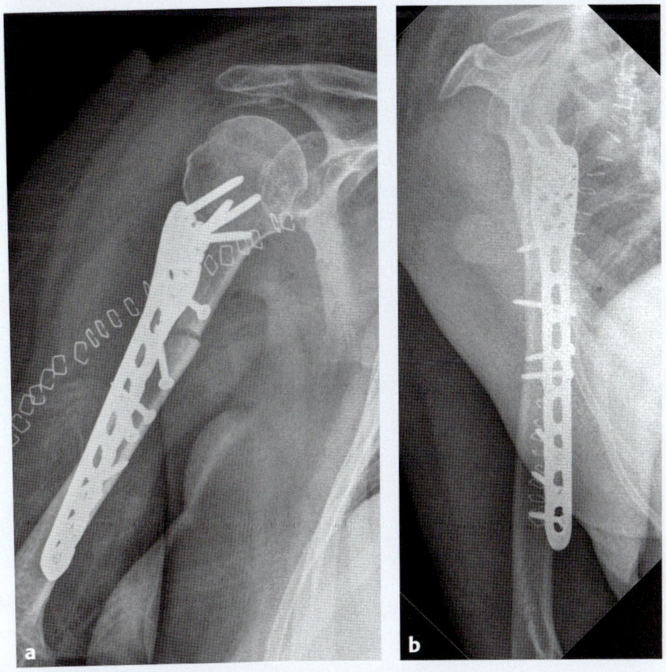

Fig 4.5-12a–b Control x-rays of the reintervention showing that the aiming device of the PHILOS plate has been removed. The reduction and stabilization of the fracture remain unchanged.

Analysis of failure and reflection

The evaluation by the surgeon responsible was correct in terms of diagnosis and treatment indication. Given that the fracture required reduction and stabilization, the radial nerve was examined to confirm that the injury was due to axonotmesis, but perhaps she or he underestimated the technical steps necessary for osteosynthesis.

Surgery requires the set of knowledge of the anatomy, of biomechanics, of patient characteristics, and of the resources available and technique for treatment. Knowledge of the different technical steps for implant placement is more complex today because of the great arsenal of resources available to surgeons.

In this case, the surgical team ignored or forgot to extract the aiming device after the proximal fixation was performed (**Fig 4.5-13**). Knowledge of all the technical steps during performance of osteosynthesis is essential for completing the procedure correctly and any slip-up may lead to the need for reintervention.

Although it does not seem possible for this to occur, this case is not an isolated incident. The authors know that it has occurred on other occasions when a surgical team has not noticed that the aiming device was not withdrawn, proceeding to finalize the intervention. In these cases, the control x-ray shows the error that must be corrected with a new intervention to remove the aiming device (**Fig 4.5-14**).

The steps of the technique for placing the PHILOS plate include the temporary fixation of the aiming device to the plate, through which the drill and screws will be directed. Once the proximal fixation of the plate is completed, the aiming device must be removed since it is not a part of the definitive implant, and it occupies space that could compromise joint mobility (**Fig 4.5-15**).

Final outcome

The postoperative course was good, both for the healing of the wound and of the soft tissues, and for the union of the bone and the articular function. At 6 months after the intervention, she recovered the extension of wrist and fingers, with just a dysesthesia in the distal territory of the radial nerve as the only sequela (**Fig 4.5-16**).

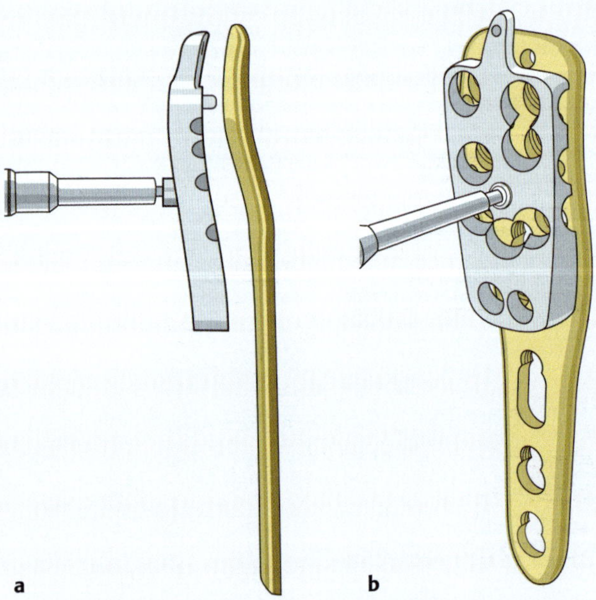

Fig 4.5-13a–b The aiming device of the PHILOS plate with the screwing mechanism that joins or separates the two pieces.

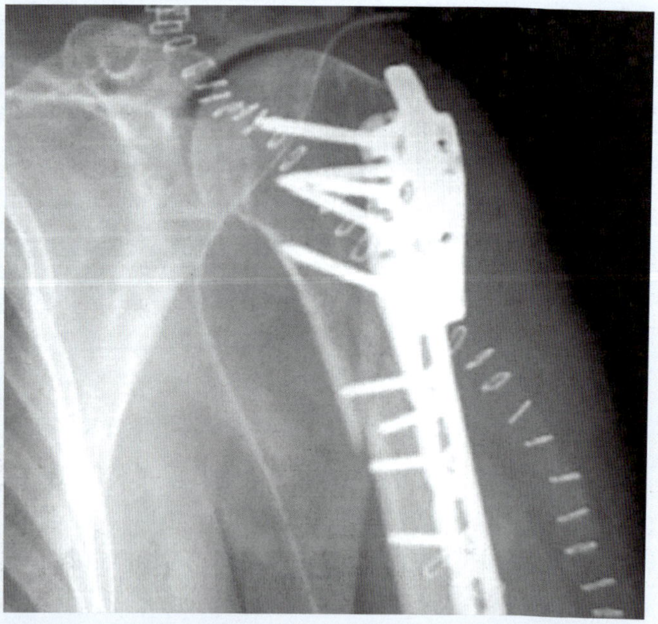

Fig 4.5-14 Postoperative control x-ray in another case where intervention was required for a proximal humeral fracture due to shear in two parts. Here too, the aiming device of the PHILOS plate was not removed during the initial intervention. The patient underwent reintervention for the extraction of the aiming device, with her fracture achieving union without further incident, with a final range of motion of 80% and a Constant score of 82 points.

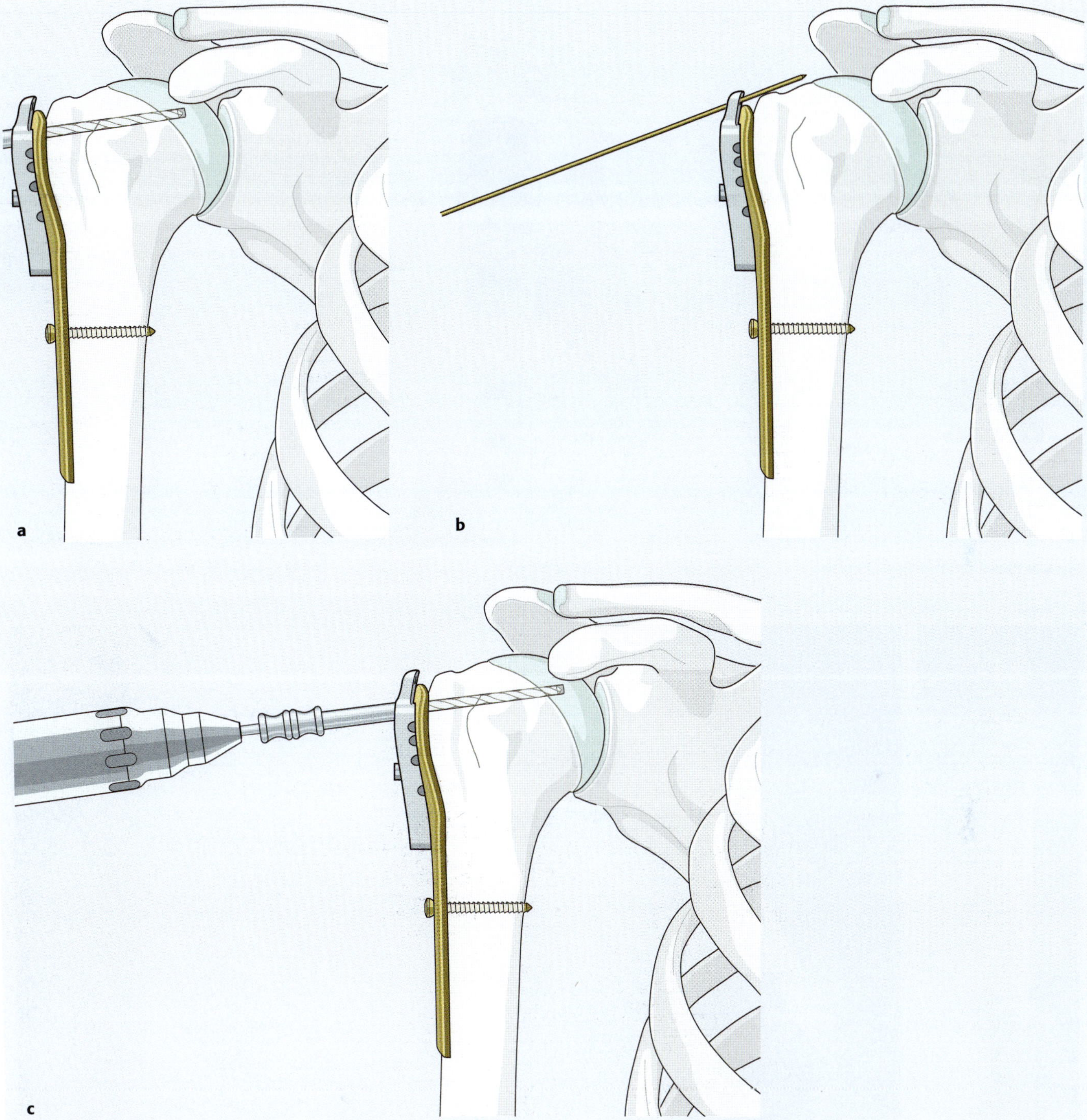

Fig 4.5-15a–e PHILOS plate.
a–c With the aiming device for screw placement.

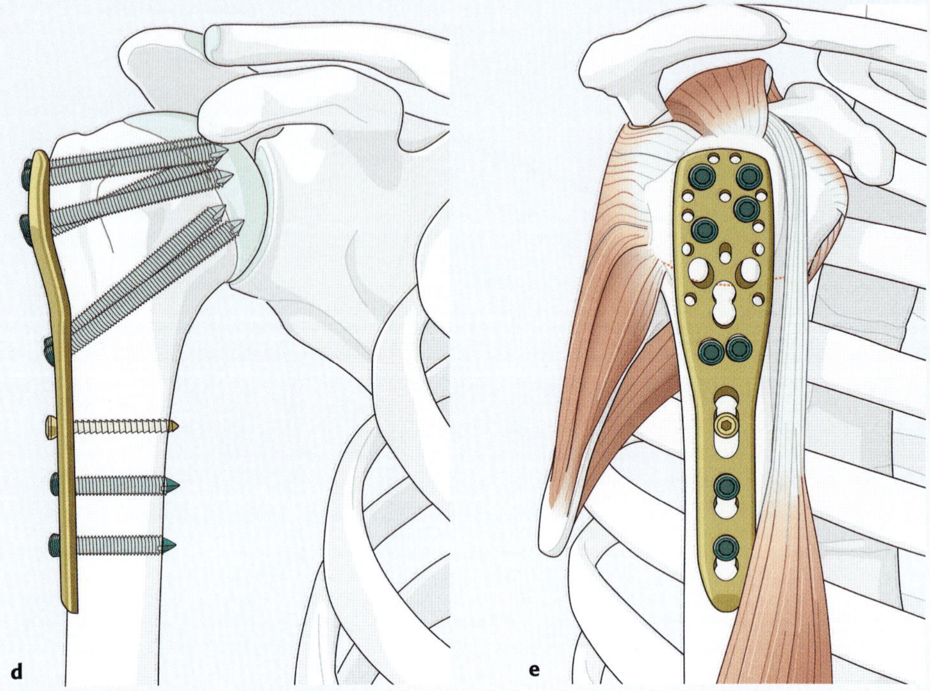

Fig 4.5-15a–e (cont) PHILOS plate.
d–e After removal of aiming device.

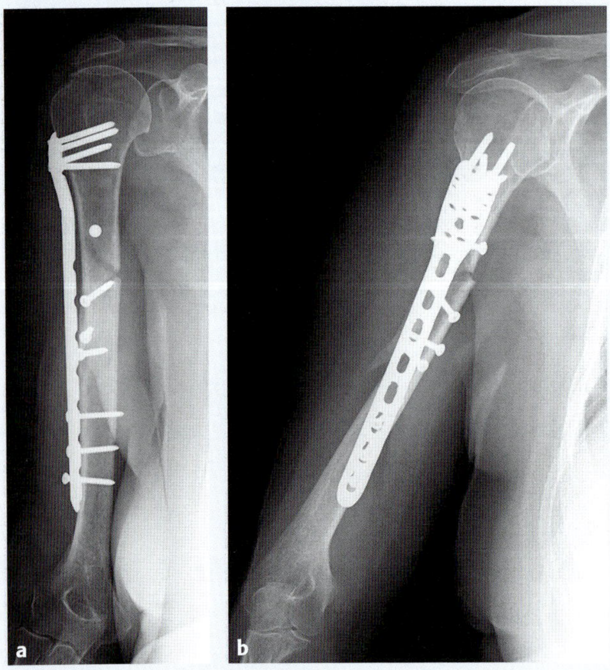

Fig 4.5-16a–b X-ray result at 6 months showing the bone continuity which is stable and evolving towards union.

Case description

An 82-year-old man suffered a casual fall in his home, with trauma at the level of the left hip, presenting with a pertrochanteric fracture of the left femur with a reverse oblique pattern (AO/OTA 31A3) (**Fig 4.5-17**).

At admission, the patient was prepared for the surgical intervention, which was to be performed the following day. Surgery was planned to reduce the fracture and stabilize it with a long intramedullary implant, positioning the patient on the operating table with traction of the limb and the contralateral limb in flexion of 90° (**Fig 4.5-18**).

Reduction before limb positioning could not be achieved due to instability of the fracture. To achieve reduction, additional maneuvers were planned through minimally invasive approaches during the intervention. Two small additional lateral incisions were made; one at the level of the proximal fragment to introduce an elevator with which this fragment was moved medially and with valgus impact; and a second incision, located on the proximal part of the diaphyseal fragment, to introduce a small bone hook to laterally move the diaphyseal fragment towards the proximal fragment, thereby achieving reduction. Such maneuvers, carried out under image intensification, enabled an anatomical reduction of the fracture followed by the introduction of the trochanteric nail during the same intervention (**Fig 4.5-19**).

While the reduction was maintained, a lateral incision was made at the trochanter to localize the entry point for the nail, carry out the perforation, and insert the nail. The nail, while advancing through the fracture site, caused the reduction to displace due to manual maneuvers. It was decided to accept the situation when the bone fragments contacted the bone fragments at the fracture site and that the good grip of the head and neck screw would maintain stability until fracture union. The intervention was completed by simply distal locking.

Postoperative control x-rays show the definitive situation following the intervention (**Fig 4.5-20**).

Four weeks after surgery, the patient could walk with the aid of a walking frame but with pain and little movement autonomy. The control x-rays showed the displacement on the AP view (**Fig 4.5-21a–b**). The lateral view (**Fig 4.5-21c**) showed the extremely posterior location of the nail entry into the trochanteric region. At the 1-month follow-up, there was shortening of the limb and the displacement was not varied (**Fig 4.5-21d**).

In control x-rays at 12 weeks, the situation had not changed and clinically, the pain when walking persisted (**Fig 4.5-22**).

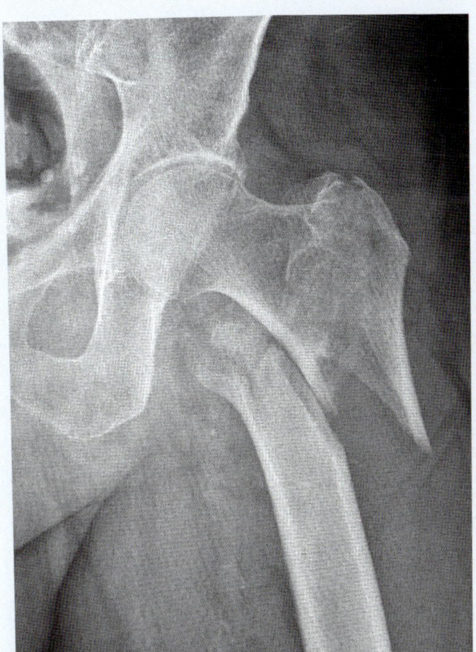

Fig 4.5-17 Preoperative AP x-ray of the pertrochanteric fracture.

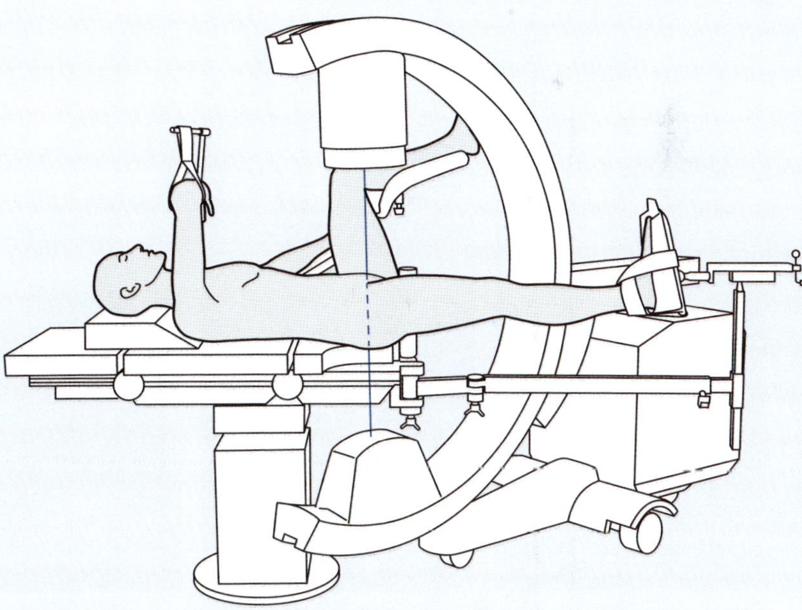

Fig 4.5-18 The patient must be correctly positioned for x-ray control with the image intensifier during surgery.

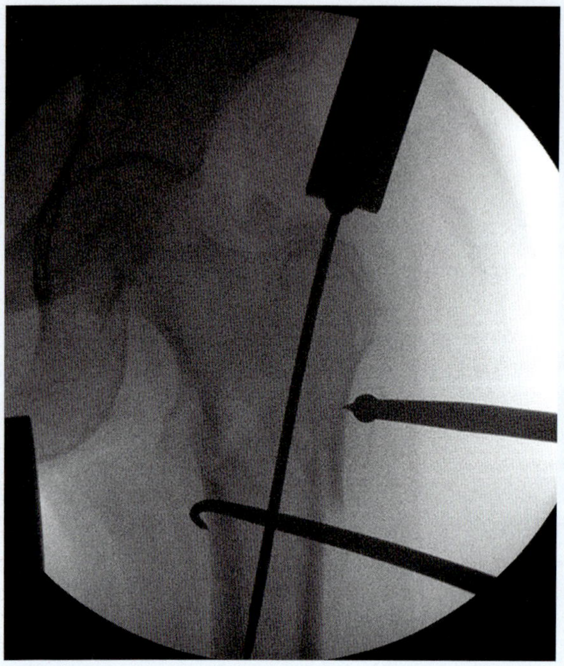

Fig 4.5-19 C-arm control image showing intraoperative reduction maneuvers. An elevator moves and reduces the proximal fragment medially, and a bone hook moves the diaphyseal fragment laterally to achieve reduction before placing the nail.

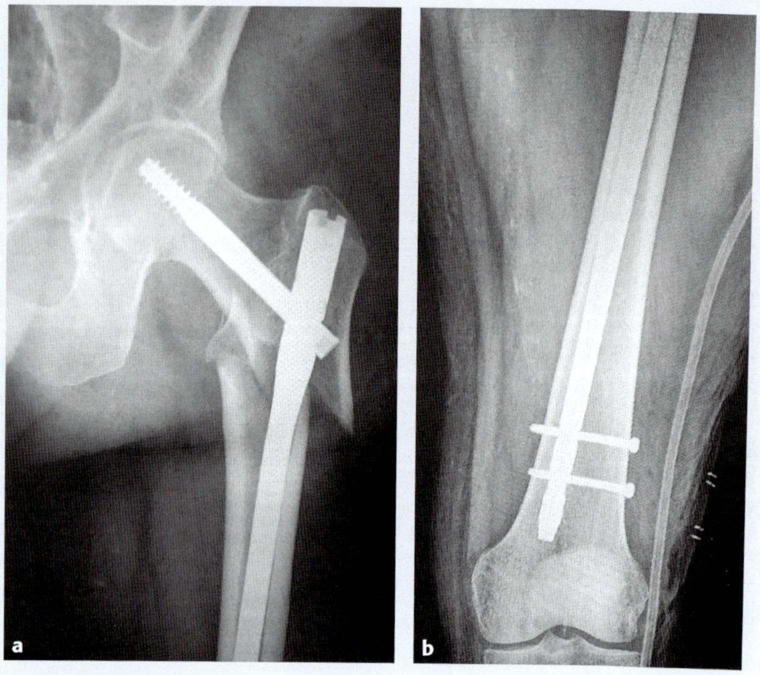

Fig 4.5-20a–b X-ray of the osteosynthesis performed in the immediate postoperative period. The fracture site is not reduced, presenting vascularization and lateral translation.

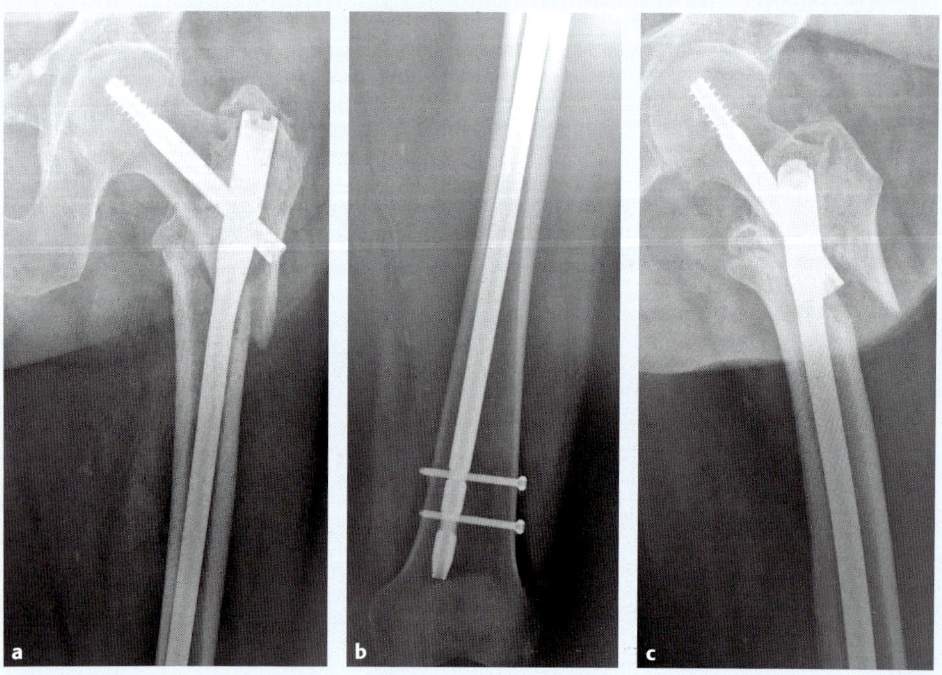

Fig 4.5-21a–d Postoperative control x-rays.
a–c At 4 weeks the fracture remains displaced in the AP view (**a–b**). In the lateral view (**c**) it is also possible to see the posterior entry in the trochanteric region.

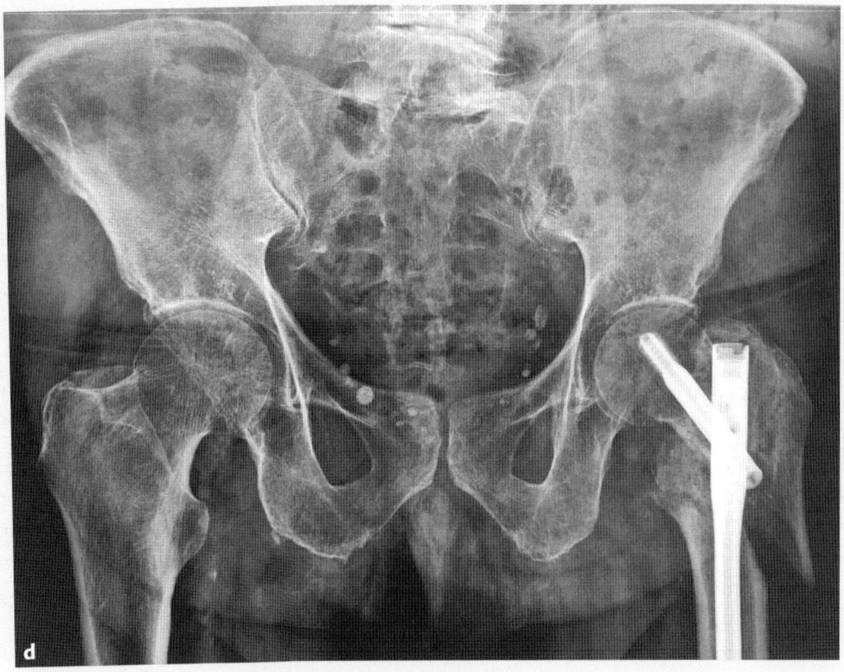

Fig 4.5-21a–d (cont) Postoperative control x-rays.
d AP x-ray of the pelvis 1 month following the intervention.

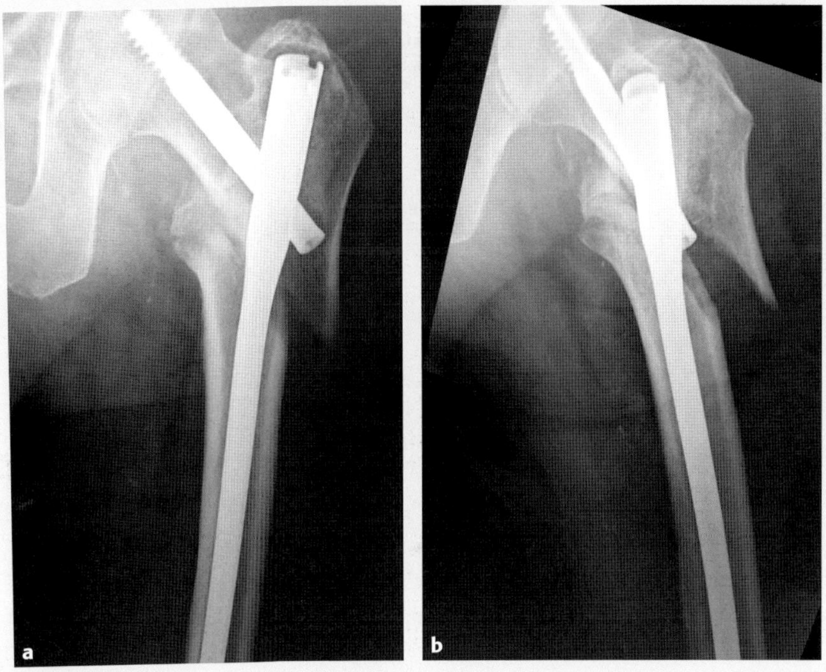

Fig 4.5-22a–b Control x-rays at 12 weeks showing no signs of union between the displaced bone fragments.

Analysis of failure and reflection

The x-ray study and the preoperative diagnosis were correct, as was the plan for medical stabilization of the patient and intervention. The decision on the type of implant, the position of the patient, and the fracture reduction, which was done intraoperatively because it had not been possible before, were all done correctly. The fractures of the trochanteric area can present significant comminution and displacements that hinder the reduction and stabilization of these fractures. In this case, for the fracture in an oblique inverted pattern (AO/OTA 31A3) the surgeon has associated difficulties in achieving an anatomical reduction. This must be achieved with added maneuvers through instruments during the intervention and prior to the placement of the intramedullary nail. However here, perhaps due to the inexperience of the surgeon or an inability to see the error, once the fracture was reduced, the entry hole that should have been created at the tip of the trochanter was displaced inadvertently towards a posterior anomalous position (**Fig 4.5-23**).

The incorrect entry of the nail in the trochanteric mass forced the displacement of the facture as it passed through the site. The attempt to manually counteract the force exercised by the nail was fruitless and the same nail, supported by the cortices and by way of a lever, forced the displacement causing additional fractures in the femoral cortices. The head and neck screw, well situated in the femoral neck, sufficiently gripped the hard nucleus of the head, therefore no cut-out occurred. If the head and neck grip of the screw is precarious due to poor positioning or reduction of bone resistance due to osteoporosis, the screw pulls out of the femoral head (cut out).

If the intervention had not continued and intraoperative analysis had been performed to check for the displacement of the fracture, it would have been possible to correct the entry of the nail and the subsequent displacement. The decision to accept an anomalous situation as satisfactory, due to fear of further breaking the trochanteric mass, to concerns for fatigue, or simply to a lack of surgical experience or excellence, can lead to inevitable repeated interventions.

The authors have detected this same failure in other cases where the location of the entry hole of the nail is poorly positioned, sometimes in the medial area, sometimes lateral, and even anterior. Special attention must be paid to this technical detail in general in all nailing since on occasion, well-planned interventions with good reductions end up with a poor result. The same thing happens with the diaphyseal nails, where depending on the implant model, they require insertion in a specific location that must be respected since the implant cannot tolerate deformation and instead forces the bone to adapt to the implant. This therefore prevents the expected reduction or causes additional fractures. The experience of the surgeon is essential but so is specific knowledge about the technical indications of each implant.

Final outcome

Given the poor clinical evolution of the patient, affected by pain and inability to walk, it was decided to perform a reintervention to achieve reduction and correct stabilization until fracture union. The removal of the intramedullary nail was planned along with an open reduction to achieve valgus bowing of the proximal femoral fragment and reduce the fracture with compression. Placement of a plate with a sliding screw was planned. The head and neck screw placed in position under the preexisting one was inserted into the plate and situated with less angulation with respect to the diaphysis, so that once the bone was reduced, the valgus bowing of the proximal fragment favored the support of loads at the fracture level and in the weakened proximal zone. Compression of the anterolateral area of the trochanter was reinforced with an additional traction screw to reduce and stabilize the previous displacement (**Fig 4.5-24**).

The patient's healing progressed well and showed fracture union in the postoperative phase. He began pain-free ambulation with a walking stick at 3 months (**Fig 4.5-25**).

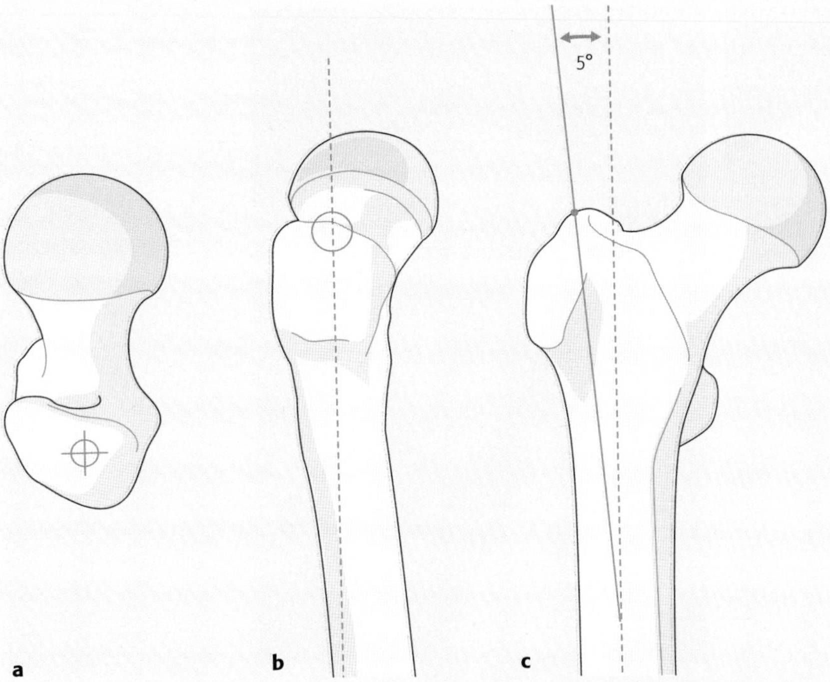

Fig 4.5-23a–c Correct location of the entry point for the trochanteric nail.

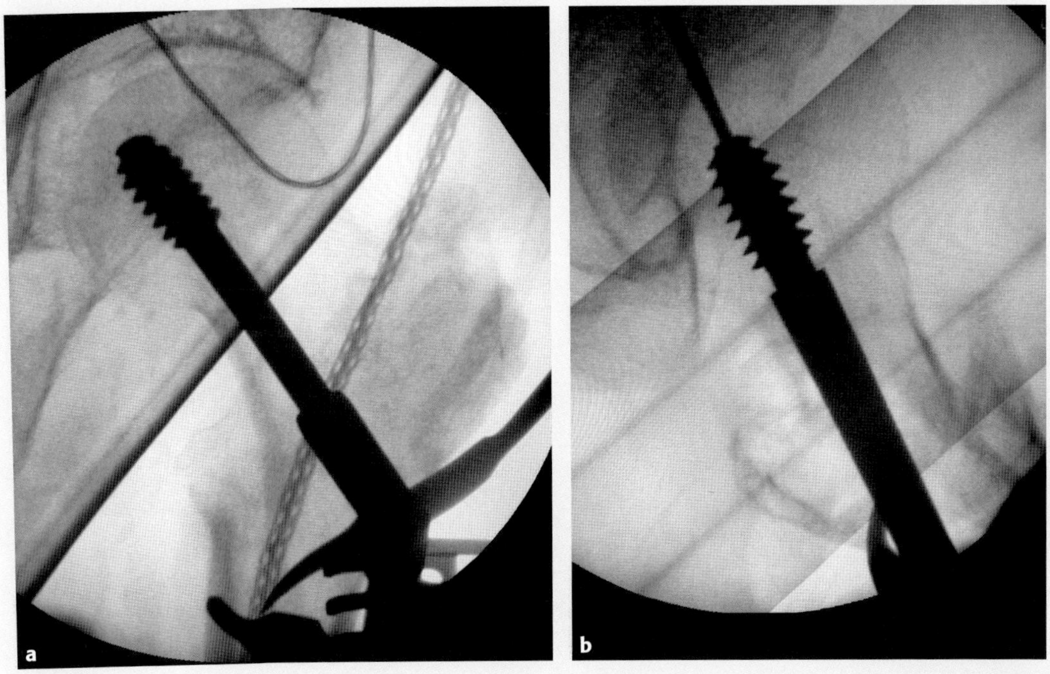

Fig 4.5-24a–e Intraoperative and postoperative images.
a–b Intraoperative C-arm images of the reintervention. Note that the cephalic screw is inserted in the lower and posterior head and neck region in order to anchor it in the healthy bone.

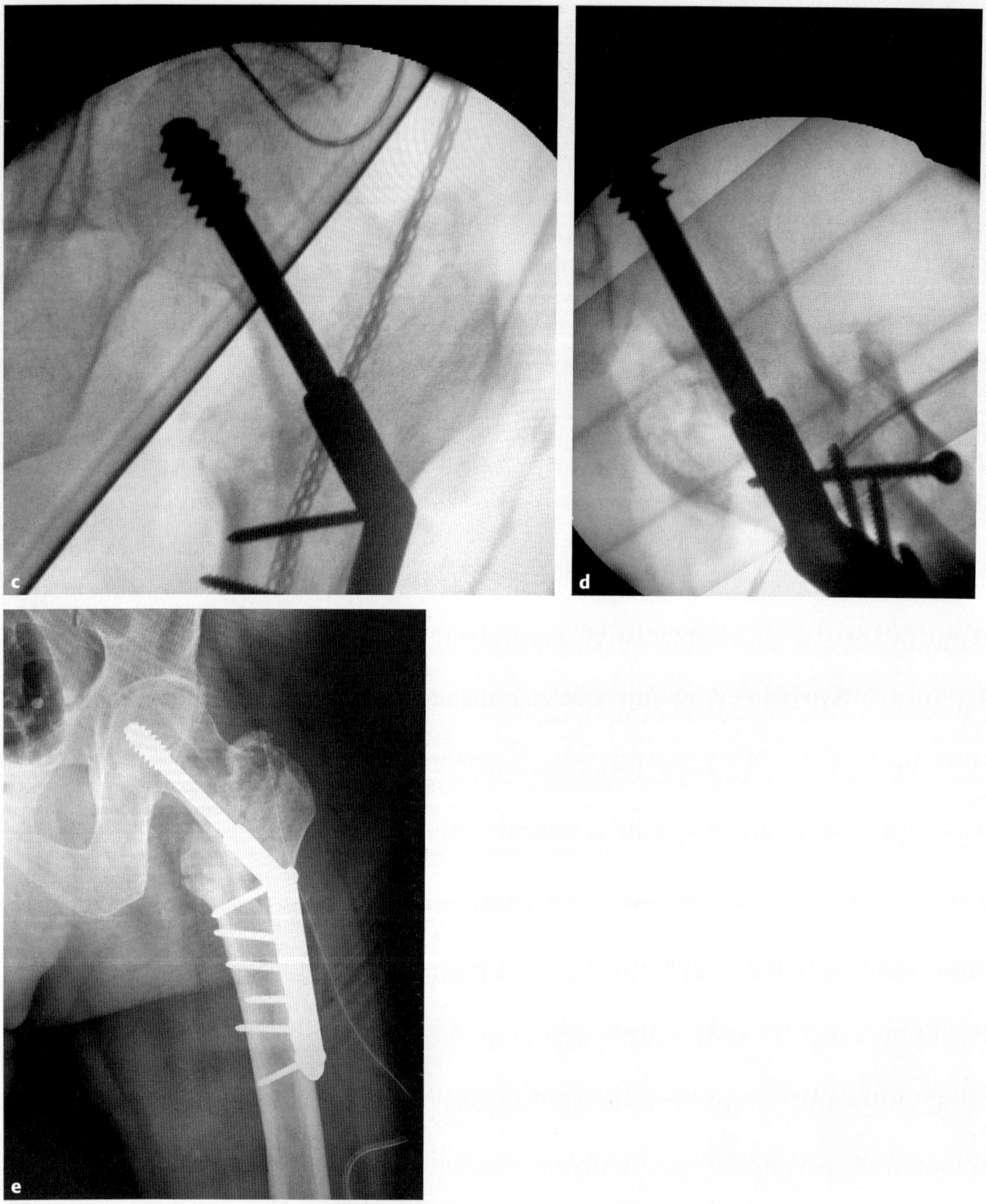

Fig 4.5-24a–e (cont) Intraoperative and postoperative image.
c–d Intraoperative C-arm images of the reintervention to achieve valgus of the proximal fragment after plate fixation. Note the valgus bowing of the site after the plate was applied to the bone.
e Control x-ray in the immediate postoperative period showing the reduction obtained and the position of the implants.

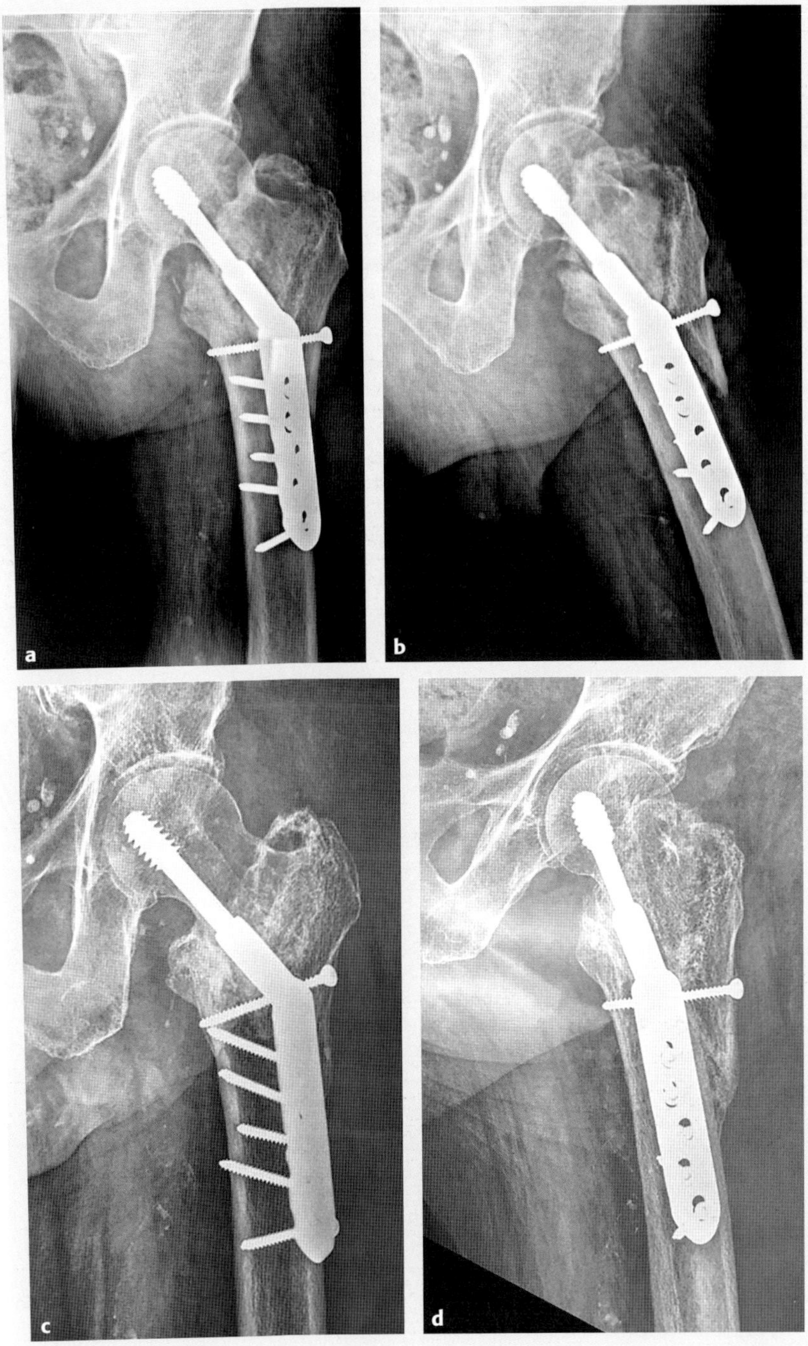

Fig 4.5-25a–d Postoperative control x-rays.

a–b Control x-rays in AP (**a**) and axial (**b**) views at 6 weeks. The reduction is maintained and the implants remain in situ, without presenting any cut-out in the femoral head.

c–d Control x-rays in AP (**c**) and axial (**d**) views 1 year after surgery. The signs of union have begun and clinically, the patient presents no pain that prevents him from walking.

Key points to remember

- The theoretical knowledge of the biological and mechanical conditions for the surgical treatment of a fracture is fundamental.
- Learning requires time and dedication to be able to perform appropriate treatments.
- Personal critical review (self-assessment) of each treatment performed is essential and helps the surgeon to assimilate concepts, know her or his own technical capacity, recognize areas that need improvement, and avoid repeating mistakes.
- The surgeon must adequately evaluate results to avoid repeating failures.
- The expertise of the surgeon needs to cover the whole process of the treatment, ie, pre-, intra-, and postoperative.
- The judicious follow-up of patients should detect any complication and therefore facilitate appropriate treatment as soon as possible.

References and suggested reading

Baumgaertner MR, Curtin SL, Lindskog DM, et al. The value of the tip-apex distance in predicting failure of fixation of peritrochanteric fractures of the hip. *J Bone Joint Surg Am.* 1995 Jul;77(7):1058–1064.

De Bruijn K, den Hartog D, Tuinebreijer W, et al. Reliability of predictors for screw cutout in intertrochanteric hip fractures. *J Bone Joint Surg Am.* 2012 Jul 18;94(14):1266–1272.

Flores SA, Woolridge A, Caroom C, et al. The Utility of the Tip-Apex Distance in Predicting Axial Migration and Cutout With the Trochanteric Fixation Nail System Helical Blade. *J Orthop Trauma.* 2016 Jun;30(6):e207–211.

Müller M, Allgöwer M, Schneider R, et al. *Manual of Internal Fixation.* 2nd ed. Berlin Heidelberg New York: Springer Verlag; 1970.

Orozco Delclós R. *Errores en la Osteosíntesis.* Barcelona: Masson; 1993. Spanish.

Orozco Delclós R. El ocaso de las placas. ¿Por qué se rompen los implantes? [The demise of plates. Why do implants break?]. *Rev Ortop Traumatol.* 2001;45(3):177–182. Spanish.

Palm H, Jacobsen S, Sonne-Holm S, et al. Integrity of the lateral femoral wall in intertrochanteric hip fractures: an important predictor of a reoperation. *J Bone Joint Surg Am.* 2007 Mar;89(3):470–475.

Vallier HA, Wang X, Moore TA, et al. Timing of orthopaedic surgery in multiple trauma patients: development of a protocol for early appropriate care. *J Orthop Trauma.* 2013 Oct;27(10):543–551.

Terry Axelrod, Suthorn Bavonratanavech, Matej Cimerman, Joan Girós Torres, Anze Kristan, Roberto Rivero Sosa, J Miquel Sales Pérez, Miquel Videla Cés

4.6 Accumulation of failures

Terry Axelrod, Suthorn Bavonratanavech, Matej Cimerman, Joan Girós Torres, Anze Kristan, Roberto Rivero Sosa, J Miquel Sales Pérez, Miquel Videla Cés

Random events tend to occur in groups.

Tylczak's Probability Postulate

We have been able to observe in the detailed study of some of the cases presented that the accumulation of more than one theoretical and/or practical failure is likely to lead to a negative result. When the failures are not significant, evolution tends towards healing, but if they are of a certain magnitude, the accumulation of several such failures in a single fracture will most certainly lead to complications that are often difficult to correct.

The accumulation of several failures is usually due to a lack of planning, which makes improvisation during surgery necessary. If the operation is not stopped when the first difficulty appears in order to consider what is happening and seek adequate solutions, a series of failures is likely to occur with consequences that are usually worse than the severity of the facture that is being treated. Occasionally, if a fracture is not reduced adequately, the implant is unlikely to achieve optimum outcome and maneuvers to try to continue with the intervention are increasingly more counterproductive, leading to an accumulation of errors and a poor outcome. Failure to comply with the osteosynthesis principles of reduction, stability, respect for vascularization, and achieving pain-free mobilization may occur for various reasons that we have progressively developed in this book. An accumulation of breaches of these principles leads to failure. In the study of cases where an accumulation of failures exists, this chain of events can usually be observed and understanding it is essential and of great educational value.

CASE 1

Case description

A 56-year-old man weighing 140 kg had a road traffic accident, presenting with a left intertrochanteric hip fracture (AO/OTA 31A3). The fracture was considered unstable in the coronal plane (**Fig 4.6-1**).

The fracture was treated with a proximal femoral locking plate. After the intervention there was a varus malreduction of 120° with the plate positioned too low. This caused the screw trajectories to be too high on the upper part of the femoral head instead of being situated in the strong inferomedial quadrant. The length of the three proximal screws was too short. All these factors contributed to the instability of the construction (**Fig 4.6-2**).

The patient began ambulation in the immediate postoperative period, but due to the instability of the fixation and the patient's heavy weight, a cut-out of the unstable implant assembly at the femoral head occurred after 3 weeks (**Fig 4.6-3**).

The removal of the implant was planned and varus correction achieved by fixation with a proximal femoral nail antirotation (PFNA)-type trochanteric nail (**Fig 4.6-4**).

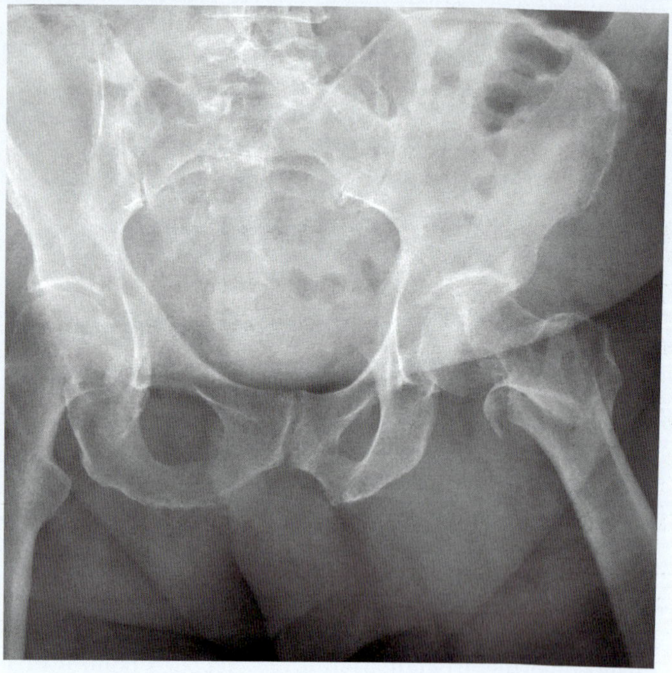

Fig 4.6-1 Preoperative x-ray of the closed intertrochanteric fracture of the left hip.

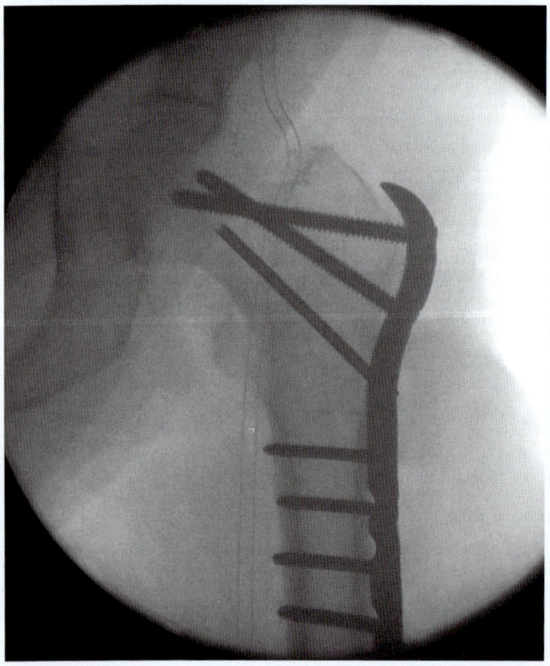

Fig 4.6-2 Intraoperative C-arm image showing a varus malposition of 120° and a plate positioning that is too low, resulting in an unstable construction.

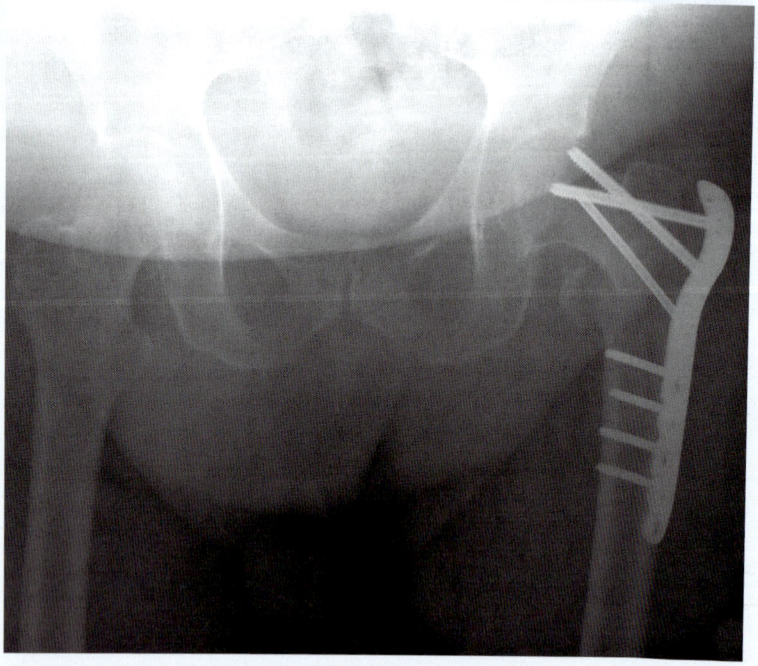

Fig 4.6-3 The unstable fixation, along with the patient's excess weight, contributed to a cut-out at the femoral head 3 weeks after the operation.

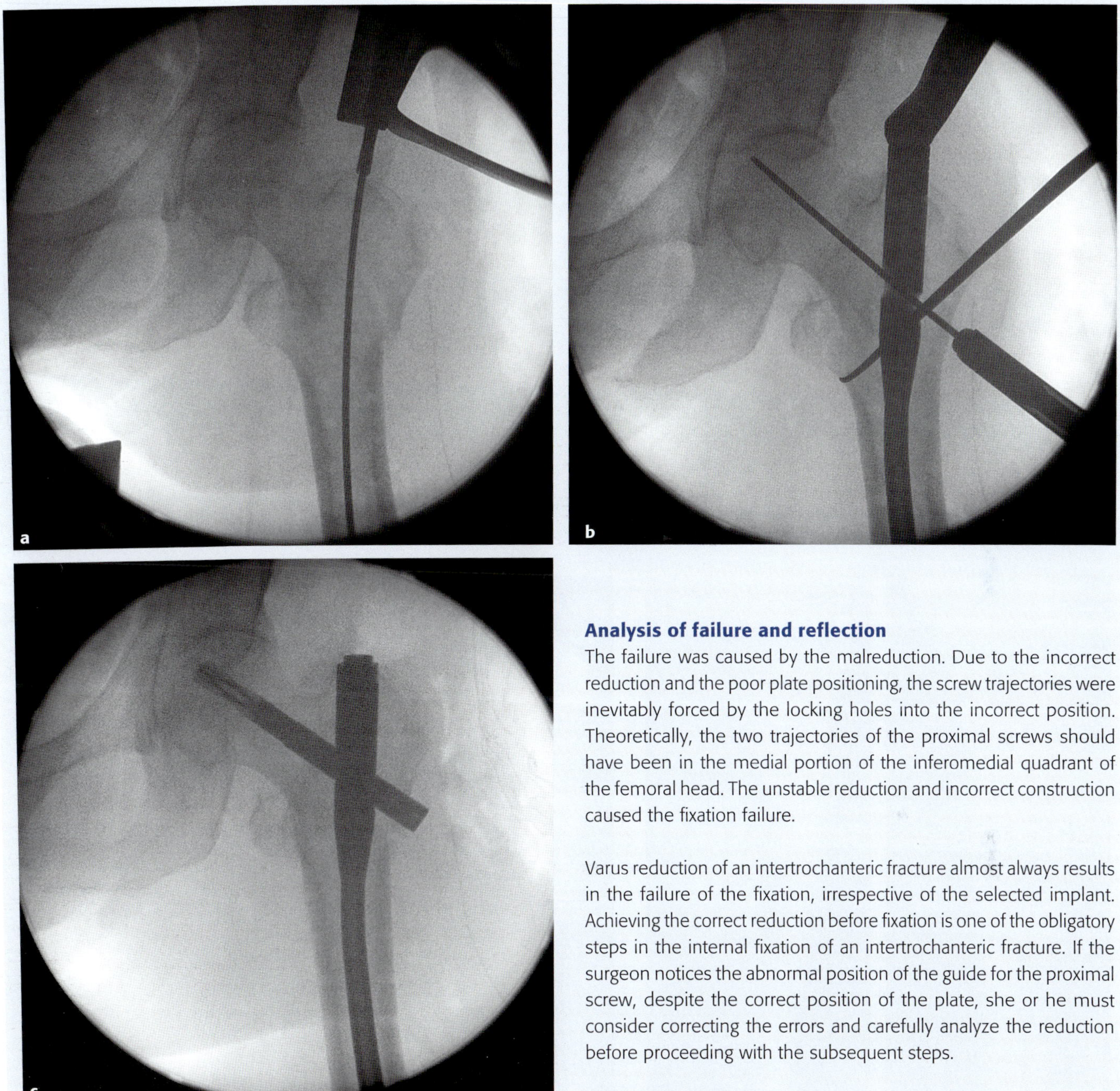

Fig 4.6-4a–c Intraoperative C-arm images.

- **a** The previous implant was removed and fixed with a proximal femoral nail antirotation (PFNA). The image shows the entry point for the trochanteric nail (ie, PFNA).
- **b** The varus reduction was corrected and maintained through traction with a bone hook.
- **c** Final reduction and fixation with the PFNA.

Analysis of failure and reflection

The failure was caused by the malreduction. Due to the incorrect reduction and the poor plate positioning, the screw trajectories were inevitably forced by the locking holes into the incorrect position. Theoretically, the two trajectories of the proximal screws should have been in the medial portion of the inferomedial quadrant of the femoral head. The unstable reduction and incorrect construction caused the fixation failure.

Varus reduction of an intertrochanteric fracture almost always results in the failure of the fixation, irrespective of the selected implant. Achieving the correct reduction before fixation is one of the obligatory steps in the internal fixation of an intertrochanteric fracture. If the surgeon notices the abnormal position of the guide for the proximal screw, despite the correct position of the plate, she or he must consider correcting the errors and carefully analyze the reduction before proceeding with the subsequent steps.

Final outcome

The varus malreduction was corrected and a PFNA was inserted. The patient was able to begin ambulation and rehabilitation in the immediate postoperative period until union in the correct position was achieved.

CASE 2

Case description

A 52-year-old man presented with a multifragmentary fracture of the right tibia after a road traffic accident with a motorbike. It was a multifragmentary segmental tibial fracture (AO/OTA 42C2), without contact between the proximal and distal fragments and with a third intermediate intercalary fragment, which was associated with a multifragmentary fibular fracture at the same level as the tibia (AO/OTA 4F2B).

High-energy fracture that is usually associated with an injury to the soft tissues occasionally requires temporary stabilization until definitive osteosynthesis can be performed. In this case, prior temporary stabilization was not required, and the condition of the soft tissues allowed for definitive osteosynthesis with a reamed intramedullary nail.

The first operation was performed using a reamed nail locked in the proximal area. A short nail which was insufficient to stabilize the distal site also presented an excessively anterior entry hole. This led to breakage of the anterior wall of the proximal tibial zone and a lack of reduction of the proximal fracture site. The ultimate position of the nail outside the proximal fragment of the tibia prevented the reduction and the nail from adequately performing its function from the biomechanical viewpoint. This was an unstable osteosynthesis causing the breakage of one of the proximal screws (**Fig 4.6-5**).

Subsequently, an attempt was made to rescue the fracture with a new unreamed nail with modern characteristics (eg, unreamed tibial nail [UTN]). This nail was longer but had the same technical defects as its predecessor: the entry point and nonreduction of the fracture (**Fig 4.6-6**).

Eventually, the shortened fibula healed and the distal site consolidated. The patient presented with pain and functional impairment despite the extensor apparatus of the knee functioning and a viable pseudarthrosis of the proximal site (**Fig 4.6-7**).

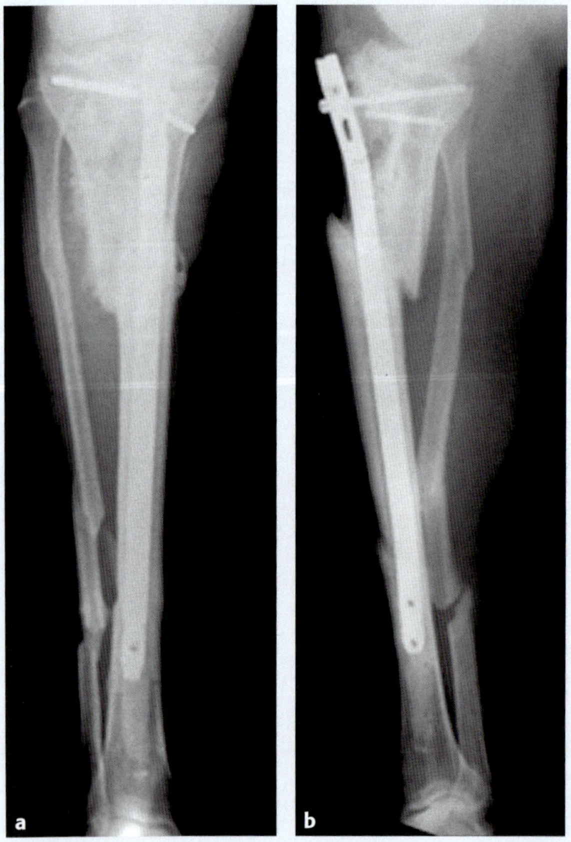

Fig 4.6-5a–b AP (**a**) and lateral (**b**) x-rays of the first nailing.

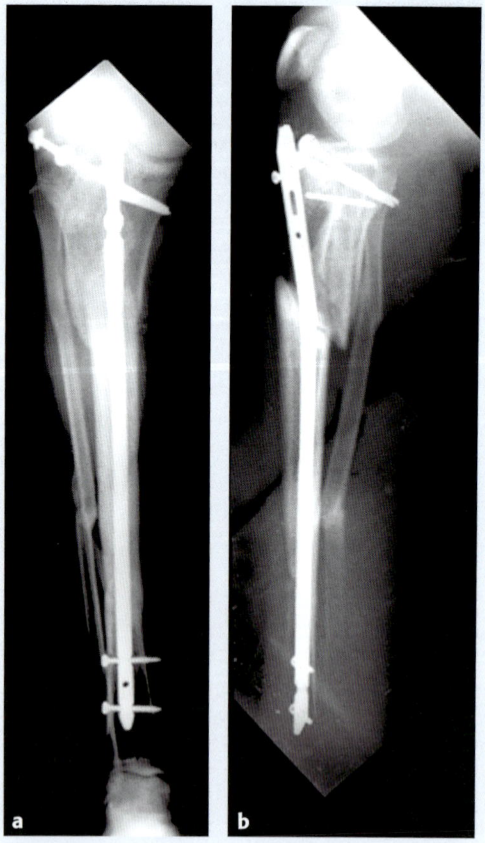

Fig 4.6-6a–b AP (**a**) and lateral (**b**) x-rays of the second nailing.

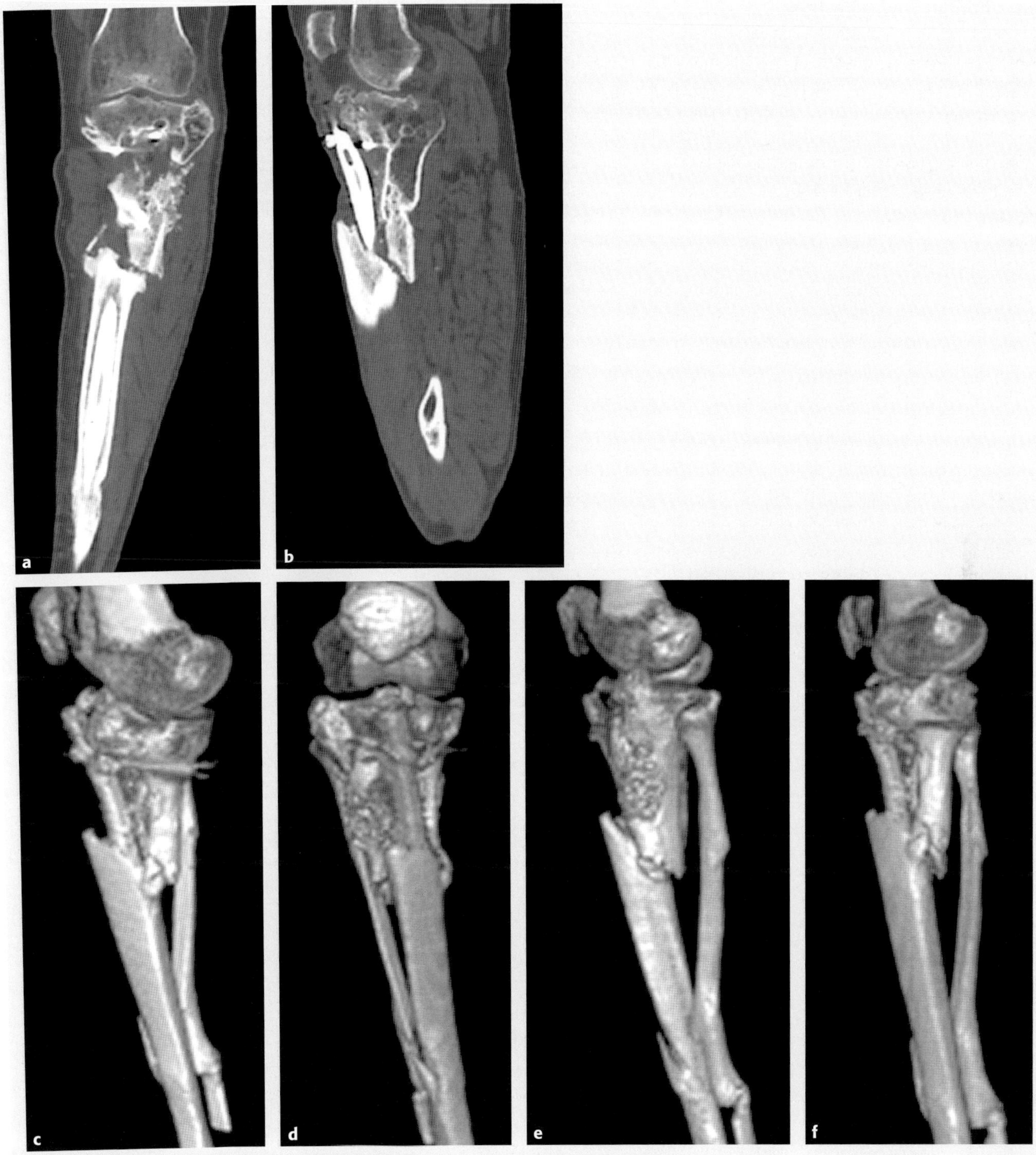

Fig 4.6-7a–f Computed tomographic scans of the fracture.
a–b Computed tomographic scans of the pseudarthrosis at the proximal fracture site.
c–f Computed tomographic scans with 3D reconstruction of the pseudarthrosis.

Analysis of failure and reflection

The indication for intramedullary nailing was correct in this case of a fracture at two levels to align and reduce the fracture, and also to act as a guide for the axial load forces. The nailing technique must be precise to avoid complications that arise if the indications are not followed correctly. The exact location for the adequate introduction of the nail means that on many occasions the nail also facilitates reduction of the fracture (**Fig 4.6-8**).

In contrast, choosing a wrong entry point can cause complications and nonreduction. The nailing technique is demanding and requires correct planning both technically and regarding the choice of the correct nail measurements. Improvising a technique that can be difficult is in itself reckless. Any unexpected event or complication that occurs during nailing must be resolved immediately by using a preplanned alternative strategy.

In this case, the attempt to rescue the first nail with another nail seems inadequate given that the lack of contact in the tibial cortex will prevent both the reduction of the fracture and its correct functioning. Substituting a reamed nail for a nonreamed one (eg, UTN), even if locked, does not provide the sufficient stability required to resolve the problem. Occasionally, as in this case, the succession of adverse effects, leads to an accumulation of failures that must be carefully analyzed to avoid adding any further setbacks.

Final outcome

A new intervention was planned for the removal of the intramedullary nail and compression of the pseudarthrosis site with two traction screws as the main osteosynthesis material, protected by a molded straight plate to maintain the correct axis of the limb. Nonweight bearing was indicated for 6 weeks after which the patient started progressive partial weight bearing until pain-free full weight bearing was achieved at 3 months. The final x-rays at 6 months showed tibial consolidation with adequate axes although with a shortening of 1.5 cm, which was compensated for by a raised insole in his footwear (**Fig 4.6-9**).

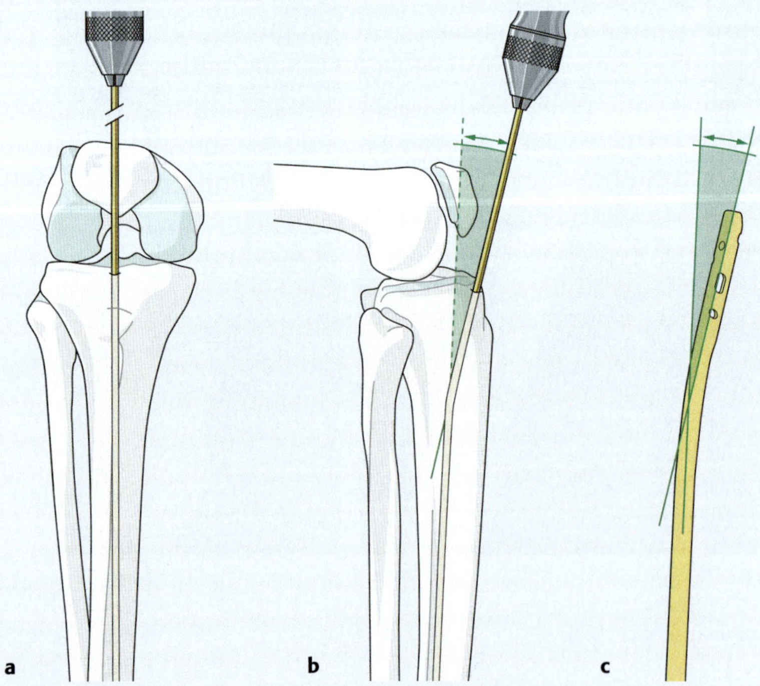

Fig 4.6-8a–f The correct entry point of the intramedullary nail in the proximal area of the tibia.

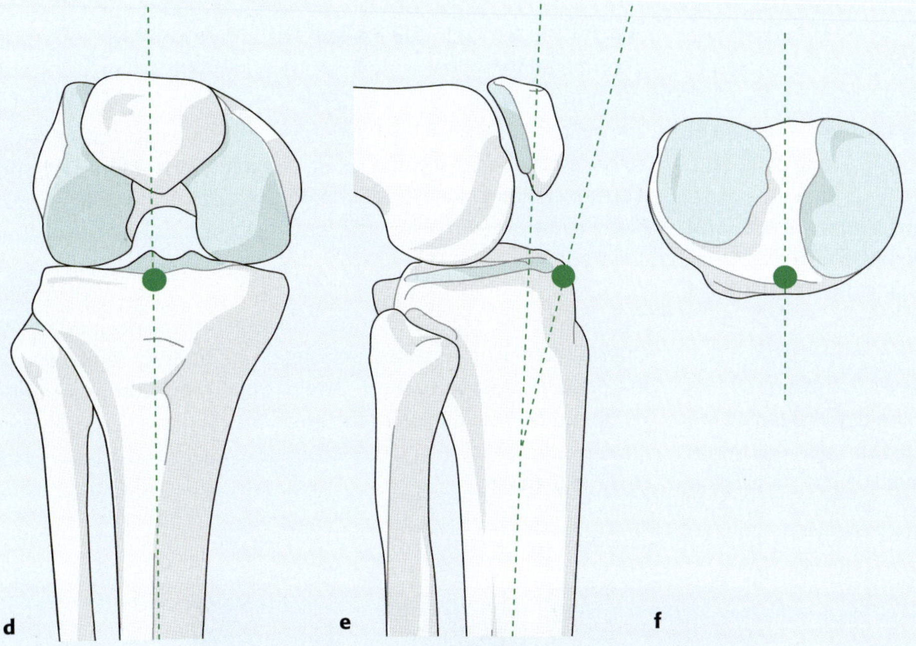

Fig 4.6-8a–f (cont) The correct entry point of the intramedullary nail in the proximal area of the tibia.

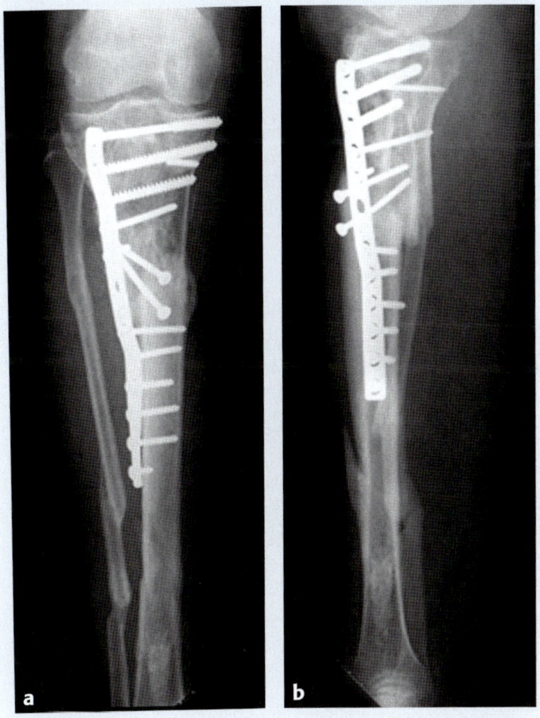

Fig 4.6-9a–b AP (**a**) and lateral (**b**) x-rays at 6 months after the definitive intervention, showing the union of the pseudarthrosis.

CASE 3

Case description

A 48-year-old woman without prior medical issues of interest was a front seat passenger when injured in a high-speed car accident.

She sustained a type C pelvic ring injury (**Fig 4.6-10a**), a fracture of the left femur (AO/OTA 32C3) (**Fig 4.6-10b**), and a lung contusion.

On the day of the accident, she underwent surgery at the local hospital for the femoral fracture with an intramedullary nail. During the femoral nailing process, another spiral fracture occurred just below the original one (**Fig 4.6-11**).

Three days after the injury, she was transferred to the author's institution for treatment of the pelvic ring. On the day of transfer, the patient was hemodynamically stable (**Fig 4.6-12**). Upon admission to the hospital, a severe deformity was observed on internal rotation of her lower left limb (**Fig 4.6-13**). The x-rays were expanded with a computed tomographic scan of the pelvis (**Fig 4.6-14**).

The patient underwent reintervention 2 days after admission to the author's hospital. Firstly, the pelvic ring injury was addressed, with a posterior fixation for the sacral injury and application of an external fixator to the anterior pelvis. The femoral torsion deformity was then checked once again (**Fig 4.6-15**).

The patient was placed on a traction table. It was decided not to change the nailing. The distal locking of the nail was removed and the fracture site approached. Careful open reduction was carried out to reduce the rotation of the fragments and two cerclage wires were used. Then the intramedullary nail was locked distally once more (**Fig 4.6-16**).

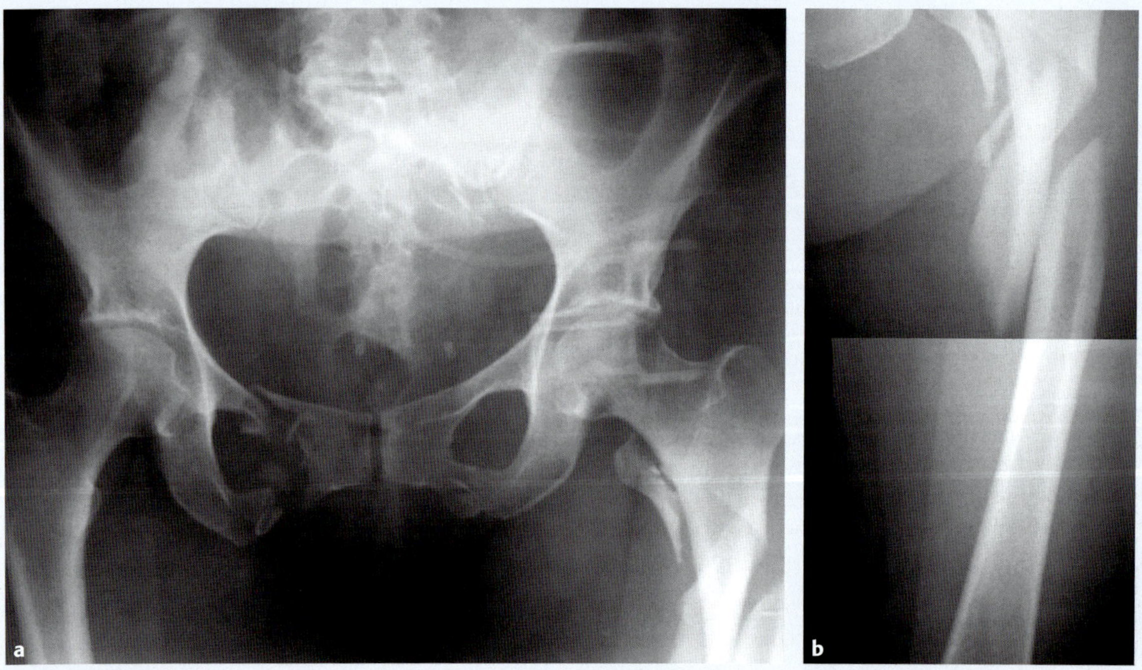

Fig 4.6-10a–b Initial injury x-rays.
a X-ray of the type C pelvic ring injury.
b X-ray of the fracture of the left femoral proximal diaphysis.

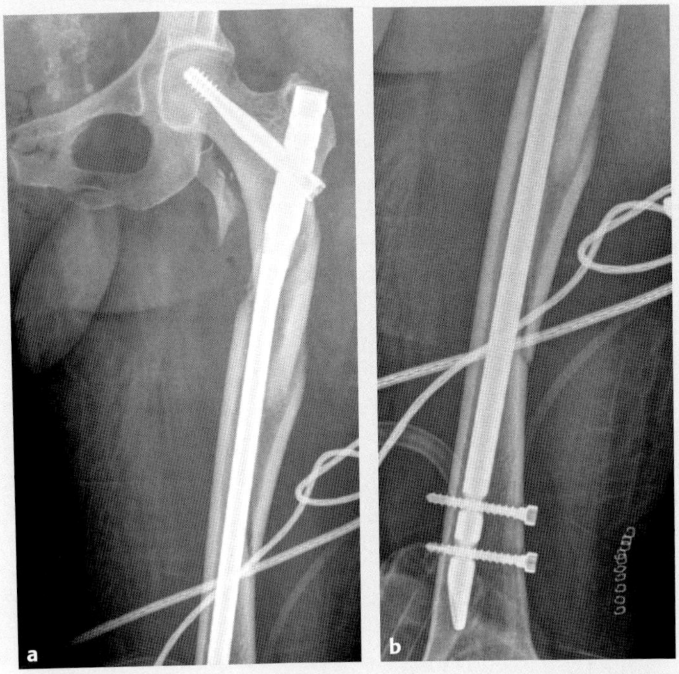

Fig 4.6-11a–b Postoperative control x-rays after the first intervention of the left femur.

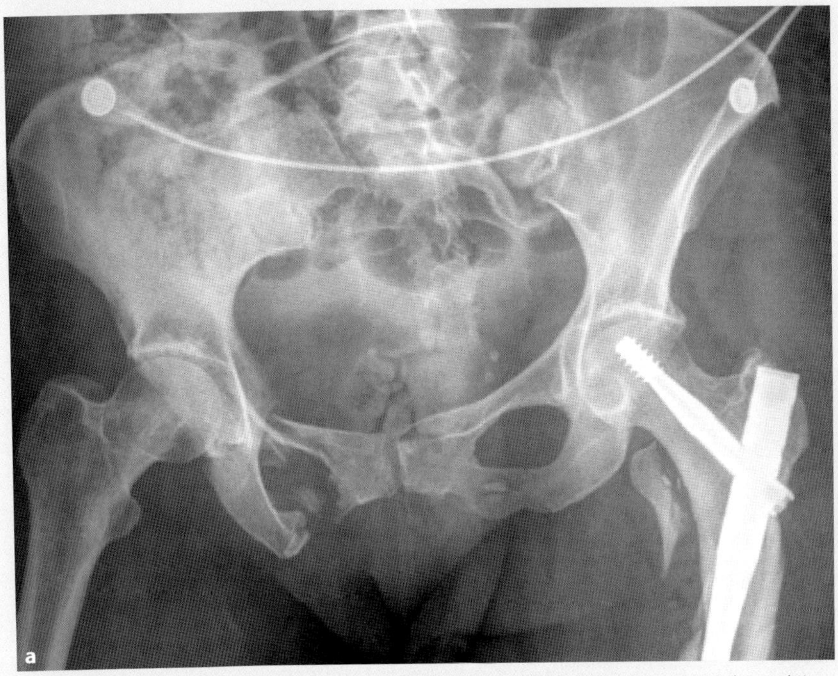

Fig 4.6-12a–c X-rays of the pelvis on the day of admission for treatment of the pelvic ring injury.

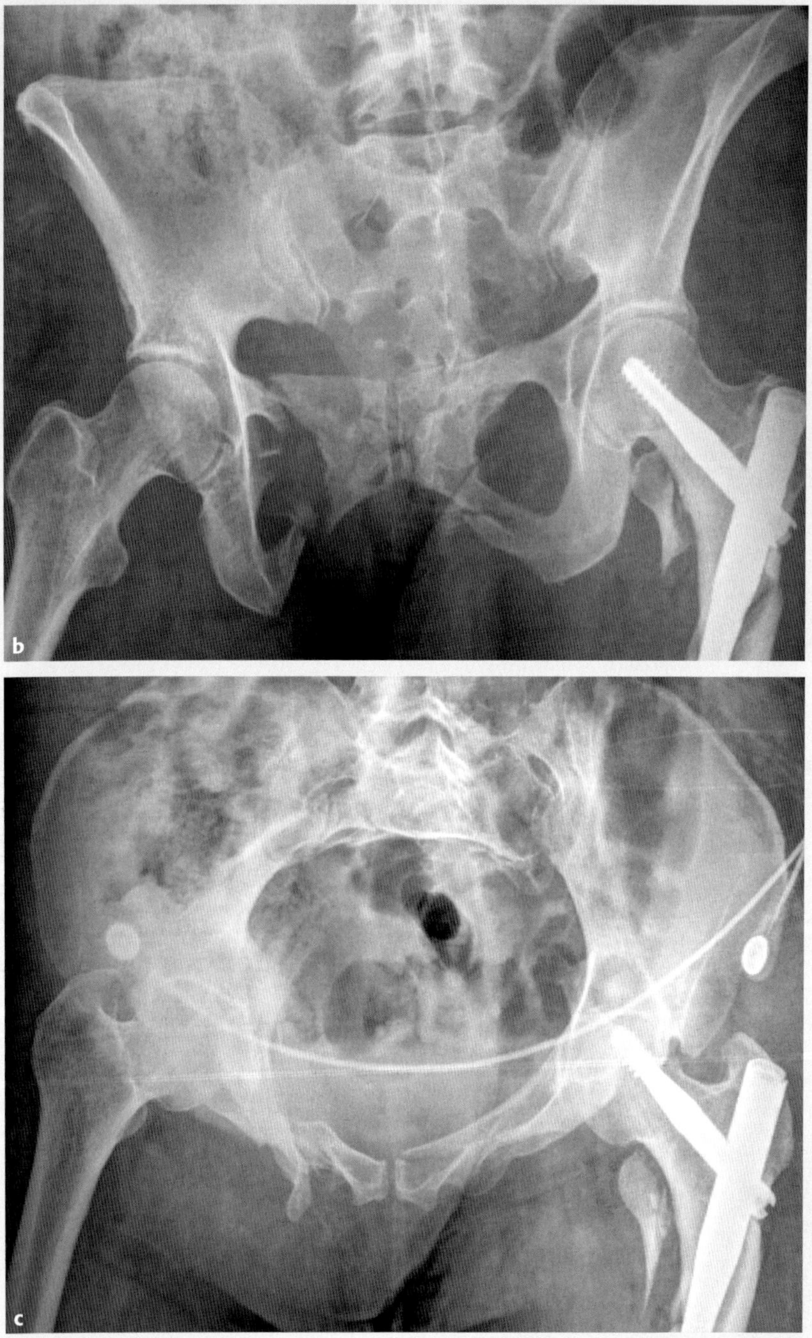

Fig 4.6-12a–c (cont) X-rays of the pelvis on the day of admission for treatment of the pelvic ring injury.

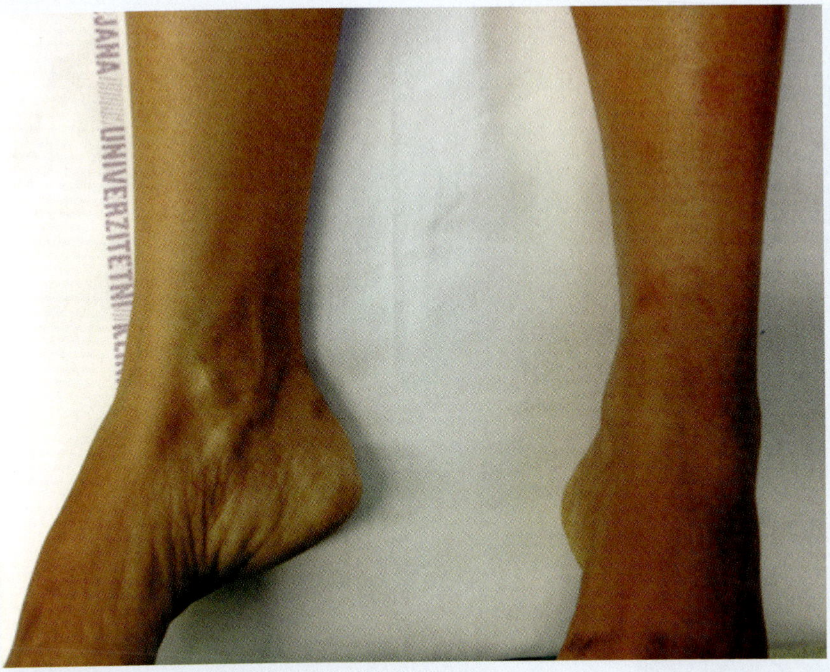

Fig 4.6-13 Torsional deformity of the lower left limb.

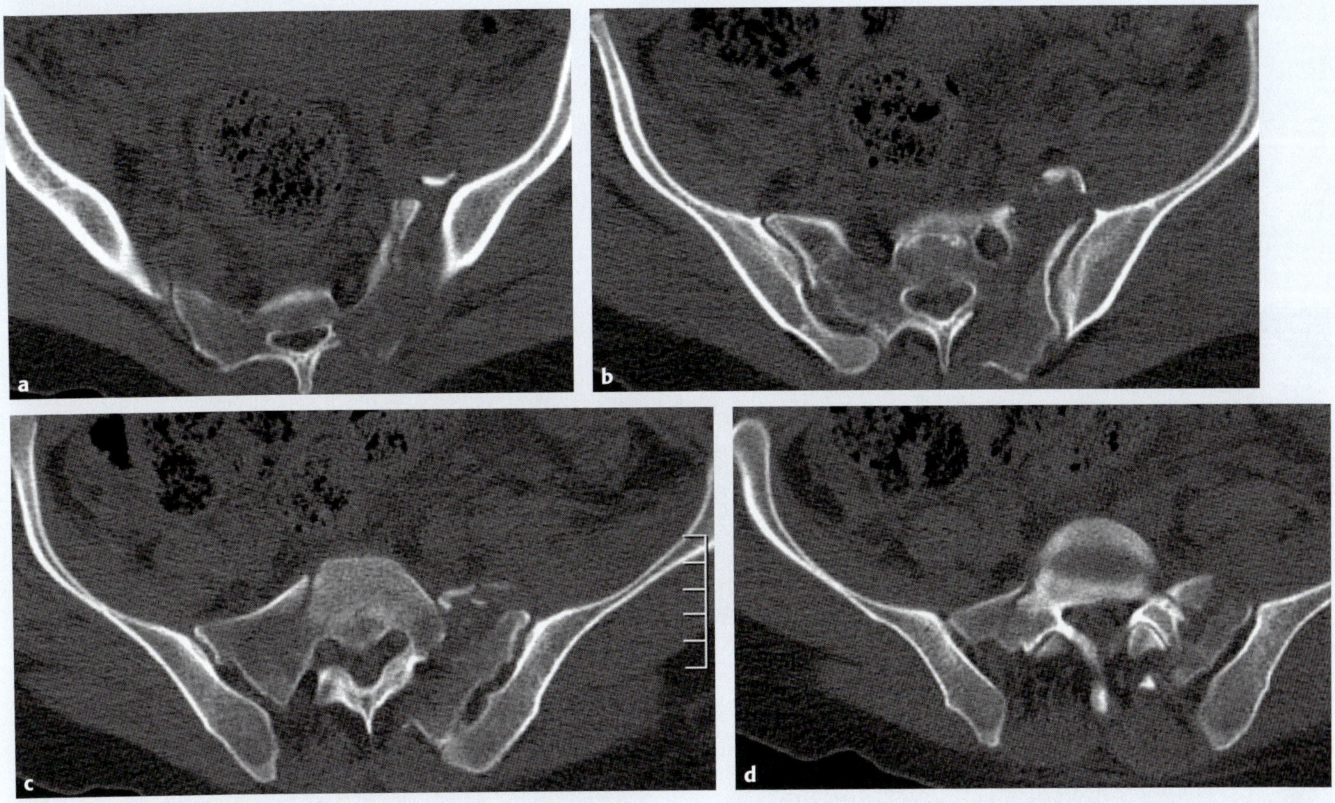

Fig 4.6-14a–i Computed tomographic scans of the sacral fracture.
a–d Axial views.

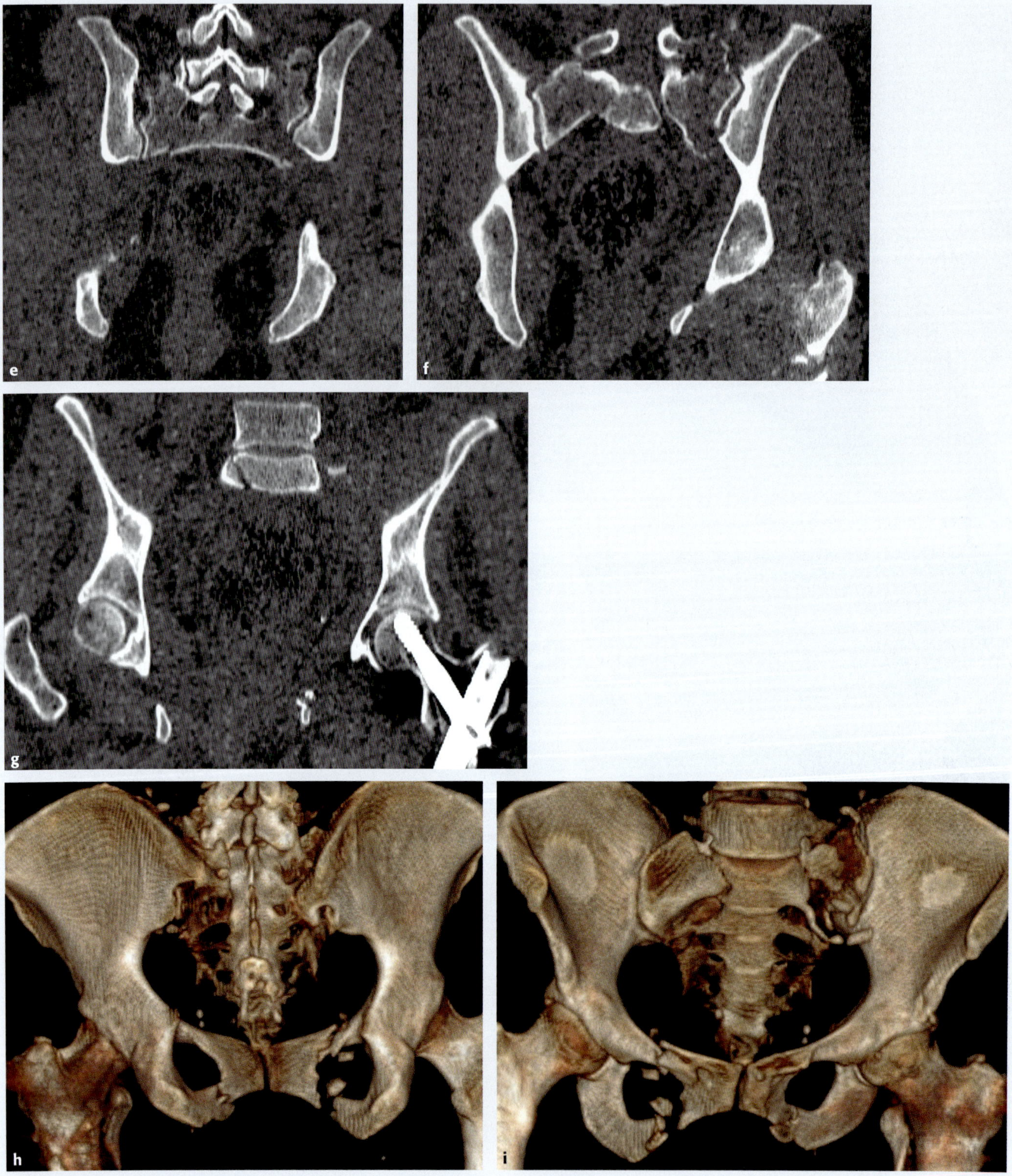

Fig 4.6-14a–i (cont) Computed tomographic scans of the sacral fracture.
e–g Coronal views.
h–i Three-dimensional reconstructions.

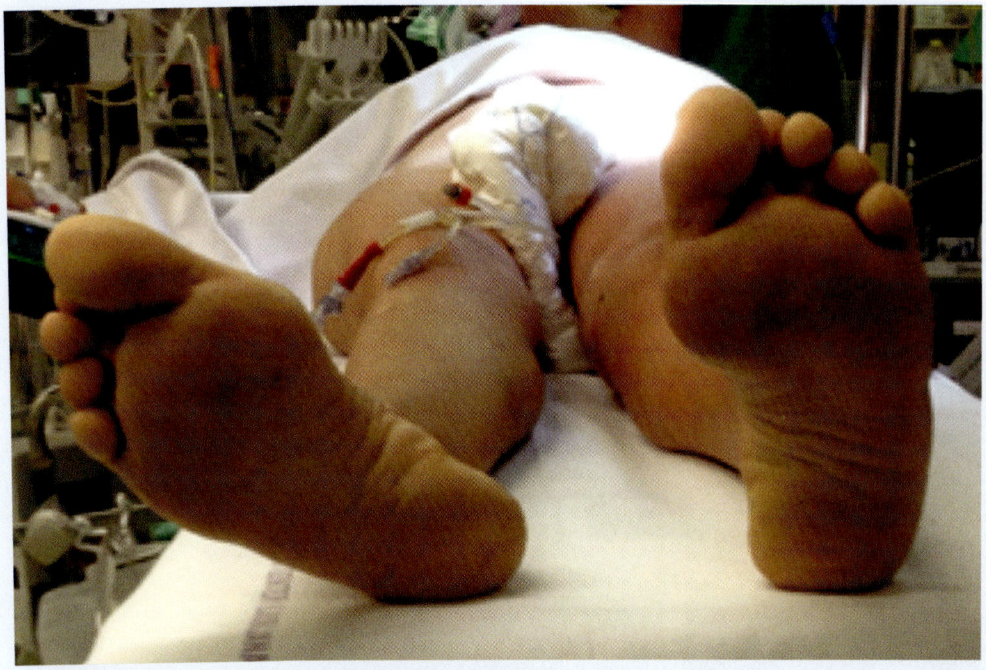

Fig 4.6-15 Torsion deformity of the lower limb after sacral fixation.

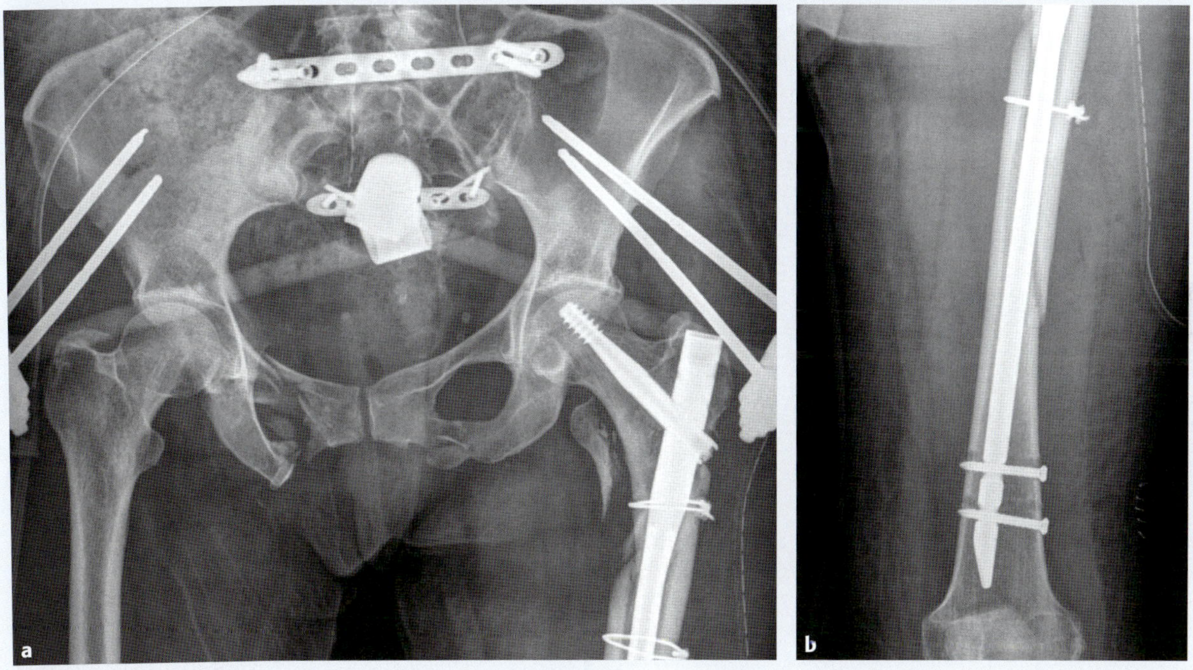

Fig 4.6-16a–b Control x-rays following the second intervention.

Analysis of failure and reflection

The first failure in this case was the treatment strategy in a severely injured patient. The woman had a lung contusion and pelvic ring injury. But the only treatment she received was stabilization of her femoral fracture. Deciding on the intramedullary fixation of the femoral fracture is extremely risky in a patient with a lung contusion. Provisional fixation of the pelvis and external fixation of the femur would have been a much safer decision, especially given that it was planned to transfer the patient to another hospital. Damage control, patient stabilization, then transfer would have been preferable.

The second failure was the malreduction of the femur. It is extremely difficult to obtain a perfect closed reduction of a type C1 diaphyseal fracture. Even more so if a deformity exists caused by the pelvic ring injury. In these cases, open reduction must be considered for optimum control of the rotation.

Final outcome

The patient was sent home 10 days after surgery. The external fixator was removed at 6 weeks. The last outpatient control was 2.5 years after surgery. The patient was able to perform her normal activities of daily living and was completely satisfied with the outcome (**Fig 4.6-17**).

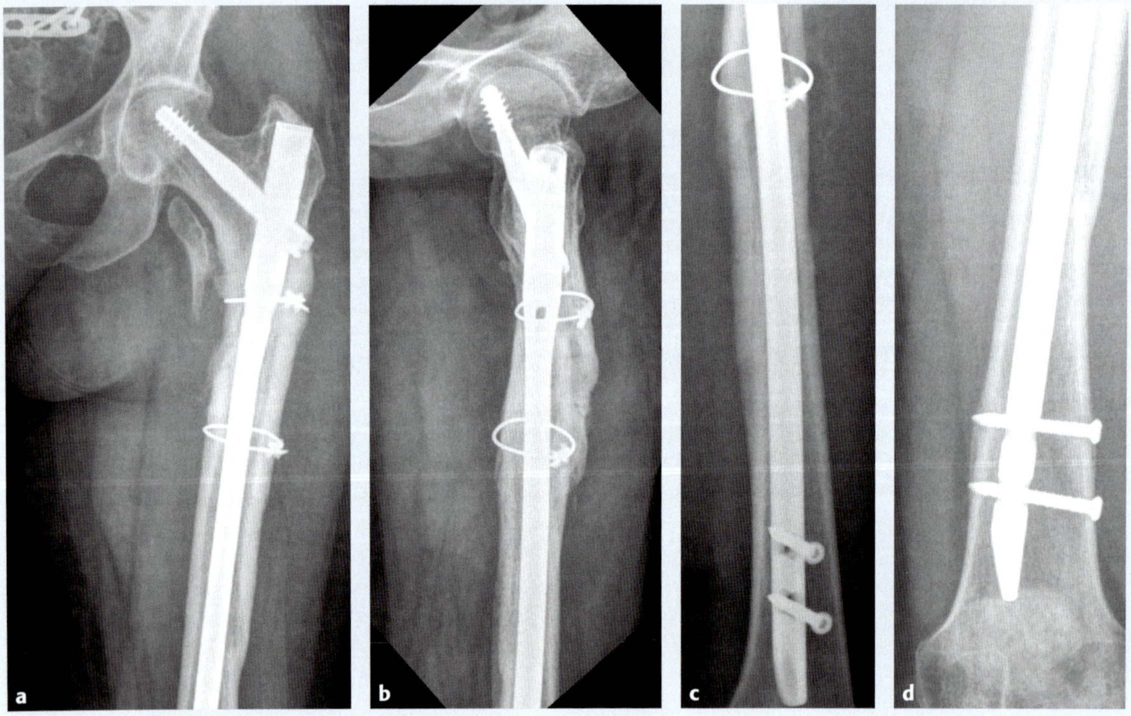

Fig 4.6-17a–f Final control x-rays.
a–d X-rays of the femur after 2 years.

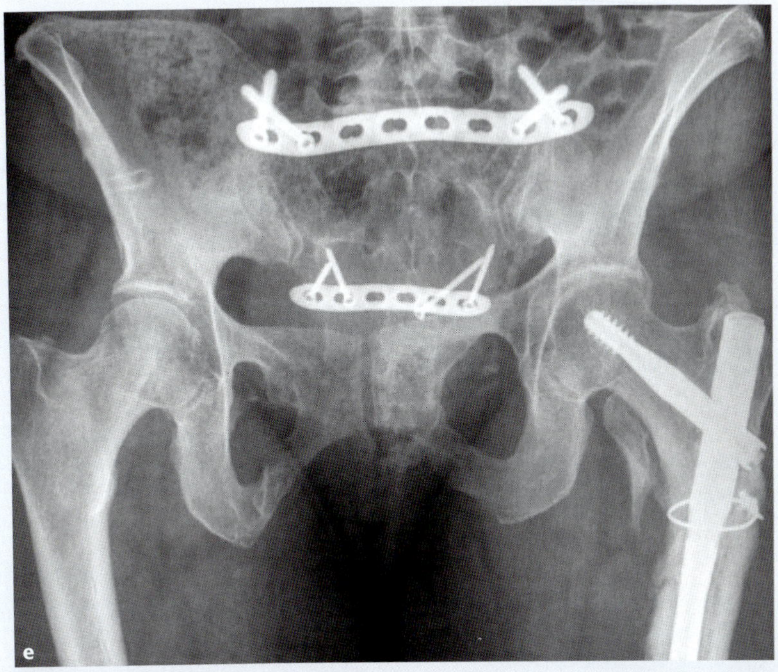

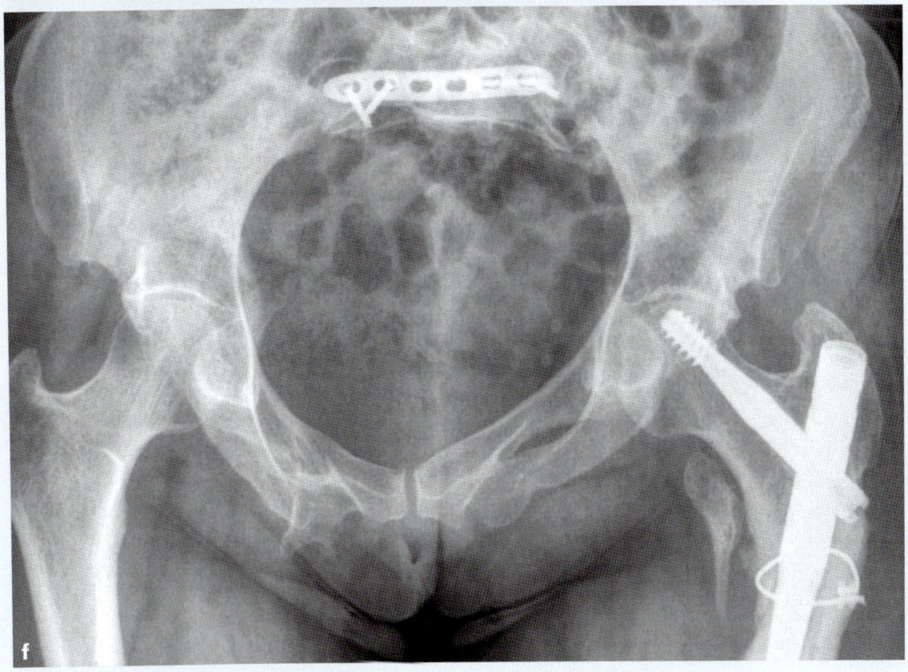

Fig 4.6-17a–f (cont) Final control x-rays.
e–f X-rays of the pelvis after 2 years.

CASE 4

Case description

This case has been authorized by Terry Axelrod for publication in this chapter. It is structured and explained differently to the other cases in this book. Since this case contains seven severe mistakes as shown in just one AP x-ray, it can be seen as a practical exercise in critical radiographic reading of a high educational value.

The x-ray in **Fig 4.6-18** shows an AP view of a complete articular distal humeral fracture (AO/OTA 13C). The surgeon made a series of errors while performing the osteosynthesis. The image shows that the reduction of the articular line is correct and the metaphyseal union with the diaphysis is acceptable in terms of their anatomical relationship. However, it shows failures in the execution of the osteosynthesis and even conceptual failures in a correct osteosynthesis that aims to follow the AO principles of fracture treatment. The internal fixation that was performed offers the reader an example of how a failure in osteosynthesis does usually not occur in isolation but is often an accumulation of failures, as shown in this case where at least seven failures were cumulatively made (**Fig 4.6-18**).

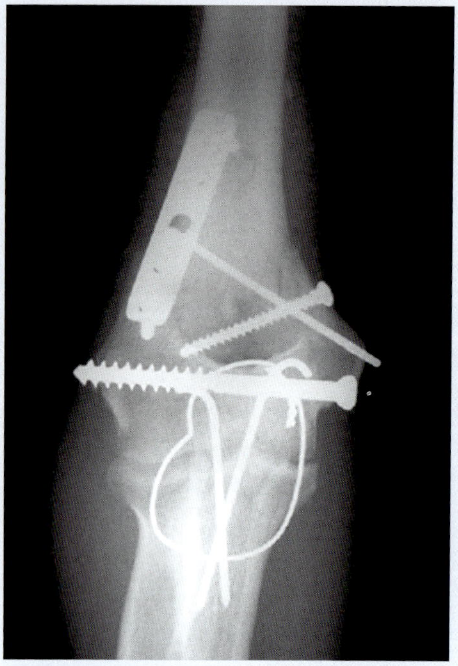

Fig 4.6-18 AP x-ray of the osteosynthesis performed on a complete articular distal humeral fracture.

Analysis of failure and reflection

First, a short cortex screw was used to attempt to compress a fracture pattern affecting the epitrochlear crest. The screw, placed so as to have a pulling effect, did not present a wider hole in the proximal orifice; therefore, the threads of the screw applied pressure at both ends of the fracture preventing it from being able to perform compression. In addition, due to its direction, the screw occupied the space of the olecranon fossa in the posterior region of the distal humeral epiphysis, hindering elbow extension (**Fig 4.6-19**, see 1).

Second, a definitive K-wire was placed percutaneously to stabilize the epitrochlear ridge. In this case, the K-wire cannot be considered more than temporary stabilization during osteosynthesis and should not be left as a definitive implant. The crossed direction of the screw described does not even allow an antirotational effect with the bone fragment screw (**Fig 4.6-19**, see 2).

Both failures should have been resolved by placing a low-profile medial plate and applying compression to the epitrochlear fragment with a traction screw placed through it and in a direction that did not invade the olecranon fossa.

Third, placing a 6.5 mm cancellous bone screw to treat the intra-articular pattern of the fracture was another failure. Aiming to compress both articular fragments is correct, as was placing the thread of the screw only in the distal fragment to achieve the traction. However, using a screw of disproportionate measure in diameter and length for this purpose shows a lack of knowledge of the material. Screws with the adequate measurements (ie, 4.0 mm) do exist and are suitable for implantation in this anatomy. The slightly proximal position and the lateral protrusion of the screw causes discomfort to the patient and may even injure the lateral ligament and/or the epicondylar muscles (**Fig 4.6-19**, see 3).

Fourth, there are crossed K-wires used in the application of a cerclage wire to close the olecranon osteotomy. The olecranon osteotomy is indicated in these fractures to facilitate visualization of the joint and achieve anatomical reduction. The crossed K-wires show poor technical execution and prevent the sliding and the compressive effect desired since they should control rotation and support the cerclage (**Fig 4.6-20**, see 4).

Fifth, the cerclage wire is arranged in a circular configuration without being crossed in the posterior area of the olecranon. Given the triangular anatomical characteristic of the olecranon with its posterior vertex, the cerclage must be crossed passing through the posterior side. When tension is applied the wire will not be displaced anteriorly, and unable to fulfil its purpose as a tension and compression band at the osteotomy site (**Fig 4.6-20**, see 5).

The situation in the patella is different, since the anterior surface is flat and does not present displacement when tension is applied. At the patella the arrangement of the cerclage wire can be carried out in a circular fashion or in a figure-of-eight, but it is always situated on the anterior side (**Fig 4.6-21**).

Sixth, a plate with little stability was placed on the lateral column of the distal humerus and the reduction was not perfectly anatomical. During its placement, technical difficulties must have occurred as a hole can be seen in the humeral cortex from fruitless attempted drilling. The plate should have been longer to apply better pressure to the articular fragment after having achieved an anatomical reduction and exercising an axial compressive force on the metaphyseal line (**Fig 4.6-20**, see 6).

Seventh, placing the K-wire percutaneously, without clearly visualizing the anatomy despite the broad exposure of the fracture, did not follow the care that would have been necessary to avoid injuring the ulnar nerve which runs along the epitrochlear-olecranon channel. The K-wire should have been removed with the nerve released during the subsequent rescue (**Fig 4.6-22**).

Final outcome

This case was fortunately resolved with revision surgery and release of the ulnar nerve, removal of the K-wire, and controlled evolution of the fracture.

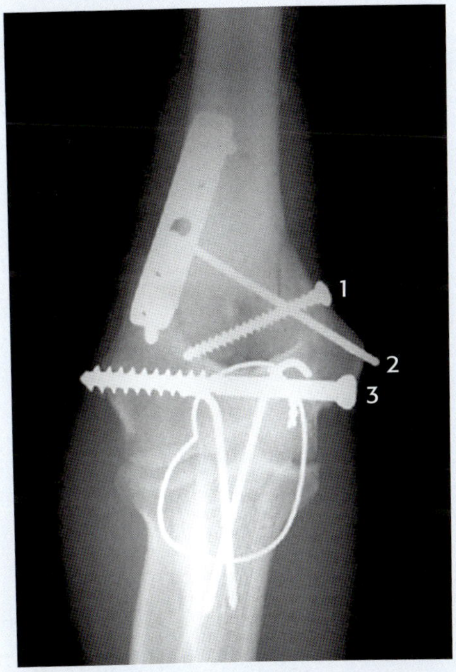

Fig 4.6-19 X-ray showing errors.

1 Cortex screw implanted to treat the epitrochlear fragment. The short screw applies pressure on both fragments of the fracture, prevents interfragmentary compression, and is poorly directed, occupying space in the posterior olecranon fossa of the distal humeral epiphysis.

2 K-wire placed percutaneously in the epitrochlear fragment to stabilize it. During osteosynthesis pins can be used temporarily to maintain the reduction and perform the definitive osteosynthesis. In this case, we cannot consider the K-wire as an implant indicated for stabilizing these fractures.

3 A 6.5 mm screw implanted with traction effect to reduce and maintain the articular line. However, its excessive diameter and length are not suitable for the fracture.

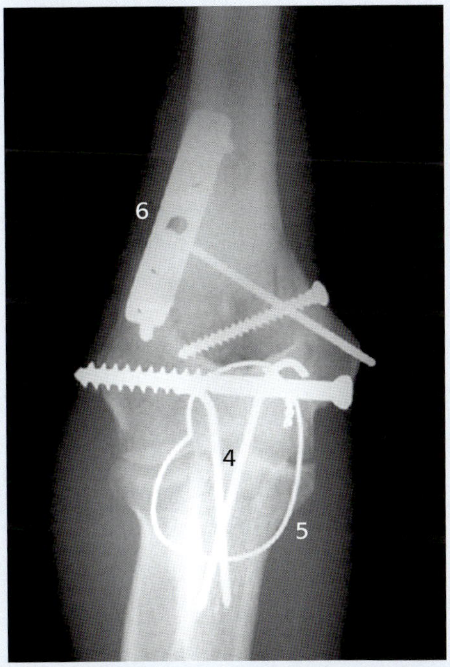

Fig 4.6-20 X-ray showing errors.

4 Crossed K-wires inserted during the application of the cerclage to close the olecranon osteotomy performed.

5 Circular arrangement of the cerclage wire, means that it loses its compressive effect at the ulna.

6 The plate on the lateral column of the distal humerus is too short for anatomical reduction.

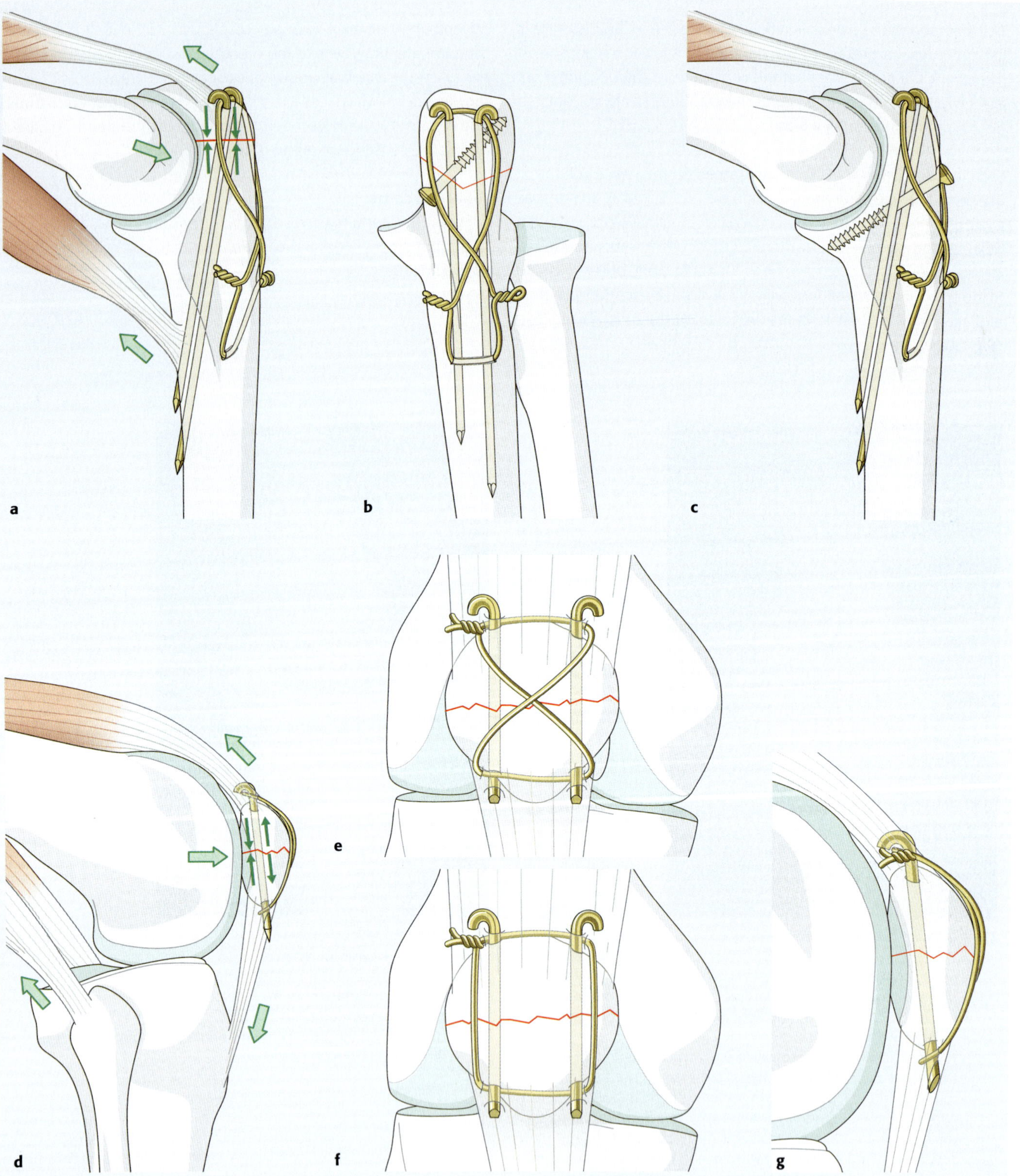

Fig 4.6-21a–g Biomechanics of a cerclage wire at the olecranon (**a–c**) and the patella (**d–g**) (in a figure-of-eight [**e**] and a circular configuration [**f**]).

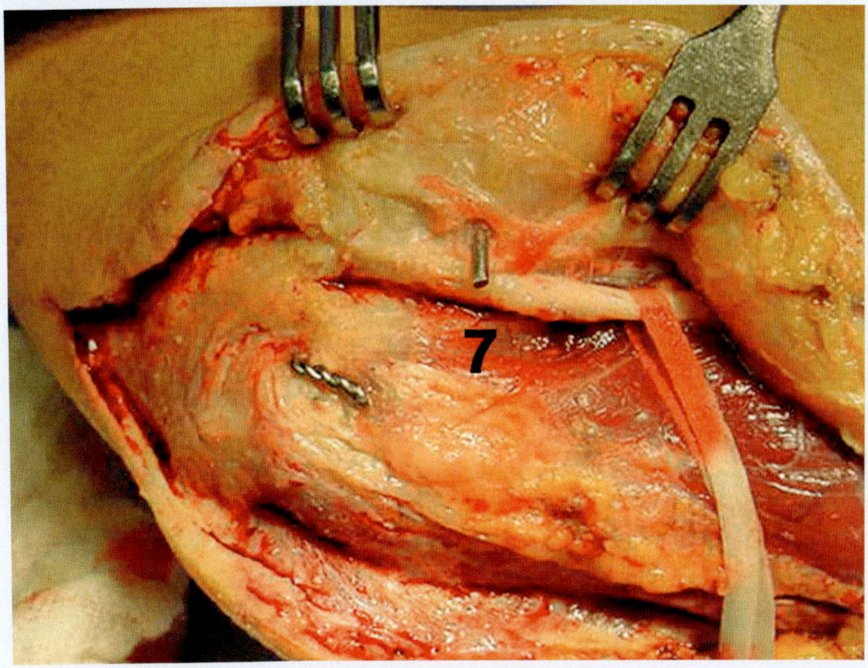

Fig 4.6-22 Intraoperative image of the rescue surgery.
7 The ulnar nerve is wrapped and compressed by fibrosis and pressed by the K-wire. Note how close the ulnar nerve is to the K-wire.

Key points to remember

- Failures in most cases are not usually isolated, and usually lead to other failures. Lack of planning and surgical improvisation usually precede a cascade of failures with serious consequences.
- The succession of failures begins after the first digression from the principles. When left uncorrected, this leads to other unplanned situations and complications.
- Inadequate planning, insufficient reduction, poor choice of implants, lack of stability, and poor technical execution lead individually or in combination to complications.

References and suggested reading

Bates DW, Gawande AA. Error in medicine: what have we learned? *Ann Intern Med.* 2000 May 2;132(9):763–767.
Haidukewych GJ. Intertrochanteric fractures: ten tips to improve results. *J Bone Joint Surg Am.* 2009 Mar 1;91(3):712–719.
Jaarsma RL, van Kampen A. Rotational malalignment after fractures of the femur. *J Bone Joint Surg Br.* 2004 Nov;86(8):1100–1104.

Section 5
Postoperative management

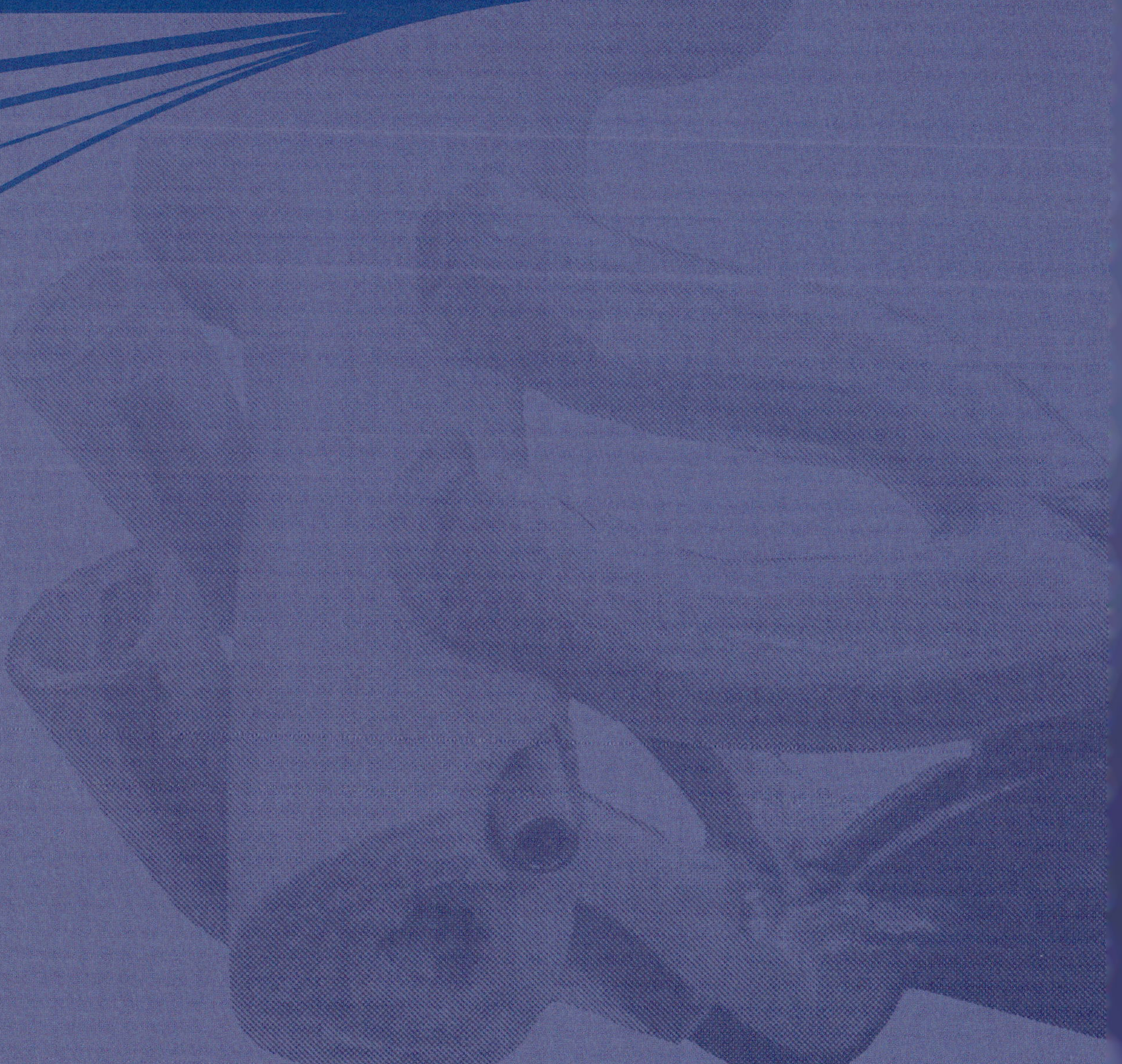

Section 5
Postoperative management

5.1 General considerations in postoperative management of internal fixation

Roberto Rivero Sosa
Joan Girós Torres, J Miquel Sales Pérez, Miquel Videla Cés

The genius begins great works, but only labor finishes them.
Joseph Joubert

When the surgical procedure has been completed, surgeons, physicians, and caregivers may relax and lower their guard, which may allow complications to occur. Postoperative management is part of comprehensive patient care and is as important as the preoperative and operative phases. Patients should therefore be informed about each phase, so they fully understand the implications. They should also be informed about all the steps that are necessary, be they surgical or medical.

According to the AO Principles of Fracture Management, the postoperative period after internal fixation is divided into three phases.

Phase 1

The goal of phase 1 is pain control, early mobilization, prevention, and early recognition of complications immediately after surgery.

Pain management is key during this phase and the whole postoperative phase. There is currently a wide array of tools available to control pain, including but not limited to, splints, casts, bandages, several types and subtypes of drugs, and nerve bundle blockage, to name but a few. Surgeons develop their own preferences within broadly applicable guidelines.

Patients who receive inappropriate pain treatment sometimes develop such a serious psychological deterioration that it can severely impact and even slow down the recovery process. If surgeons understand this, they can easily conclude that a properly adjusted analgesic treatment will allow the patient to perform better during physical therapy and speed up recovery.

The most widely used and recommended drugs in pain management are nonsteroidal antiinflammatory drugs (NSAIDs), selective cyclooxygenase 2 (COX-2) inhibitor; the surgeon may always employ opioids, neuromodulating drugs, or N-methyl-D-aspartate receptor antagonists, depending on her or his preference and following international pain management protocols and guidelines.

The surgeon must always explain to the patient and relatives the medication(s) prescribed and how long the treatment will last. This is vital, as the patient needs to realize the importance of correct adherence to the treatment, including dosage and duration, and that infratherapeutic levels or pharmacological interactions and overdose must be avoided.

Surgical wound care, which is equally essential in this phase, must be tailored to each case, and the healing progress of the wound must be correctly documented in the patient's medical history. This needs to be done to prevent or correctly and quickly diagnose possible complications, such as infection, hematoma, secondary damage due to splints or casts, pressure ulcers, nerve damage, vascular damage, or undesirable pharmacological effects.

Surgeons should communicate with patients and relatives on a regular basis, reporting clinical status, progression, and estimated recovery time.

Phase 2

Once the patient has been discharged from hospital, care should aim to reintegrate the patient into her or his social environment and regain full mobility.

The medical team should establish a protocol for patient follow-up visits after hospital discharge, which must include but not be limited to medical check-ups, radiological control, supervision, control and documentation of wound healing, as well as adherence to rehabilitation and therapeutic recommendations and measures.

In this phase, the medical team should also identify patients who are or may be noncompliant with the postoperative follow-ups, whether voluntarily or involuntarily (eg, drug and substance abusers, psychiatric patients, elderly people, or children), and develop a strategy for adherence, if needed. This point is particularly important for patients with internal fixation of the lower extremities or the pelvis who are allowed either no or only partial load bearing of the lower extremities.

Finally, during phase 2 the surgeon must be careful to correctly diagnose serious complications like wound-site infection, rigidity, complex regional pain syndrome, refractures, or failure to consolidate, and also be prepared to intervene and treat any of these pathologies if they arise.

Phase 3

In this final phase of treatment, the patients should, if possible, regain the same functional capacity as they enjoyed prior to their injury.

This phase can last several months. A correct protocol must be established to reintroduce high-demand physical activities, be they sport- or work-related, and to also establish limits if required.

In some cases, removal of the osteosynthesis material represents the end of the patients' treatment; however, this must be evaluated for each patient and case. The surgeon, or her or his team, must also verify good bone consolidation with at least two different x-ray views and be absolutely sure that removal of the implanted material is necessary. All of this should be done taking into account the patient's expectations and correctly informing them of the benefits, risks, and possible complications of surgical extraction of implants. If the patient decides in favor of this last step, then she or he must also undergo postoperative care and follow-up as in any other orthopedic surgery.

Key points to remember

- Establish a thorough and individualized postoperative check-up.
- Be familiar with all the phases of postoperative management and be prepared to deal with any complications that may arise.
- Tell the patient that her or his active participation in this process is essential to recovery.
- Prevent and/or rapidly treat possible complications.
- Identify patients with risk of noncompliance to postoperative management and establish strategies to help patients adhere to the treatment.
- Update the patient and relatives regularly about her or his clinical state, expected postoperative progress, and estimated time to recovery.

References and suggested reading

American Orthopaedic Foot & Ankle Society. *Removal of Hardware. A step in the right direction* [Internet]. Available at: legacy.aofas.org/footcaremd/treatments/Pages/Removal-of-Hardware.aspx. Accessed May 2019.

Bruder AM, Shields N, Dodd KJ, et al. Prescribed exercise programs may not be effective in reducing impairments and improving activity during upper limb fracture rehabilitation: a systematic review. *J Physiother.* 2017 Oct;63(4):205–220.

Buckley RE. Fracture healing: Does hardware removal enhance patient outcomes? *Orthopedic Trauma Directions.* 2009;7(06):1–9.

Chao EY, Inoue N, Koo TK, et al. Biomechanical considerations of fracture treatment and bone quality maintenance in elderly patients and patients with osteoporosis. *Clin Orthop Relat Res.* 2004 Aug(425):12–25.

Colton CL, Orson J. *Plates—Form and function. Basic Principles of Fracture Management for ORP.* Dübendorf: AOTrauma, 2013.

Gohy B, Ali E, Van den Bergh R, et al. Early physical and functional rehabilitation of trauma patients in the Medecins Sans Frontieres trauma centre in Kunduz, Afghanistan: luxury or necessity? *Int Health.* 2016 Nov;8(6):381–389.

Haidukewych G, J,, Lyons S, Bernasek T. Treatment of periprosthetic fractures around a total knee arthroplasty. In: Scott WN, eds. *Insall & Scott surgery of the knee.* 5th ed. Philadelphia: Elsevier Churchill Livingstone; 2012. 799–807.

Hall AJ, Watkins R, Lang IA, et al. The experiences of physiotherapists treating people with dementia who fracture their hip. *BMC Geriatr.* 2017 Apr 20;17(1):91.

Hanson B, van der Werken C, Stengel D. Surgeons' beliefs and perceptions about removal of orthopaedic implants. *BMC Musculoskelet Disord.* 2008 May 24;9:73.

Jansen H, Jordan M, Frey S, et al. Active controlled motion in early rehabilitation improves outcome after ankle fractures: a randomized controlled trial. *Clin Rehabil.* 2018 Mar;32(3):312–318.

Langford JR, Jacofsky DJ, Haidukewydh GJ. Tibial plateau fractures. In: Scott WN, eds. *Insall & Scott surgery of the knee.* 5th ed. Philadelphia: Elsevier Churchill Livingstone; 2012. 773–784.

Lin CW, Donkers NA, Refshauge KM, et al. Rehabilitation for ankle fractures in adults. *Cochrane Database Syst Rev.* 2012 Nov 14;11:Cd005595.

Lindvall EM, F. IA, Sanders R. Distal femur fractures. In: Scott WN, eds. *Insall & Scott surery of the knee.* 5th ed. Philadelphia: Elsevier Churchill Livingstone; 2012:762–771.

Liporace JR, Langford JR, Haidukewych GJ. Fracture of the patella. In: Scott WN, eds. *Insall & Scott surgery of the knee.* 5th ed. Philadelphia: Elsevier Churchill Livingstone; 2012:786–797.

Orozco Delclós R, Sales J, Videla M. *Atlas de osteosíntesis fracturas de los huesos largos. Clasificación y prólogo de M.E Müller, Revisión de 54.280 fracturas.* Barcelona: Masson; 1993.

Raschke MJ, Kittl C, Domnick C. Partial proximal tibia fractures. *EFORT Open Rev.* 2017 May;2(5):241–249.

Rockwood CA, Matsen FA, A WM, et al. *Fracturas del húmero proximal (chapter 9). Hombro.* 4th ed. Madrid; 2014:273–306.

Ryf C, Weymann A, Matter P. Postoperative management: general considerations. In: Rüedi TP, Murphy WM, ed. *AO Principles of Fracture Management.* Stuttgart New York: George Thieme Verlag; 2001:723–731.

Sherrington C, Fairhall N, Kirkham C, et al. Exercise and fall prevention self-management to reduce mobility-related disability and falls after fall-related lower limb fracture in older people: protocol for the RESTORE (Recovery Exercises and STepping On afteR fracturE) randomised controlled trial. *BMC Geriatr.* 2016 Feb 2;16:34.

Sociedad Española de Cirugía Ortopédica y Traumatología (SECOT). Hombro. In: SECOT. *Manual de Cirugía Ortopédica y Traumatología.* 2nd ed. Madrid; 2010. Available at: www.medicapanamericana.com/libro/manual-de-cirugia-ortopedica-y-traumatologia-2-tomos. Accessed May 2019.

Sociedad Española de Cirugía Ortopédica y Traumatología (SECOT). Brazo. In: SECOT. *Manual de Cirugía Ortopédica y Traumatología.* 2nd ed. Madrid; 2010. Available at: www.medicapanamericana.com/libro/manual-de-cirugia-ortopedica-y-traumatologia-2-tomos. Accessed May 2019.

Sociedad Española de Cirugía Ortopédica y Traumatología (SECOT). Codo. In: SECOT. *Manual de Cirugía Ortopédica y Traumatología.* 2nd ed. Madrid; 2010. Available at: www.medicapanamericana.com/libro/manual-de-cirugia-ortopedica-y-traumatologia-2-tomos. Accessed May 2019.

Sociedad Española de Cirugía Ortopédica y Traumatología (SECOT). Fracturas diafisarias del cúbito y radio. In: SECOT. *Manual de Cirugía Ortopédica y Traumatología.* 2nd ed. Madrid; 2010. Available at: www.medicapanamericana.com/libro/manual-de-cirugia-ortopedica-y-traumatologia-2-tomos. Accessed May 2019.

Sociedad Española de Cirugía Ortopédica y Traumatología (SECOT). Fracturas distales del radio. In: SECOT. *Manual de Cirugía Ortopédica y Traumatología.* 2nd ed. Madrid; 2010. Available at: www.medicapanamericana.com/libro/manual-de-cirugia-ortopedica-y-traumatologia-2-tomos. Accessed May 2019.

Sociedad Española de Cirugía Ortopédica y Traumatología (SECOT). Fracturas de metacarpianos y falanges. In: SECOT. *Manual de Cirugía Ortopédica y Traumatología. 2nd ed. Madrid;* 2010. Available at: www.medicapanamericana.com/libro/manual-de-cirugia-ortopedica-y-traumatologia-2-tomos. Accessed May 2019.

Sociedad Española de Cirugía Ortopédica y Traumatología (SECOT). Pelvis y cadera. In: SECOT. *Manual de Cirugía Ortopédica y Traumatología.* 2nd ed. Madrid; 2010. Available at: www.medicapanamericana.com/libro/manual-de-cirugia-ortopedica-y-traumatologia-2-tomos. Accessed May 2019.

Sociedad Española de Cirugía Ortopédica y Traumatología (SECOT). Muslo. In: SECOT. *Manual de Cirugía Ortopédica y Traumatología.* 2nd ed. Madrid; 2010. Available at: www.medicapanamericana.com/libro/manual-de-cirugia-ortopedica-y-traumatologia-2-tomos. Accessed May 2019.

Sociedad Española de Cirugía Ortopédica y Traumatología (SECOT). Fracturas de la extremidad distal del fémur. In: SECOT. *Manual de Cirugía Ortopédica y Traumatología.* 2nd ed. Madrid; 2010. Available at: www.medicapanamericana.com/libro/manual-de-cirugia-ortopedica-y-traumatologia-2-tomos. Accessed May 2019.

Sociedad Española de Cirugía Ortopédica y Traumatología (SECOT). Rotura del aparato extensor de la rodilla. In: SECOT. *Manual de Cirugía Ortopédica y Traumatología.* 2nd ed. Madrid; 2010. Available at: www.medicapanamericana.com/libro/manual-de-cirugia-ortopedica-y-traumatologia-2-tomos. Accessed May 2019.

Sociedad Española de Cirugía Ortopédica y Traumatología (SECOT). Fracturas diafisarias de tibia y peroné. In: SECOT. *Manual de Cirugía Ortopédica y Traumatología. 2nd ed. Madrid;* 2010. Available at: www.medicapanamericana.com/libro/manual-de-cirugia-ortopedica-y-traumatologia-2-tomos. Accessed May 2019.

Sociedad Española de Cirugía Ortopédica y Traumatología (SECOT). Fracturas y luxaciones del tobillo. In: SECOT. *Manual de Cirugía Ortopédica y Traumatología.* 2nd ed. Madrid; 2010. Available at: www.medicapanamericana.com/libro/manual-de-cirugia-ortopedica-y-traumatologia-2-tomos. Accessed May 2019.

Sociedad Española de Cirugía Ortopédica y Traumatología (SECOT). Fracturas y luxaciones de los huesos del tarso. In: SECOT. *Manual de Cirugía Ortopédica y Traumatología.* 2nd ed. Madrid; 2010. Available at: www.medicapanamericana.com/libro/manual-de-cirugia-ortopedica-y-traumatologia-2-tomos. Accessed May 2019.

Sociedad Española de Cirugía Ortopédica y Traumatología (SECOT). Fracturas de los metatarsianos. In: SECOT. *Manual de Cirugía Ortopédica y Traumatología.* 2nd ed. Madrid; 2010. Available at: www.medicapanamericana.com/libro/manual-de-cirugia-ortopedica-y-traumatologia-2-tomos. Accessed May 2019.

Twaddle B. Implant removal. Dübendorf: AOTrauma; 2013.

Voegeli AV, Pericé RV. Traumatismos del antepié. In: Voegeli AV, Pericé RV, Pericé AVVRnV, eds. *20 lecciones sobre patología del pie.* Barcelona: Mayo Ediciones; 2009:285.

5.2 Physiotherapy

Matej Cimerman, Joan Girós Torres, Roberto Rivero Sosa, J Miquel Sales Pérez, Matevž Tomaževič, Miquel Videla Cés

No pain, no gain.
Benjamin Franklin

The basic principles of osteosynthesis are anatomical reduction, stable osteosynthesis, preservation of vascularization, and early mobilization. Ideally, mobilization should start as early after surgery as possible. It should be active, painless, and safe for both the injured area and the patient as a whole. These principles play a fundamental role in the patient's complete recovery after a fracture.

The general aims of physiotherapy are to encourage fracture union, treat the affected soft tissues, reduce the effects of immobilization, and avoid and prevent complications.

It has been confirmed during the evolution of the fracture treatment that prolonged immobilization and absence of weight bearing on a fractured limb leads to joint stiffness, circulatory dysfunction, and muscular as well as cutaneous atrophy.

Early mobilization is desirable to minimize the harmful effects of nonweight bearing. It enables the musculature and blood flow to be restored as soon as possible to their normal parameters. Prolonged immobilization, ie, longer than 6 weeks, does not improve the chances of fracture union, but it does favor the appearance of complications, such as "fracture disease", also known as Sudeck's atrophy or chronic complex regional pain syndrome (**Fig 5.2-1**).

Postoperative management must be planned by the surgical and physiotherapy teams that are in charge of the patient follow-up and may have to be adapted to the needs of both patient and injury. At the beginning of the recovery process, the estimated time for starting physiotherapy must be established. Mobilization should start on the first day after surgery unless there are complications or other associated injuries.

Verifying the condition of the soft tissues is mandatory when requesting and initiating rehabilitation. The correct healing of the surgical wound is fundamental. Active physiotherapy should be started only if the surgical wound is healed.

It is also important to take into account the location and function of the fractured bone, the fracture pattern, the type of fracture, and the resulting stability following osteosynthesis.

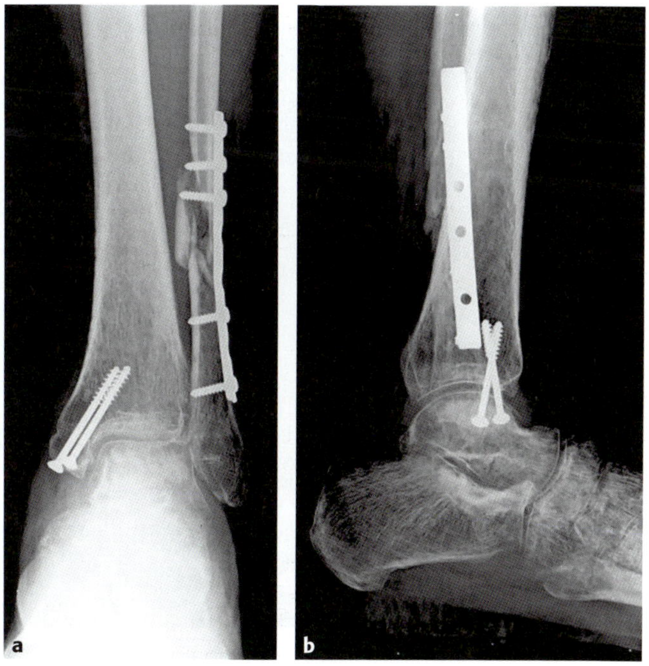

Fig 5.2-1a–b AP (**a**) and lateral (**b**) control x-rays of an ankle fracture showing osteopenia due to prolonged immobilization.

Diaphyseal fractures

In diaphyseal fractures, anatomical reduction of all the fragments is not necessary to restore the normal limb function. The goal is to regain the preinjury length, alignment of the bone fragments, and physiological rotation. In the lower limb, the physiological axes must be recovered, since shortening, angulation, and malrotation are not well tolerated. Considered acceptable are a dissymmetry of a maximum of 1 cm, varus or valgus of less than 5°, and up to 10° anteroposterior inclination.

In the upper limb, the humeral diaphyseal fracture tolerates axis variations better due to the great mobility of the shoulder joint. Meanwhile, in diaphyseal fractures of the radius and ulna, anatomical reduction is necessary to recover their function, as they are part of the forearm articulations complex.

In the postoperative period of diaphyseal factures, the determining factor for starting mobilization and weight bearing is the evaluation of the resulting stability, taking into account the fracture and the fixation technique used. Whenever possible, the bone-implant interface should allow load transfer on the fracture site, as this represents an excellent stimulus for union.

Joint fractures

Our goal in joint fractures must be to restore the anatomy and the articular congruity, to favor stability, and to achieve active and painless mobilization (AO/OTA 44B2) (**Fig 5.2-2a–c**). Generally, this can only be obtained through open reduction and internal fixation (**Fig 5.2-2d–e**).

Immobilization of articular fractures leads to stiffness. The combination of anatomical reduction and stable internal fixation is necessary to restore the articular congruity, enabling early mobilization of the joint. This begins with passive and active movements and isometric exercises, supervised by a physiotherapist until the recovery of function is progressively achieved.

It is common for lower limb, articular, periarticular, and pelvic ring fractures to require nonweight bearing for a determined period of time. Continuous passive mobilization is recommended for fractures around the knee. This helps to reduce inflammation and gain articular balance.

Fractures that are pathological, osteoporotic, or involve a significant loss of bone tissue are likely to benefit from nonweight bearing during rehabilitation. In multifragmentary metaphyseal, or diaphyseal fractures treated by

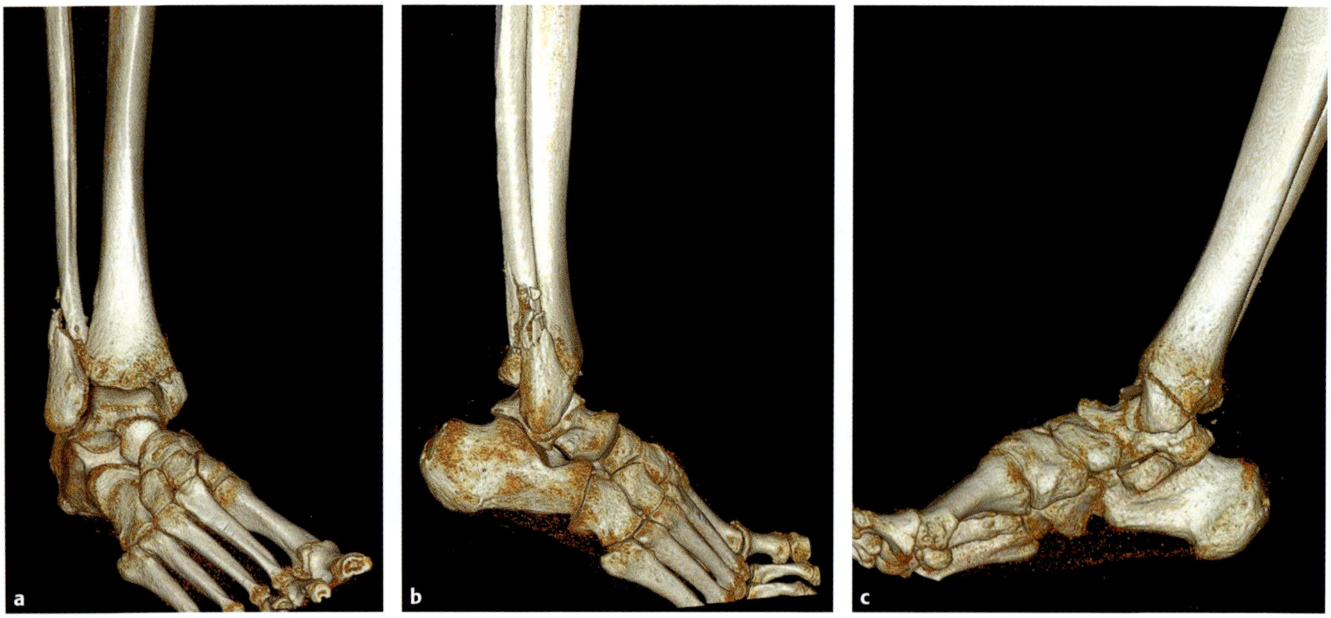

Fig 5.2-2a–e Computed tomographic (CT) scans of the ankle fracture.
a–c AP (**a**), lateral (**b**), and medial (**c**) views.

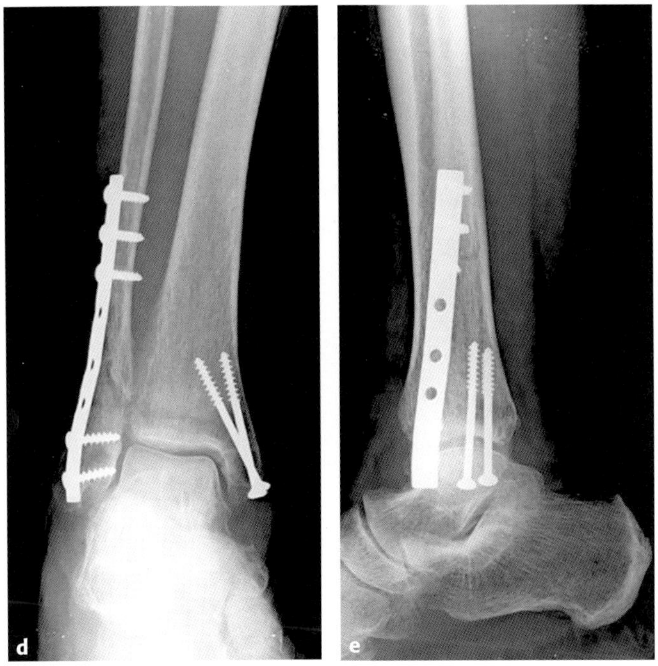

Fig 5.2-2a–e (cont) Computed tomographic (CT) scans of the ankle fracture.
d–e AP (**d**) and lateral (**d**) control x-rays showing the restoration of articular congruity.

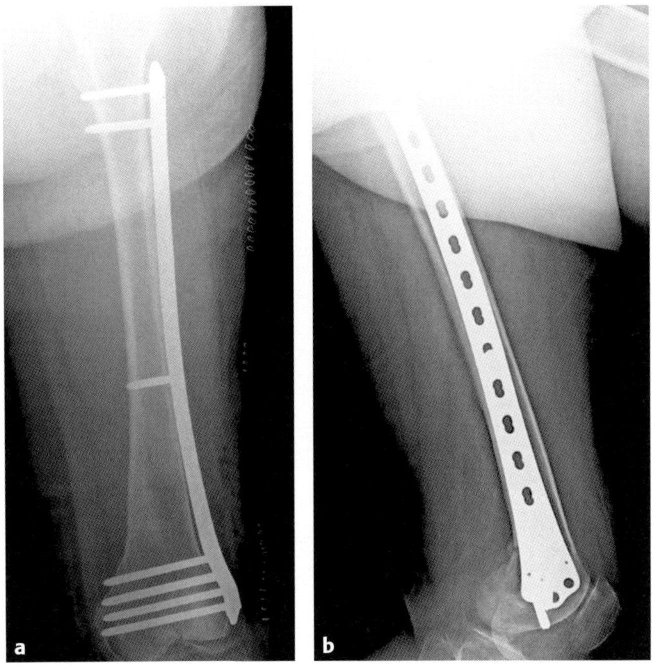

Fig 5.2-3a–b AP (**a**) and lateral (**b**) x-rays of the supraintercondylar fracture of the femur stabilized with an angular stable plate. The fracture is stable for mobility but not for immediate weight bearing.

extramedullary osteosynthesis, it is necessary to "protect" the synthesis by avoiding weight bearing until fracture union has been achieved.

With regard to stability after osteosynthesis, it would be a mistake to relate absolute stability with weight bearing during rehabilitation. Achieving absolute stability after surgery does not always enable the patient to bear weight during the immediate postoperative period. It is necessary to define whether the synthesis is stable for weight bearing or only for mobility. For example, in supraintercondylar fractures of the femur (AO/OTA 33C1) stabilized with an angular stable plate (**Fig 5.2-3**) where anatomical reduction has been achieved, the osteosynthesis is stable for mobility but not for weight bearing; full weight bearing must not start until after fracture consolidation. In some cases it is possible to evaluate partial progressive weight bearing after a reasonable period of time. This all depends on the patient's needs and the results visible on her or his control x-rays.

Conversely, some fractures treated by applying the relative stability criteria benefit from weight bearing, such as diaphyseal fractures of the femur or tibia, where a locked intramedullary nail was implanted. These parameters must be evaluated by the orthopedic surgeon, and be communicated to the patient, family, rehabilitation physician, and physiotherapist.

The rehabilitation protocol must be based on objectives to be met by the patient within a period of time. Recording progression during the recovery period allows us to compile data that will help to identify possible problems. It also helps to improve these patients' follow-up. In rehabilitation after the osteosynthesis, there are numerous factors which can influence its evolution. The purpose of a rehabilitation program is basically the same, although the form of execution differs. The rehabilitation protocol for a proximal humeral fracture is different from that for an ankle fracture. Surgeons must pay attention to every detail and listen to the patient, rehabilitation physician, and physiotherapist. It is necessary to establish a follow-up control suited to each patient, emphasize the importance of complying with the established protocol, and report on the progress achieved at each visit.

Special care must be taken with fragile patients, including elderly people and those affected by chronic disorders of the musculoskeletal system, multiple chronic conditions, and psychiatric disorders.

Keeping patients and their family members motivated always helps. Motivated patients with good family support will certainly deal better with the rehabilitation process.

It is very important during the postoperative and recovery process that the patient understands and takes responsibility for her or his prescribed treatment. Communication and feedback between patient, rehabilitation physician, physiotherapist, and orthopedic surgeon is fundamental for the correct follow-up and the patient's complete recovery.

Case description

An 89-year-old woman living with her daughter, with a history of arterial hypertension and chronic asthmatic bronchitis, fell on her right leg after tripping on the ground at home. She presented with a spiral fracture with a butterfly fragment of the distal third of the right femoral diaphysis (AO/OTA 32B2) (**Fig 5.2-4**).

Open reduction and internal fixation with a less invasive stabilization system-distal femoral (LISS DF) plate was performed, splinting almost the entire femoral diaphysis (**Fig 5.2-5**). Excellent postoperative progress was made, leaving the patient pain free and restoring mobility of the knee and hip. She was discharged and returned to her family home with daily home-based rehabilitation. The physiotherapist authorized ambulation with full weight bearing.

At the 3-month postoperative follow-up, the patient had ceased ambulation due to pain in her thigh. The control x-rays showed all the diaphyseal holding screws had broken, resulting in the loosening of the plate (**Fig 5.2-6**).

The patient underwent reintervention 3 months after the first surgery (**Fig 5.2-7**). Given the patient's age and comorbidity, the decision was to use a less aggressive surgical technique. Minimally invasive surgery was performed without removing the implant material but instead reanchoring the plate to the diaphysis.

Rehabilitation of the leg with nonweight bearing for 4 weeks was started. At the x-ray control 2 months after the rescue surgery, there were signs of consolidation with the formation of periosteal callus on the medial surface of the distal femur (**Fig 5.2-8**).

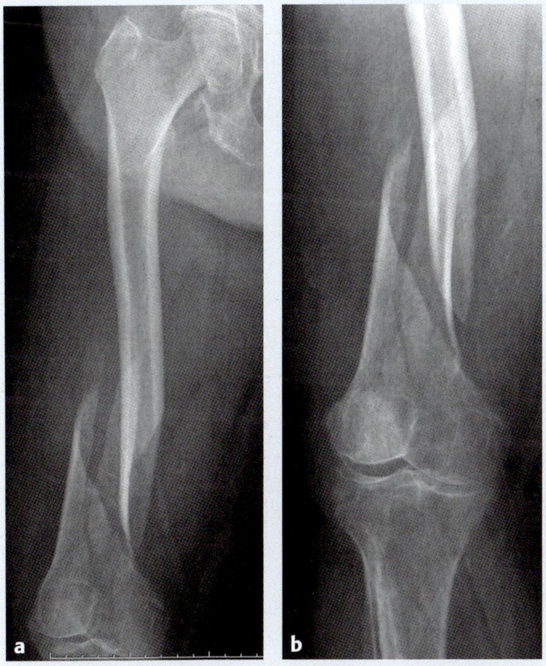

Fig 5.2-4a–b The spiral diaphyseal fracture with a butterfly fragment of the right femur.

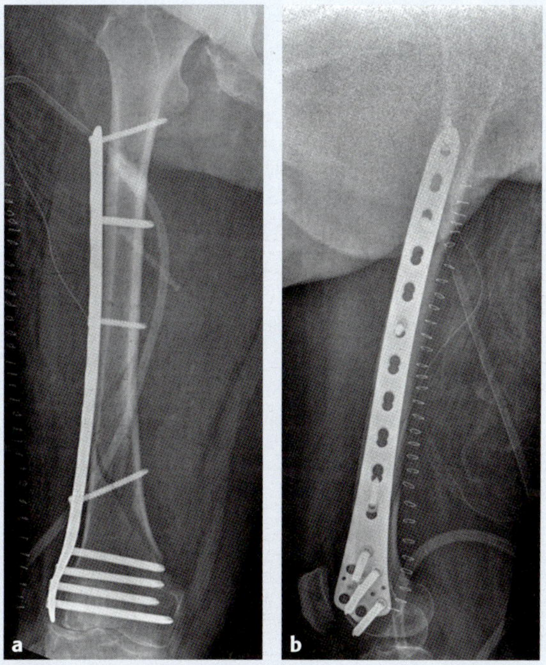

Fig 5.2-5a–b Postoperative x-rays showing correct reduction. Note the splinting of the femoral diaphysis and the use of an interfragmentary compression screw in the butterfly fragment.

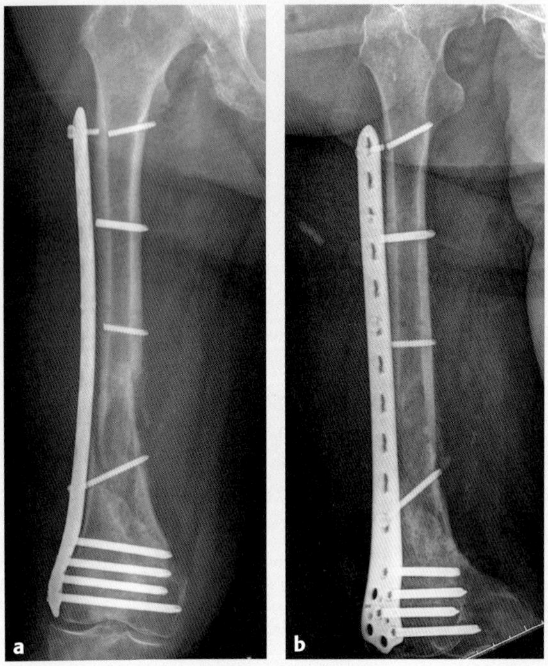

Fig 5.2-6a–b X-rays at 3 months showing moderate impaction of the fracture site. The alignment and reduction are maintained, but there has been breakage of the cortex screws and locking screws, which have a greater diameter than the cortex screws, resulting in loosening of the less invasive stabilization system-distal femoral (LISS DF) plate. This was due to too much weight bearing on the limb, since she felt no pain, had good joint function of the knee and hip, and was authorized to walk with full weight bearing.

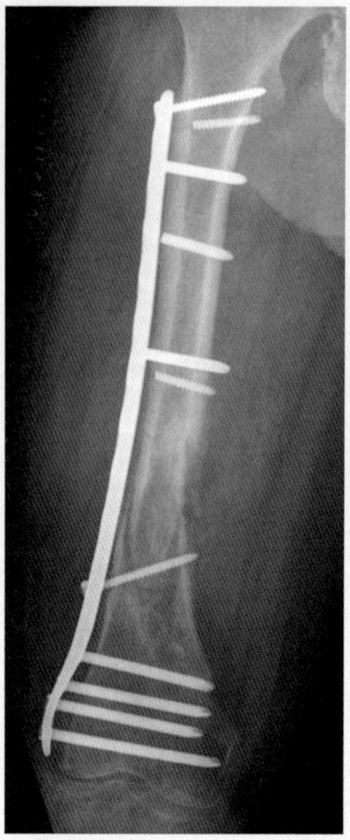

Fig 5.2-7 Rescue surgery 3 months after the first surgery. Minimally invasive surgery was performed without removal of the material. The plate was reanchored in the diaphysis.

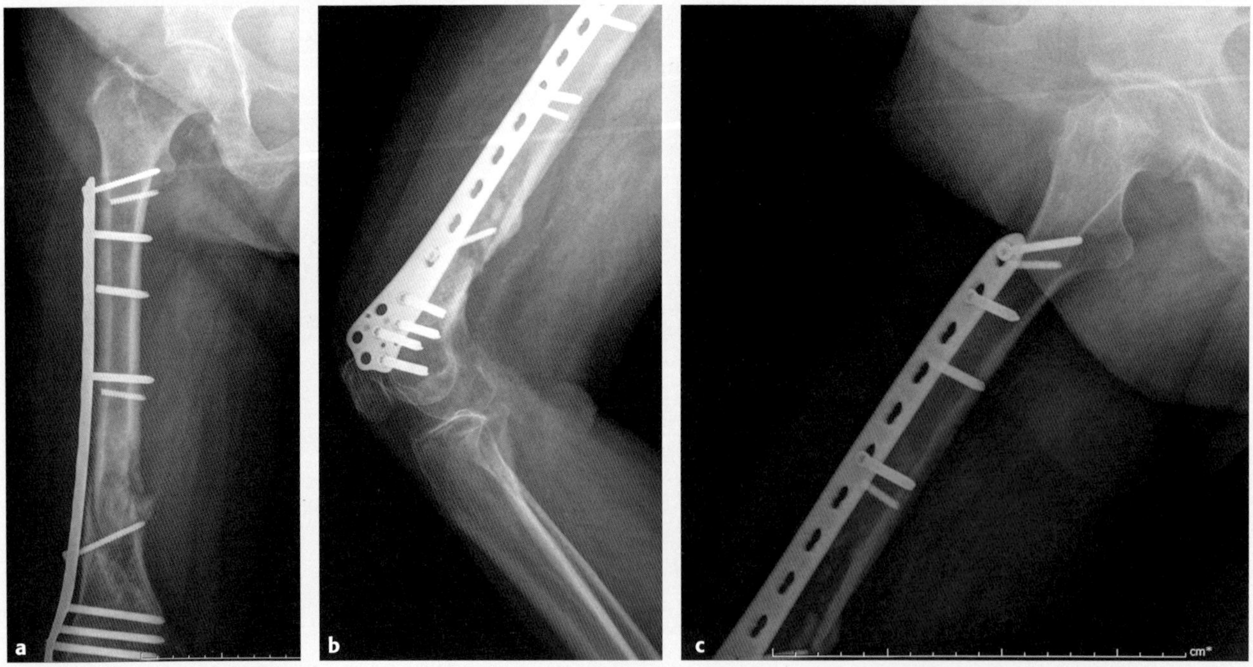

Fig 5.2-8a–c Control x-rays at 2 months after reintervention. Radiological signs of fracture consolidation can be observed with the presence of a posteromedial callus and the absence of periimplant bone lysis.

Analysis of failure and reflection

Despite having performed interfragmentary compression with the butterfly fragment of the fracture and having splinted practically the whole femur, the assembly was sufficiently stable to permit movement but not weight bearing. The absence of pain during active mobilization of the hip and knee led the physiotherapist to think that it was a sufficiently stable osteosynthesis to allow the patient to perform exercises with weight bearing. He recommended assisted ambulation with weight bearing approximately 6 weeks after the first surgery.

The elderly and weak patient shows total physical incapacity to perform ambulation with partial weight bearing. This incapacity is not voluntary but physical, which means despite instructions not to bear weight, patients will nonetheless perform weight-bearing ambulation.

In theory, replacement of the material with the aim of carrying out effective, short, and biologically less aggressive surgery is indicated. However, in very old and fragile patients surgeons should try to be less aggressive, for example, by not removing all the implant material but rather reanchoring the plate to the diaphysis through minimally invasive means. The advantage here is that there is no interference between the new screws and the broken screws, which can be left in situ.

Final outcome

The fracture was consolidated and the patient recovered her autonomy, achieving ambulation with the help of walking aids.

CASE 2

Case description

A 25-year-old male sound technician was hit by a large and heavy loudspeaker. He sustained an unstable injury of the left hemipelvis: symphysiolysis and rami fracture on the right side, and sacral fracture on the left side with vertical and posterior dislocation of the left hemipelvis (AO/OTA 61C1) (**Fig 5.2-9**).

After careful preoperative planning (**Fig 5.2-10**), the unstable left hemipelvis was treated by closed reduction (**Fig 5.2-11**) and internal fixation (**Fig 5.2-12**). The patient was discharged after 6 days and was instructed to use crutches without weight bearing on the left lower limb.

He came to the outpatient clinic after 4 weeks and complained of pain in the left sacral region. AP, inlet, and outlet views of the pelvis were taken (**Fig 5.2-13**). A clear posterior dislocation was seen, especially on the inlet view (**Fig 5.2-13a**).

The patient said that he always used crutches as advised by the surgeon, but he visited a physiotherapist who recommended he perform various muscle exercises, especially planks (**Fig 5.2-13c**).

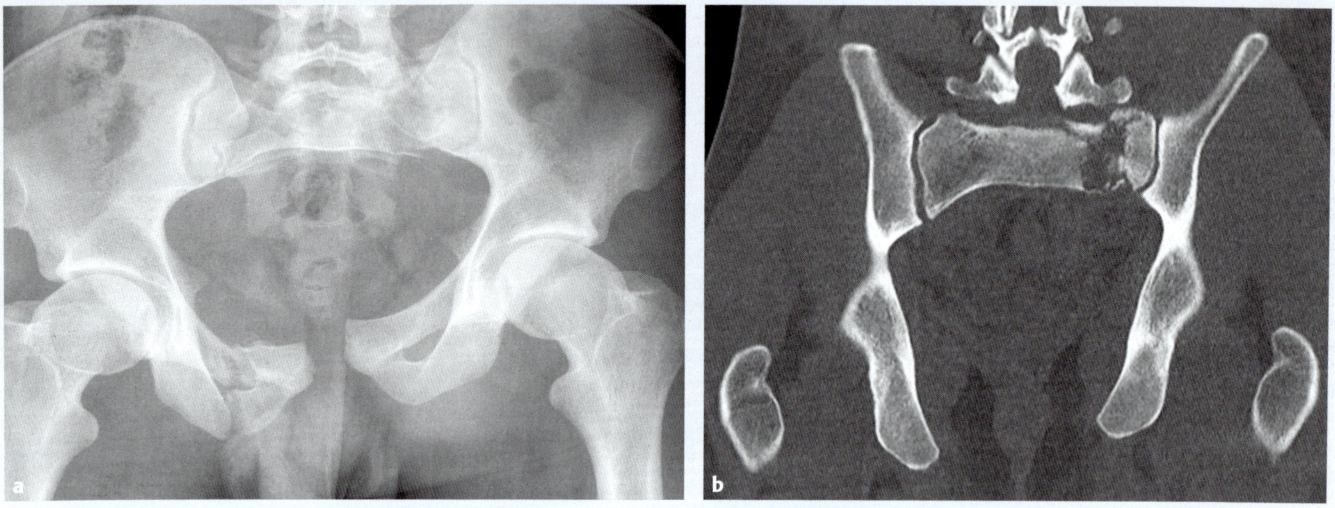

Fig 5.2-9a–b X-ray and computed tomographic (CT) scan of the unstable pelvic fracture.
a AP view x-ray of the injured pelvis.
b The CT image showing a sacral fracture on the left side.

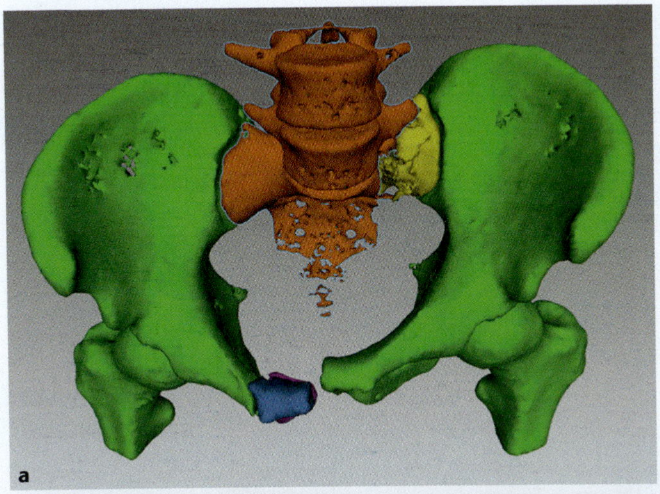

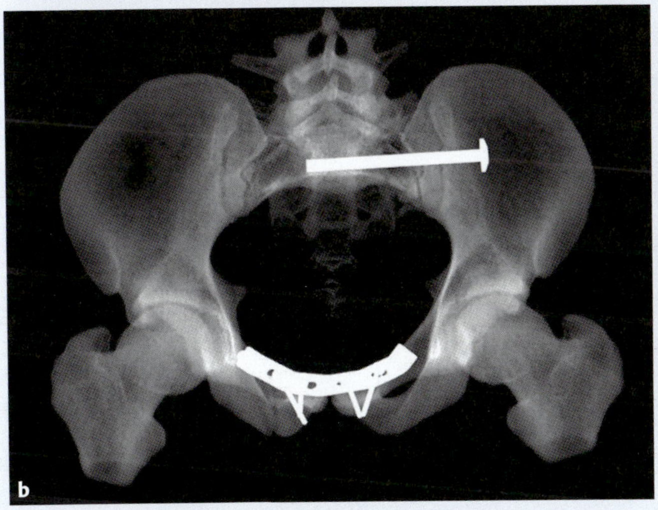

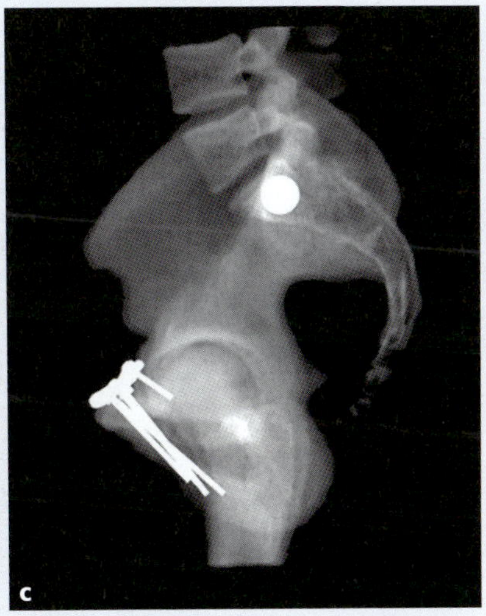

Fig 5.2-10a–c Preoperative planning.
a The segmentation of the fractures.
b Internal fixation in AP view.
c Internal fixation in lateral view.

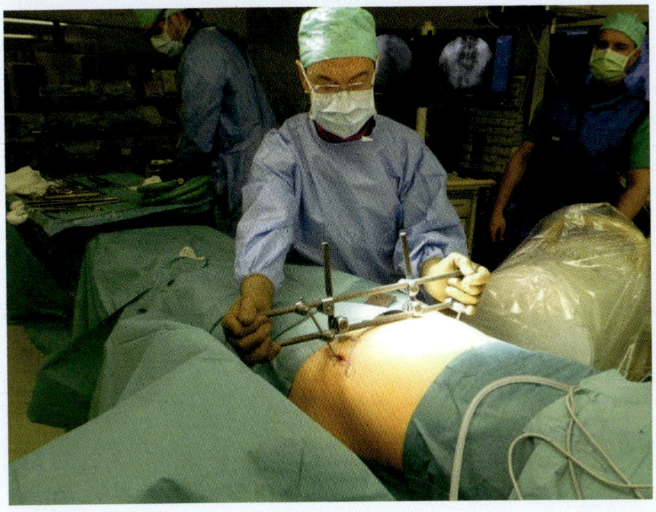

Fig 5.2-11 Closed reduction of the displaced left hemipelvis using a temporary external fixator.

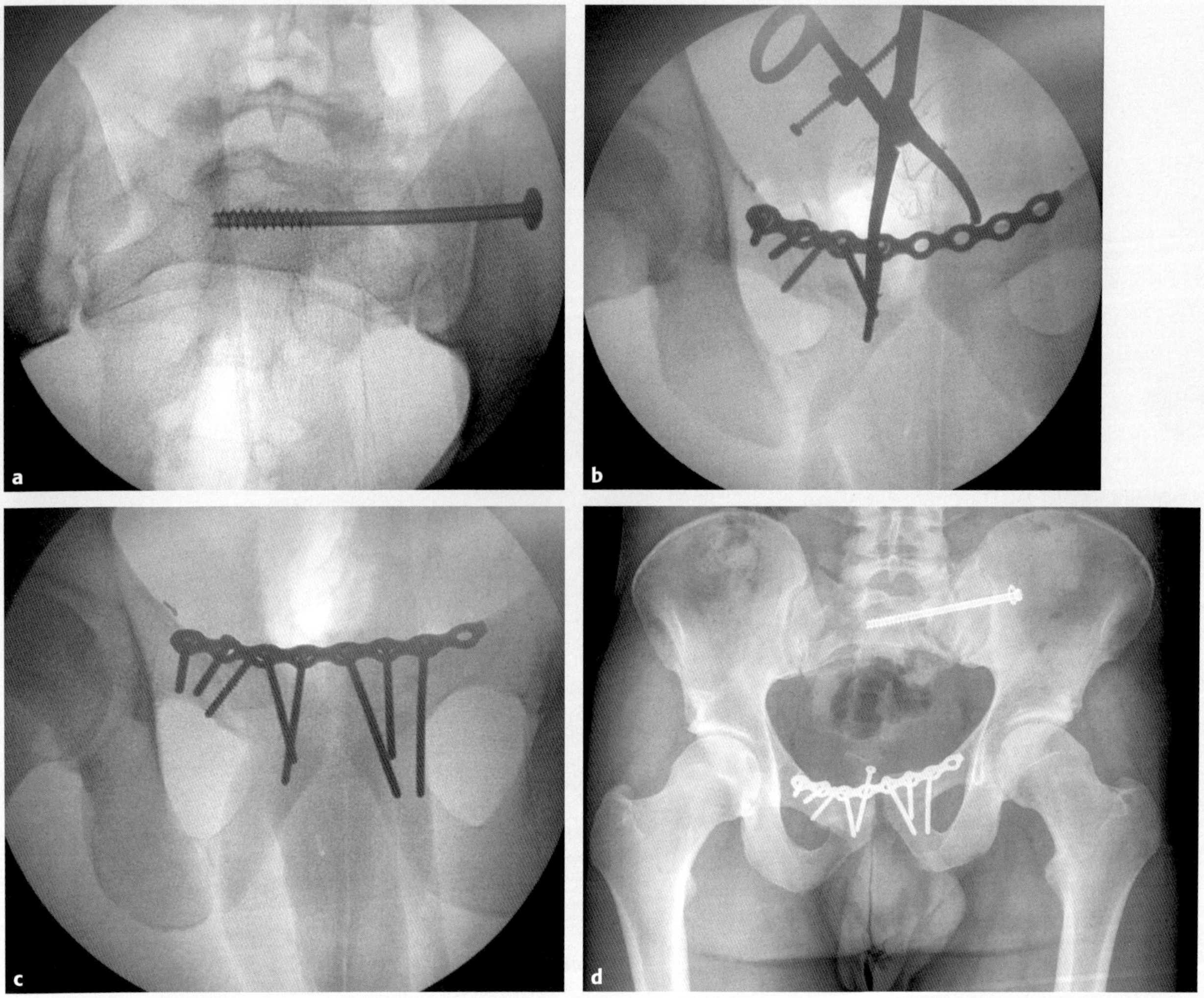

Fig 5.2-12a–d Images during and after surgery.

- **a** Intraoperative view of reduction and fixation of the sacral fracture.
- **b** Intraoperative view of reduction of the symphysiolysis.
- **c** Intraoperative view of reduction and fixation of the anterior pelvis.
- **d** AP view of the pelvis 4 weeks after discharge.

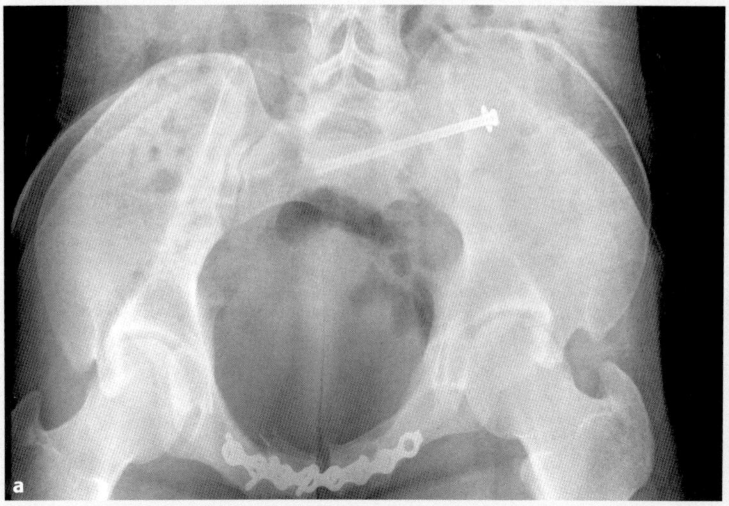

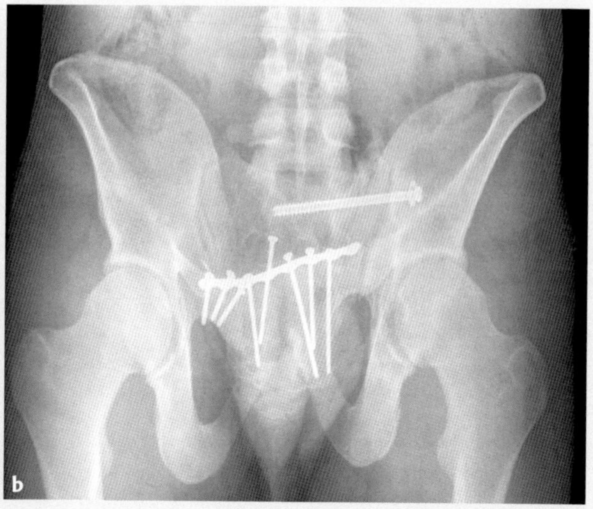

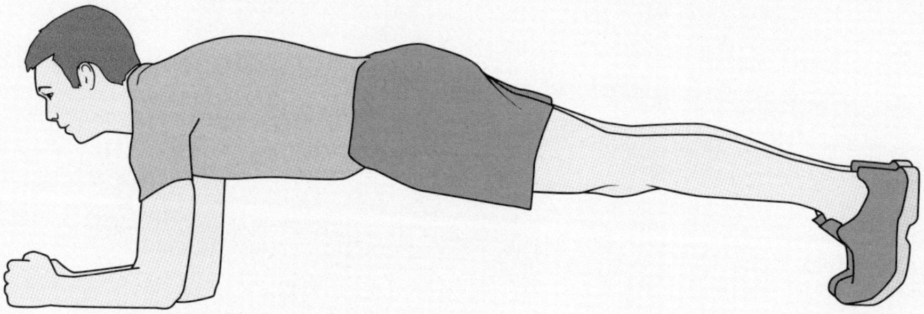

c

Fig 5.2-13a–c Postoperative x-rays and physical exercise.
a Inlet view of the pelvis 4 weeks after discharge.
b Outlet view of the pelvis 4 weeks after discharge.
c Patient doing a plank exercise.

Analysis of failure and reflection

The biomechanical role of the pelvis is the transfer of gravitational forces from the axial skeleton to the lower limbs. If the pelvis is unstable (type C injury), this transfer is completely interrupted. After reduction and fixation, the injured hemipelvis should be protected from immediate weight bearing with crutches. That is exactly what the patient did. However, the physiotherapist did not realize that doing planks loaded the pelvis as much as weight bearing but in an anteroposterior direction. The human pelvis is designed for vertical load (ie, walking) and is very sensitive to horizontal loading, for instance, as in planks.

Final outcome

The patient immediately stopped doing planks and the pain ceased. After 6 weeks he started with partial weight bearing and after another 6 weeks with normal walking. After 2 years, he had fully recovered and regained his preinjury level of activity (**Fig 5.2-14**).

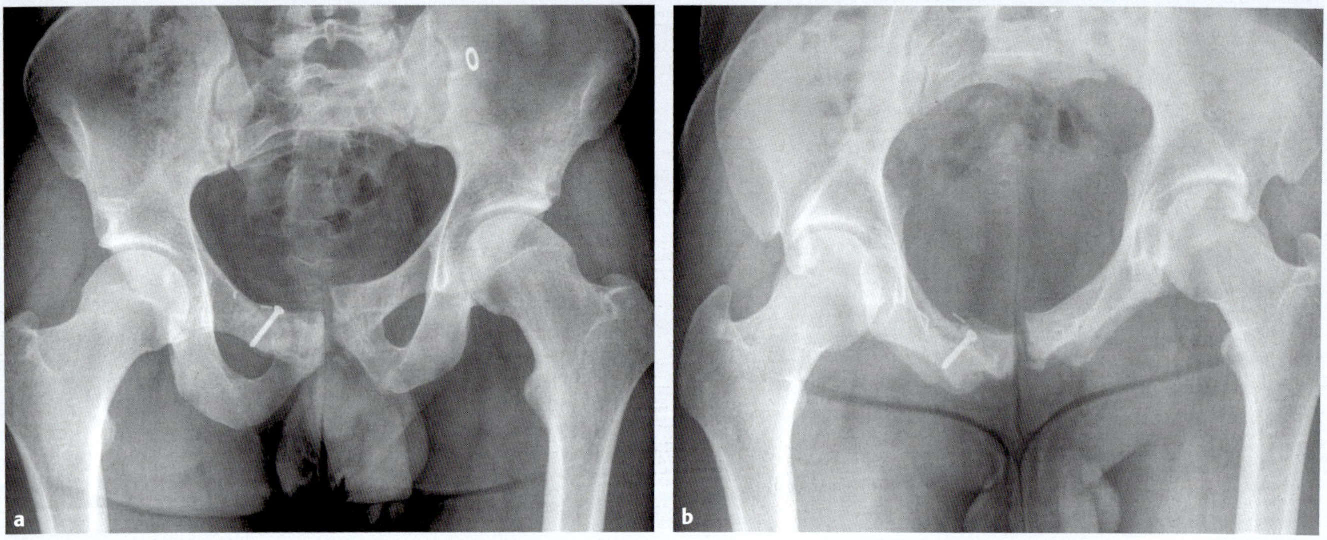

Fig 5.2-14a–b AP (**a**) and inlet (**b**) view of pelvis after 2 years.

Key points to remember

- Always define in each case whether the resulting synthesis is stable for movement only or for movement and weight bearing.
- Postoperative management and follow-up of the patient must be jointly planned by the surgical team and the rehabilitation specialist(s).
- Identify any risk factors that might negatively influence the recovery process, such as senility, osteoporosis, obesity, or psychiatric pathologies.
- Establish an individualized rehabilitation protocol, ensuring that the osteosynthesis patient understands the importance of rigorously adhering to the established protocol and giving the patient the responsibility for a good outcome.
- Start mobilization and weight bearing early and safely, where appropriate, taking into account the patient's specific circumstances, type of fracture, soft tissue, and fixation technique used.
- Patients with pathological or osteoporosis-related fractures or with fractures involving a substantial loss of bone tissue should engage in nonweight-bearing rehabilitation during the first weeks to preserve mobility and musculature.
- Keep the patient and her or his family members motivated throughout the rehabilitation process.
- Establish an effective feedback system between the surgeon, rehabilitation specialist, physical therapist, and patient.

References and suggested reading

Brink PRG, Verleisdonk E, Blokhuis TJ. [Earlier weight-bearing mobilisation after fracture fixation]. *Ned Tijdschr Geneeskd.* 2017;161:D1533.

Buckley RE, Moran CG, Apivatthakakul T. *AO Principles of Fracture Management.* 3rd ed. Stuttgart New York: Thieme; 2017.

Gangavalli AK, Malige A, Rehman S, et al. Patient Comprehension and Compliance Survey to Assess Postoperative Pain Regimens in the Orthopaedic Trauma Population. *J Orthop Trauma.* 2017 Jun;31(6):e190–e194.

Hall AJ, Watkins R, Lang IA, et al. The experiences of physiotherapists treating people with dementia who fracture their hip. *BMC Geriatr.* 2017 Apr 20;17(1):91.

Kuyucu E, Kocyigit F, Ciftci L. The importance of patient compliance in nonunion of forearm fracture. *Int J Surg Case Rep.* 2014;5(9):598–600.

Meinberg EG, Agel J, Roberts CS, et al. Fracture and Dislocation Classification Compendium-2018. *J Orthop Trauma.* 2018 Jan;32 Suppl 1:S1–s170.

Orozco Delclós R. *Errores en la Osteosíntesis.* Barcelona: Masson; 1993.

Sirkin M, Sanders R, DiPasquale T, et al. A staged protocol for soft tissue management in the treatment of complex pilon fractures. *J Orthop Trauma.* 2004 Sep;18(8 Suppl):S32–38.

5.3 Implant removal

Peter A Cole, Anthony J Dugarte, Joan Girós Torres, Jose Mendoza-Vera, Roberto Rivero Sosa, J Miquel Sales Pérez, Eladio Saura-Sanchez, Francisco Saura-Sanchez, Mariano Saura-Sanchez, Miquel Videla Cés

Sometimes the remedy is worse than the disease.

Virgil, The Aeneid, Book XII,16

Implant removal consists of extracting any device that was implanted into the bone to treat an injury. The main objective is to prevent complications that may develop in the host bone in the medium or long term, such as pain or discomfort, because of the material used. Initially, it can be considered a simple, fast, and relatively unattractive operation for the experienced orthopedic surgeon and is therefore frequently performed by the least experienced surgeon on the team. The indication for implant removal is not manifold and a vacuum exists in terms of scientific evidence. In children, it may be necessary to avoid complications in their growing skeleton or in anticipation of future reconstructive surgery after skeletal maturity is reached.

Historically, the need to remove an implant has been widely discussed. There is no universal protocol for surgery of removing material, but every country, region, or hospital may have different protocols. And not all implants must be removed. Legal, cultural, and individual differences all have an influence on the decision regarding the need to remove an implant. Every hospital should have its own directives when it comes to recommendations and performance of this type of intervention.

Surgery for implant removal has been compared to using fishing hooks: so easy to put in but difficult to take out. There is also a common saying when performing this type of intervention: "You know when you will enter the operating room but you don't know when you will leave". Surgery for the removal of such material should never be underestimated.

For some patients the removal of osteosynthesis material represents the last step in the process of recovery from their injury. Attention must be paid to patient expectations, the cost of surgery, its usefulness, and the remaining risks of removing the material, including the possibility of aggressive surgery. All these variables must be evaluated globally and clearly communicated to the patient.

Prior to such surgery, it is necessary to obtain imaging such as x-rays in at least two planes to confirm the union of the fracture and evaluate the type, condition, and exact location of the implant. Preoperative planning plays a fundamental role when considering implant removal surgery. The entire surgical team must know the procedure to be performed and be prepared for unforeseen incidents.

When a primary osteosynthesis is to be performed, it is important to bear in mind that the implant may need to be removed in the future. Performing surgery with respect for the principles of osteosynthesis, orienting the screws correctly and locking them adequately if working with an angular stable locking system is crucial (**Fig 5.3-1**). It is imperative to respect areas of connection between the implant and the device for its placement, the correct use of material for insertion, as well as applying the necessary force for its fixation. These details help to avoid wear, deformation, or breakage of the instruments and the implant, in the hope that the extraction surgery in many cases is more predictable and less problematic.

The surgeon must bear in mind that the usual techniques described for the extraction of a specific piece of material may not work, preventing removal at the first attempt and leading to improvisation and failure. It is always necessary to have a plan B before surgery begins.

Patients must be correctly informed about the possibility of surgeons having to perform aggressive surgery to remove the implanted material. This surgery has a high percentage of minor complications, and occasionally, serious complications arise resulting, in some cases, in the lengthening of the recovery period anticipated by the patient, or some permanent damage.

It is vital for surgeons to have all the necessary surgical instruments and information about the implant to be removed. However, experienced surgeons frequently have their own or unconventional instruments for these types of surgery to assist with removal.

The orthopedic surgeon must analyze each case in detail and prepare for surgery in advance. The following five questions may be helpful when planning implant removal surgery (**Fig 5.3-2**):

1. Which implant must be removed?
2. Why must the implant be removed?
3. When was it implanted?
4. Where is the implant located?
5. Who will perform the surgery?

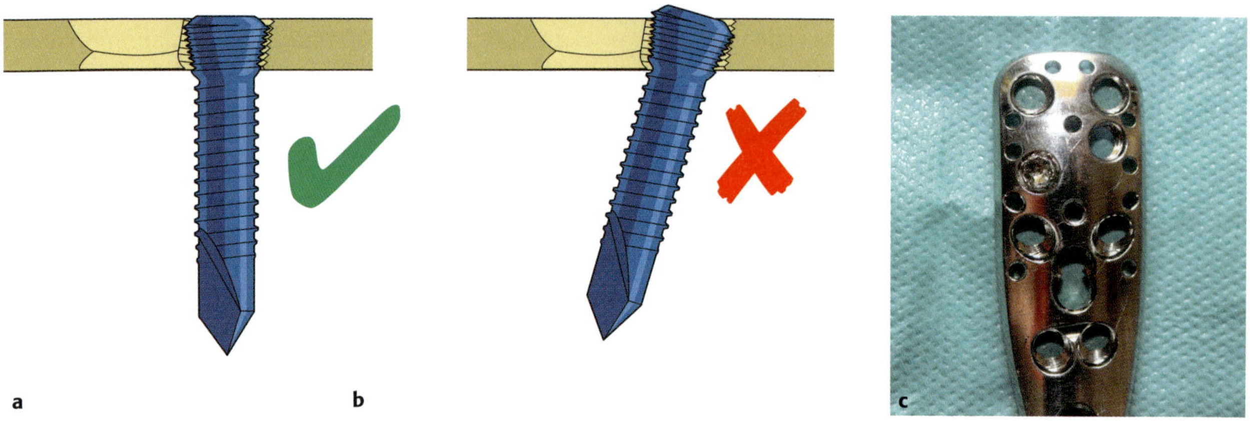

a b c

Fig 5.3-1a–c Screws and angular stable plate.
a–b Locking screws must be carefully placed. Best angular stability is achieved by inserting the screws at 90° (**a**). Illustration (**b**) shows incorrect insertion of the locking screw.
c Intraoperative photograph of a deformed screw.

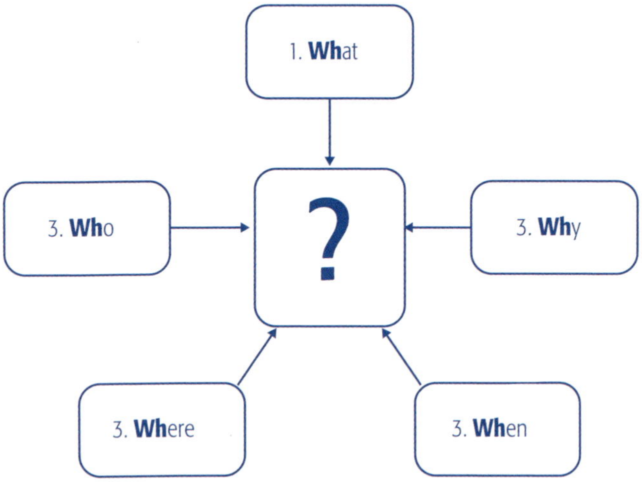

Fig 5.3-2 Rule of **wh**-questions.

Generally, the answer to the first question is obvious. The surgeon must be clear about which material is to be extracted, its characteristics, measurements, type of alloy, and commercial brand, as in some cases the material for removal is specific to the company that designed and manufactured the piece.

Numerous reasons exist that would justify implant removal. Implants that delay mobilization or the healing of a fracture must be removed before 6–8 weeks after insertion, such as screws with a positioning effect, syndesmotic screws, or static bolts used to compress the fracture sites in intramedullary (IM) nailing.

In general, the fixation must be kept in acute infections for a maximum of 4 weeks and the implants do usually not need to be removed when the infection has passed. However, if the implants are loose, they must be extracted at any stage. It seems that in most cases, stability is more important than the negative effects of the foreign body (ie, implant) on the host's defense mechanisms. Only during the course of some types of infections caused by *Pseudomonas aeruginosa*, for instance, must the material be removed.

Late implant removal is more common in young patients, lower limbs, especially at the patella, and in the malleolar region. In the upper extremity, implant extraction is generally not necessary or recommended. For implants that are found in areas with a high risk of iatrogenesis (eg, forearm, humeral diaphysis, pelvis) their removal is not advisable. As a universal rule, the implants in elderly patients must not be extracted unless infected or unstable.

Pain caused by soft-tissue damage due to the presence of osteosynthesis material is the most common complication. Other causes may be late infection, injury, or nerve compression (**Fig 5.3-3**), allergy to implants, periimplant fracture, delayed union, or pseudarthrosis. Delayed union and pseudarthrosis frequently occur with fatigue-related implant breakage (**Fig 5.3-4**).

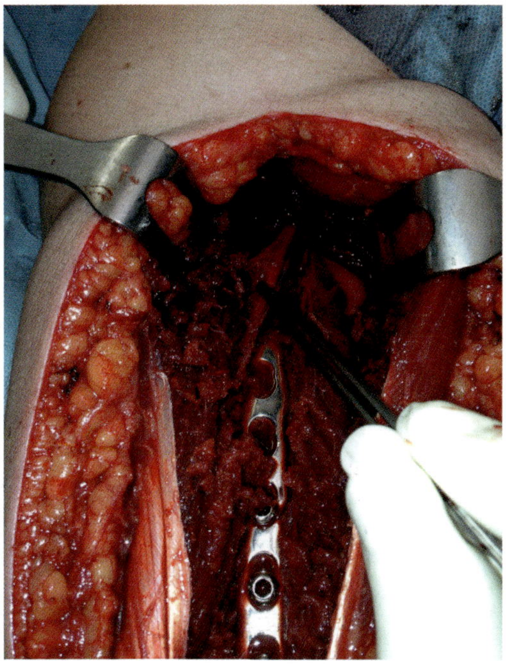

Fig 5.3-3 Intraoperative photograph of osteosynthesis of a diaphyseal humeral fracture, showing the implanted plate and its proximity to the radial nerve.

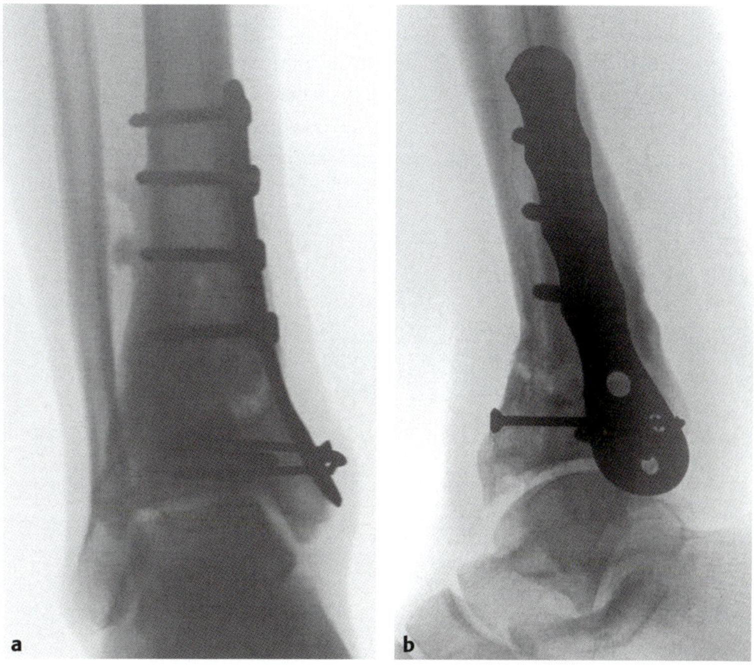

Fig 5.3-4a–b AP (**a**) and lateral (**b**) images of pseudarthrosis in the tibial pilon fracture, which makes implant removal necessary.

Another factor that indicates the necessity of removing the material is metallosis: in some patients, ions of nickel, chrome, and cobalt (cobaltism) are released over time into the bloodstream (**Fig 5.3-5**). Despite potential toxicity, this side effect has not been confirmed in clinical practice yet.

Timing of implant removal surgery is important, as the process of fracture union must be complete. If we are dealing with a case where we want to favor compression of the fracture site by early extraction of the static bolt from an IM nail, the intervention must be performed when the probability of compression of the site is favorable, which is generally before the third month after surgery.

In the case of proposing the removal of plates and/or nails implanted in long bones, eg, periarticular plates or IM nails, it is necessary to wait at least 18 months after the initial surgery. The more time that passes since the primary osteosynthesis, the more laborious the implant removal is made by bone integration of the material, corrosion, and scar tissue, especially if the implant is made of titanium.

Knowledge regarding the location of the implant is essential to perform adequate preoperative planning. Knowing where the implant is located enables us to place the patient in the correct position on the operating table and choose the surgical approach route. Ideally, the surgeon who performed the initial surgery should also be the one who does the follow-up, makes the decision to remove the implant, and executes the removal of the material. This surgeon knows whether there were difficulties at the time of the intervention and the local relationship between anatomical structures in that particular patient.

Before entering the operating room, the surgeon must know whom to call if any serious complication arises during the operation, preferably an experienced surgeon. Making "wrong" decisions may lead to mistakes. The consequences may be minor or may have a major impact on the patient, such as difficulty in wound healing, devascularization or infection of the soft tissues, vascular or nerve damage, or bone fragility which may result in refractures.

A few days after surgical extraction, and once soft-tissue healing has been achieved, complete functioning and weight bearing can recommence, depending on the location and type of implant removed. In general, a period of partial weight bearing is recommended in extramedullary implants extracted from lower limbs.

It is always important to consider the risks and benefits for each patient, although this is not always easy to determine. As Hippocrates, the ancient Greek physician and father of medicine, said "primum non nocere", ie, first, do no harm.

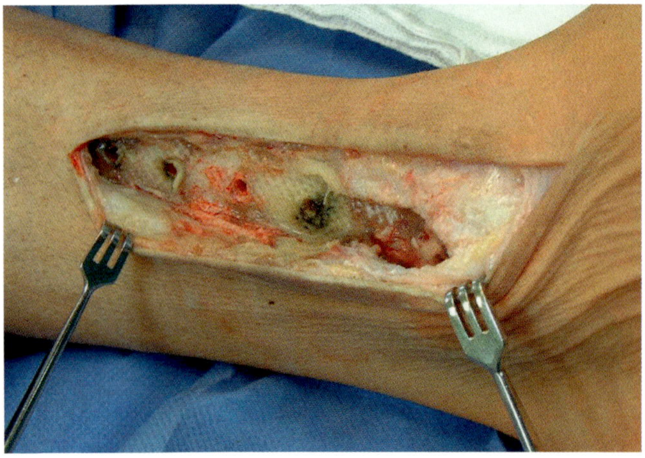

Fig 5.3-5 Extraction of osteosynthesis material at 15 months, showing the resulting metallosis.

Peter A Cole, Anthony J Dugarte, Joan Girós Torres, Jose Mendoza-Vera, Roberto Rivero Sosa, J Miquel Sales Pérez, Eladio Saura-Sanchez, Francisco Saura-Sanchez, Mariano Saura-Sanchez, Miquel Videla Cés

Case description

A 58-year-old builder received a direct blow while working, sustaining a Gustilo type I tibial shaft fracture in his right leg with the fibula still intact (AO/OTA 42A2). He was initially treated in the author's hospital the same day with a titanium unreamed tibial nail (UTN) through a standard transpatellar approach without reaming the canal and with static locking. Secondary dynamization of the nail at 2 months by removing the proximal static bolt resulted in uneventful fracture healing (**Fig 5.3-6**).

Twenty-five months after fixation, the surgeon decided to remove the nail after the patient complained of anterior knee pain. After removing the locking bolts and while trying to extract the nail, the connecting piece of the extraction device broke and the surgeon left it in situ. Any attempt at extracting the nail was unsuccessful (**Fig 5.3-7**).

When the implant producer was told about this complication, they informed the surgeon that the broken fragment should be removed from the patient because it was a "nonimplantable device" and the combination of two different materials could have adverse effects. They sent an expert to remove the nail with a recently designed extractor, but when they analyzed the x-rays, they realized that the nail could not be removed with the extractor because the broken piece was stuck in the dynamic hole (**Fig 5.3-7**).

The patient was informed, and in agreement with the hospital, advisors from the company who created the implant, and his lawyer, decided to remove the nail anyway. Six months after the first removal attempt, the surgeons performed a new surgery with several options planned and the firm conviction that the nail must be removed. The first option engaged the nail proximally through the free-locking holes with some instruments that were designed specifically for that surgery. All the trials failed, though (**Fig 5.3-8**).

The second preoperative plan was a new technique which coupled (interlocked) the proximal part of the titanium nail with a custom-made IM tibial nail. This new attempt failed and worsened the situation because repeated back hammering caused the interlocked stainless steel nail to break and remain attached to the UTN (**Fig 5.3-9**).

After a 3.5-hour intervention, it was clear that the nail was stuck in the bone. Finally, a tailored anteromedial tibial strut of almost its whole length was cut with an oscillating saw and removed, leaving the proximal metaphyseal block intact (**Fig 5.3-10**). Complete osteointegration between the titanium nail and the surrounding bone was seen. The nail had to be extracted from the remaining bone in the diaphyseal and distal areas with a chisel. To avoid further damage to the proximal tibial segment, both nails were disengaged first by removing the interlocking bolts. Once uncoupled, the UTN was removed from distal and the remaining broken piece of the custom-made IM stainless steel tibial nail was taken from the proximal incision (**Fig 5.3-11**). A reposition of the tibial wall graft was fixed with four stainless steel lag screws (**Fig 5.3-12**). When analyzing the removed nail, bone ingrowth inside the dynamic hole was also seen (**Fig 5.3-13**).

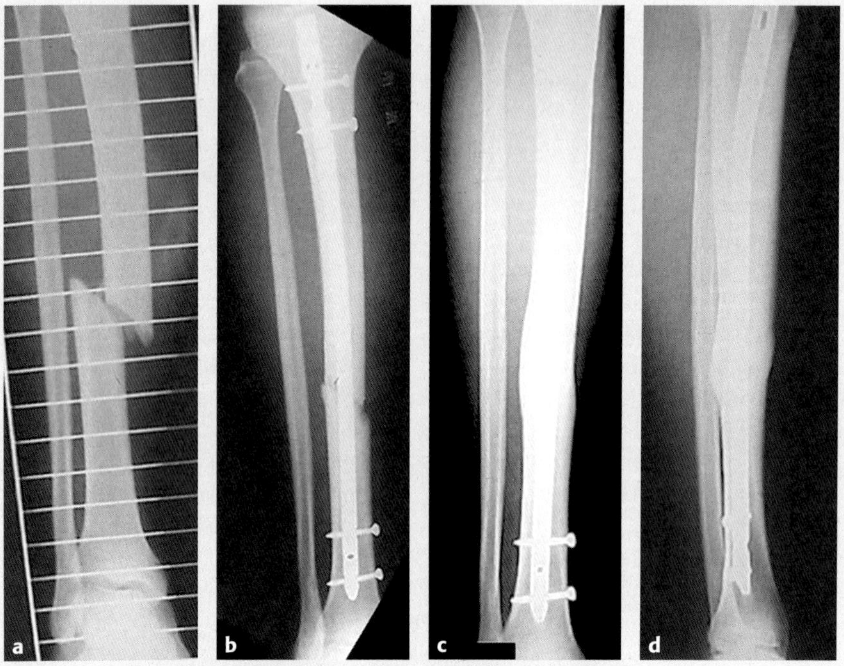

Fig 5.3-6a–d X-rays of the oblique Gustilo type I tibial shaft fracture.

- **a** Gustilo type I tibial fracture.
- **b** Postoperative AP x-ray.
- **c** AP x-ray 25 months after surgery showing fracture healing.
- **d** Lateral x-ray 25 months after surgery showing uneventful healing.

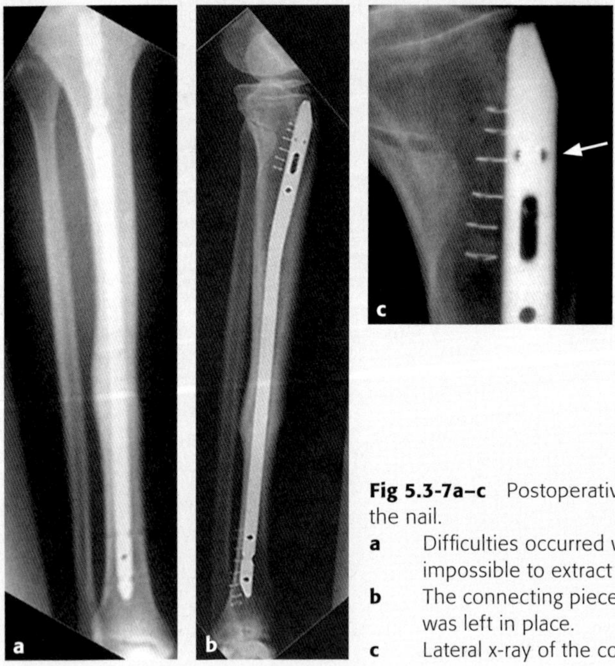

Fig 5.3-7a–c Postoperative x-rays after the first attempt at removing the nail.

- **a** Difficulties occurred while removing the implant. As it was impossible to extract it, only the locking bolts were removed.
- **b** The connecting piece of the extraction device broke, so the nail was left in place.
- **c** Lateral x-ray of the connecting piece inside the proximal tibial nail.

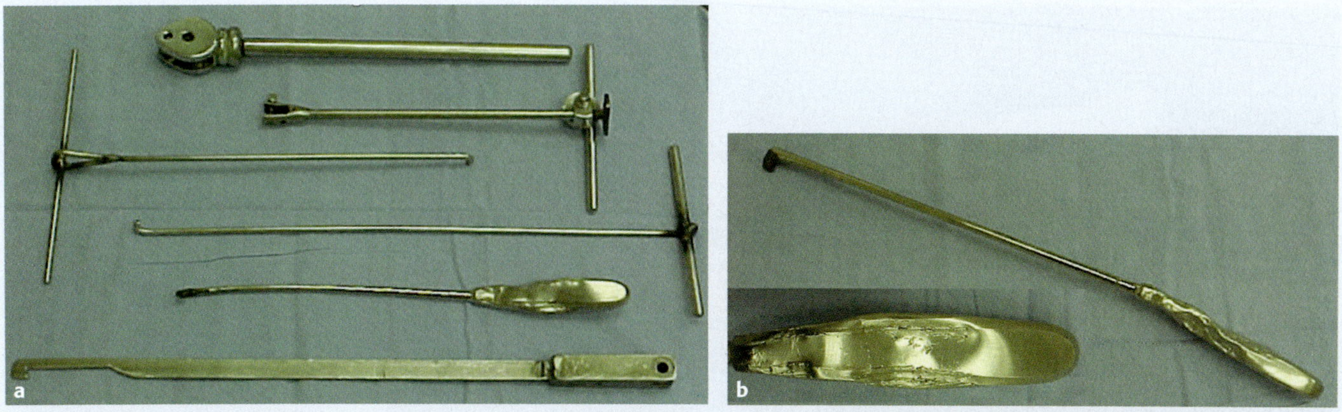

Fig 5.3-8a–b Some of the instruments designed specifically for this removal surgery which failed (first option). Note the damage to the device caused while trying to extract the nail.

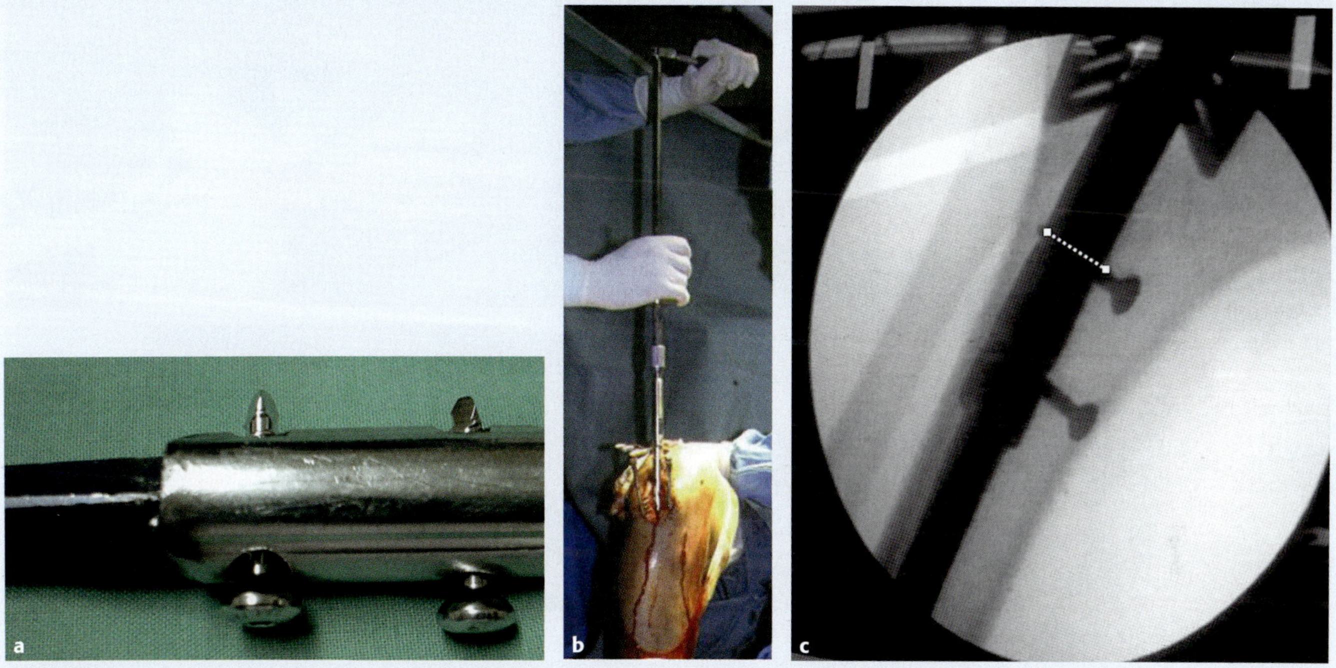

Fig 5.3-9a–c Interlocking of the proximal part of the titanium nail with a custom-made intramedullary (IM) tibial nail (second plan).

a Clinical image depicting the coupling of implants in a sample prior to surgery. New distal holes drilled in the custom-made IM tibial nail and matched with the standard unreamed tibial nail (UTN).

b Intraoperative image during repeated back hammering the interlocked stainless steel nail.

c Dotted line in the intraoperative C-arm image shows the rupture zone of the custom-made IM tibial nail (proximal interlocking hole) whose distal part remained attached to the UTN (**c**).

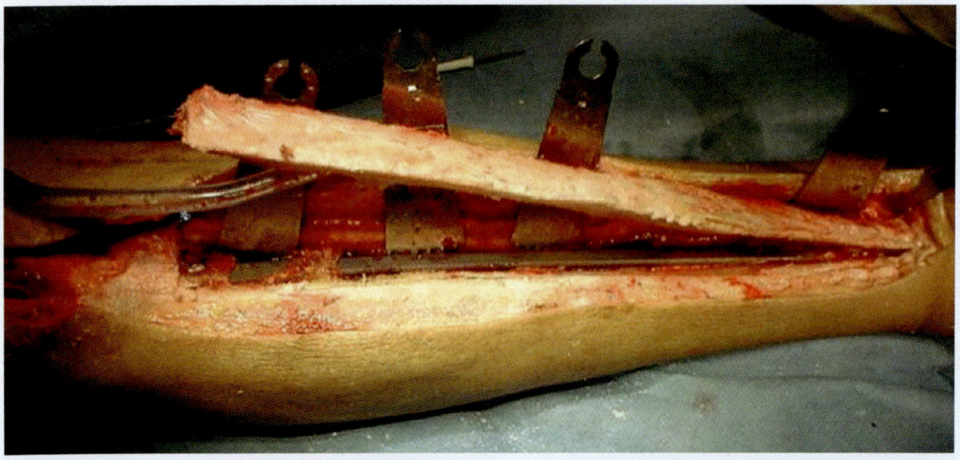

Fig 5.3-10 Opening of the anteromedial tibial strut of almost its whole length leaving the proximal metaphyseal block intact and close to the tip of the nail. Notice the osteointegration with bone overgrowth surrounding the titanium nail.

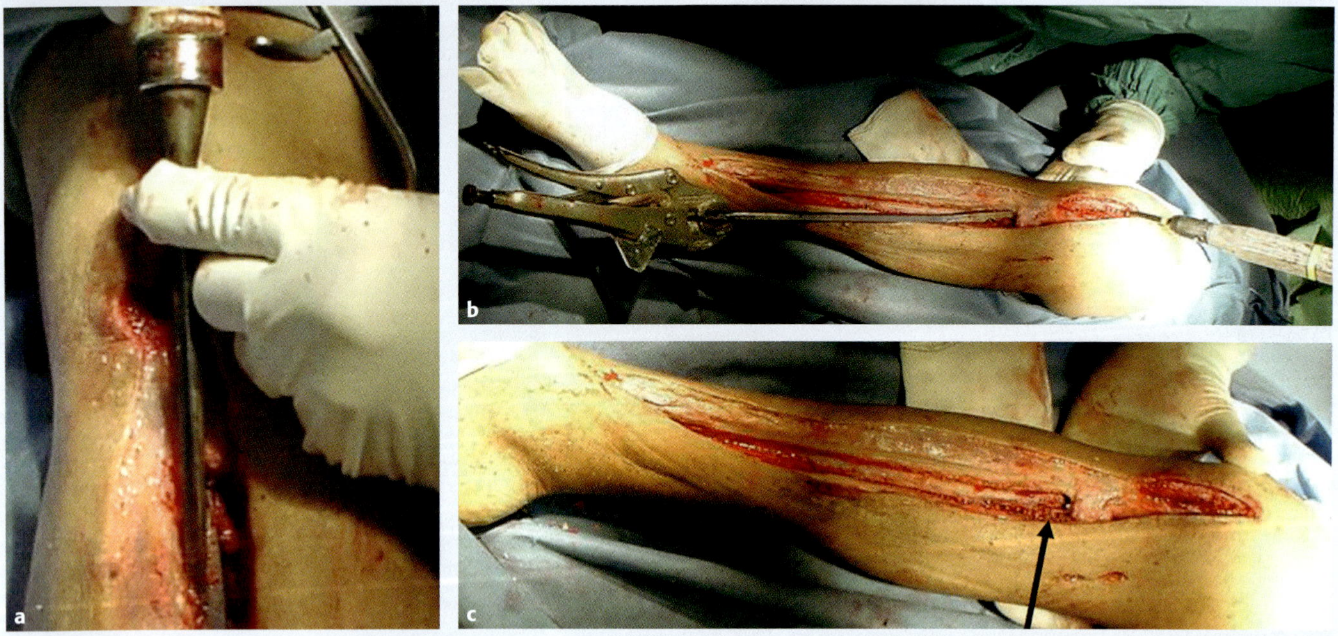

Fig 5.3-11a–c Removal of the osteointegrated nail.
a Separating the unreamed tibial nail from the cortical diaphyseal bone with a chisel.
b–c After removing the proximal interlocking bolts, the titanium nail was removed distally and the remaining part of the broken custom-made stainless steel nail was taken from proximally (**b**). Note the remaining proximal piece of broken nail (**c**).

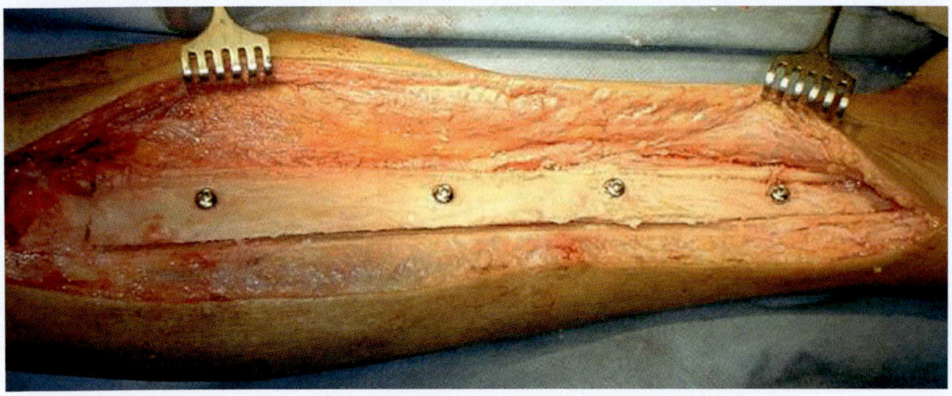

Fig 5.3-12 Repositioning of the "tibial flap" and fixation with four lag screws.

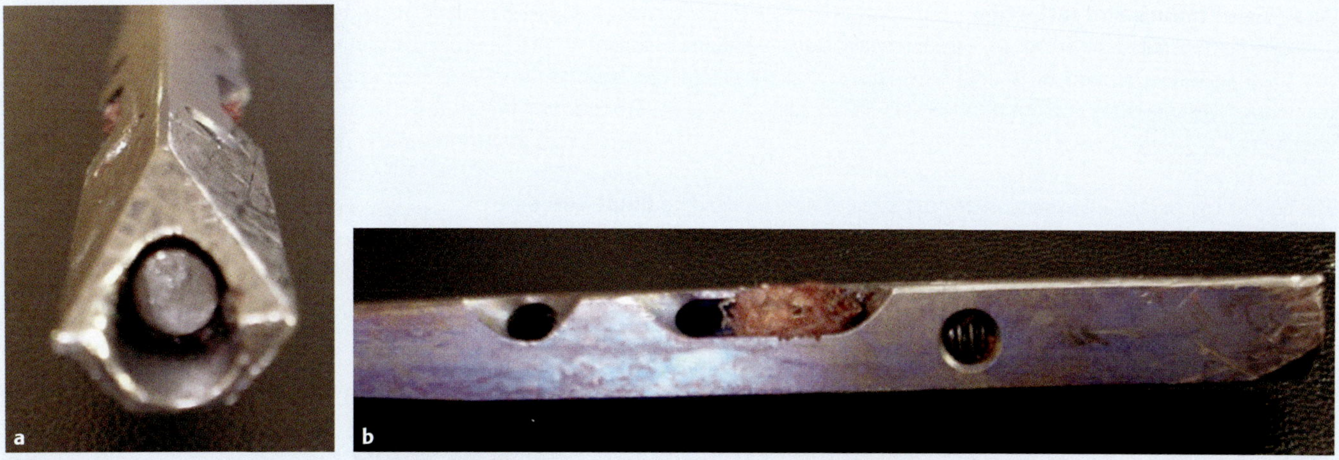

Fig 5.3-13a–b Details of the removed titanium nail. Notice the remaining bone in the dynamic hole and the broken piece of the extraction device inside the nail.

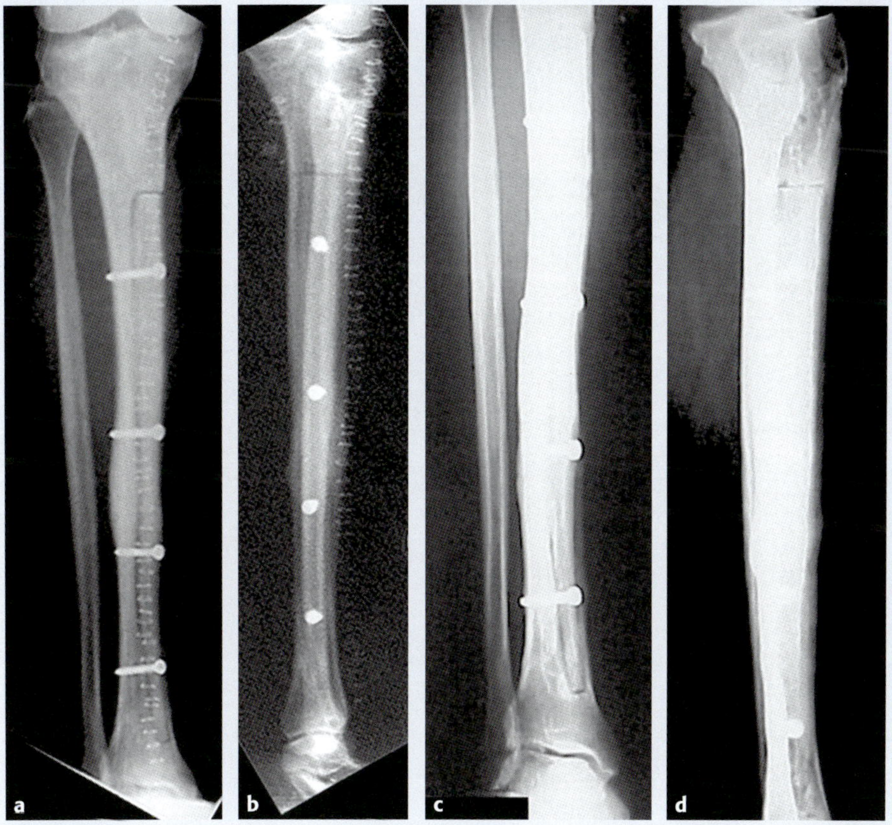

Fig 5.3-14a–h Follow-up x-rays.
a–d Postoperative x-rays on day 1 (**a–b**) and at 3 months showing consolidation (**c–d**).

Analysis of failure and reflection

This case demonstrated the existence of titanium nail osteointegration in a tibial fracture. The surgeon should have known that standard techniques described for implant removal may fail in case of true integration.

The correct use of implant extraction devices is mandatory to avoid problems later, because the need to extract the nail was related to the broken nonimplantable piece of the extraction device rather than the knee pain itself. Patients must be informed that aggressive surgery may be required if the nail has to be removed. As is usual in stem revision surgeries, opening the canal is the only way to remove well-integrated implants, although it is not a standard approach in implant removal surgery.

Final outcome

The patient's clinical course was good with no wound complications and final bone healing of the anterior tibial bone wall (**Fig 5.3-14**).

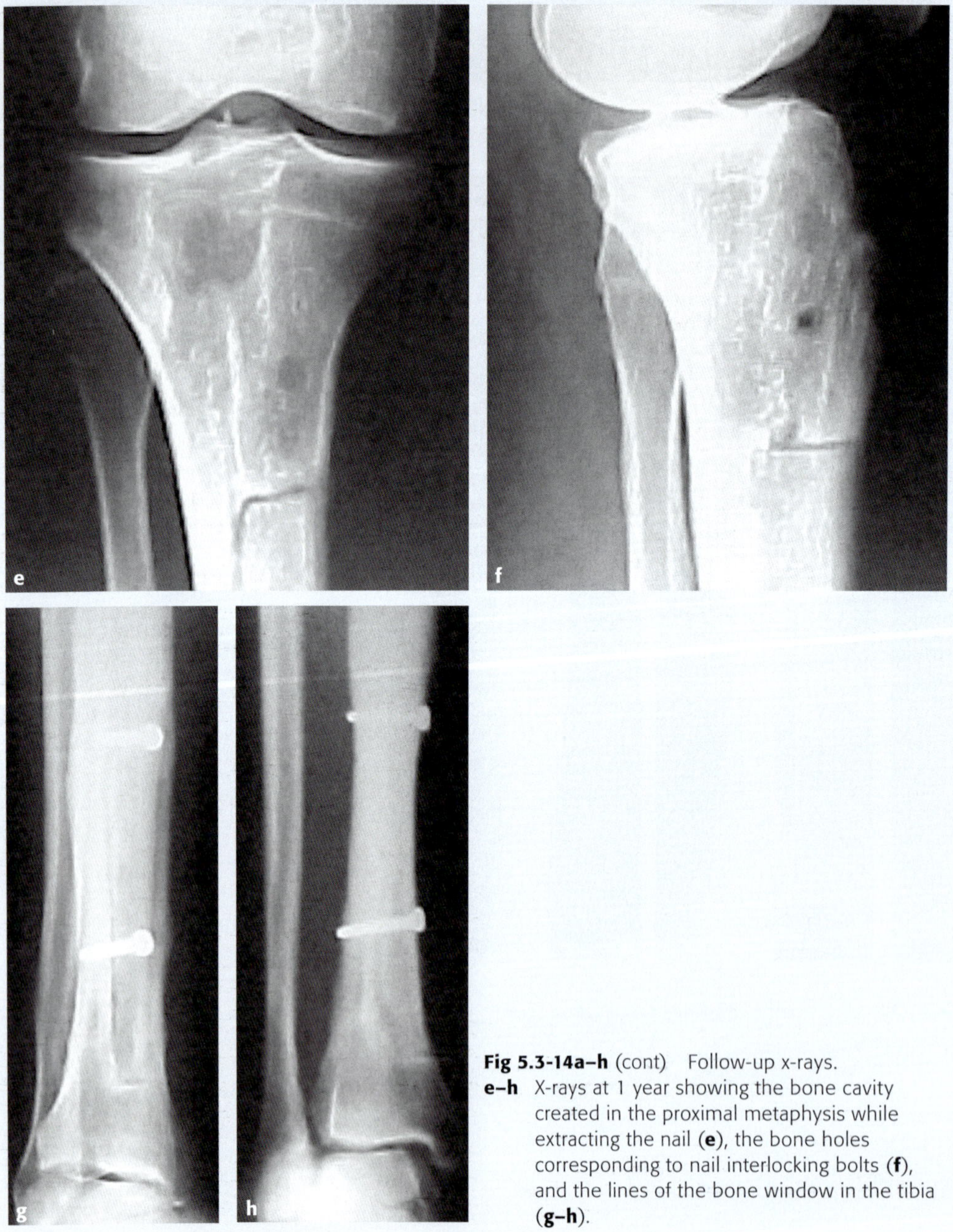

Fig 5.3-14a–h (cont) Follow-up x-rays.
e–h X-rays at 1 year showing the bone cavity created in the proximal metaphysis while extracting the nail (**e**), the bone holes corresponding to nail interlocking bolts (**f**), and the lines of the bone window in the tibia (**g–h**).

Peter A Cole, Anthony J Dugarte, Joan Girós Torres, Jose Mendoza-Vera, Roberto Rivero Sosa, J Miquel Sales Pérez, Eladio Saura-Sanchez, Francisco Saura-Sanchez, Mariano Saura-Sanchez, Miquel Videla Cés

Case description

A 16-year-old boy, who was an athlete at school, had a high-energy motorbike accident in 2005. Due to a direct impact on his left leg, he sustained a closed supraintercondylar fracture of the distal femur (AO/OTA 33C2). It was an isolated injury with no neurovascular damage. He was treated in the hospital with a minimally invasive technique, using lag screw fixation of the condylar fracture and a titanium less invasive stabilization system (LISS) plate to bridge the complex metaphyseal area. Good clinical results and consolidation were obtained (**Fig 5.3-15**).

Two years after surgery the patient started university. He had a good range of motion in his left knee but complained of pain in the lateral part of his knee close to the scar. There was a bulky mass in the anterior zone of his thigh, corresponding to a healed femoral fracture fragment, with no associated pain (**Fig 5.3-16**). He requested an implant removal because he wanted to increase his sports activity.

Surgery was performed 26 months after the initial fixation under general anesthesia without tourniquet, with the patient in a standard supine position. The same approach as in the first surgery was used. When using the hexagonal screwdriver to remove the screws, some of the distal locking screws lost their purchase and the conical extraction device designed for this situation (ie, damaged screw recess) had to be used (**Fig 5.3-17**). After successfully extracting some screws, the surgeons found it difficult to remove those remaining, and too much force was applied to unscrew the jammed screws. As a result, the extraction device broke in the purchase of one of the locked screws (**Fig 5.3-18**), making it impossible to pull that screw out because its head was locked by a nonimplantable hard material.

A spherical diamond burr failed to remove that piece because it was made of stainless steel. The final option was to remove the jammed screws by using a diamond saw to cut them through the plate (**Fig 5.3-19**). The first cuts aimed to remove the "problematic hole". As other screws could not be removed either, the surgeons decided to detach the distal part of the plate. A second cut in the plate was needed to remove the distal third that may have been the initial cause of pain (**Fig 5.3-20**). To prevent further complications, no attempt was made to remove the proximal diaphyseal screws. Extensive metallic debris had to be cleaned from surrounding soft tissues despite using dressings around the plate to avoid it spreading (**Fig 5.3-21**).

Some jammed screws were cut from their shaft (next to the plate) to keep their heads fixed to the plate so the interface could be analyzed by electron microscopy. Their screw shafts were removed from the metaphyseal area without any problems with the standard technique and specific instrumentation (ie, hollow reamer, extraction bolt, and pliers depending on the situation). Several conical extraction devices were used because some broke and others stuck inside the purchase of the extracted screw (**Fig 5.3-22**).

Postoperative x-rays taken at the 1-year follow-up showed no complications. The patient was able to engage in his preinjury activities without knee pain, and there were no changes in the range of knee movement (**Fig 5.3-23**). Postoperative analysis of the removed plate was performed at the Mechanical Engineering Department of the Polytechnic University of Cartagena, Spain. The interface between the plate and the head of the screw (titanium–titanium) and the interface between the screw head and the broken metallic piece that remained inside the deformed screw shape at purchase, mixing titanium (screw head) and stainless steel (screw driver) were studied.

Electron microscope images showed almost fused surfaces between the implants. This could explain the great difficulty during removal. Deformation of the titanium screw head due to the force applied to the extraction device may also have explained its breakage. The absence of space between titanium surfaces of plate–locking head screw (titanium interface) resembled a cold fusion process (**Fig 5.3-24** and **Fig 5.3-25**). Clinically, there was no doubt that a cold fusion process had developed.

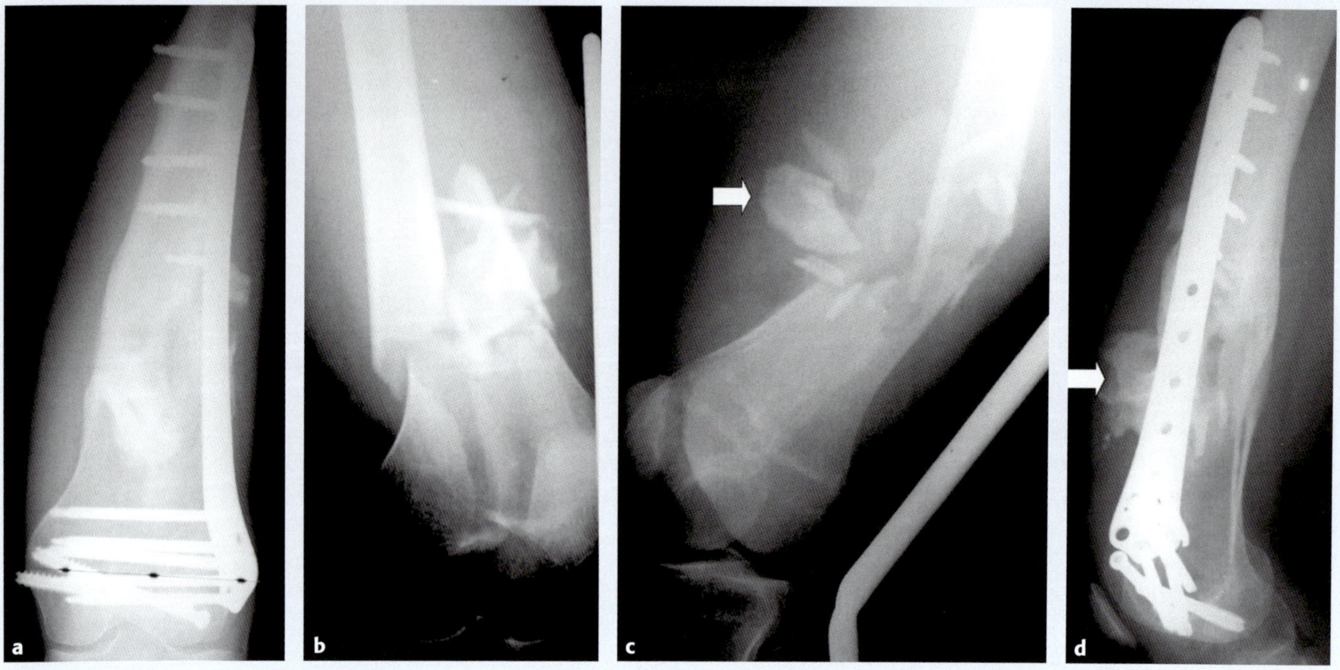

Fig 5.3-15a–d X-rays showing the initial fracture and final result with complete bone healing 25 months after surgery. The fracture was treated with a less invasive stabilization system in a minimally invasive procedure. White arrows (in **c–d**) depict the anterior diaphyseal femoral fragment that remained untouched.

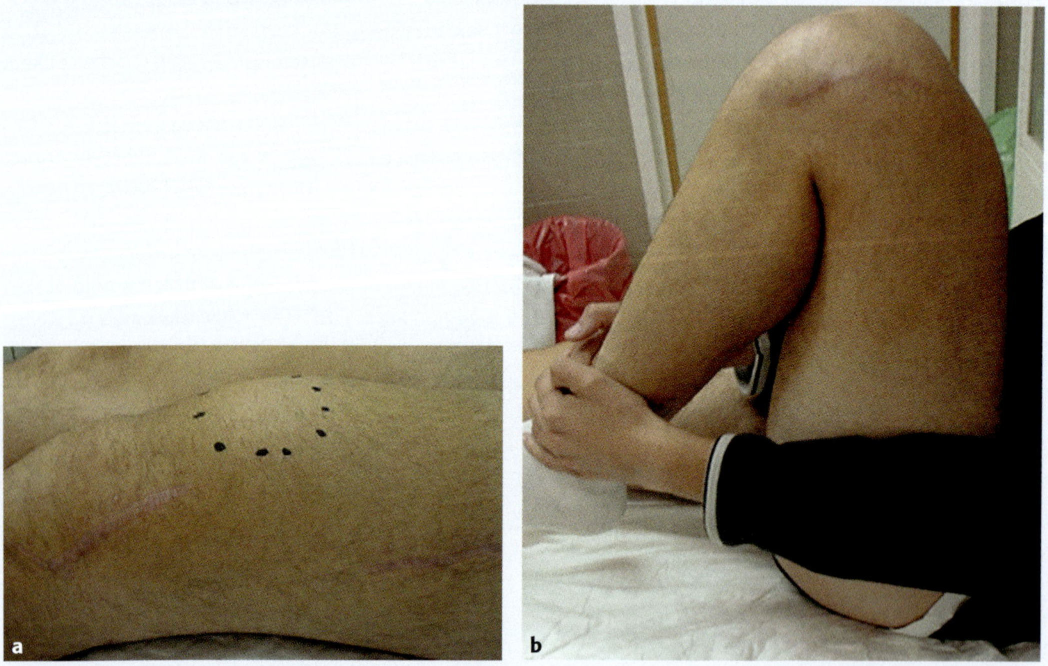

Fig 5.3-16a–b Clinical exploration. Note the bulky mass in the anterior part of the patient's leg. Pain related to the lateral part of the knee when flexed close to the surgical scar (iliotibial band) which corresponds to the white arrows shown in **Fig 5.3-15c–d**.

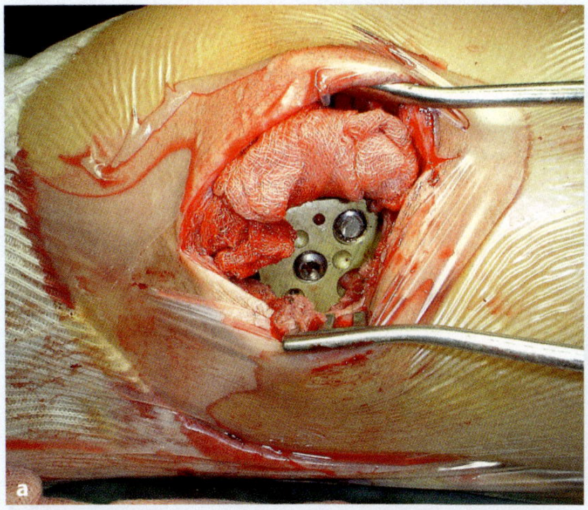

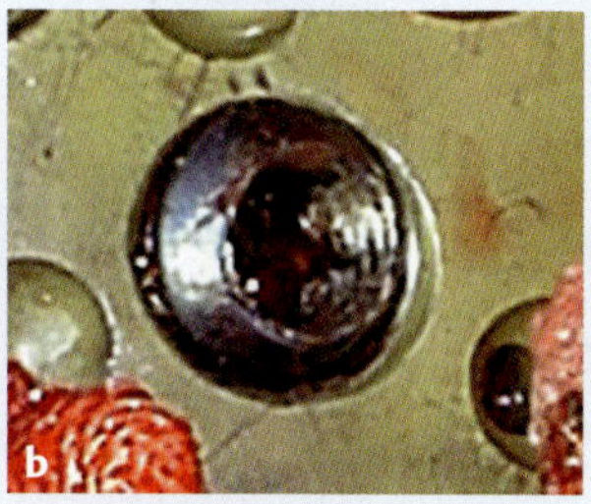

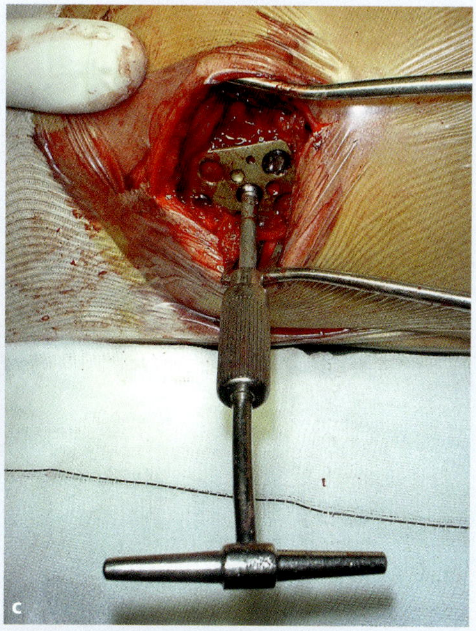

Fig 5.3-17a–c Intraoperative clinical images.

a–b The screwdriver purchase was lost at the head recess of the screw while removing it from the distal plate, eroding its surface, and rendering the screwdriver useless.

c To remove the screws with a damaged screw recess, a conical extraction screw must be used and turned anticlockwise. Some of the distal screws could be removed with this device.

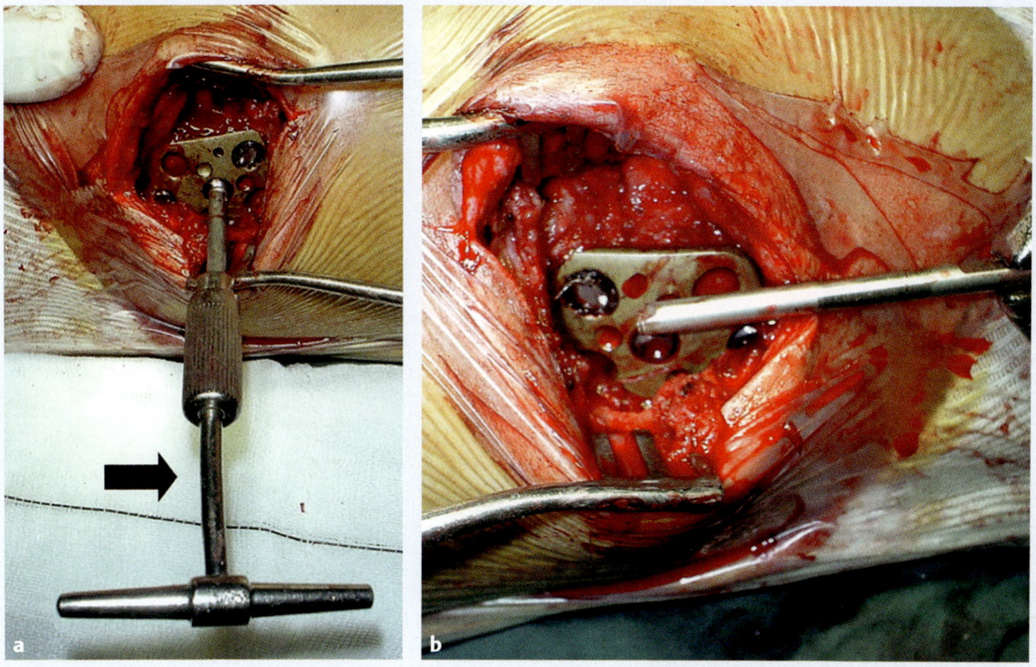

Fig 5.3-18a–b Breakage of the extraction device. Too much force was applied to remove some of the distal locking screws. Note the deformity of the quick coupling T-handle (black arrow in **a**). The final breakage of the conical extraction screw left its tip locked in the head of the screw making its extraction impossible.

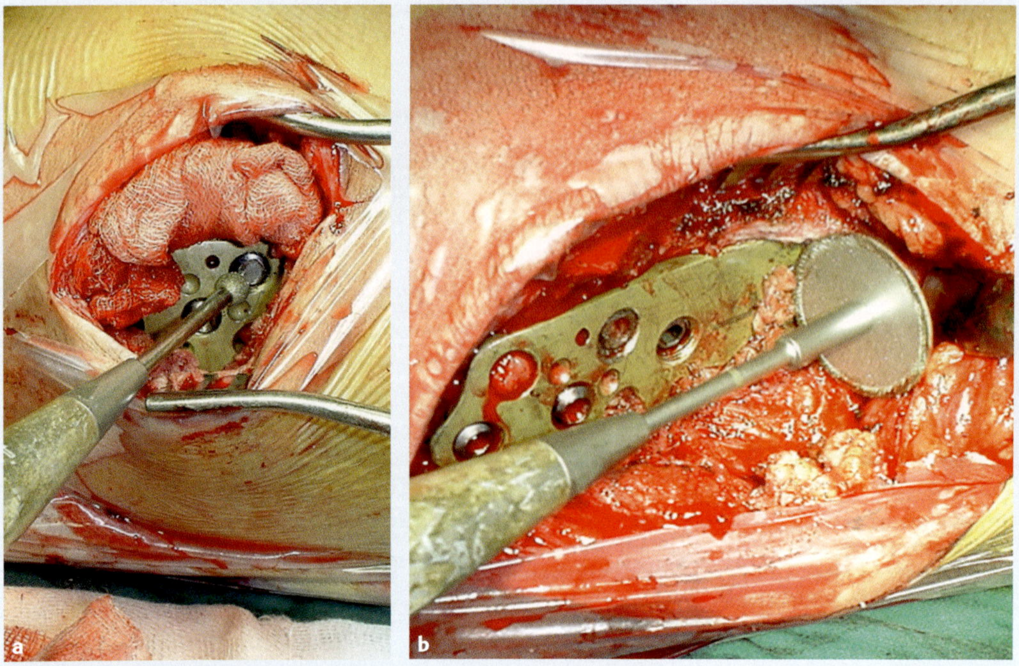

Fig 5.3-19a–b Since the broken piece made of stainless steel could not be removed by the sphere diamond burr (**a**), the plate had to be cut with a diamond saw (final option) (**b**).

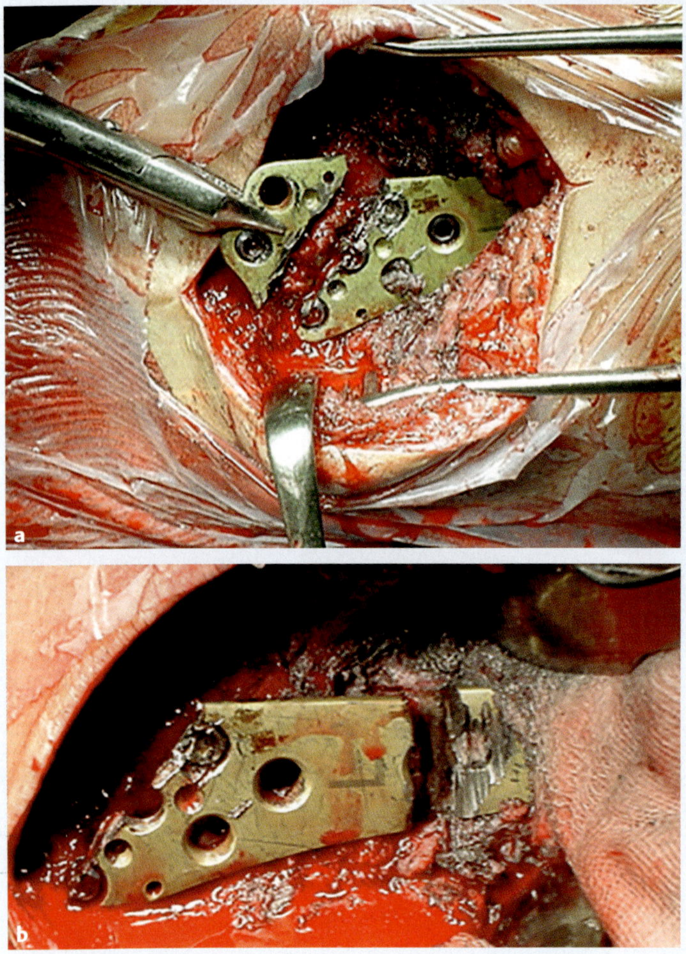

Fig 5.3-20a–b Intraoperative images showing the plate being cut in two to remove the plate.

- **a** First the plate is cut to remove the screws.
- **b** The plate is cut a second time more proximally to remove the distal part of the plate that was the initial cause of pain. No attempt was made to remove the proximal diaphyseal screws, to prevent further complications.

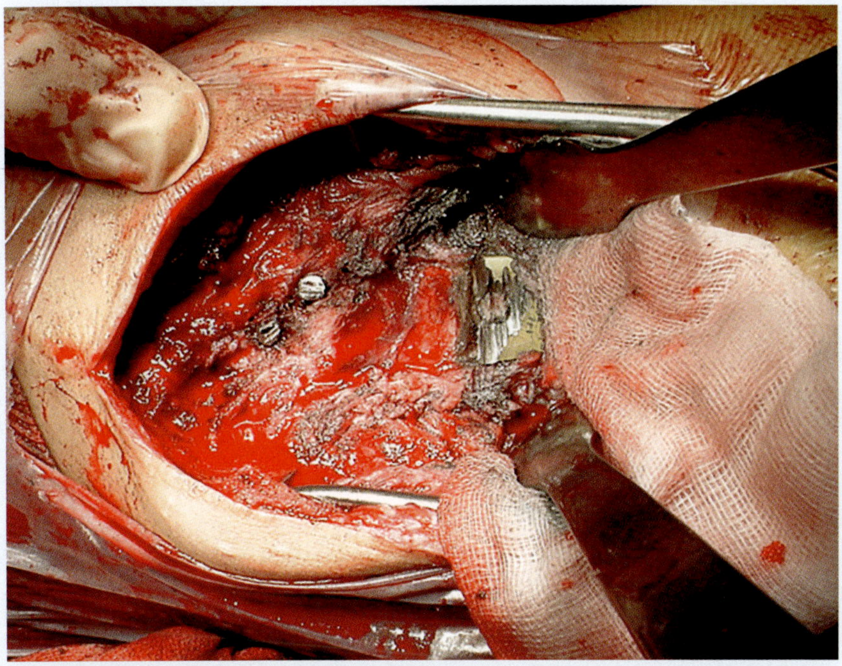

Fig 5.3-21 The soft tissues after partial plate removal. Note the metallic debris despite the dressings used. Some screws were cut from their shafts to keep their jammed heads in the plate for later analysis.

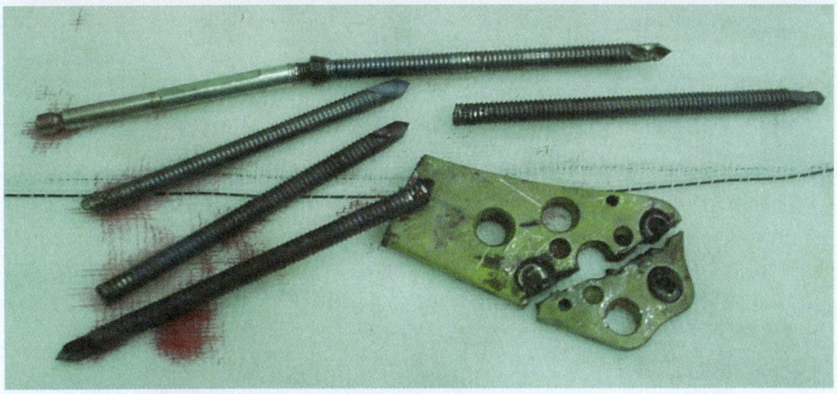

Fig 5.3-22 The removed material. Note some conical extraction screws remain stuck in the removed screws.

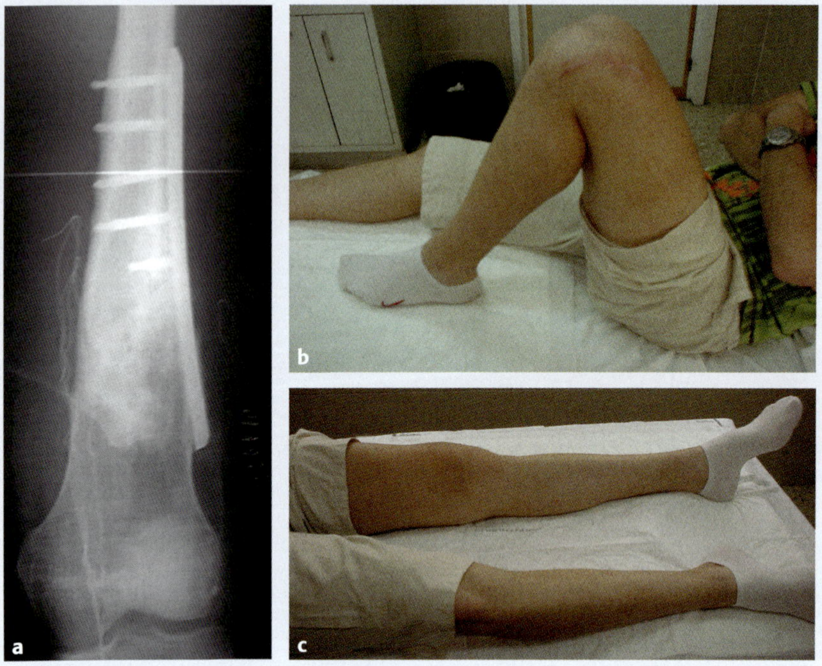

Fig 5.3-23a–c Final postoperative x-ray (**a**) showing the level at which the plate was cut. Follow-up at 1 year (**b–c**): the patient experienced no knee pain and was able to achieve the desired level of sports activity.

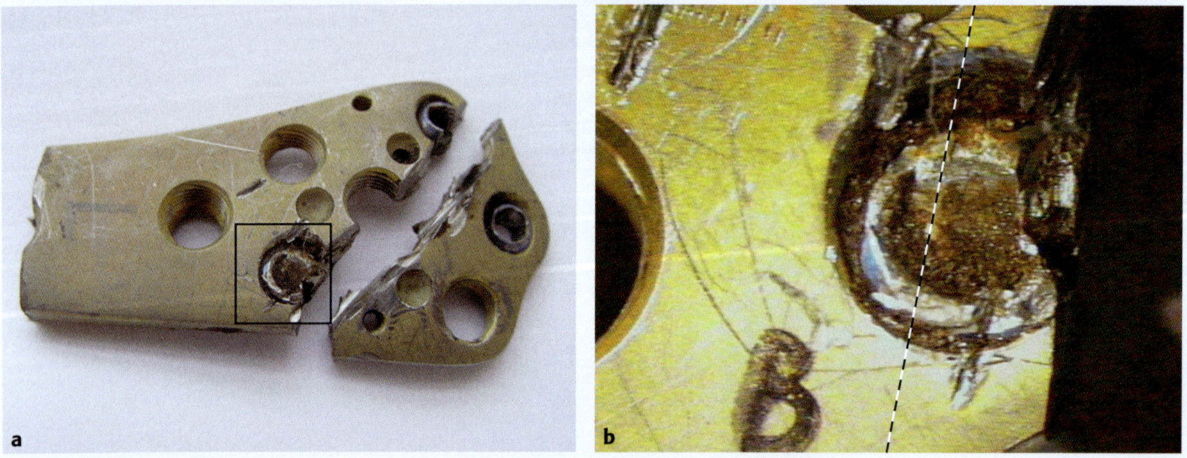

Fig 5.3-24a–b Macroscopic image of the removed plate (**a**) centered on analysis of the plate hole with the broken extraction piece inside (**b**). The dotted line shows the cutting line made to study the interfaces between plate and screw head (titanium–titanium) and the interface between the screw head and the broken metallic piece of the extraction device left in place (titanium–stainless steel).

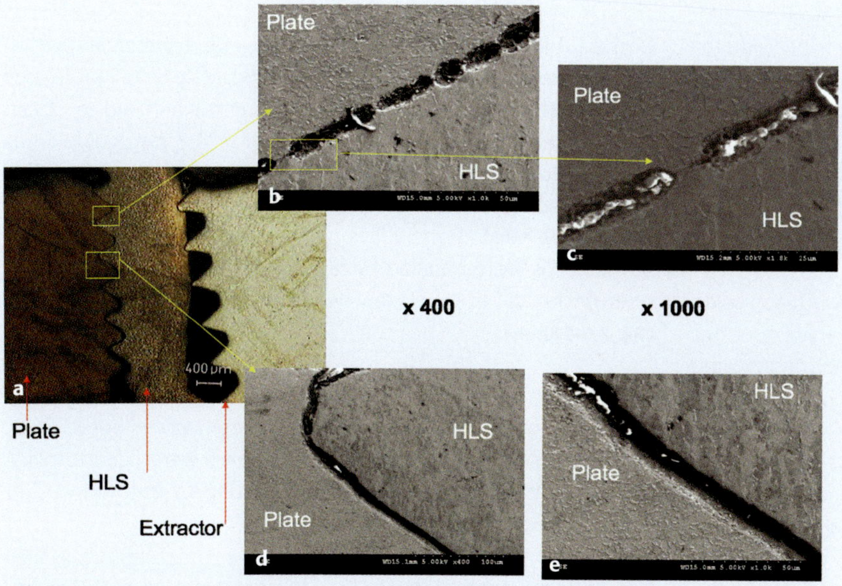

Fig 5.3-25a–e Electron microscope images (magnified 400 [**b**, **d**] and 1,000 [**c**, **e**] times) to study the interfaces between implants. The magnified images (**b–c**) show some areas of "fusion" between the titanium surface of the plate and the head of the locked screw (HLS). Image (**a**) shows how the conical stainless steel extractor deforms the inner surface of the titanium HLS.

Analysis of failure and reflection

This case shows some problems that may occur when removing titanium locking plate implants and describes a complication from a time when the first LISS was used in Spain. At that time self-drilling and self-tapping screws were recommended. Hexagonal locking head screws were also standard. Reporting clinical cases like this one may push the industry to develop new recommended implant removal techniques and devices. Today, with the "stardrive" design fewer complications are seen during implant removal procedures. Improvements in removal sets facilitate these surgeries (eg, stronger and better grasping T-handles, carbide drill bits).

The surgeon must avoid situations that may result in complications when removing a locked screw. Prevention is crucial. Screw insertion must be strictly perpendicular to its axis (nominal angle) when a fixed-angle plate is chosen. It is important to avoid penetrating the distal (far) cortex with self-drilling screws because they can increase damage and periosteal bone formation around the tip of the screw. Inserting the screws by hand reduces the risk of producing cold fusion between the implants. Torque-limiting instruments should always be used at low speed. Some surgeons choose stainless steel implants because titanium implants are more difficult to extract due to better bone integration.

Use brand new screwdrivers, and if the extraction device has to be used, never force it until it breaks because such a difficult problem as shown here may occur. The correct use of implant extraction devices is mandatory to avoid future problems. Having a diamond saw available is strongly recommended. Today, carbide drill bits have been developed to overcome this specific situation and the surgeon can destroy this broken locked piece of metal inside the purchase, but it takes a lot of time and generates a huge amount of metallic debris.

Patients must be informed that aggressive surgery may be required if the plate needs to be removed. Further investigation should be done when complications with implant removal appear, trying to coordinate clinical and mechanical analysis when possible to extensively investigate the cold fusion process.

Final outcome

One year after surgery, the patient was able to engage in his pre-injury activities. He had no knee pain and there were no changes in the range of knee movement (**Fig 5.3-23**).

CASE 3

Case description

A 44-year-old man sustained an unstable pelvic ring injury (anteroposterior compression [APC] Young-Burgess type III; AO/OTA 61C2) and underwent bilateral percutaneous iliosacral (IS) fixation and pubic symphyseal plating (**Fig 5.3-26a–b**) **[Dalal et al, 1989]**. Eight months after surgery, the patient complained of weakness in the right leg and a severe limp. Imaging revealed two broken IS screws and a failed symphyseal plate (**Fig 5.3-26c**).

Though we use the failure of posterior pelvic IS screw fixation as an illustrative example, the problem we are seeking to solve does not relate to the failure of pelvic fixation but to the challenge of removing retained broken cannulated screw parts, and their corresponding washers. Removal of these devices is awkward and time-consuming. Many attempts have failed, resulting in frustration.

Two techniques are demonstrated: one for the removal of cannulated screws and their pieces and one for the removal of their corresponding washers. Each technique is distinct; technique 1 utilizes a reverse-threaded trephine (**Fig 5.3-27** and **Fig 5.3-28**) while technique 2 uses a large Kocher clamp (**Fig 5.3-29**). The C-arm was used to obtain perfect inlet and outlet views. Placement of 2.7 mm guide wires into the heads of the 7.3 mm cannulated screws was achieved. This is often quite challenging due to the ingrowth of bone and scar tissue. A cannulated screwdriver was seated over each guide wire, screw heads were impaled by tapping the end of the cannulated screwdriver, and broken screw heads were backed out one by one (**Fig 5.3-28a–b**).

The screws tend to simply turn in the bone. An osteotome larger than 0.5 cm can be used to free up overgrowth of bone. Once removed, inlet and outlet views of the pelvis were used to place the tip of the Kocher jaws into the washer (**Fig 5.3-29**). The washer was clamped and removed.

Next, a screw removal device was advanced into each of the cannulated screw tips under C-arm guidance (**Fig 5.3-28c–d**). Once seated, it is helpful to tap the end of the trephine into the screw head so it "cuts and grabs" the metal, and then it is reversed a turn while pushing hard.

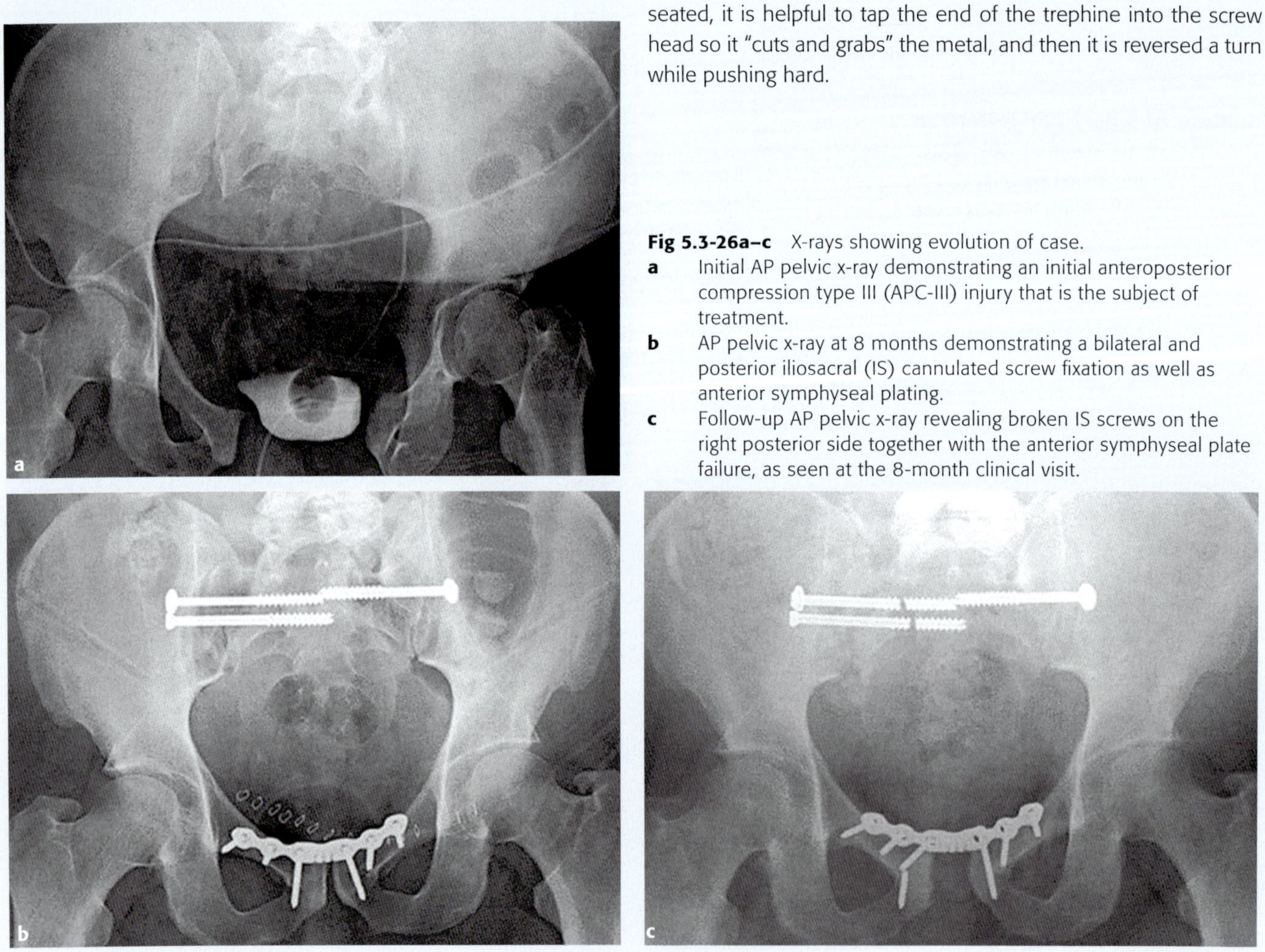

Fig 5.3-26a–c X-rays showing evolution of case.
- **a** Initial AP pelvic x-ray demonstrating an initial anteroposterior compression type III (APC-III) injury that is the subject of treatment.
- **b** AP pelvic x-ray at 8 months demonstrating a bilateral and posterior iliosacral (IS) cannulated screw fixation as well as anterior symphyseal plating.
- **c** Follow-up AP pelvic x-ray revealing broken IS screws on the right posterior side together with the anterior symphyseal plate failure, as seen at the 8-month clinical visit.

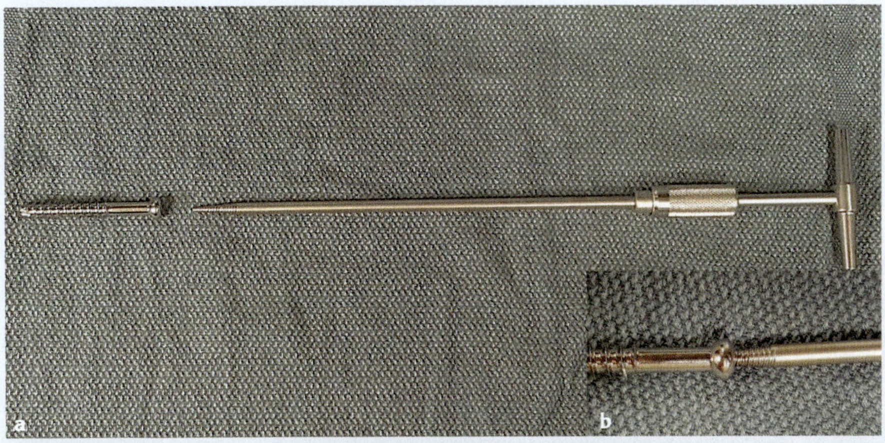

Fig 5.3-27a–b The assembled reverse-threaded trephine (**a**), with the sharp trephine inside of a cannulated screw head (**b**).

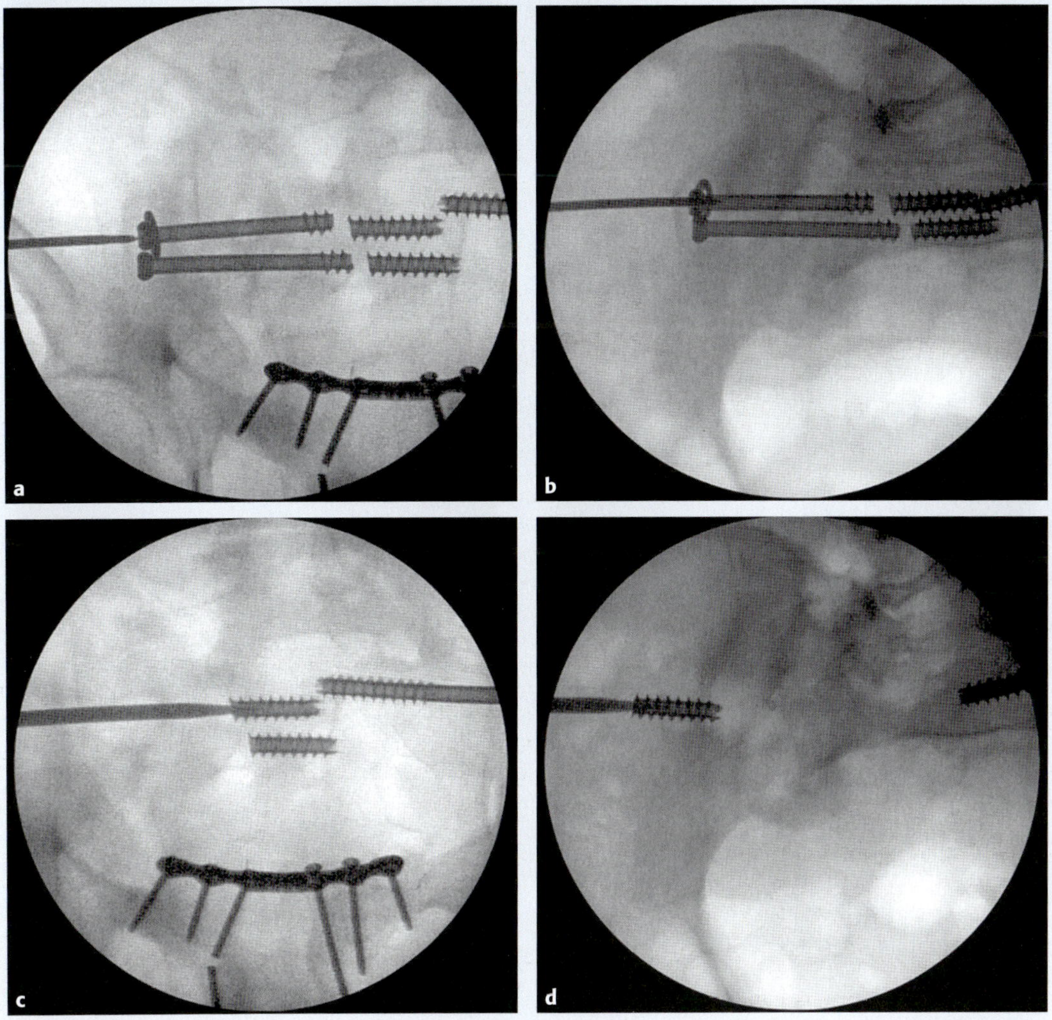

Fig 5.3-28a–d Technique 1: intraoperative C-arm imaging of the removal of broken cannulated screws using a reverse-threaded trephine from a broken screw removal set.

- **a** The sharp trephine inside the pelvis, zeroing in on the screw head.
- **b** The trephine engaged with the screw head.
- **c** The trephine inside of the broken cannulated screw tip.
- **d** The trephine backing the broken screw tip out into the buttock soft tissue.

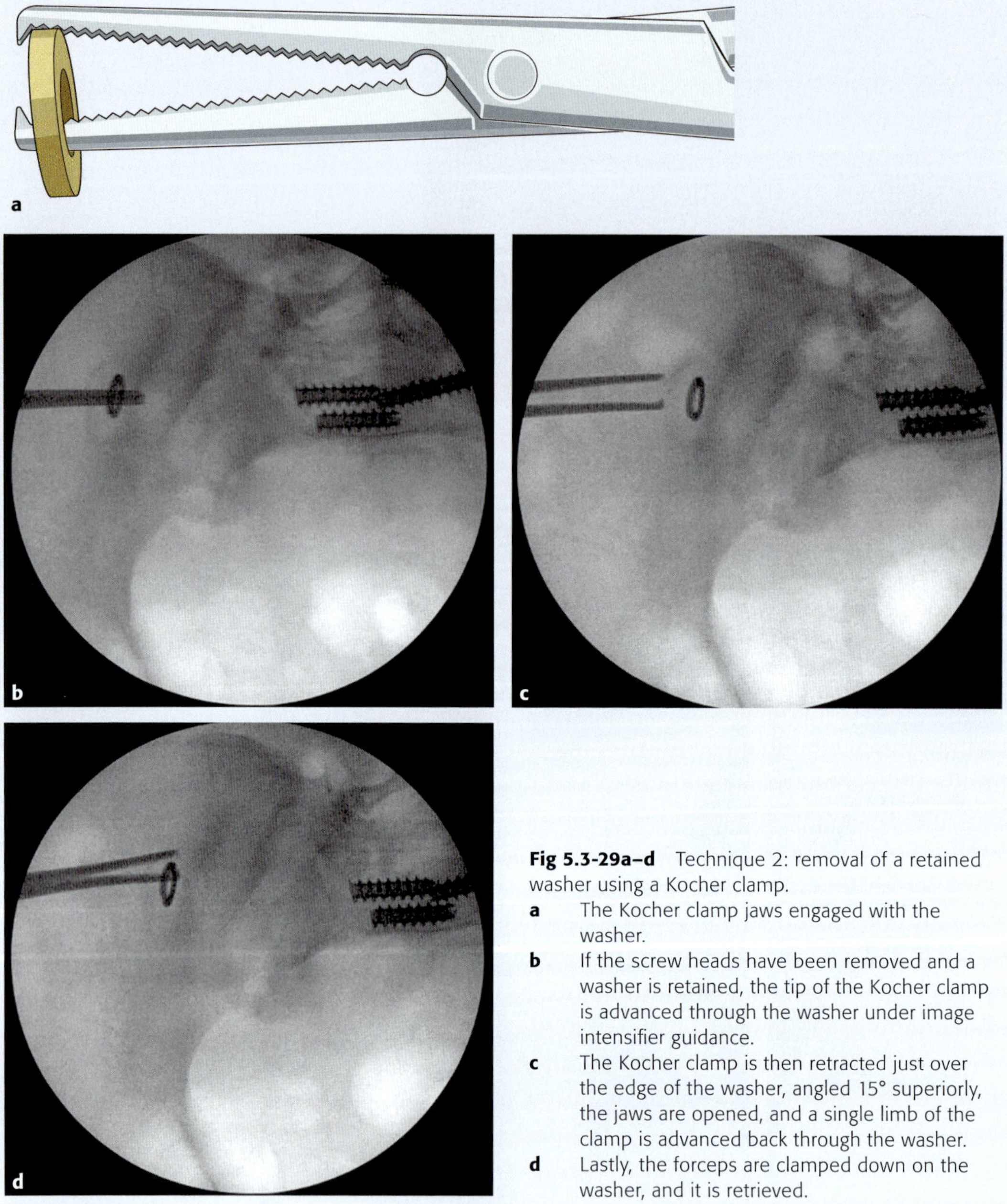

Fig 5.3-29a–d Technique 2: removal of a retained washer using a Kocher clamp.

- **a** The Kocher clamp jaws engaged with the washer.
- **b** If the screw heads have been removed and a washer is retained, the tip of the Kocher clamp is advanced through the washer under image intensifier guidance.
- **c** The Kocher clamp is then retracted just over the edge of the washer, angled 15° superiorly, the jaws are opened, and a single limb of the clamp is advanced back through the washer.
- **d** Lastly, the forceps are clamped down on the washer, and it is retrieved.

Analysis of failure and reflection

Orthopedic management of unstable pelvic fractures requires appropriate reduction and stabilization to provide the best means for union **[Georgiadis et al, 2004]**. Due to technological advances and enhanced understanding of pelvic ring anatomy, percutaneous IS screw placement has become popular **[Hinsche et al, 2002]**. Commonly, these screws are supplemented with washers for compression and to avoid overpenetration. Even with percutaneous fixation under image intensifier guidance, malunions and implant failures still occur. Reports have shown screw malposition rates ranging from 2% to 15% **[Matta and Saucedo, 1989; Pattison et al, 1999]**, with revision rates as high as 19% **[Routt et al, 2000]**. Screw removal strategies have been developed **[Templeman et al, 1996; Weil et al, 2007; Zwingmann et al, 2013]**; however, there are no published techniques describing the removal of percutaneously applied washers in the pelvis, nor broken screw tips inside the sacral bodies.

The patient was referred for failure of hardware and pelvic malunion, but the problem we wish to demonstrate in our two techniques has to do with the retrieval of this hardware. This is time-consuming and difficult to accomplish, often resulting in the decision to simply leave the problematic hardware in place.

Thus, we offer an effective method for removing broken screws and retained washers using image intensification and a Kocher clamp, both of which are available in most operating rooms. This method is recognized as a safe and reliable means of washer removal, with minimal blood loss and operative time, and without associated complications.

Final outcome

At the 2-year follow-up, the patient had returned to work, was pain free, had a normal gate, full strength throughout both lower extremities, and normal sensation distally. AP pelvic x-rays revealed a well-aligned, symmetrical pelvis without evidence of hardware loosening (**Fig 5.3-30**).

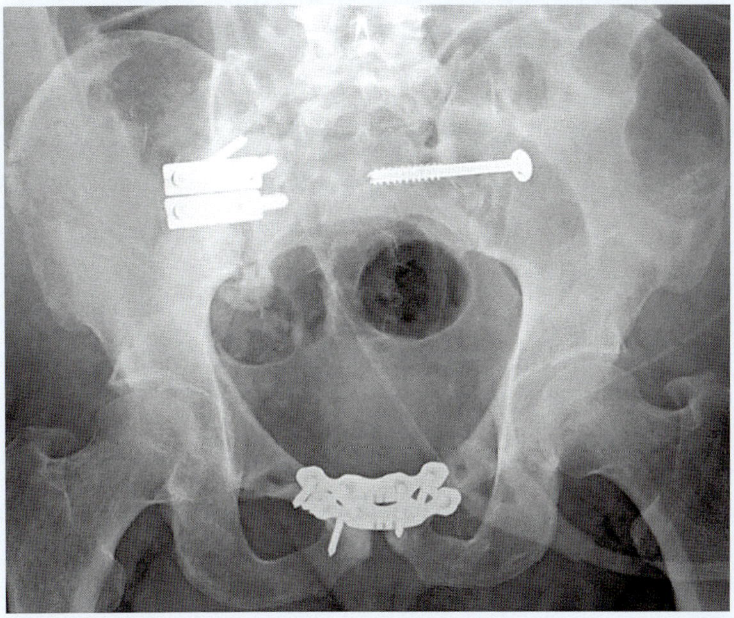

Fig 5.3-30 After removal, the surgeon reconstructed the pelvis using a dual open plating technique of the right sacroiliac joint and symphysis pubis. This AP pelvic x-ray was taken 6 months postoperatively.

Key points to remember

- All hardware removal must be justified by pain, restricted range of motion, or risk of periimplant fracture. Hardware must never be removed for aesthetic reasons or due to the whims of the patient.
- Determine the right moment to carry out the removal surgery, in keeping with the recommendation and aim of the intervention.
- Inform the patient and her or his family of the treatment options, explaining the risks and possible complications of the surgery. Explain that it may not be possible to remove the implant.
- Adhere to the established postoperative times for keeping the implant, which can be removed between 18 and 24 months after surgery.
- Obtain as much information as possible about the surgery performed to apply the hardware (eg, means of surgical access, type of fracture, implant used, incidents, complications).
- Create a comprehensive preoperative plan, including two different x-ray views to confirm the consolidation of the fracture, identify the implant, locate the hardware material, and determine whether it is whole or broken.
- Know the technique for the removal of the material. Have several alternative plans in place to complete the removal, in case the "plan A" technique fails.
- The surgery must be supervised or carried out by an expert surgical team.
- Be sure to have all the necessary conventional and specific materials for the hardware removal surgery as well as unconventional or customized materials to facilitate the surgery.
- Define the moment at which the intervention should be deemed finished, assessing the risks in relation to the benefits during a complex hardware removal surgery.

References and suggested reading

Brown OL, Dirschl DR, Obremskey WT. Incidence of hardware-related pain and its effect on functional outcomes after open reduction and internal fixation of ankle fractures. *J Orthop Trauma.* 2001 May;15(4):271–274.
Buckley RE, Moran CG, Apivatthakakul T. *AO Principles of Fracture Management.* 3rd ed. Stuttgart New York: Thieme; 2017.
Buckley RE. Fracture healing: Does hardware removal enhance patient outcomes? *Orthopedic Trauma Directions.* 2009;7(06):1–9.
Dalal SA, Burgess AR, Siegel JH, et al. Pelvic fracture in multiple trauma: classification by mechanism is key to pattern of organ injury, resuscitative requirements, and outcome. *J Trauma.* 1989 Jul;29(7):981–1000; discussion 1000–1002.
Georgiadis GM, Gove NK, Smith AD, et al. Removal of the less invasive stabilization system. *J Orthop Trauma.* 2004 Sep;18(8):562–564.
Golbakhsh M, Sadaat M, Noughani F, et al. The Impact of Psychological Factors on Device Removal Surgery. *Trauma Mon.* 2016 May;21(2):e25871.
Hinsche AF, Giannoudis PV, Smith RM. Fluoroscopy-based multiplanar image guidance for insertion of sacroiliac screws. *Clin Orthop Relat Res.* 2002 Feb(395):135–144.
Matta JM, Saucedo T. Internal fixation of pelvic ring fractures. *Clin Orthop Relat Res.* 1989 May(242):83–97.
Meinberg EG, Agel J, Roberts CS, et al. Fracture and Dislocation Classification Compendium-2018. *J Orthop Trauma.* 2018 Jan;32 Suppl 1:S1–s170.
Orozco Delclós R. *Errores en la Osteosíntesis.* Barcelona: Masson; 1993. Spanish.
Pattison G, Reynolds J, Hardy J. Salvaging a stripped drive connection when removing screws. *Injury.* 1999 Jan;30(1):74–75.
Routt ML Jr, Nork SE, Mills WJ. Percutaneous fixation of pelvic ring disruptions. *Clin Orthop Relat Res.* 2000 Jun(375):15–29.
Templeman D, Schmidt A, Freese J, et al. Proximity of iliosacral screws to neurovascular structures after internal fixation. *Clin Orthop Relat Res.* 1996 Aug(329):194–198.
Twaddle B. *Implant removal.* Dübendorf: AOTrauma; 2013.
Weil YA, Nousiainen MT, Helfet DL. Removal of an iliosacral screw entrapping the L5 nerve root after failed posterior pelvic ring fixation: a case report. *J Orthop Trauma.* 2007 Jul;21(6):414–417.
Zwingmann J, Sudkamp NP, Konig B, et al. Intra- and postoperative complications of navigated and conventional techniques in percutaneous iliosacral screw fixation after pelvic fractures: Results from the German Pelvic Trauma Registry. *Injury.* 2013 Dec;44(12):1765–1772.

Section 6
Patient compliance

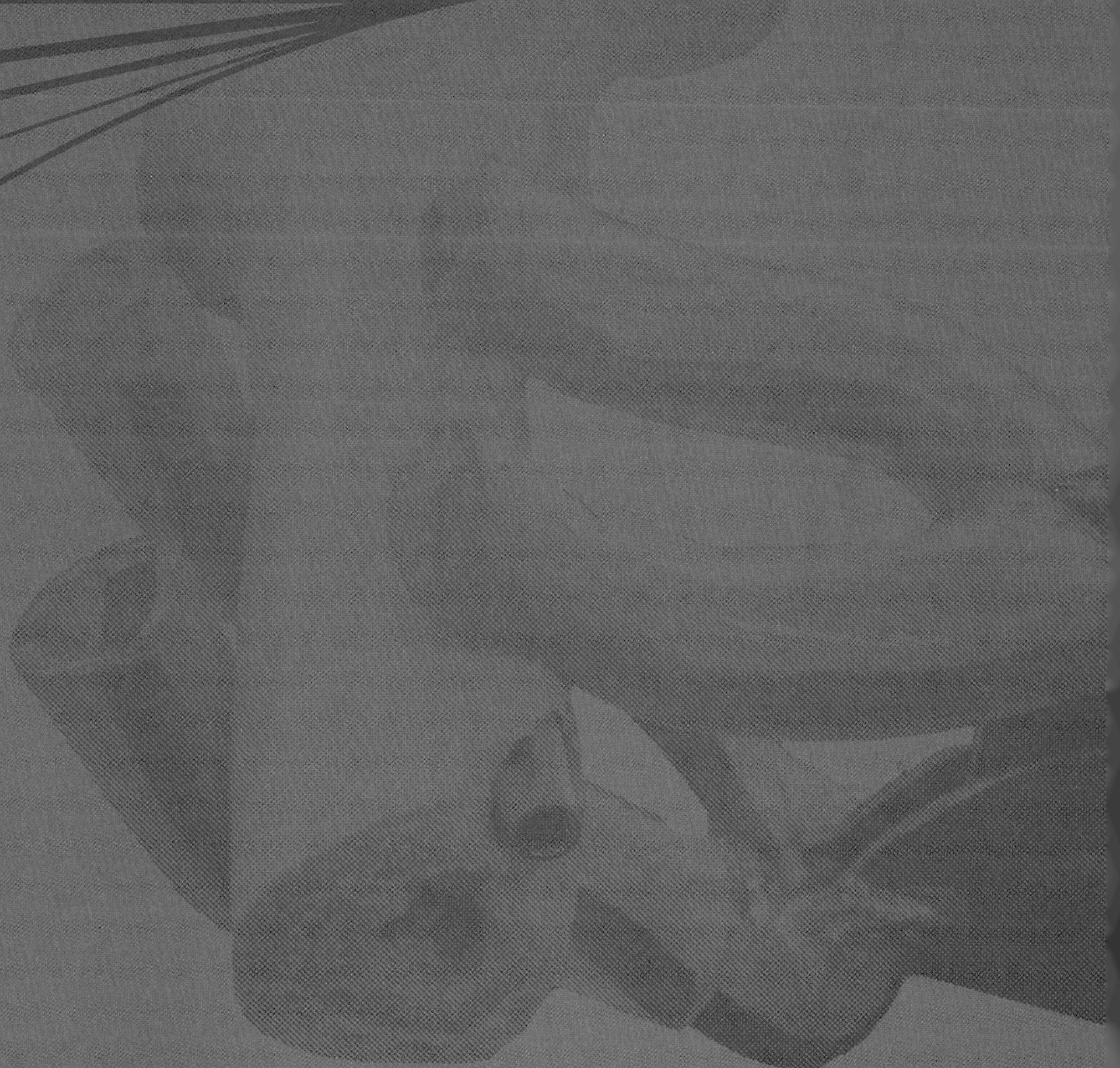

Section 6
Patient compliance

Roberto Rivero Sosa
Reto Babst, Christopher A Becker, Frank Beeres, Joan Girós Torres, Christian Kammerlander, Björn Link, Bianka Rubenbauer,
J Miquel Sales Pérez, Miquel Videla Cés

6.1 Failures unrelated to the healthcare team but related to patient compliance

Roberto Rivero Sosa
Reto Babst, Christopher A Becker, Frank Beeres, Joan Girós Torres, Christian Kammerlander, Björn Link, Bianka Rubenbauer, J Miquel Sales Pérez, Miquel Videla Cés

I've decided to do what I like because it's good for my health.

Voltaire

The patient plays an important part in the healing process, and is generally overlooked but undoubtedly has significant responsibility for the results of the osteosynthesis. The patient's active and responsible participation in the rehabilitation process subsequent to a surgical intervention for a fracture is indispensable for achieving a complete and satisfactory recovery.

Patients also commit "errors" in the care and protection of their osteosynthesis, generally involuntarily, and due to a lack of knowledge about the healing process, and their excessive confidence in the painless stability of their recently operated fracture.

Every bone, every fracture, and every osteosynthesis has its own evolution and requires protection adequate to its characteristics, ie, in relation to location, type of fracture, means of fixation, etc. Only the surgeon can evaluate the weight and type of loading that a fracture treated by osteosynthesis will tolerate. It is necessary to establish an individualized action protocol. All the phases of the rehabilitation process must be communicated to the patient with full clarity and any doubts that the patient or family may have must be clarified. It is important to clearly articulate what the patient must and must not do and ensure that this is understood. Throughout the recovery period, the patient, family members, rehabilitation physician, physiotherapist, and orthopedic surgeon should give and receive effective feedback.

Osteosynthesis may be contraindicated in patients with mental illness or disability as well as in patients with a history of drug or alcohol abuse. The appropriateness of osteosynthesis should be well evaluated in children, elderly people, patients with physical disabilities, and amputees. Certain risk factors exist, such as age, osteoporosis, and obesity, that must be taken into account when dictating the rules for the postoperative period. In elderly patients, special precaution must be taken when indicating rehabilitation with partial weight bearing. These patients may have physical limitations due to weakness associated with senility and may not be capable of complying effectively. This can result in serious complications or falls and may occasionally even need a new surgical intervention, which can be disastrous considering the problems this poses for a fragile patient. Obese patients may have difficulties walking or performing some exercises due to their inability to control their weight.

The probability for patient compliance with postoperative management often influences the surgical technique to be developed. Literature contains numerous articles that aim to relate uncooperative patients with the final outcome after fracture treatment. Fong et al published a study in 2007 in which they showed that the rate of infections and failures of osteosynthesis was 0% for patients complying with the rehabilitation rules.

Patients' noncompliance with postoperative appointments continues to be a common problem in trauma and orthopedic departments. The lack of adherence to rehabilitation is directly related to the lack of attendance at follow-up appointments. Men, smokers, patients without health insurance coverage, and illegal drug addicts have a high risk of abandoning the rehabilitation plan and failing to attend follow-up appointments. Early identification of patients who are unlikely to comply with guidelines in the recovery process may lead to additional measures being taken to try to guarantee the correct adherence to the rehabilitation protocol and prevent complications.

Patients with psychiatric disorders must have a more restrictive monitoring plan, because they frequently have to be readmitted to the acute care hospital in order to channel their rehabilitation or treat medical or mechanical complications. It is necessary to create strategies to maximize these patients' active participation in their recovery and their attendance at postoperative control appointments. Motivation for the patient and family environment is fundamental.

The physiotherapist must adapt the therapy according to the rehabilitation potential of patients with dementia. For the physiotherapist it is a challenge and can be frustrating because rehabilitation does not progress as expected. Hall et al [2017] report that up to 40% of people with dementia could not perform physical therapy exercises after a hip fracture.

At the beginning of treatment, physiotherapists must take time to earn the patient's trust, build a positive relationship, and express themselves clearly using short and simple sentences. Nonverbal communication is another tool. Adequate use of body language and visual contact helps the interaction between patient (especially those with dementia) and physiotherapist and reduces difficult and aggressive behavior. The standard physical therapy guides are not adapted to patients with intellectual disabilities; evaluation forms can therefore not be applied to this population.

As discussed in chapter 5.2 Physiotherapy, patient involvement in their own recovery process is essential to obtain satisfactory results. In cases where patients voluntarily or involuntarily do not take responsibility for their treatment, monitoring their treatment can become cumbersome for the healthcare team, and the consequences can be serious for all, in addition to the high costs associated with treating any complications.

Roberto Rivero Sosa
Reto Babst, Christopher A Becker, Frank Beeres, Joan Girós Torres, Christian Kammerlander, Björn Link, Bianka Rubenbauer, J Miquel Sales Pérez, Miquel Videla Cés

Case description

A 48-year-old man had a skiing accident and was treated for a left extraarticular distal lower left leg fracture (AO/OTA 42B2,4F2A) in a local hospital (**Fig 6.1-1**). On admission, the skin was intact and the neurovascular status normal. Minimally invasive plate osteosynthesis (MIPO) was performed using the metaphyseal locking compression plate (LCP) for the distal tibia (**Fig 6.1-2**).

Five days postoperatively, the patient accidentally put more than the permitted partial weight on the operated limb causing the plate to deform (**Fig 6.1-3**). Reoperation was performed applying a similar plate and adding screws to provide stability (**Fig 6.1-4**).

Three months postoperatively at a larger outpatient department, the patient presented with symptomatic valgus malunion (**Fig 6.1-5**).

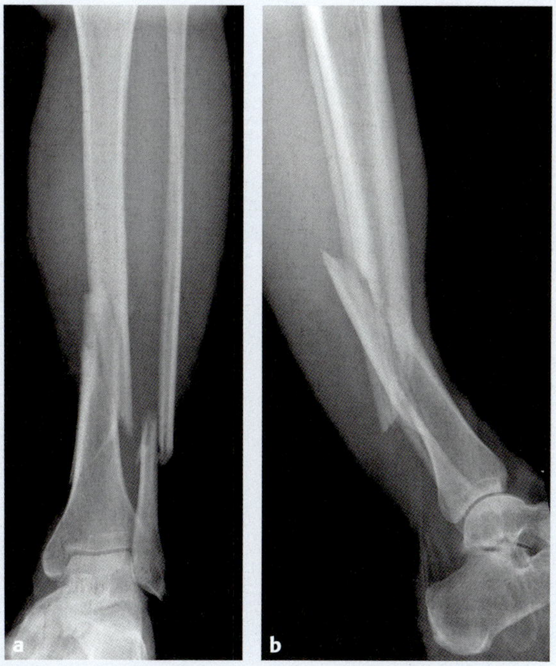

Fig 6.1-1a–b X-rays showing the extraarticular fracture of the distal tibia and fibula. Note that the medial wedge fragment of the tibia is also fractured.

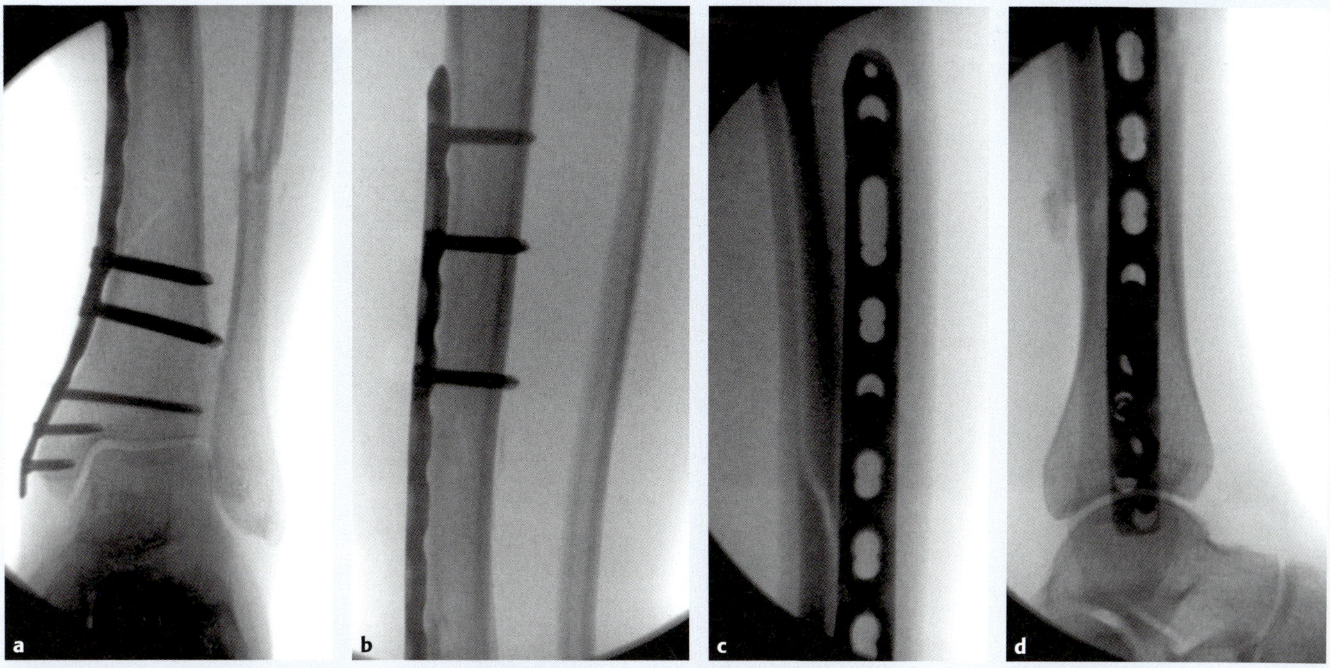

Fig 6.1-2a–f Intraoperative and postoperative images.
a–d Intraoperative C-arm images taken under image intensifier showing minimally invasive plate osteosynthesis (MIPO) of the distal tibia. A metaphyseal locking compression plate for the distal medial tibia was used to bridge the fracture area.

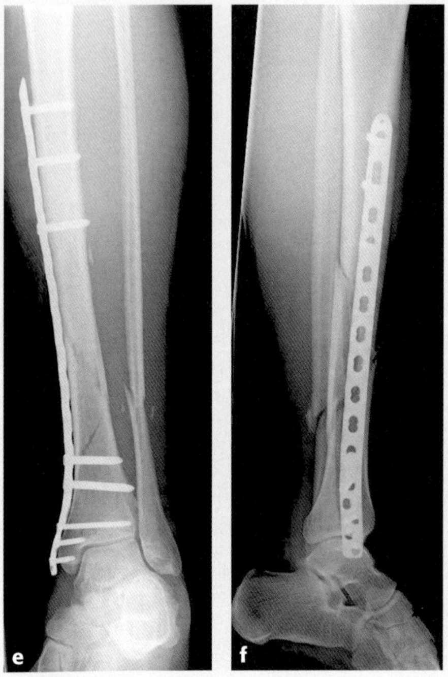

Fig 6.1-2a–f (cont) Intraoperative and postoperative images.
e–f Postoperative x-rays showing an adequate MIPO result.

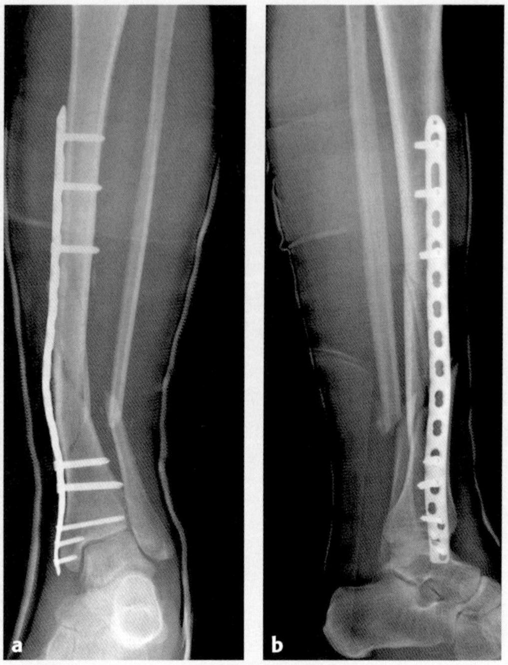

Fig 6.1-3a–b X-rays taken on the fifth postoperative day showing the deformed plate caused by excessive weight bearing on the operated limb.

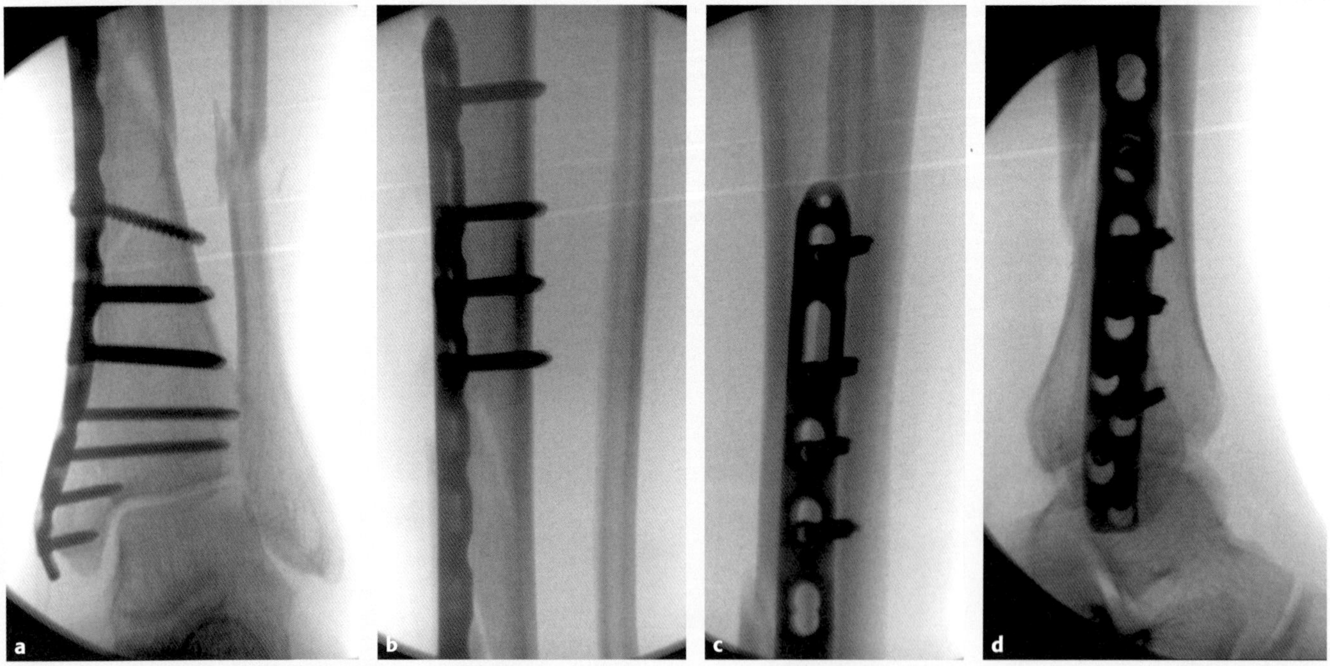

Fig 6.1-4a–j Postoperative x-rays of the revision surgery.
a–d Revision surgery was performed using an identical plate. To supplement stability, a lag screw was placed through the plate to apply interfragmentary compression, thereby fixing the distal part of the wedge fragment to the metaphysis. Furthermore, additional locking screws were used both proximally and distally. Note the valgus alignment of the fibula indicating a problem with the orientation of the tibia as well (**a**).

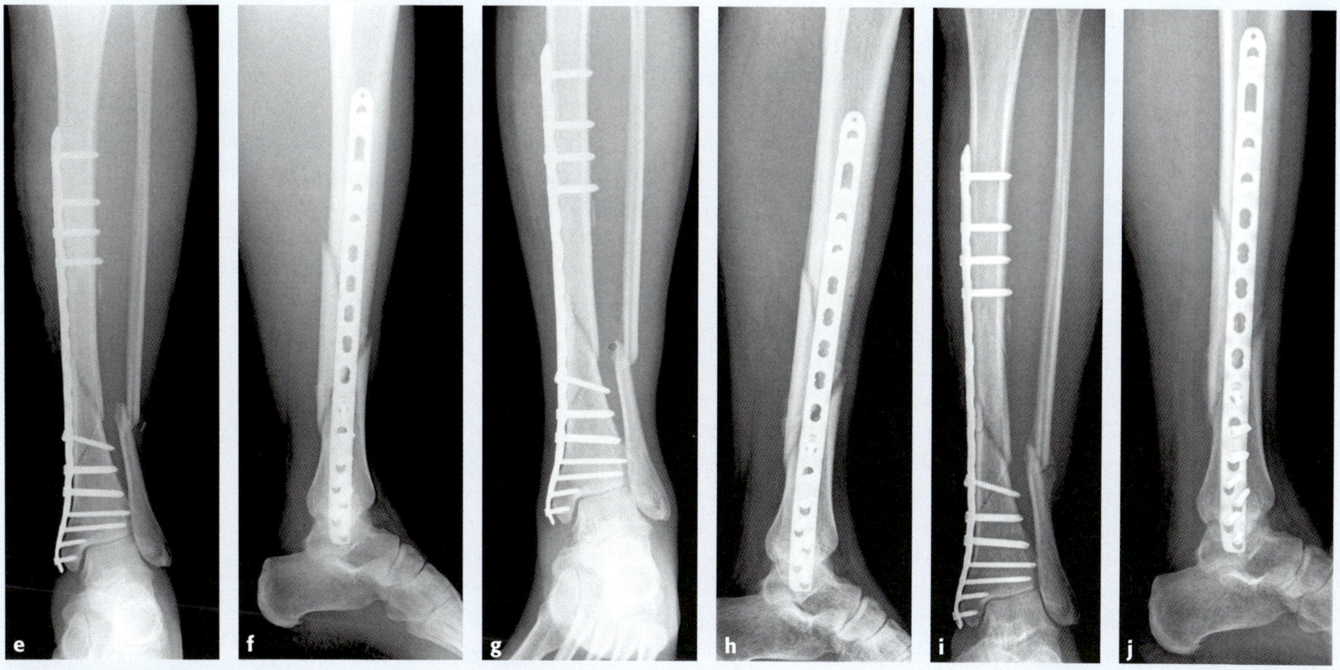

Fig 6.1-4a–j (cont) Postoperative x-rays of the revision surgery.
e–f Note the valgus malpositioning of the fracture of more than 10°.
g–h Six weeks postoperatively, callus is visible at the fibula. No secondary displacement occurred.
i–j Ten weeks postoperatively, the fibular fracture has healed with bridging callus. The distal fracture line of the tibia shows signs of callus formation as well.

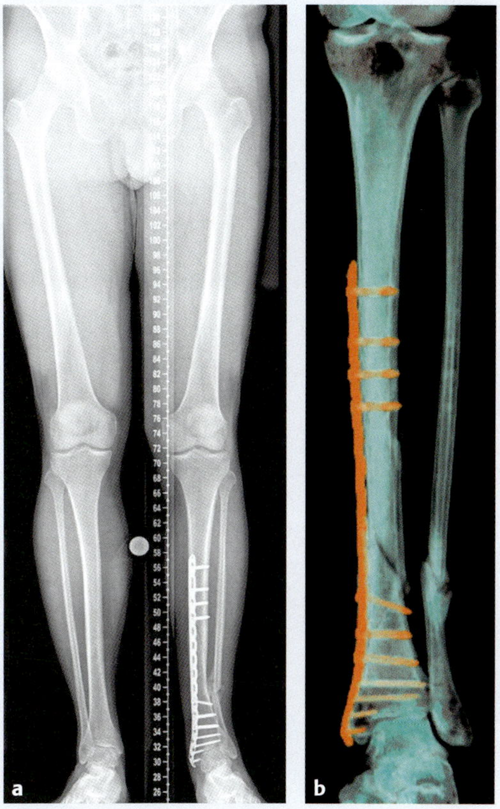

Fig 6.1-5a–b Twelve weeks postoperatively, the patient presented with persistent pain at the fracture site. The long-leg standing x-ray clearly showed the valgus malalignment of the lower leg of 12° (**a**). A computed tomographic scan of the lower leg showed healed fractures of the fibula and distal tibia (**b**). The proximal fracture lines were atrophic. Due to these results, plate removal, corrective osteotomy of the fibula, and reamed intramedullary nailing of the tibia were planned to revise the valgus malalignment and to promote bony union.

Analysis of failure and reflection

Minimally invasive bridge plating for a multifragmentary fracture of the distal tibia is a reasonable approach (**Fig 6.1-6**). As described by Gautier and Sommer **[2003]**, plate length and positioning of screws were adequate. Partial weight bearing for at least 6 weeks postoperatively was advised because of the long working length of the nail (**Fig 6.1-7**). However, the large comminuted fracture zone was bridged by a rather flexible implant and because the fibular fracture was not fixed, it provided no additional lateral support.

In this case, patient compliance proved difficult 5 days after the initial operation. Consequently, an alternative approach in the revision surgery should have aimed to provide more stability or even allowed for full weight bearing. The revision surgery addressed this problem only partially, by applying a lag screw in the distal fragment to reduce the working length of the nail. However, absolute stability in the proximal part of the fracture was not obtained. The placement of the additional locking screws, both proximally and distally, increases the plate-screw density. It does not, however, increase axial stiffness **[Stoffel et al, 2003]** and is therefore unnecessary. In addition, after deformation of the plate clearly demonstrated the excessive flexibility of the implant in this fracture configuration, the fibula was not fixed to increase stability of the construct. Plating the fibula would have prevented the tibial valgus deformity of more than 10° that was caused by the revision surgery.

Final outcome

To address the valgus malpositioning of the fracture and the delayed union or impending nonunion, the implant was removed, an osteotomy of the fibula with subsequent plating was performed, and reamed intramedullary nailing of the tibia was completed. To correct the alignment, a blocking screw was placed distally to maintain the planned nail position in the distal tibia. The fibula was plated after osteotomy to provide additional support against valgus deforming forces. With the intramedullary reaming, potential biological shortcomings of the fracture area were avoided.

Twelve weeks after revision osteosynthesis the fractures had healed (**Fig 6.1-8**), the patient could bear full weight without walking aids and was able to perform unrestricted activities of daily living (**Fig 6.1-9**).

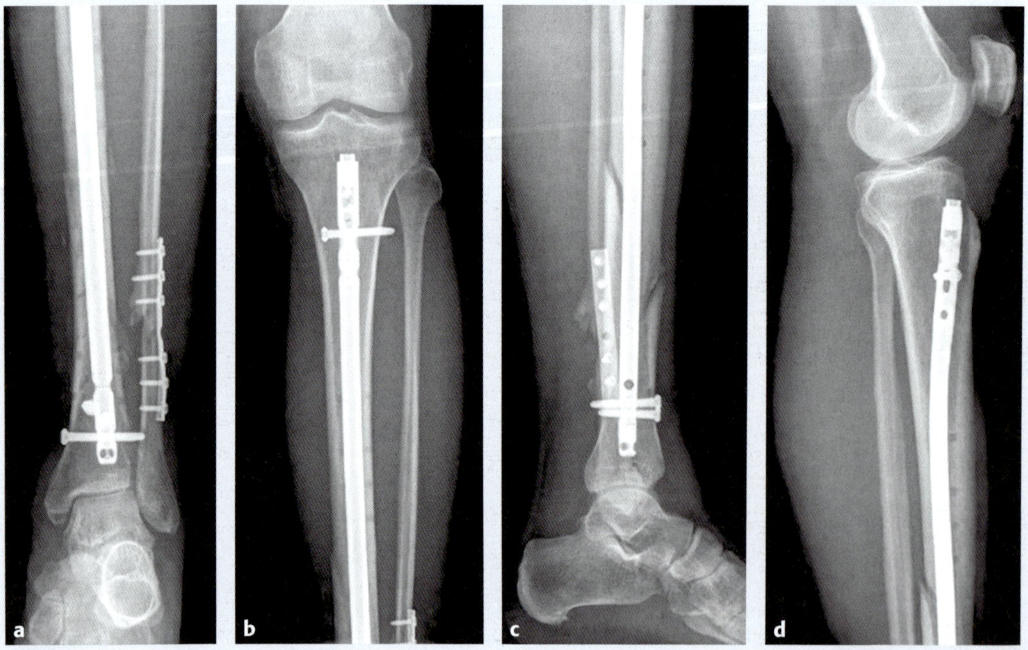

Fig 6.1-6a–d Postrevision x-rays showing the corrected alignment of the lower leg. A distal blocking screw was placed to facilitate adequate positioning of the nail to correct the axis. Plating of the fibula was implemented to provide support against valgus deforming forces.

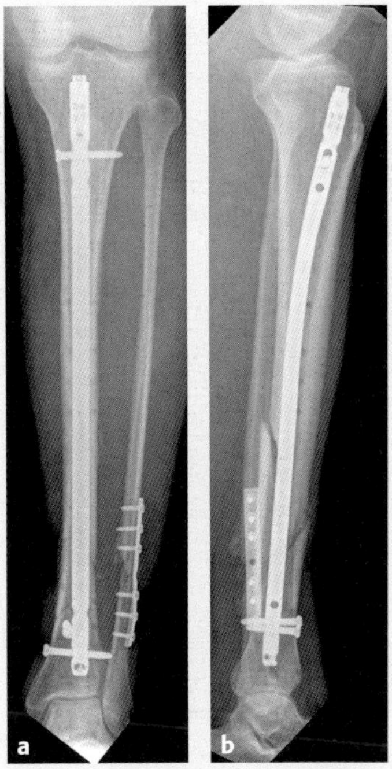

Fig 6.1-7a–b Six weeks after revision.

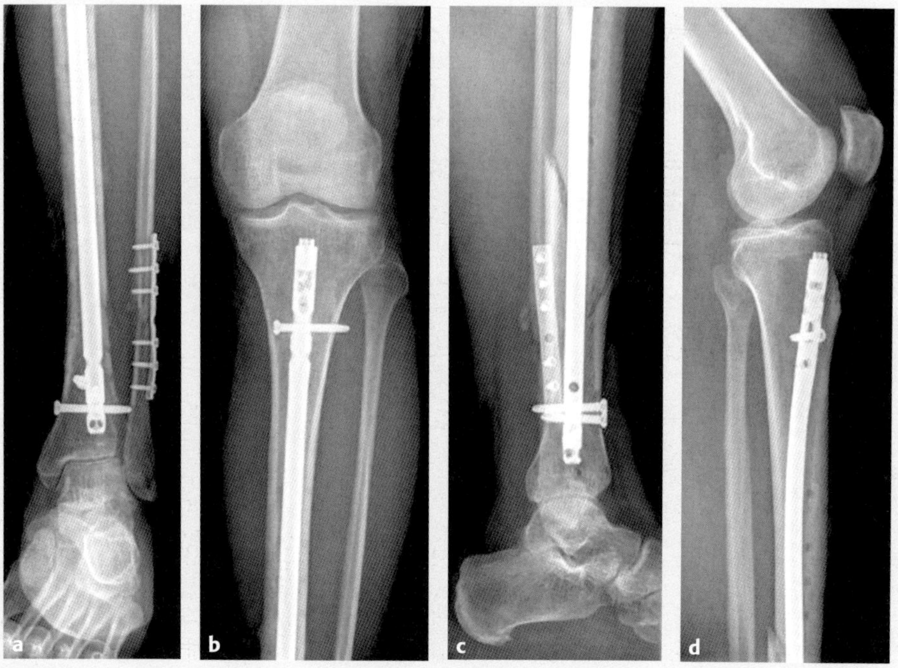

Fig 6.1-8a–d X-rays of the healed fracture 12 weeks after revision surgery, showing callus formation at all fracture lines.

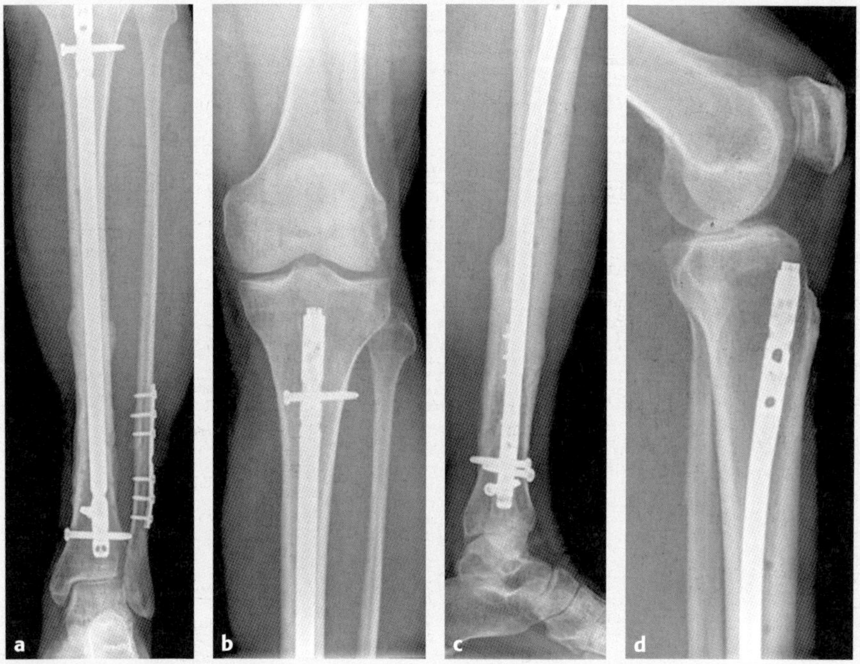

Fig 6.1–9a–h Follow-up x-rays after revision surgery.
a–d Six months after revision surgery.

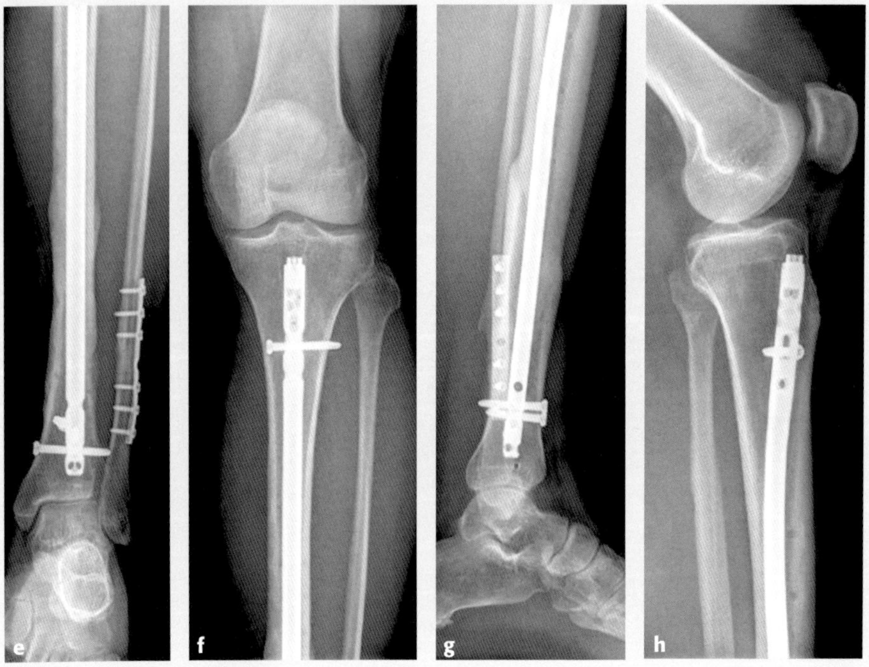

Fig 6.1-9a–h (cont) Follow-up x-rays after revision surgery.
e–h Final outcome 1 year after the revision operation and 17 months after the accident.

Roberto Rivero Sosa
Reto Babst, Christopher A Becker, Frank Beeres, Joan Girós Torres, Christian Kammerlander, Björn Link, Bianka Rubenbauer, J Miquel Sales Pérez, Miquel Videla Cés

Case description

A 42-year-old man with a medical history of compulsive smoking and severe schizophrenia of the bipolar subtype who required various admissions to the psychiatric hospital. The patient had previously made several suicide attempts.

He fell from a height of 8 m when making another suicide attempt, which resulted in head trauma, rib fractures, multiple contusions, and Gustilo type II fracture of the distal tibia and fibula (AO/OTA 43B2) (**Fig 6.1-10**).

In the emergency department the wounds underwent surgical cleaning, debridement, open reduction and internal fixation of the fibular fracture, open reduction of the articular fracture of the tibial pilon, and external fixation for the distal tibial fracture. Nonweight-bearing instructions were established.

In the postoperative period, the patient's mental health decompensated and he presented with paranoid ideation, agitation, and lack of discipline, which required his transfer to an acute psychiatric center (**Fig 6.1-11**). The patient did not comply with the nonweight-bearing recommendation but was bearing full weight while walking, despite still wearing an external fixator. He presented with a progressive varus and recurvatum deformity.

The patient underwent reintervention 8 weeks after the first surgery (**Fig 6.1-12**). The external fixator was removed and a below-the-knee plaster cast applied that was left in place for another 2 months (**Fig 6.1-13**). During this period the patient's psychiatric condition did not improve, and he continued to walk bearing full weight. He did not attend the recommended follow-up appointments. The varus and recurvatum deformities in the distal tibia and fibula continued to progress to the point of preventing him from walking and requiring a wheelchair for mobilization (**Fig 6.1-14**).

Eight months after the first surgery (**Fig 6.1-15**), he consulted another hospital regarding his leg deformity and inability to walk. At that point his psychiatric disorder was under control.

The patient was scheduled for surgery to remove the broken fibular plate, with a triplane osteotomy of the distal tibia, osteosynthesis of the fibula with a locking compression plate (LCP) 3.5/4.0, and osteotomy of the distal tibia with an LCP for the medial distal tibia (**Fig 6.1-16**). He was put on a personalized rehabilitation program with close control of weight bearing and gait reeducation. The follow-up visits were scheduled at 6 weeks, 4 months, and 1 year following the operations (**Fig 6.1-17**).

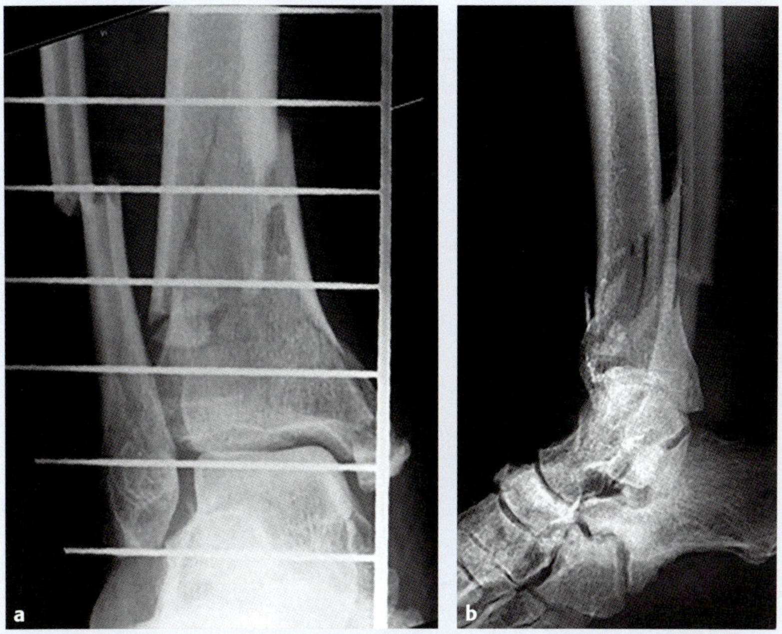

Fig 6.1-10a–b AP (**a**) and lateral (**b**) x-rays of the Gustilo type II comminuted fracture of the distal tibia and fibula.

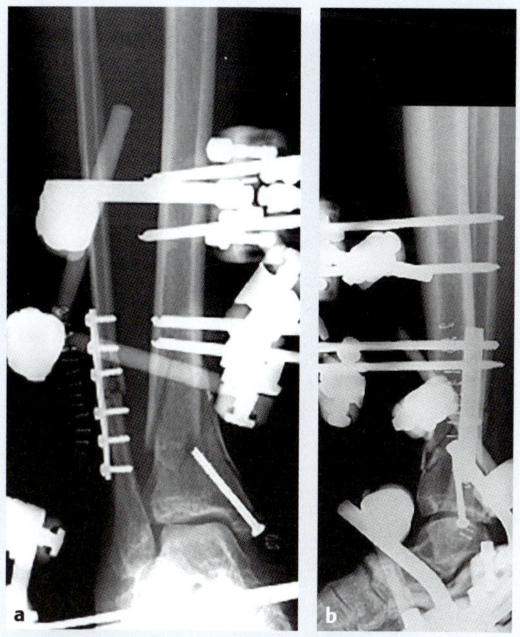

Fig 6.1-11a–b Postoperative x-rays showing malreduction of the transverse fibular fracture that caused a moderate varus deformity of the fibular malleolus, also leading to the axial varus malalignment of the tibial pilon.

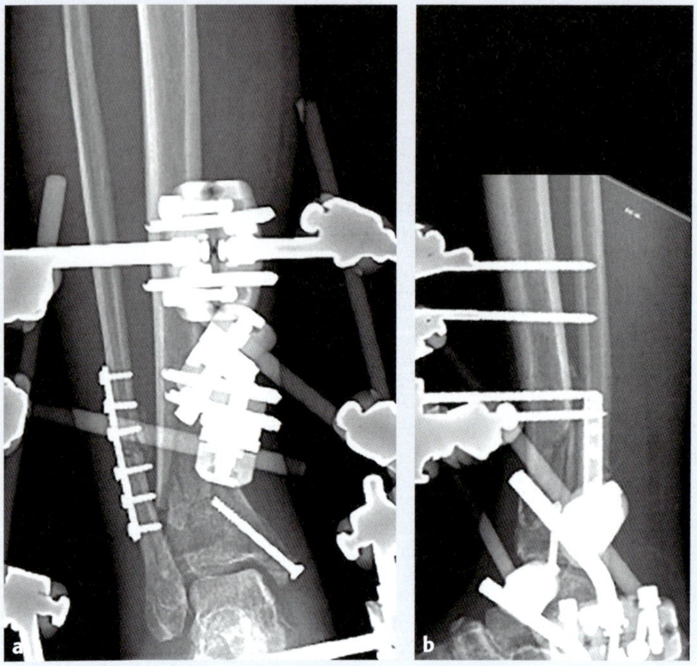

Fig 6.1-12a–b X-rays at 8 weeks showing a loss of reduction with an increase of the varus deviation of the fibula and of the tibial pilon; this is due to the patient putting full weight on the limb because of his lack of discipline in physiotherapy as a consequence of his psychiatric disorder.

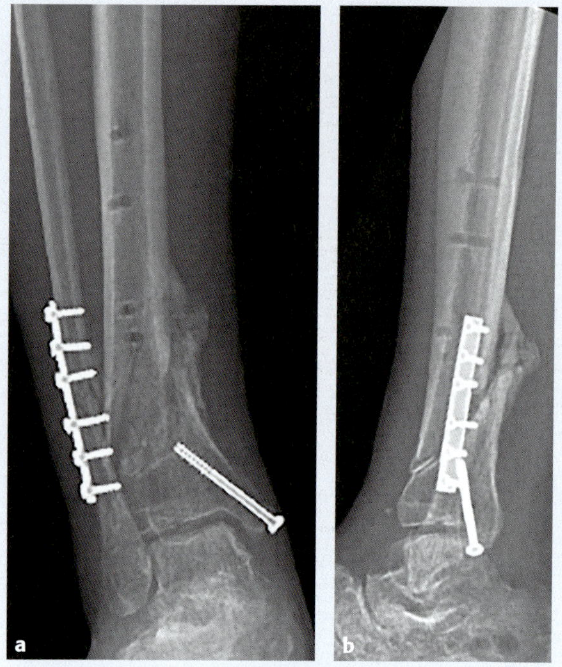

Fig 6.1-13a–b X-rays of the ankle 2 months after removal of the external fixator and immediately after removal of the plaster cast. The involuntary lack of discipline due to his worsening psychiatric condition meant that the patient continued walking bearing full weight, which led to the genu varum (ie, bow leg) and recurvatum malunion.

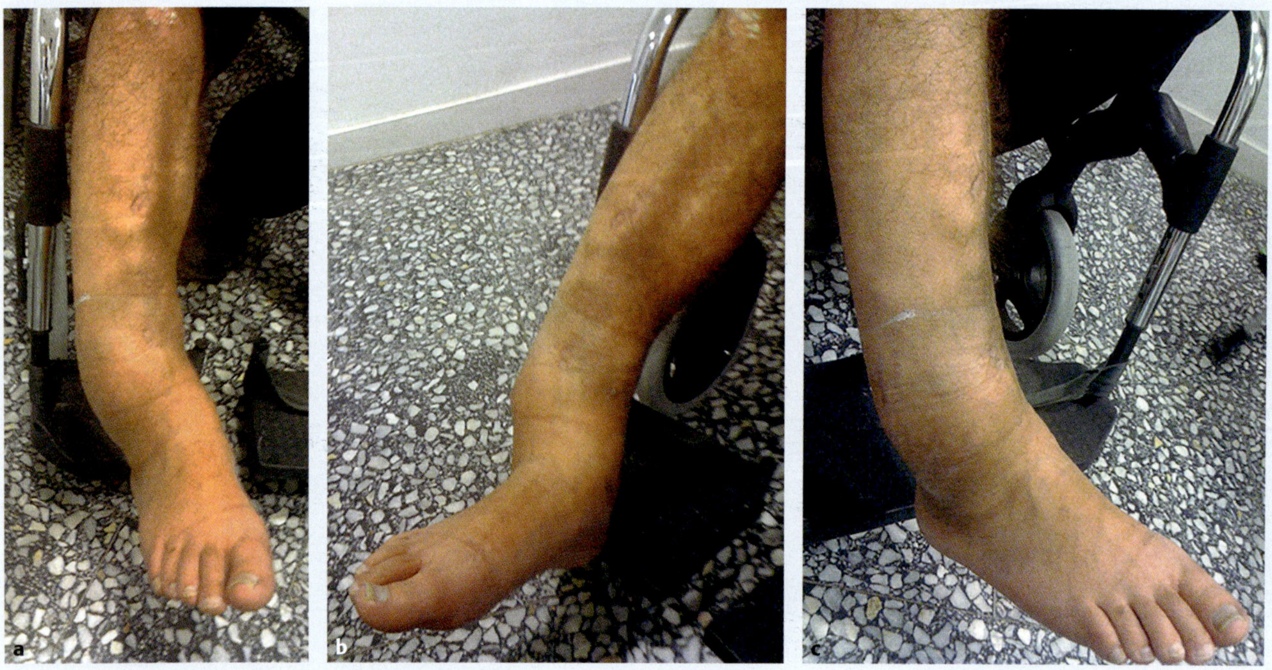

Fig 6.1-14a–c The leg deformity made walking impossible and required the patient to use a wheelchair for mobility.

Roberto Rivero Sosa
Reto Babst, Christopher A Becker, Frank Beeres, Joan Girós Torres, Christian Kammerlander, Björn Link, Bianka Rubenbauer,
J Miquel Sales Pérez, Miquel Videla Cés

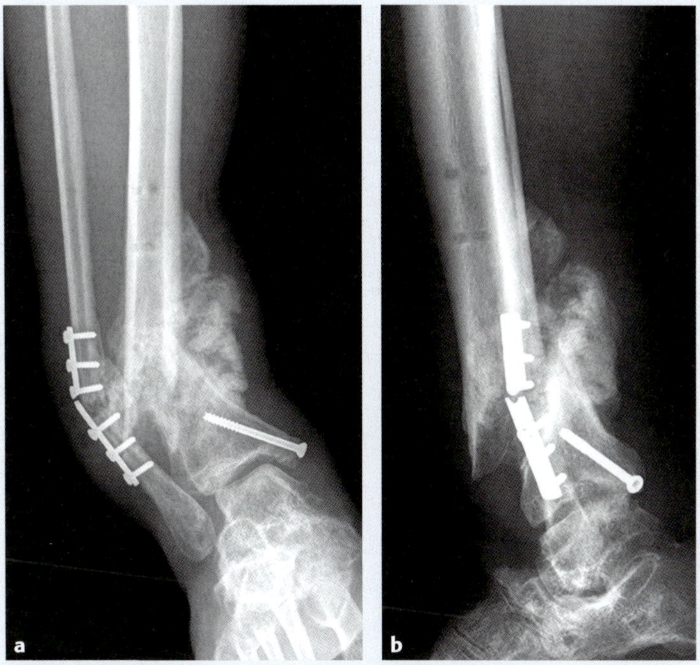

Fig 6.1-15a–b Control AP (**a**) and lateral (**b**) x-rays at 8 months after the accident. The genu varum and recurvatum malunion of the fracture is observed with exuberant callus on the medial and posterior faces of the tibia and fibula. The x-rays also show breakage of the fibular plate.

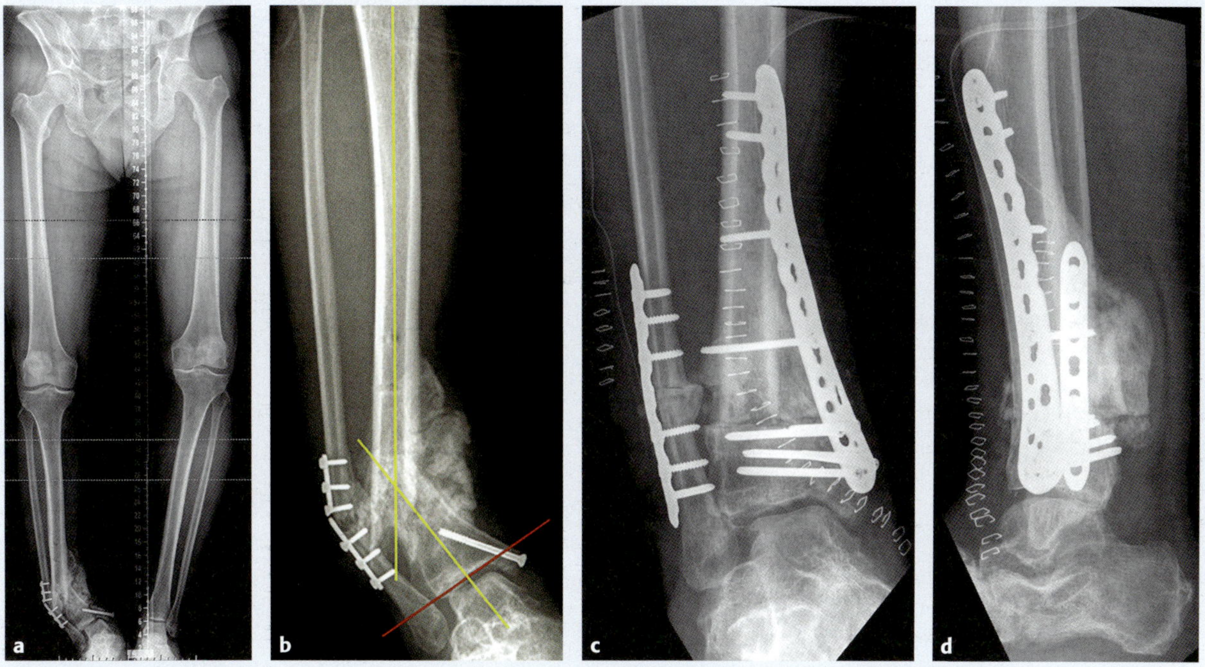

Fig 6.1-16a–d X-rays showing the left leg deformity and postoperative corrective osteotomy.

a Telemetry showing the dissymmetry of the lower right limb which is shortened due to the varus malunion of the right tibial pilon.

b Planning the calculation of the angles for the corrective osteotomy.

c–d X-rays of the rescue surgery in which the surgeon removed the broken fibular plate and performed a triplane osteotomy of the distal tibia and osteosynthesis of the fibula with a locking compression plate (LCP) 3.5/4.0 and an osteotomy of the distal tibia with an LCP for the distal medial tibia.

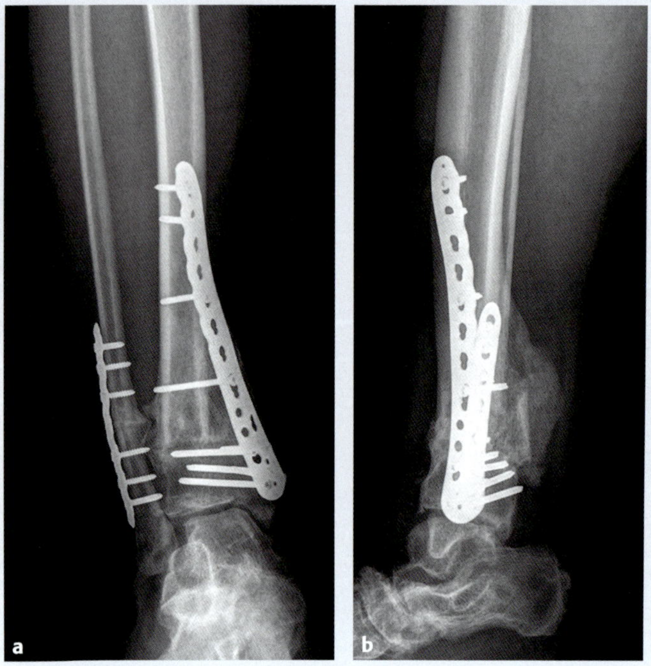

Fig 6.1-17a–b Radiological consolidation at the control 1 year after the osteotomy showing no fatigue of the osteosynthesis material. The moderate varus deviation observed, which does not affect limb function, is due to a planned undercorrection in the execution of the osteotomy.

Analysis of failure and reflection

When deciding on the type of fracture treatment, it is essential to include a comprehensive assessment of the patient, ie, not only the physical comorbidity but also the psychological status and degree of discipline and cooperation in the pre- and postoperative periods. Damage control cannot be questioned in a high-energy polytrauma patient as in this case since it was a fall from a height of more than 8 m. However, leaving an external fixator that offers little stability as definitive treatment could be questioned.

After the first control phase of the soft tissues, definitive treatment of the intraarticular tibial pilon fracture should have been considered. In the first phase of the sequential fracture treatment, synthesis of the fibula to avoid shortening, debridement, approaching the soft tissues, and immobilization of the tibial component with an external fixator is recommended. Once the soft tissues allow a safe surgical approach, the medial component of the fracture is reconstructed in a second phase **[Sirkin et al, 2004]**.

Open reduction and internal fixation is the "gold standard" for the definitive treatment of intraarticular tibial pilon fractures. The new generations of intramedullary nails with very distal locking holes at the ends of the implant allow their use in very distal tibial fractures with good results. These intramedullary devices better tolerate loads without affecting the fracture reduction; so it is a treatment option for patients with little discipline or willingness to undertake physiotherapy with controlled weight bearing.

Final outcome

Ultimately, the osteotomy achieved union and the axis of the leg, and the functional capacity of the ankle as well as the ability to walk were recovered 1 year after the rescue surgery (**Fig 6.1-18**). The moderate residual varus resulting from an undercorrection in relation to the preoperative planning had no consequences in terms of pain or clinical deformity.

Roberto Rivero Sosa
Reto Babst, Christopher A Becker, Frank Beeres, Joan Girós Torres, Christian Kammerlander, Björn Link, Bianka Rubenbauer, J Miquel Sales Pérez, Miquel Videla Cés

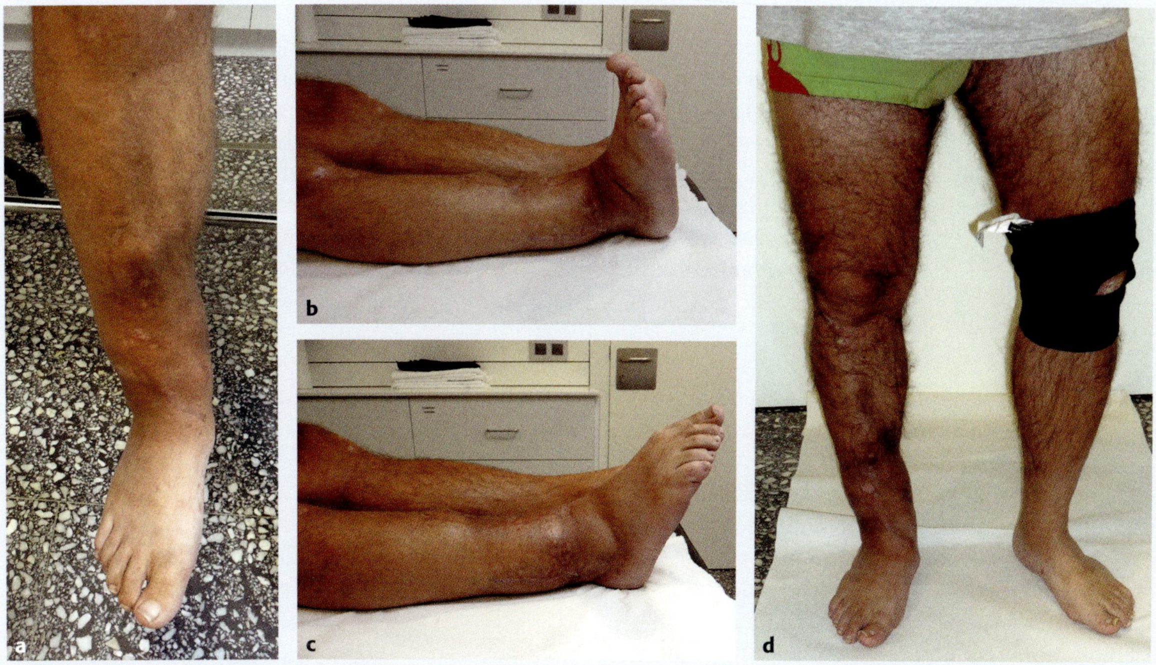

Fig 6.1-18a–d At the control visit 1 year after the corrective osteotomy, the patient's ankle range of motion is 0–40°.

a View of corrected axis of the leg.

b–c The functional capacity of the ankle 1 year after the osteotomy shows the range of movement possible with only minimal limitation of plantar flexion.

d Clinical image 1 year following the osteotomy. The patient maintains bipedal weight bearing without difficulty and walks without walking aids.

CASE 3

Case description

An 85-year-old woman, who had sustained a subcapital right femoral fracture 4 years previously that was treated with a head and neck prosthesis, had a fall in the nursing home resulting in trauma to the left hip. The x-ray revealed a fracture of the left femoral trochanteric region (AO/OTA 31A3) (**Fig 6.1-19**) without further traumatic injuries.

To rule out that the fracture might also have affected the femoral head region, a computed tomographic (CT) scan was performed (**Fig 6.1-20**).

Surgery with a trochanteric nail was planned. The postoperative control x-ray showed a lack of reduction of the fracture site and the head and neck screw centered in the femoral neck region (**Fig 6.1-21**).

Given that the screw was centered, ambulation with crutches and full weight bearing was authorized. Wound healing was satisfactory, but the patient presented with psychomotor agitation at night, sustaining a new fall with increased pain and functional deficit 6 weeks after surgery. The x-rays showed a screw cut-out in the upper region of the femoral head (**Fig 6.1-22**).

A reintervention was planned to remove the intramedullary (IM) nail, reduce the fracture, achieve valgus alignment of the proximal fragment, and stabilize it with a sliding dynamic hip screw (DHS) and plate. During surgery using image intensifier control, the proximal plate screw was inserted and centered in the head and neck region. This screw was longer than the previous one and achieved a good grip in the hard core of the femoral head. Postoperative x-rays showed satisfactory reduction and the correct position of the implant (**Fig 6.1-23**).

Physical restraint was recommended to avoid further falls until the agitation symptoms were under control, but the patient's family refused. The patient had another three falls during the recovery period. After the last fall, the patient returned to the hospital and presented with pain and inability to walk. New x-rays were taken that showed a new cut-out of the head screw (**Fig 6.1-24**).

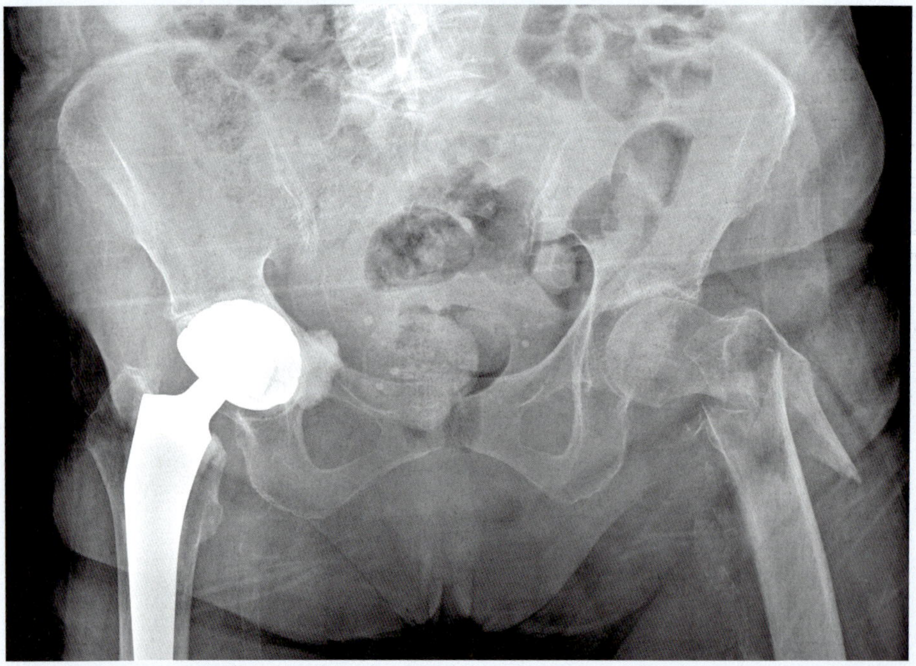

Fig 6.1-19 Preoperative AP x-ray of the pelvis. Fracture with an inverted fracture line that affects the trochanteric mass of the left femur. The right hip shows the head and neck prosthesis implanted previously.

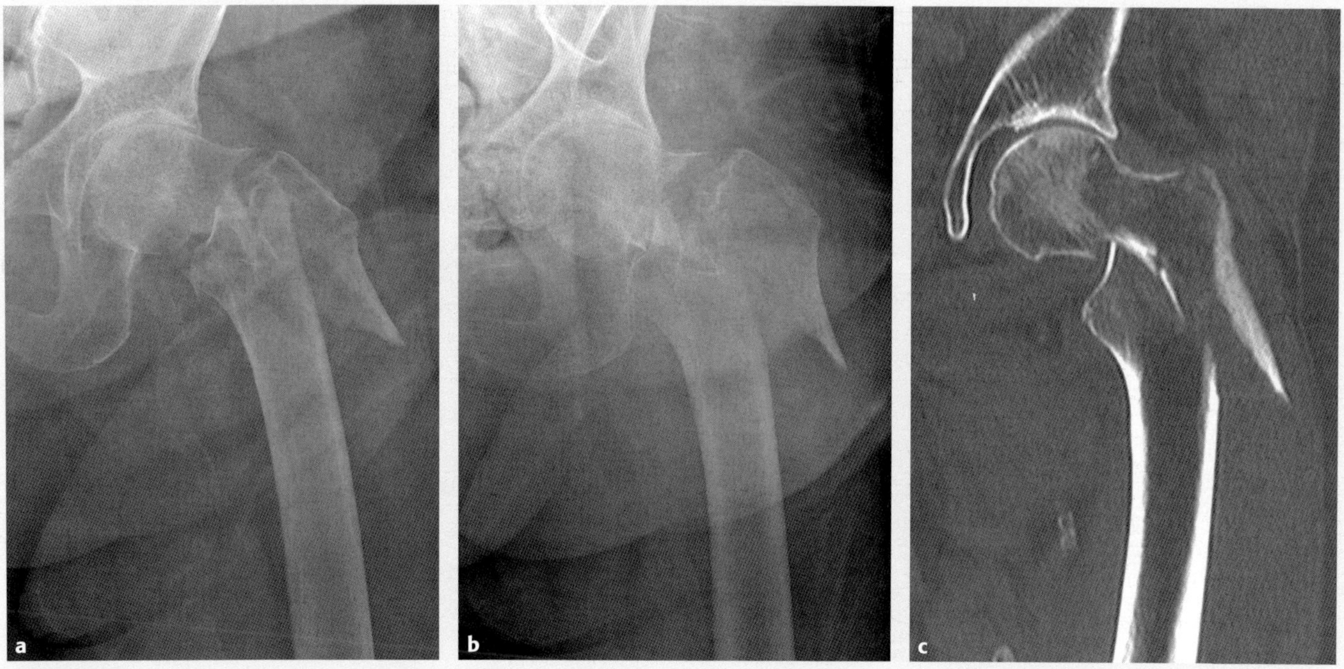

Fig 6.1-20a–c Preoperative x-rays of the left hip (**a–b**) and a computed tomographic scan to rule out a combined fracture in the femoral neck region (**c**).

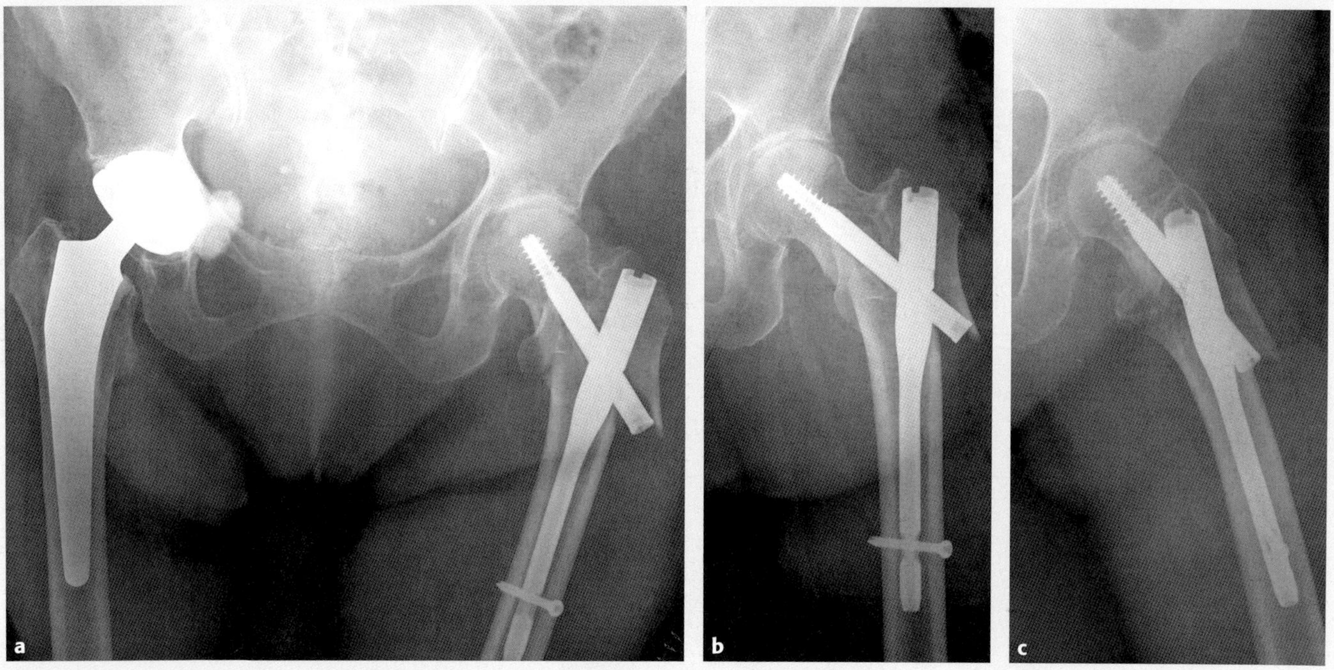

Fig 6.1-21a–c Postoperative and control x-rays.
a Immediate postoperative AP x-ray.
b–c AP (**b**) and lateral (**c**) x-rays of the left hip 1 month after surgical intervention.

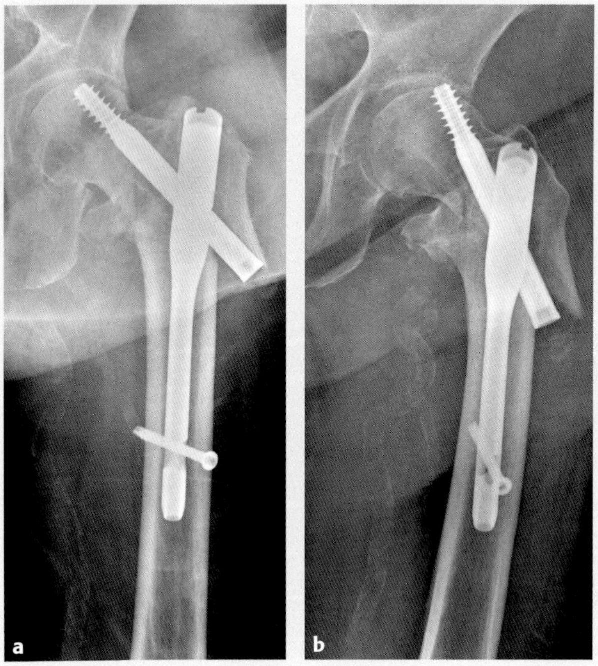

Fig 6.1-22a–b Control x-rays in AP (**a**) and axial (**b**) views of the left hip following the patient's second fall. The cut-out can be seen in the upper region of the femoral head.

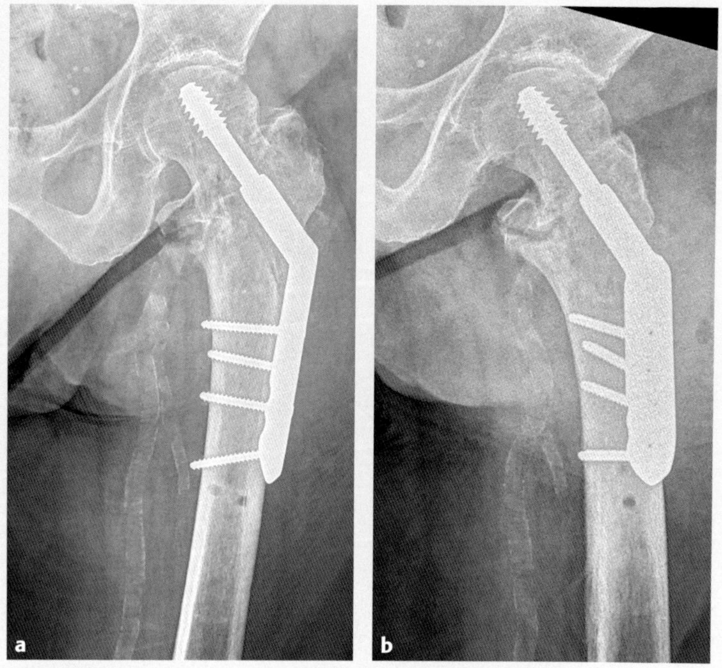

Fig 6.1-23a–b Postoperative control x-rays of the reintervention (ie, removal of the intramedullary nail, valgus alignment of the head and neck fragment, and implantation of the sliding dynamic hip screw with plate). The x-rays show correct reduction of the fracture through valgus alignment. The head and neck screw is properly positioned.

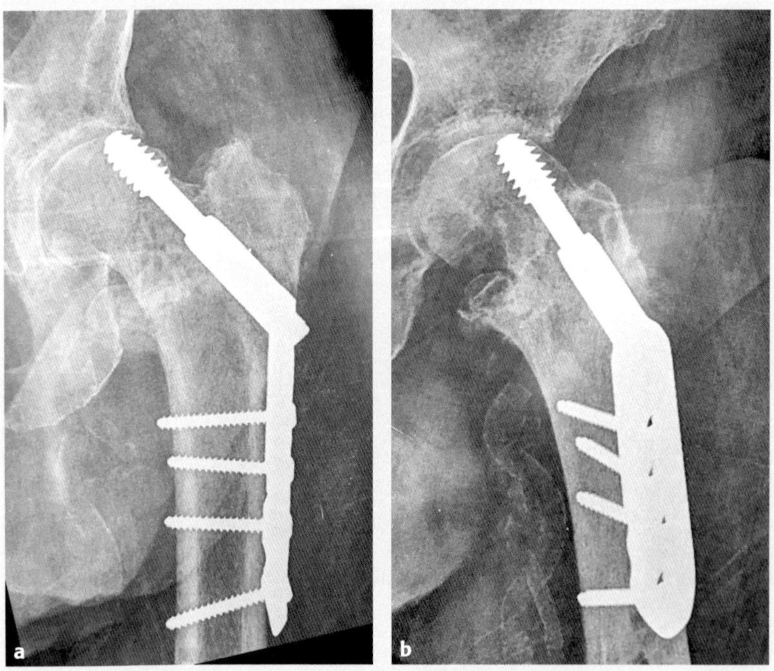

Fig 6.1-24a–b Control x-rays of the left hip after three new falls on the extremity; although the fracture remains reduced, a new cut-out of the screw occured in the upper region of the femoral head.

Roberto Rivero Sosa
Reto Babst, Christopher A Becker, Frank Beeres, Joan Girós Torres, Christian Kammerlander, Björn Link, Bianka Rubenbauer, J Miquel Sales Pérez, Miquel Videla Cés

Analysis of failure and reflection

The diagnosis of this patient was correct and the CT scan taken allowed the surgeon to rule out a combined fracture of the neck and trochanteric region **[Videla-Cés et al, 2017]**. In cases where two fractures occur in the same bone segment, the treatment must take into accout increasing instability due to the affected bone mass.

The osteosynthesis was done on an unreduced fracture; thus, the bone did not participate in stabilizing the fracture and the implant had to bear the entire load. In a patient with motor agitation, treatment with IM osteosynthesis is indicated, because a screwed plate could present breakage or weakening of the screws as it needs to bear the entire load in an unreduced fracture.

The rescue of the first cut-out of the IM nail screw was correct since it allowed open reduction of the fracture site and valgus alignment of the proximal segment to improve the biomechanical situation. If perforation of the femoral head occurs due to cut-out, the augmentation technique where liquid cement is injected into the bone to improve or increase bone quality should not be used because of the risk of cement leaking into the joint. Even so, correct evaluation of the patient is fundamental when faced with possible noncompliance.

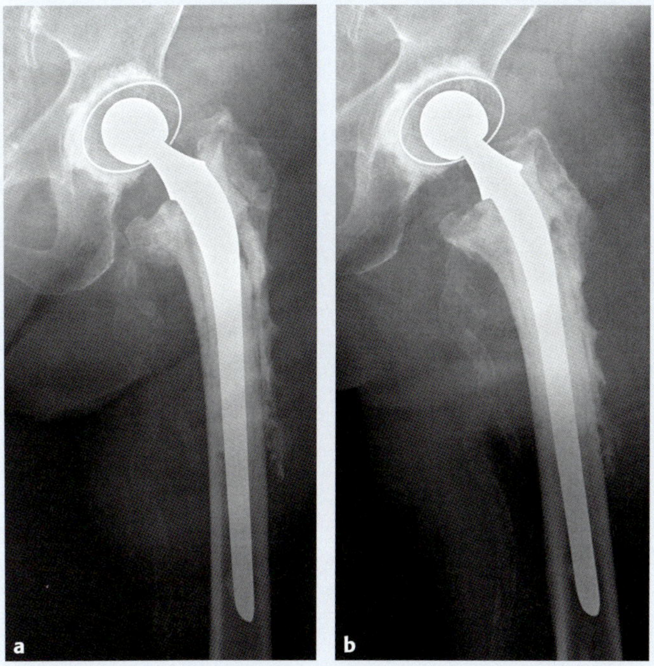

Fig 6.1-25a–b Postoperative control x-rays after a new intervention to remove the sliding dynamic hip screw and plate and perform total hip arthroplasty with a long-stem prosthesis.

Final outcome

Due to the absence of bone in the femoral head region and the cut-out contraindicating the use of bone augmentation, the decision was made to remove the osteosynthesis material and opt for total hip arthroplasty using a cemented long stem. This avoids new fractures in the femoral diaphysis already weakened by numerous drillings during previous interventions. The patient's psychiatric situation stabilized, and she is now able to ambulate with the aid of a walking frame or crutches (**Fig 6.1-25**).

CASE 4

Case description

A 49-year-old man fell on his right shoulder while playing football. He sustained a diaphyseal fracture of the right clavicle (AO/OTA 15.2B) (**Fig 6.1-26**). It was treated with open reduction and internal fixation using absolute stability criteria, and an interfragmentary compression screw and a precontoured protection plate were applied to the upper surface of the clavicle. Surgery was performed 7 days after the injury. The postoperative control x-ray clearly showed that the most medial screw was too long due to a mistake made when measuring for the screw (**Fig 6.1-27**).

Since the patient was pain free and had no functional limitations in the postoperative period, he decided to ride his motorbike, but reported pain symptoms and functional deficit of the right arm at 4 weeks. The x-rays showed a loss of reduction with loosening of the plate and mobilization of the screws (**Fig 6.1-28**).

The patient underwent reintervention 6 weeks after the first surgery. The implants were removed, a new reduction and decortication performed, autogenous bone grafting obtained from the iliac crest was applied, and new osteosynthesis with a contoured locking compression plate (LCP) applied to the anterior surface of the clavicle (**Fig 6.1-29**). The patient was immobilized with a sling for 3 weeks after which active rehabilitation was initiated.

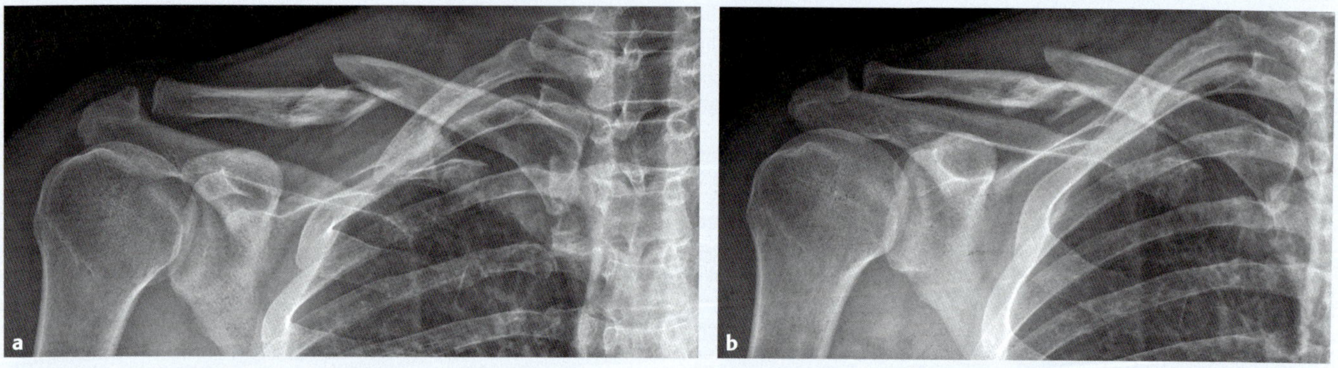

Fig 6.1-26a–b AP (**a**) and cephalic (**b**) x-rays of the comminuted diaphyseal fracture of the right clavicle (dominant arm).

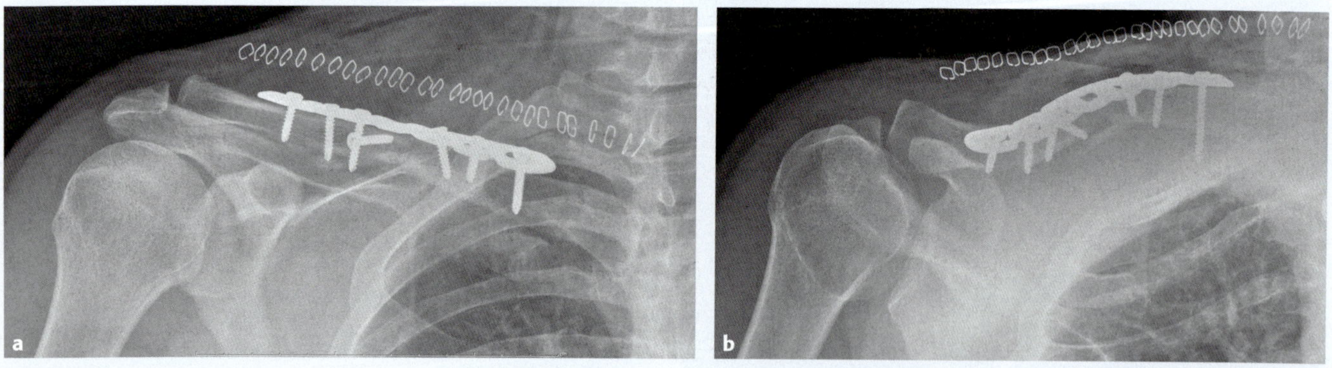

Fig 6.1-27a–b Postoperative x-rays in which we can observe correct reduction. Note the oversized most medial screw which is probably due to a measuring error.

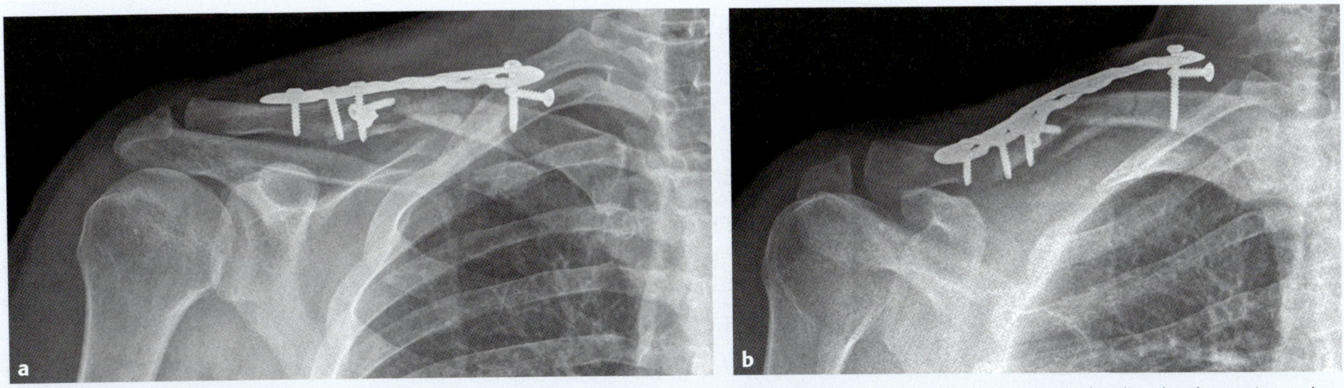

Fig 6.1-28a–b X-rays at 4 weeks showing a loss of reduction and loosening of the material, which was due to overloading by the patient who decided to ride his powerful motorbike 2 weeks postoperatively.

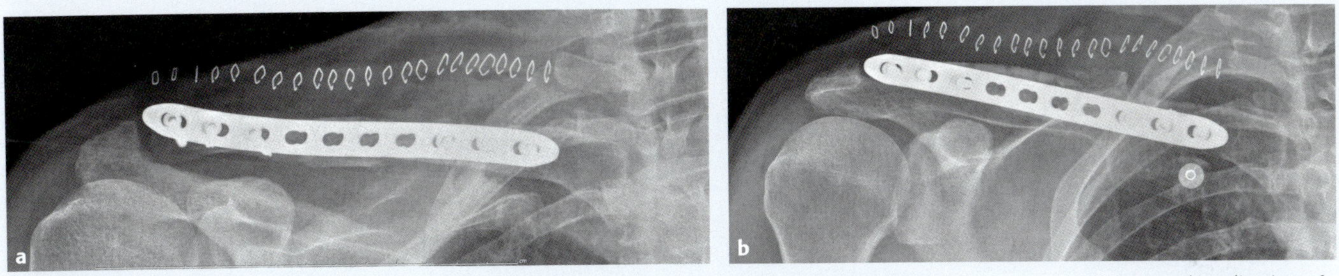

Fig 6.1-29a–b Rescue surgery 6 weeks after the first surgery with removal of the material, a new reduction, decortication, and application of autogenous grafting obtained from the iliac crest, and new osteosynthesis with a precontoured locking compression plate (LCP) applied to the anterior surface of the clavicle.

Analysis of failure and reflection

Despite the technical error in the measurement of the most medial screw in the plate, the osteosynthesis was considered sufficiently stable; therefore, the patient was not immobilized in the immediate postoperative period.

The absence of pain after actively mobilizing the arm led the patient to assume that the osteosynthesis was sufficiently stable to carry out load-bearing exercise. He started riding his powerful motorbike as soon as the sutures were removed.

Although the clavicle is not a load-bearing bone, it does receive axial load as a component of the kinetic chain of the upper limb. Mechanically, the clavicle is subject to a rotational movement around its axis. In the absence of fracture consolidation, this micromovement is transmitted to the material causing it to loosen and therefore leading to failure of the osteosynthesis and loss of reduction.

Final outcome

The fracture finally consolidated and arm function was recovered after a long period of rehabilitation (**Fig 6.1-30**). Distally, the anterior plate is in contact with the acromioclavicular joint, and the authors will wait until 18 months after the intervention to propose implant removal.

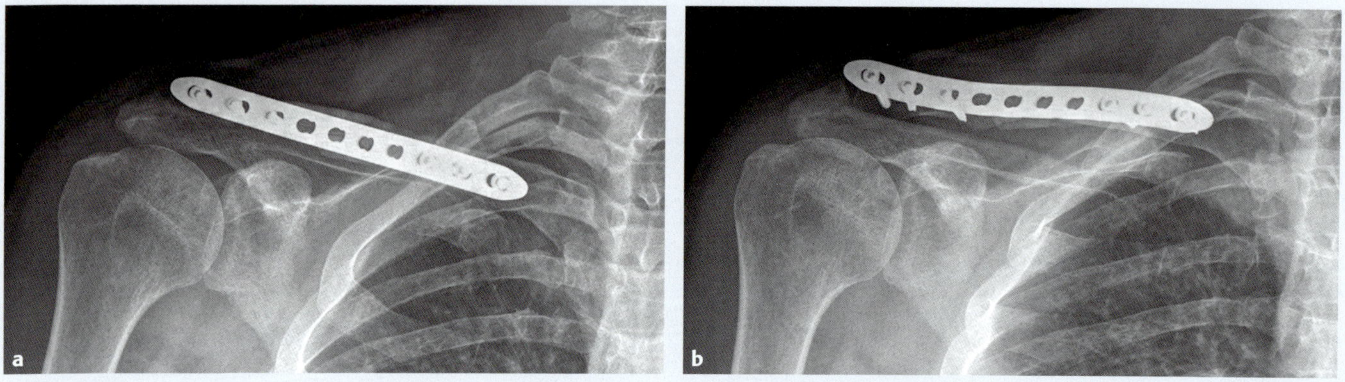

Fig 6.1-30a–b Control x-rays at 6 months after the intervention showing radiographic consolidation of the fracture.

Roberto Rivero Sosa
Reto Babst, Christopher A Becker, Frank Beeres, Joan Girós Torres, Christian Kammerlander, Björn Link, Bianka Rubenbauer, J Miquel Sales Pérez, Miquel Videla Cés

Case description

A 76-year-old woman with obesity stumbled and fell at home. The patient was formerly living independently and was able to manage her activities of daily living. After admission to the emergency department, an x-ray and computed tomographic (CT) scans were obtained showing an anterior and posterior column acetabular fracture (AO/OTA 62C) (**Fig 6.1-31**). The indication for open reduction and internal fixation was given and the surgeons performed an anterior angular stable plate osteosynthesis with a 14-hole reconstruction plate through an ilioinguinal approach. The intraoperative x-rays showed an anatomical reduction with a single posterior screw addressing the dorsal column of the acetabulum (**Fig 6.1-32**).

Postoperatively, the left leg was externally rotated. An x-ray and CT scan showed the failed osteosynthesis (**Fig 6.1-33**). The patient was informed of the necessity to perform a second operation for the acetabular fracture. In this operation a total hip arthroplasty with a revision cup was inserted in the left hip.

The second intervention took place 12 days after the initial operation. This second procedure was performed through an anterolateral approach to the left hip. The revision cup for the acetabulum was fixed with a lick (ie, a metal buttstrap or metal link of the revision cup for the fixation of the cup to the iliac bone with screws) attaching the cup construction to the iliac bone. An inner component of the revision cup is attached with angular stability to the metal ring and a lateralized inlay provides a better offset of the hip. A size 9 hip stem was used to finalize the total hip arthroplasty (**Fig 6.1-34**).

After the second operation, the patient started and practised full weight bearing with physiotherapists. Eight days after the second operation, the patient was discharged and transferred to the rehabilitation unit. Six weeks after discharge the patient did not report any pain or any other problems. The flexion/extension was 110°/0°/20° for the left hip and the gait was normal without hobbling. Internal and external rotation of the left hip was complete. There was no difference in leg length.

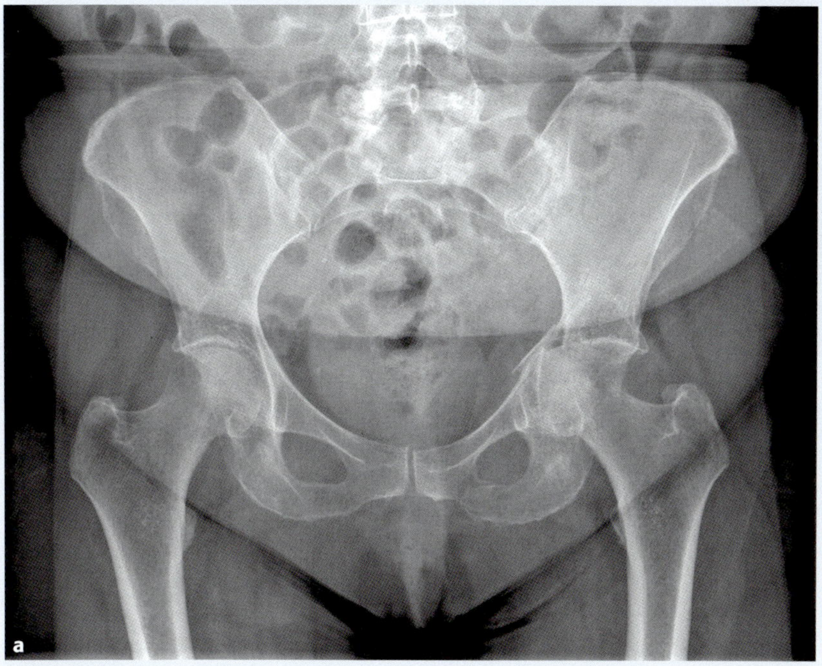

Fig 6.1-31a–e Preoperative images.
a X-ray showing a left acetabular fracture with protrusion of the left hip.

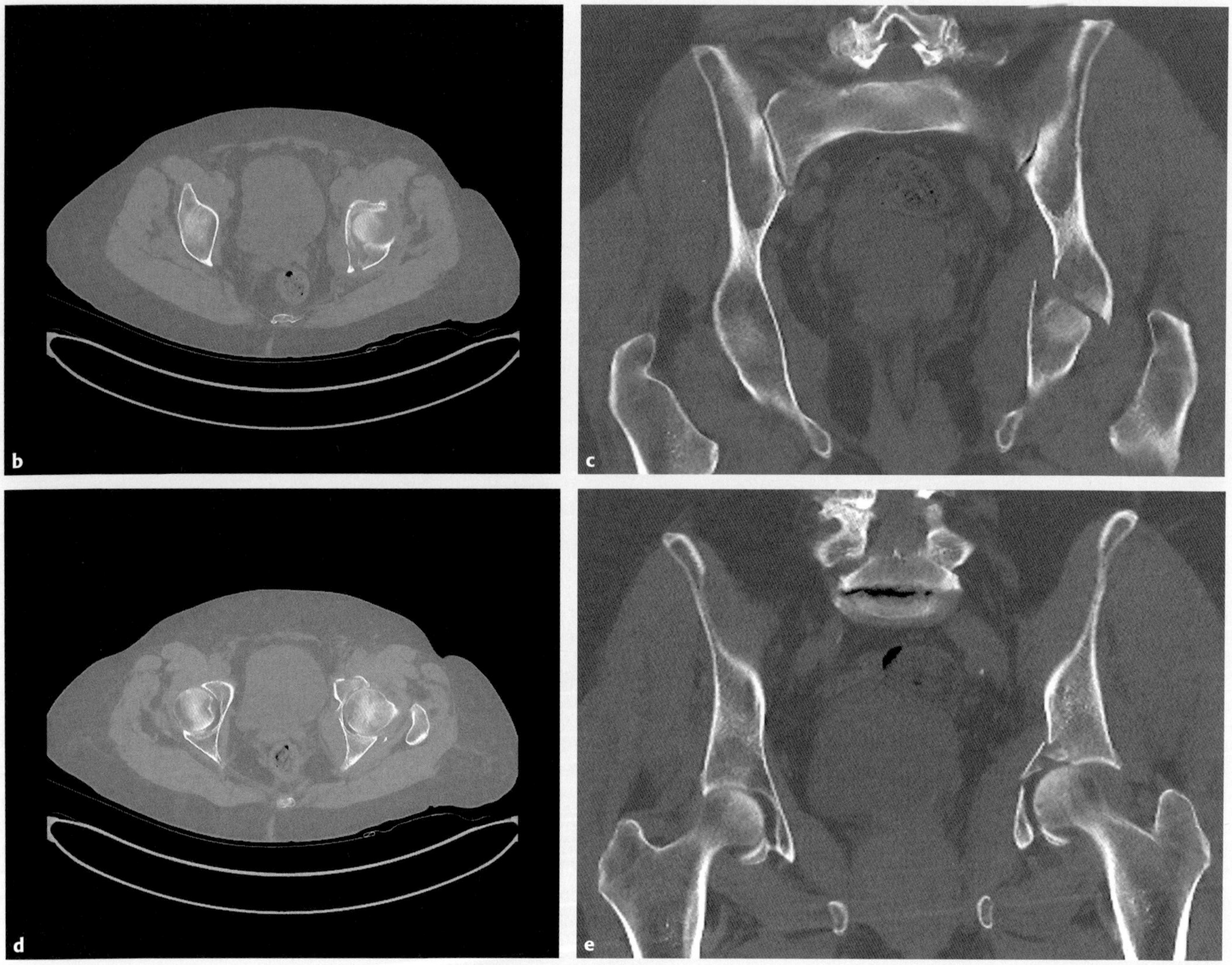

Fig 6.1-31a–e (cont) Preoperative images.
b–e The CT scans show an anterior and posterior column fracture (anterior column and posterior hemitransverse fracture) of the left acetabulum.

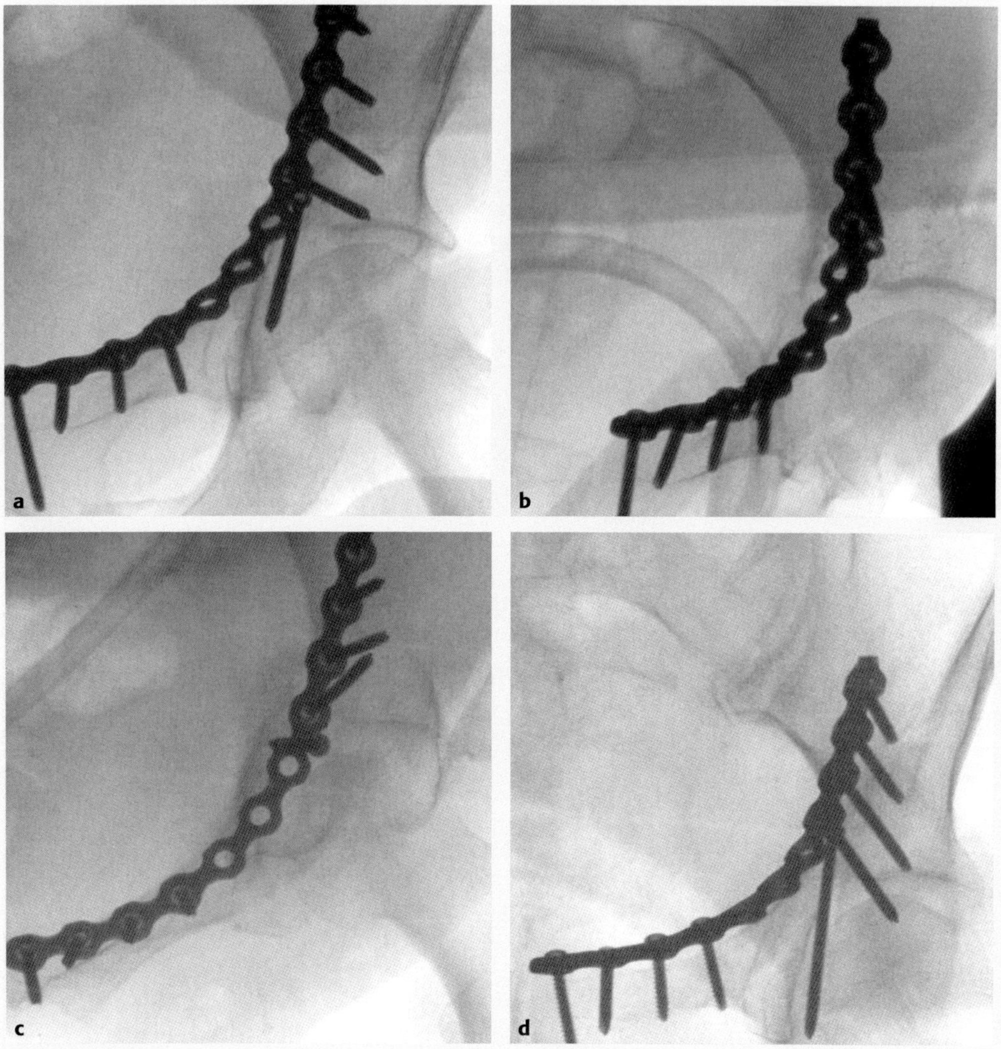

Fig 6.1-32a–d Intraoperative C-arm images of the first surgery.

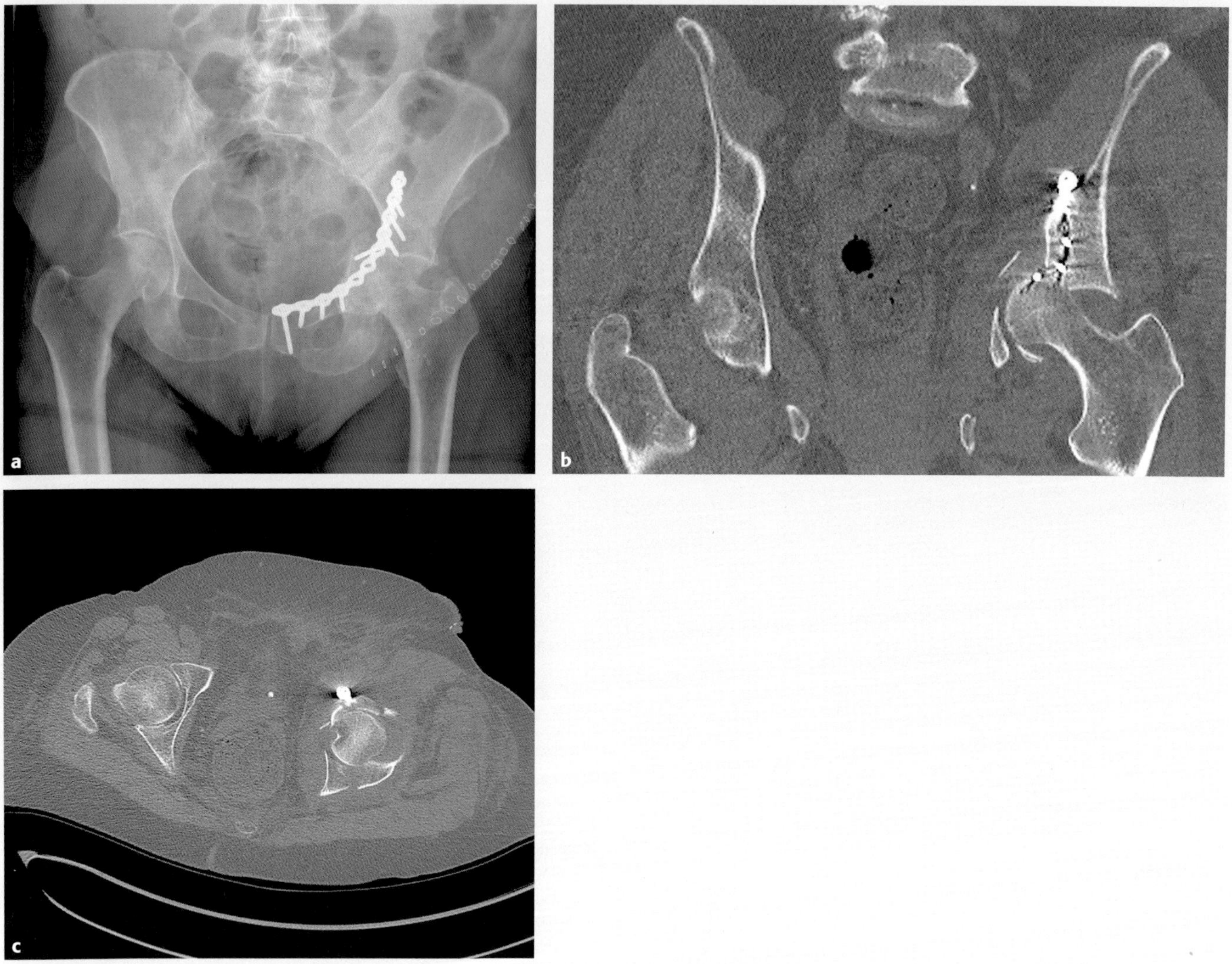

Fig 6.1-33a–c X-ray (**a**) and computed tomographic scans (**b–c**) after the first operation showing protrusion of the left hip and failed lag screw of the posterior column.

Analysis of failure and reflection

The initial problem of the surgeons' management plan was that they did not consider the patient's inability to manage even partial weight bearing after the first surgery, which led to the osteosynthesis failure. Other aggravating factors were the presence of osteoporosis and obesity.

The posterior column of the acetabulum was not adequalety addressed with only one screw. While performing the first operation, the reduction of the acetabular fracture was anatomical (**Fig 6.1-32**). For a patient who is able to manage at least partial weight bearing, the reduction and fixation of the fracture would be sufficient. But this patient was noncompliant during the entire hospital stay and had other risk factors for osteosynthesis failures (obesity, severe osteoporosis).

The posterior part of the acetabulum should have been fixed with another plate osteosynthesis to prevent a secondary dislocation, because one lag screw does not provide enough stability for this combined acetabular fracture. Preventing protrusion of the femoral head into the inner pelvis, which destroyed the quadrilateral surface, was not possible using an anterior plate osteosynthesis with an additional lag screw.

This case shows the necessity to evaluate each patient's risk factors for osteosynthesis failure in advance to provide an osteosynthesis with maximum stability. Perhaps one should immediately perform stable osteosynthesis in geriatric patients to allow full weight bearing, especially if they are obese and noncompliant. For acetabular fractures, a total hip replacement provides the best stability for this patient cohort.

Final outcome

One year after discharge from the hospital, the patient can lead a normal life and manage her activities of daily living only using crutches for longer walks.

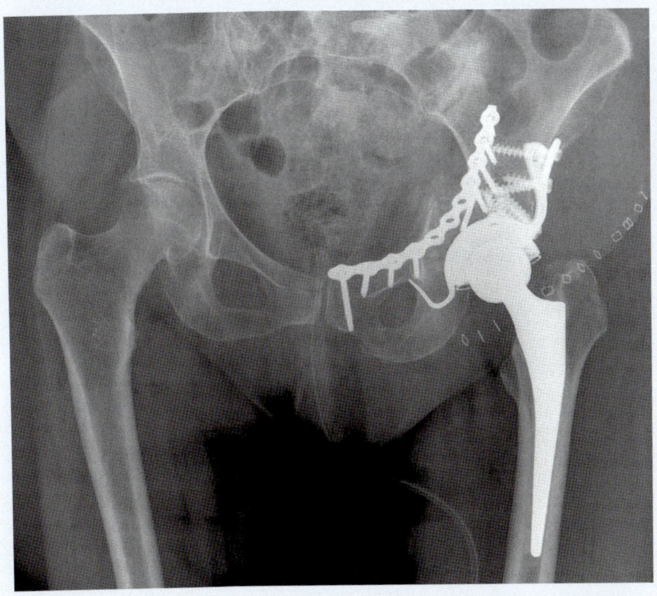

Fig 6.1-34 X-ray after the second operation.

Key points to remember

- Identify patients with a risk of noncompliance with the postoperative protocol.
- In patients with a risk of noncompliance, whether voluntary or involuntary, adjust the advisability of surgery, evaluating other possibilities.
- Plan an osteosynthesis that allows for immediate mobility and weight bearing, where appropriate.
- Be sure that the patient understands that her or his active and responsible participation in the postoperative phase is fundamental for a complete recovery.
- Establish an individualized postoperative protocol and clearly explain each phase of the protocol to the patient. Explain what the patient can do and what she or he must not do.
- Take additional measures to guarantee adherence to the treatment and prevent complications, for each case.
- Adjust the postoperative control for noncompliant patients and for those who are elderly, obese, children, patients with psychiatric pathologies, and amputees.

References and suggested reading

Basamania CJ, Rockwood CA, Jr. Fractures of the Clavicle. In: Rockwood CA Jr, Matsen FA, eds. *The Shoulder.* 4th ed. Philadelphia: Saunders Elsevier; 2009:381–452.
Bisaccia M, Meccariello L, Rinonapoli G, et al. Comparison of Plate, Nail and External Fixation in the Management of Diaphyseal Fractures of the Humerus. *Med Arch.* 2017 Apr;71(2):97–102.
Brink PRG, Verleisdonk E, Blokhuis TJ. [Earlier weight-bearing mobilisation after fracture fixation]. *Ned Tijdschr Geneeskd.* 2017;161:D1533.
Buckley RE, Moran CG, Apivatthakakul T. *AO Principles of Fracture Management.* 3rd ed. Stuttgart New York: Thieme; 2017.
Fong W, Acevedo JI, Stone RG, et al. The treatment of unstable ankle fractures in patients over eighty years of age. *Foot Ankle Int.* 2007 Dec;28(12):1256–1259.
Gautier E, Sommer C. Guidelines for the clinical application of the LCP. *Injury.* 2003 Nov;34 Suppl 2:B63–76.
Hall AJ, Watkins R, Lang IA, et al. The experiences of physiotherapists treating people with dementia who fracture their hip. *BMC Geriatr.* 2017 Apr 20;17(1):91.
Hall RF Jr. Treatment of metacarpal and phalangeal fractures in noncompliant patients. *Clin Orthop Relat Res.* 1987 Jan(214):31–36.
Kuyucu E, Kocyigit F, Ciftci L. The importance of patient compliance in nonunion of forearm fracture. *Int J Surg Case Rep.* 2014;5(9):598–600.
Lin CW, Donkers NA, Refshauge KM, et al. Rehabilitation for ankle fractures in adults. *Cochrane Database Syst Rev.* 2012 Nov 14;11:Cd005595.
Meinberg EG, Agel J, Roberts CS, et al. Fracture and Dislocation Classification Compendium-2018. *J Orthop Trauma.* 2018 Jan;32 Suppl 1:S1–s170.
Orozco Delclós R. *Errores en la Osteosíntesis.* Barcelona: Masson; 1993.
Seitz DP, Gill SS, Austin PC, et al. Rehabilitation of Older Adults with Dementia After Hip Fracture. *J Am Geriatr Soc.* 2016 Jan;64(1):47–54.
Sirkin M, Sanders R, DiPasquale T, et al. A staged protocol for soft tissue management in the treatment of complex pilon fractures. *J Orthop Trauma.* 2004 Sep;18(8 Suppl):S32–38.
Snowdon DA, Leggat SG, Taylor NF. Does clinical supervision of healthcare professionals improve effectiveness of care and patient experience? A systematic review. *BMC Health Serv Res.* 2017 Nov 28;17(1):786.
Stoffel K, Dieter U, Stachowiak G, et al. Biomechanical testing of the LCP—how can stability in locked internal fixators be controlled? *Injury.* 2003 Nov;34 Suppl 2:B11–19.
Videla-Cés M, Sales-Pérez JM, Girós-Torres J, et al. A retrospective cohort study of concomitant ipsilateral extra-capsular and intra-capsular fractures of the proximal femur. Are they casual findings or an undervalued reality? *Injury.* 2017 Jul;48(7):1558–1564.
Zelle BA, Buttacavoli FA, Shroff JB, et al. Loss of Follow-up in Orthopaedic Trauma: Who Is Getting Lost to Follow-up? *J Orthop Trauma.* 2015 Nov;29(11):510–515.

Section 7
Failure recognition and timing

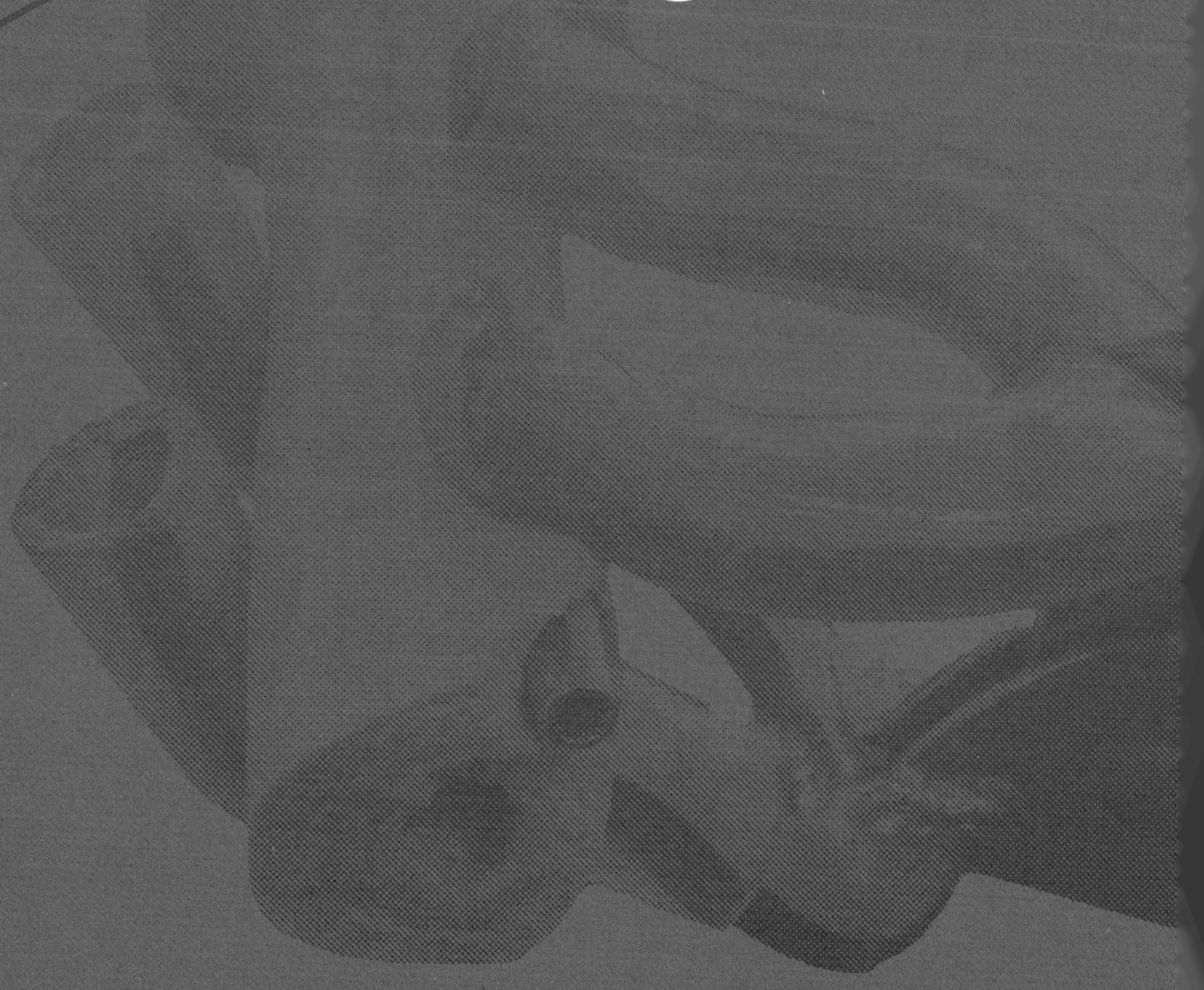

Section 7
Failure recognition and timing

7.1 Early recognition of failures

Joan Girós Torres
Jordi Bertrán Padrós, Roberto Rivero Sosa, J Miquel Sales Pérez, Juan Carlos Serfaty Soler, Miquel Videla Cés

If what you're doing works, carry on doing it.
If what you're doing doesn't work, don't do it.
If you don't know what you're doing, don't do anything.
Anonymous

The process that encompasses the surgical treatment of a bone injury does not end with the patient leaving the operating room. It starts at admission to the emergency department and ends when the definitive healing of the injured bone is complete. An overall assessment of the patient and correct planning can avoid many failures. General clinical condition, bone quality, and soft-tissue status must be evaluated before proceeding to the therapeutic indication. Failure to plan means planning to fail.

The clinical and x-ray evaluation must be carefully analyzed, and great attention must be paid to patients' comments, because "the patient must also have a say" [Orozco Delclós, 1993:199], together with scrupulous and critical observation of the radiographical results and their evolution. Any clinical change in the evolution of the healing process contrasting with the consecutive radiographical images must raise suspicion. Surgeons analyzing an x-ray that contains one failure will almost always detect another failure. Early recognition is essential because it gives them, at least in some cases, the opportunity to remedy the mistake more easily than if the failure is discovered later.

Loosening of some implants used in osteosynthesis, such as one or several screws with bone osteolysis around them in an extramedullary assembly, or the movement of a blade or dynamic screw at the level of the proximal femur together with a loss of fracture reduction, is a warning sign of a possible osteosynthesis failure in the short term. Breakage of distal bolts in an intramedullary nail can also be a warning sign or alternatively, a sign of spontaneous nail dynamization.

Axis or rotational defects that can be confirmed in the immediate postoperative period require a solution, otherwise this results in an overload of the neighboring joints. In joint fractures it is necessary to be stricter. Residual step-offs cause posttraumatic osteoarthritis of the joint.

The formation of hard callus should be observed through a series of control x-rays that show the evolution in the expected healing process and depends on the stability applied. Any anomaly such as halt or lack of progress of hard callus consolidation in two successive control x-rays or the appearance of a cloudy or "irritation" callus after an interfragmentary compression are signs of poor evolution of the healing process and a pseudarthrosis is likely to develop.

It is always upsetting for surgeons to have to tell patients that the result of the surgery was not as satisfactory as hoped and that it must be remedied by another intervention. In many cases, patients have difficulty understanding the surgical situation, but the ethical requirement is to reoperate to obtain the optimum solution.

CASE 1

Case description

A 76-year-old woman without severe comorbidity fell at home from standing height. She sustained an intertrochanteric fracture (AO/OTA 31A3) and treatment was planned with a proximal femoral nail antirotation (PFNA) (**Fig 7.1-1**).

In the postoperative control x-ray, the spiral blade was placed in a center–center position with a tip-apex distance a little larger than 2.5 cm. The rotational forces in the femoral neck were in conflict with the spiral blade which made movement into the bone possible, causing bone loss and loosening of the spiral blade and leading to the cut-out (**Fig 7.1-2**).

At the 2-week follow-up, an initial loosening of the spiral blade and the cranial migration of the PFNA was seen, which led the surgeons to think that reoperation was preferable to a cut-out (**Fig 7.1-3**).

The patient was reoperated 6 weeks after the first surgery. The spiral blade was changed and placed in a lower position in the femoral neck. To improve the spiral blade attachment to the bone, cement augmentation was performed. The surgeons focused on checking radiologically to ensure the correct placement of the new implant, avoiding joint penetration to facilitate the augmentation process (**Fig 7.1-4**). The patient was authorized to bear full weight in the immediate postoperative period after the second surgery.

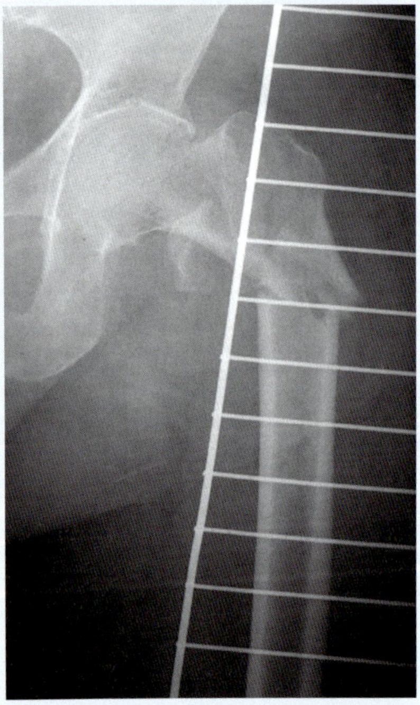

Fig 7.1-1 AP x-ray of the intertrochanteric left femoral fracture.

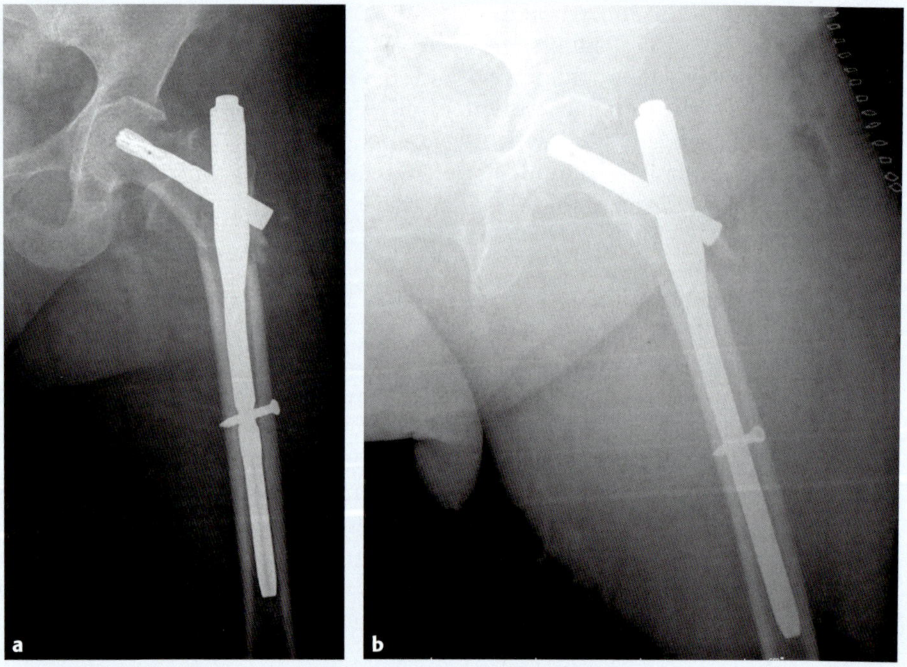

Fig 7.1-2a–b Postoperative AP (**a**) and lateral (**b**) control x-rays showing the spiral blade in a center-center position with a tip-apex distance of more than 2.5 cm. The excessive tip-apex distance is more visible in the AP view.

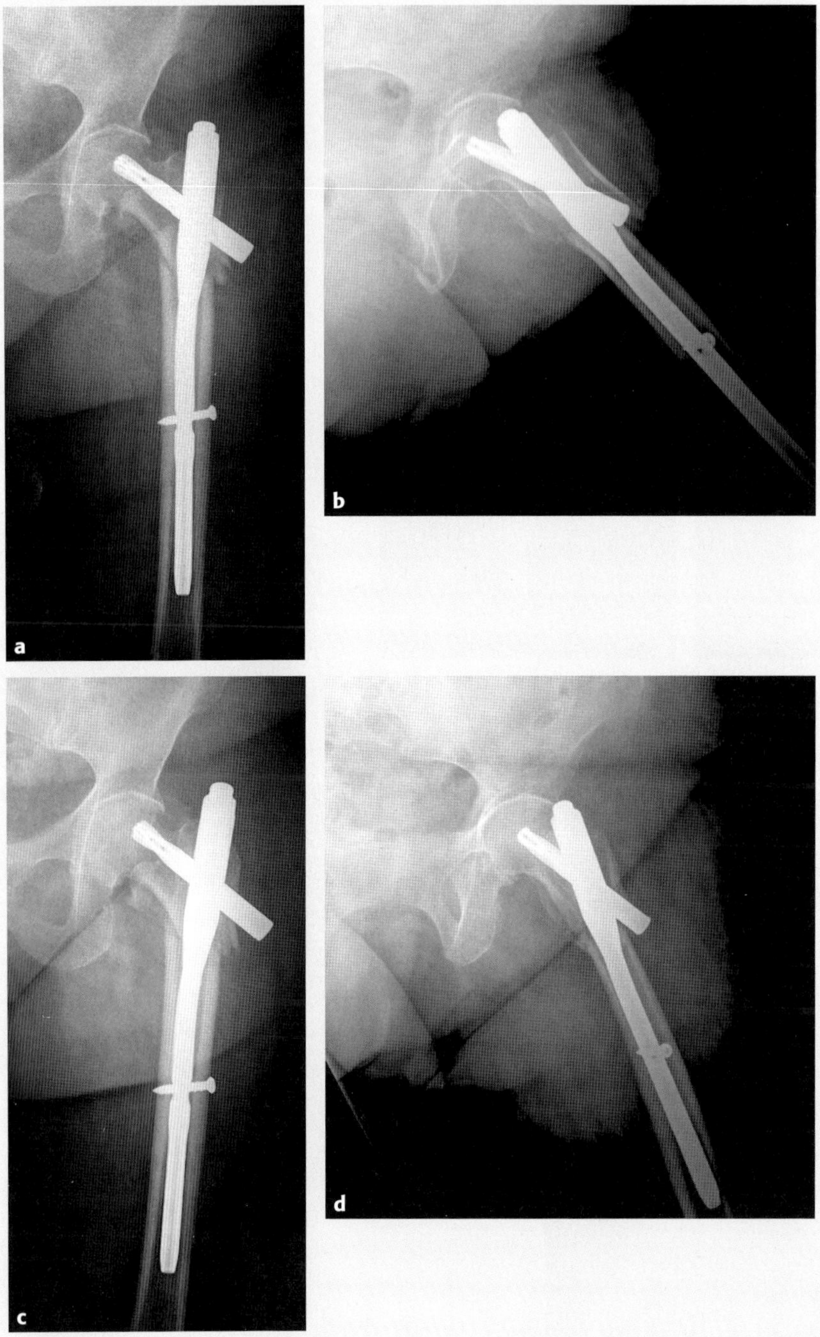

Fig 7.1-3a–g Postoperative control x-rays.
a–b AP (**a**) and axial (**b**) x-ray follow-up control at 2 weeks.
c–d AP (**c**) and axial (**d**) x-ray follow-up control at 6 weeks.

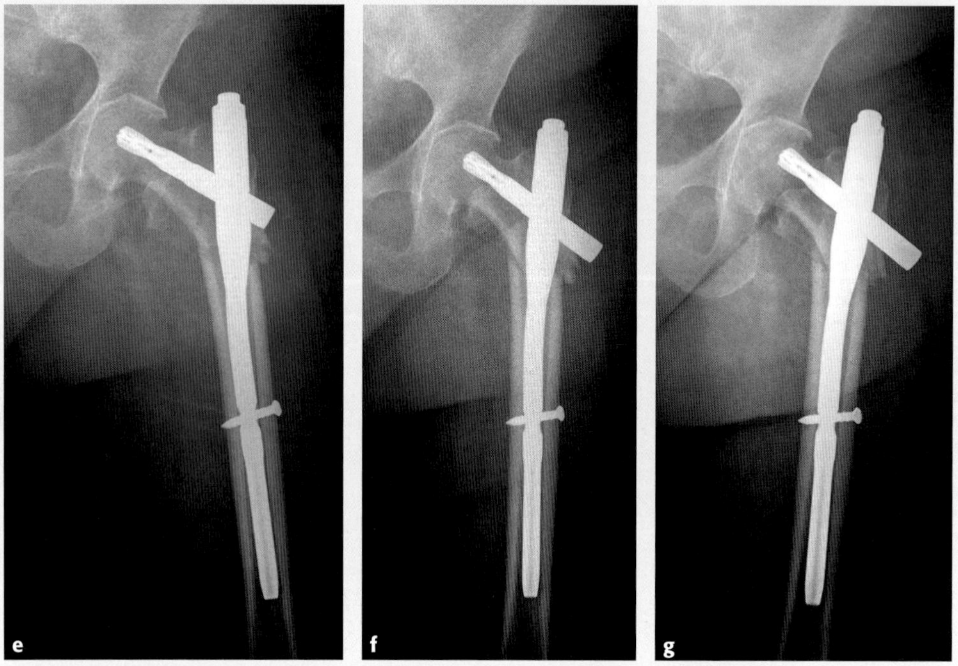

Fig 7.1-3a–g (cont) Postoperative control x-rays.
e–g Comparative postoperative AP (**e**) views at 2 (**f**) and 6 (**g**) weeks showing the lateral and cranial migration of the proximal femoral nail antirotation blade.

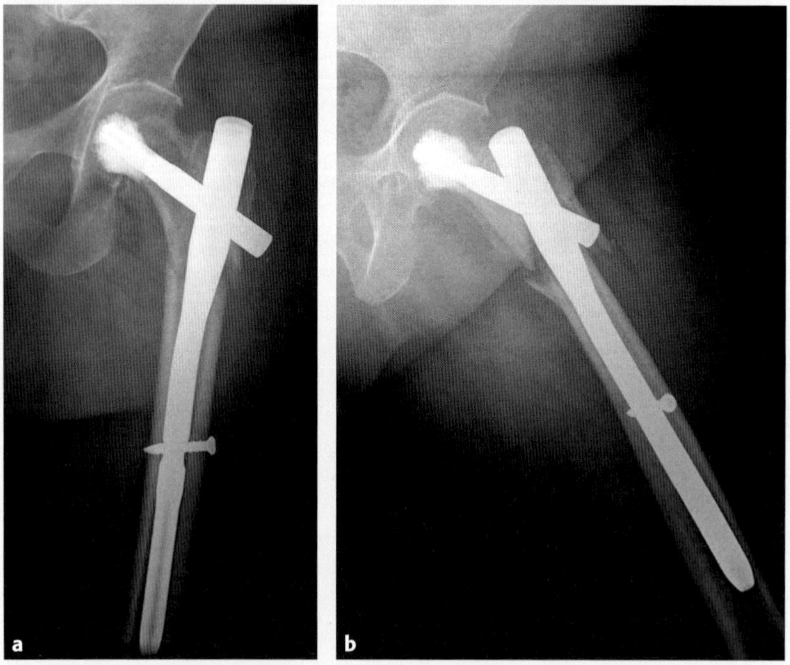

Fig 7.1-4a–b Postoperative AP (**a**) and axial (**b**) x-rays of the reoperation. The proximal femoral nail antirotation spiral blade was placed subchondral and posteroinferior in the neck and femoral head with cement augmentation.

Analysis of failure and reflection

The poor bone quality in the cervicocephalic region of the femur may have been the cause of the precarious anchorage of the spiral blade. The spiral blade was introduced by hammering into osteoporotic bone. In young patients with good bone quality, only the use of the drill bit is recommended.

Seeing changes in the x-ray in the first weeks, such as a lateral and cranial migration of the PFNA blade, should have indicated that a reoperation was a better choice than a cut-out.

Augmentation techniques are very helpful. Augmentation can be done with cement or allograft/autograft. The aim is to fill the empty zone to improve the anchorage of the blade or the screw. Planning the rescue surgery does not have to increase the morbidity. Delaying the reoperation after it has been detected will not improve an adverse situation.

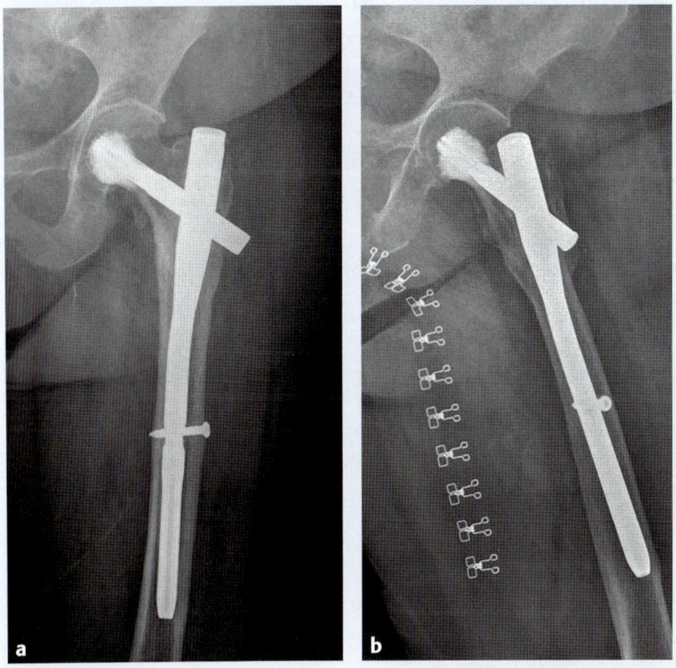

Fig 7.1-5a–b AP (**a**) and axial (**b**) x-rays showing the proximal femoral nail antirotation spiral blade in place without loosening.

Final outcome

The fracture healed completely. The patient recovered the ability to walk without crutches. She recovered complete functionality and quality of life in the first year postfracture (**Fig 7.1-5**).

CASE 2

Case description

A 49-year-old man had a workplace accident and presented with a closed diaphyseal fracture of the tibia and fibula of the right leg. It was a simple oblique (> 30°) fracture of the tibia (AO/OTA 42A2) and of the fibula (AO/OTA 4F2B).

The fracture was treated with reamed intramedullary nailing locked in the proximal and distal zones. The surgical intervention proceeded uneventfully, but a deficient reduction with separation of the fragments and valgus position of the ankle was detected in the postoperative control x-rays (**Fig 7.1-6a–b**). The clinical examination also showed the distal deviation of the tibia (**Fig 7.1-6c**).

The patient underwent a subsequent surgical intervention, and the proximal and distal locking bolts of the intramedullary nail were extracted. The nail, assembled on the aiming device, partially moved to the area near the fracture site (**Fig 7.1-7** and **Fig 7.1-8a–b**). Manual reduction of the valgus was performed under image intensifier control. The axis of the distal tibial fragment and the angle of the fracture were determined and two Steinmann pins were temporarily placed at the level of the concave angulation close to the fracture site to avoid placing the guide and nail in the wrong position again (**Fig 7.1-8c–d**). In this way, centering the nail in relation to the axial axis of the tibia was achieved. The pins were replaced by two definitive screws to avoid secondary displacements (**Fig 7.1-8e–h**, and **Fig 7.1-9**).

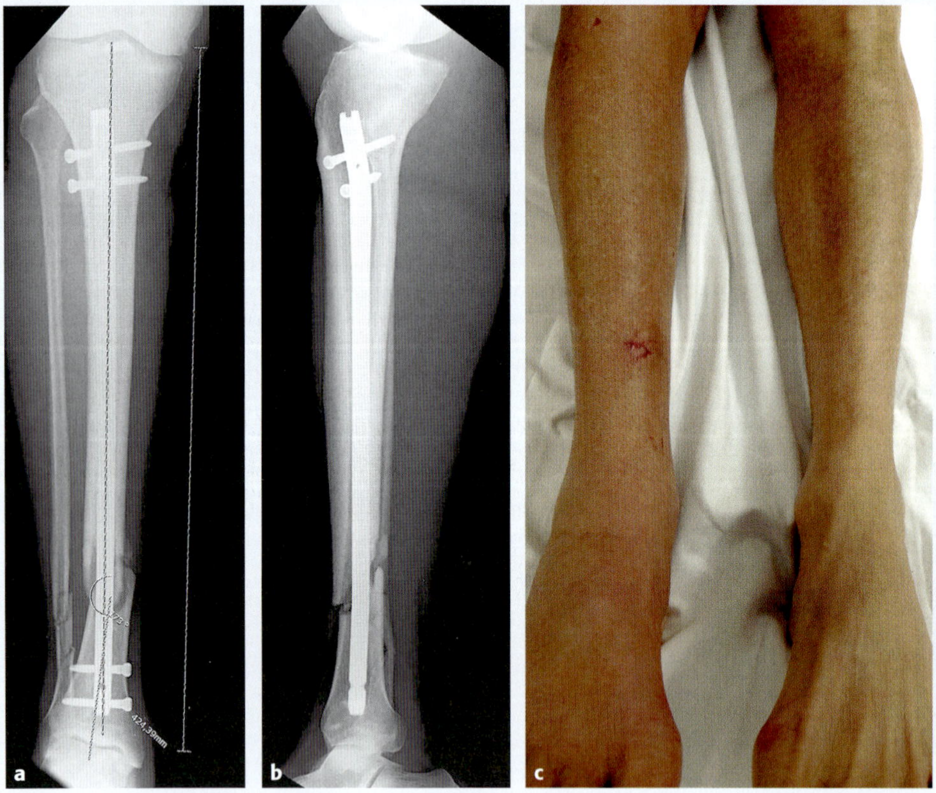

Fig 7.1-6a–c Postoperative images.
a–b Immediate postoperative AP (**a**) and lateral (**b**) control x-rays of the tibia.
c Postoperative clinical photograph showing the ankle valgus.

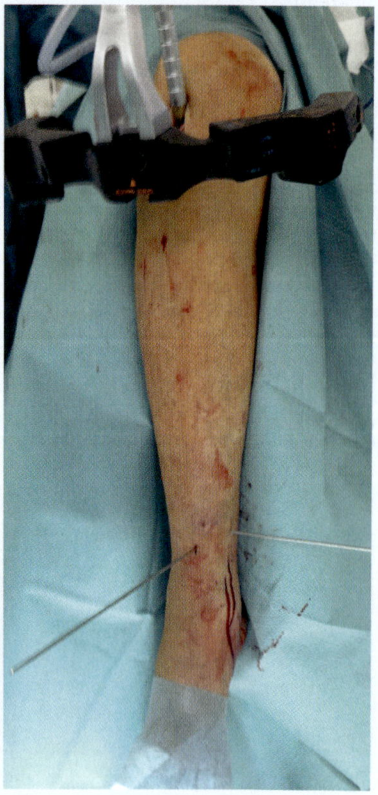

Fig 7.1-7 The rescue surgery.

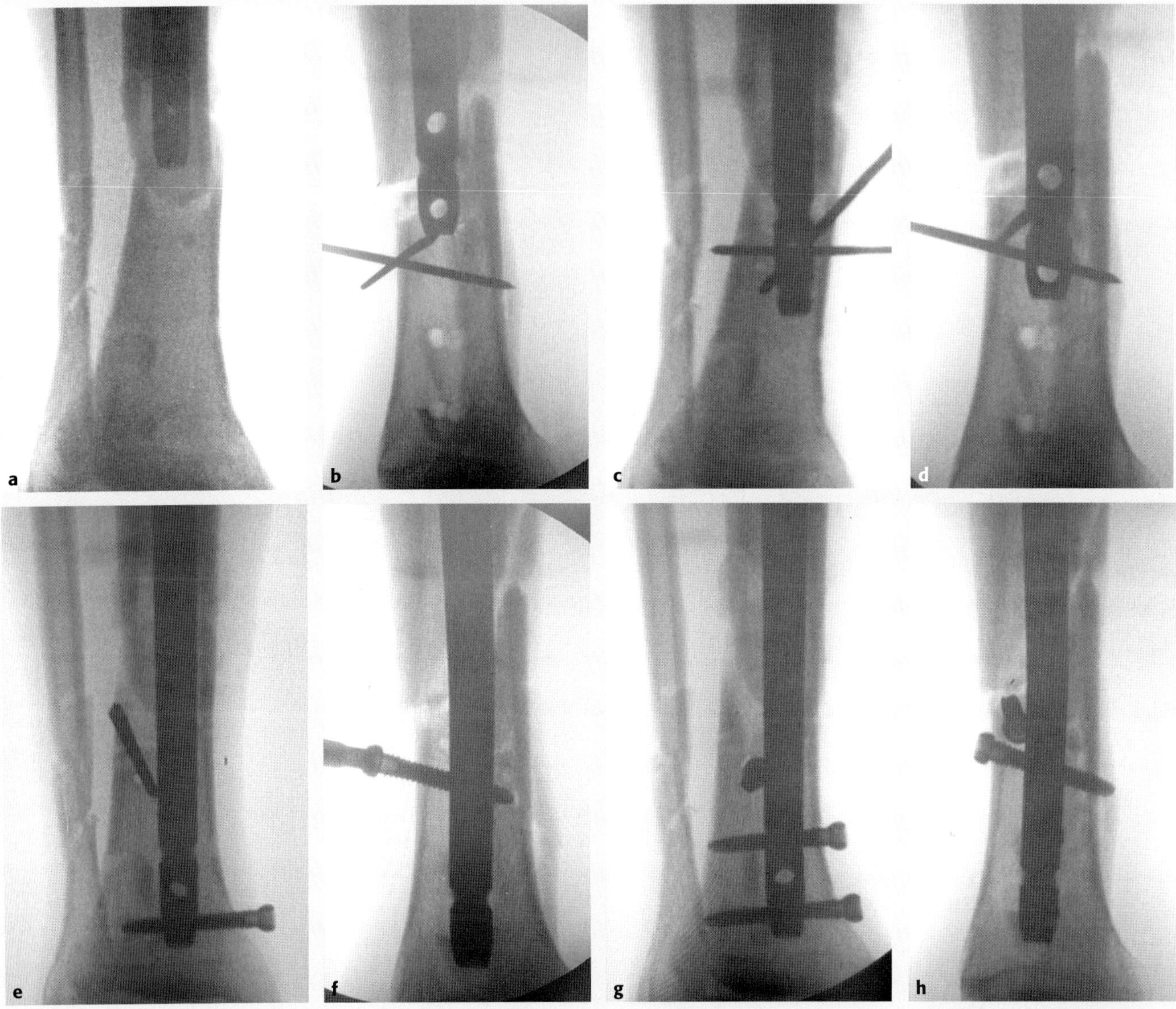

Fig 7.1-8a–h Intraoperative C-arm images showing the original nails after partial extraction.
a–b AP and lateral views.
c–d AP and lateral views.
e–f AP and lateral views.
g–h AP and lateral views.

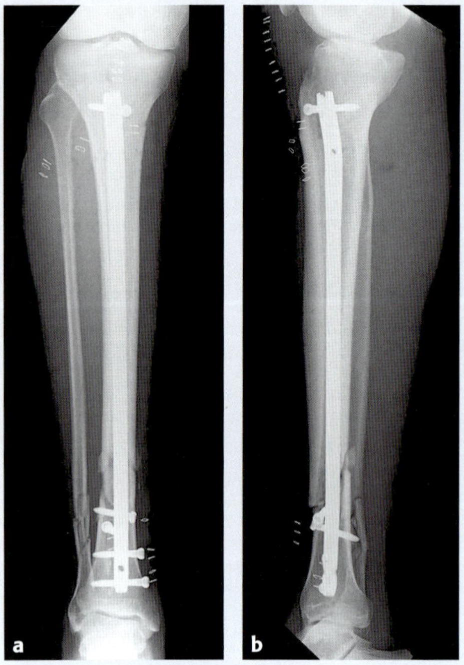

Fig 7.1-9a–b AP (**a**) and lateral (**b**) control x-rays of the tibia in the immediate postoperative period following reintervention.

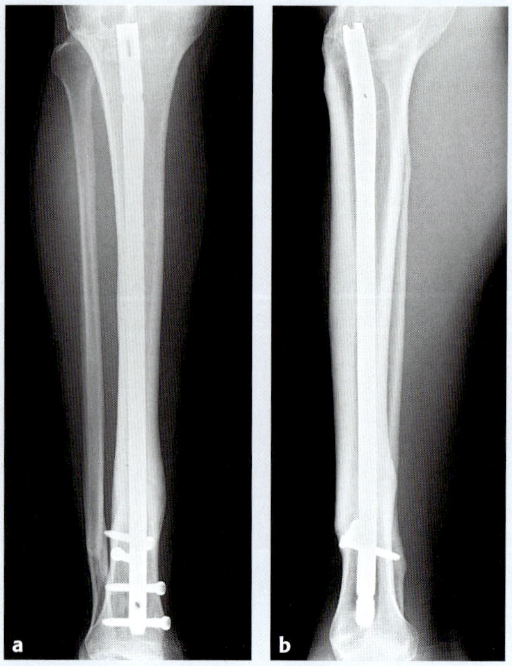

Fig 7.1-10a–b Final AP (**a**) and lateral (**b**) control x-rays of the tibia.

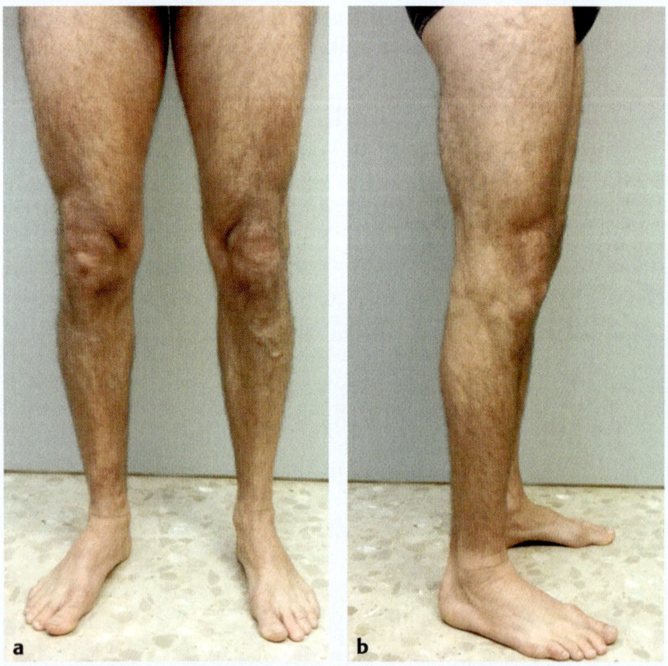

Fig 7.1-11a–b Final clinical photographs showing a good outcome.

Analysis of failure and reflection

The tibial fractures were unstable because the fibula was fractured at the same level. The treatment indication was reamed intramedullary nailing, locked in the proximal and distal zone. Frequently in transverse and oblique tibial fractures, contact of the nail with the intramedullary surface of the proximal and distal fragments ensures the reduction, stability, and dynamic compression along the axial axis when the fracture is subjected to weight bearing. When the fracture is located in the distal diaphyseal zone, the widened intramedullary metaphyseal zone may not come into contact with the nail, and the bone-implant ensemble may be angulated with regard to the axial axis, with the bone fragment displaced and without achieving fracture reduction.

These fractures must be locked in the distal zone to achieve sufficient grip in the widest part of the tibia. Before performing distal fixation with locked intramedullary nails, varus or valgus of the ankle must be prevented to avoid fixing the distal tibial fragment with malalignment. The introduction of the supplementary screws (eg, Poller screws) act as a limit in case the nail has been inserted at an angle; this is a technical tip that surgeons must know and use to help reduce the fracture, avoid the angulated introduction of the nail, and prevent varus or valgus of the ankle. These supplementary screws enable controlled fracture reduction in two planes and are placed before nail insertion, at the side of the nail and perpendicular to the direction in which the nail could move and be displaced in the metaphysis. They allow the channel to be narrowed and increase the stability of the system, reducing any lateral or frontal movement by avoiding angulation and secondary displacement.

If malalignment is detected in the postoperative phase, the deficiency must be recognized and early reintervention should be carried out to achieve the correct reduction and alignment before union takes place.

If the soft tissues are amenable to surgery, anatomical reduction and internal fixation with a traction screw and protection by a molded plate according to the criteria of absolute stability would also be a correct indication of treatment in this type of fracture; in that case weight bearing must be delayed.

Final outcome

The fracture thus reduced and stabilized with control of the axes healed uneventfully, enabling early weight bearing (**Fig 7.1-10** and **Fig 7.1-11**).

CASE 3

Case description

A 45-year-old man fell from a height of 2 m and presented with a subtrochanteric fracture of the right femur. The fracture had an inverted descending intertrochanteric line that was associated with a line in the direction of the greater trochanter and with a posteromedial cortical fragment detachment at the level of the lesser trochanter (AO/OTA 31A3) (**Fig 7.1-12**).

This case was initially treated using a long intramedullary nail with femoral head and neck fixation with two screws through the nail and distal locking with two bolts, one of them in a dynamic position and the other in a static position. The intervention was performed respecting the soft tissues (**Fig 7.1-13**).

The immediate postoperative clinical phase developed satisfactorily, allowing the patient to soon start walking with weight bearing using crutches but presenting pain with weight bearing at the level of the proximal femoral area. The control x-rays showed a discrete lack of contact between the fragments at the fracture site level without signs of radiographic union for up to 3 months (**Fig 7.1-14**).

In this situation and given that pain persisted, it was decided that dynamization of the assembly would be performed by removing the two distal bolts (**Fig 7.1-15a–b**). Radiologically, some compression was observed at the fracture site level, but clinically the pain persisted during rotation and weight bearing, which indicated instability of the assembly (**Fig 7.1-15c**).

Five months after the fracture, it was decided to perform a new intervention to achieve better stabilization and to improve the biological conditions of the site. In the reintervention, the surgeon opened the fracture site through an osteoperiosteal decortication to improve the local biological conditions (**Fig 7.1-16**).

Stabilization was performed with an impacted locking compression hook plate for proximal femur with axial compression and fixation with a locking attachment plate distal to the site and a proximal monocortical screw (**Fig 7.1-17**). During the closure of the surgical site, autogenous bone graft was obtained from the patient's iliac crest and added. Obtaining the autogenous graft should be the first step in the intervention.

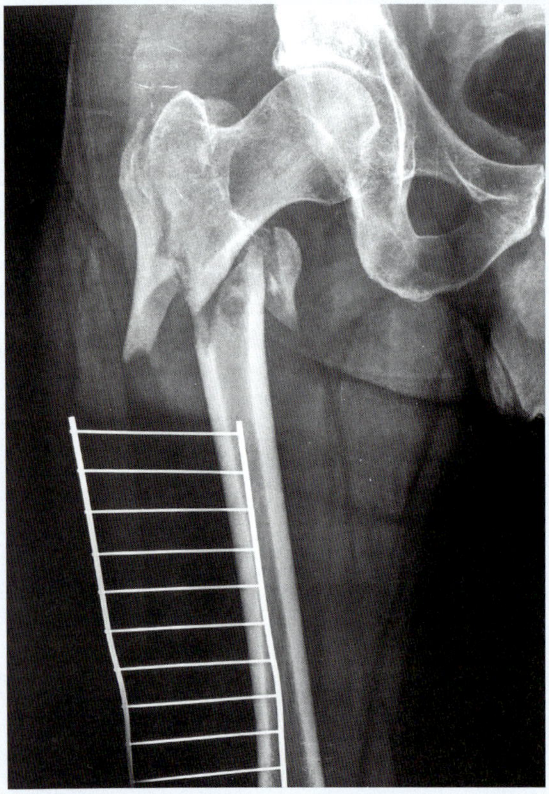

Fig 7.1-12 X-ray of the subtrochanteric right femoral fracture.

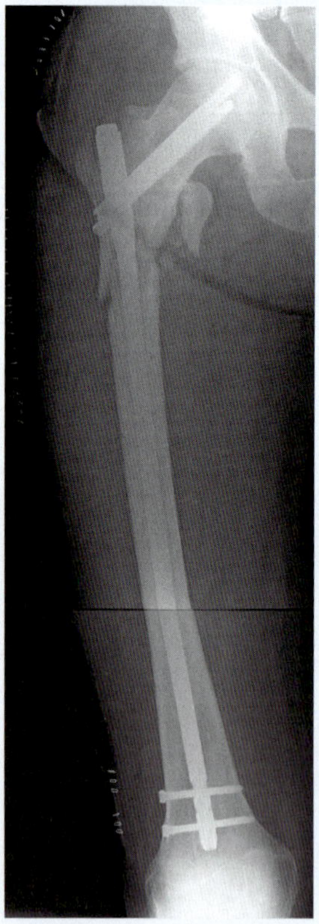

Fig 7.1-13 Immediate postoperative x-ray.

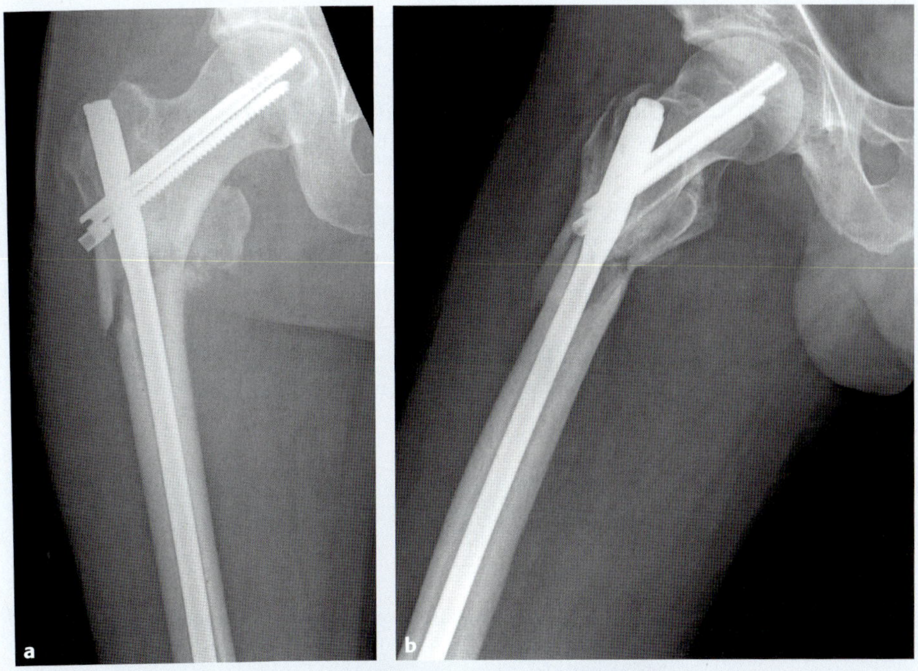

Fig 7.1-14a–b AP (**a**) and axial (**b**) x-rays at 4 months after the surgical intervention.

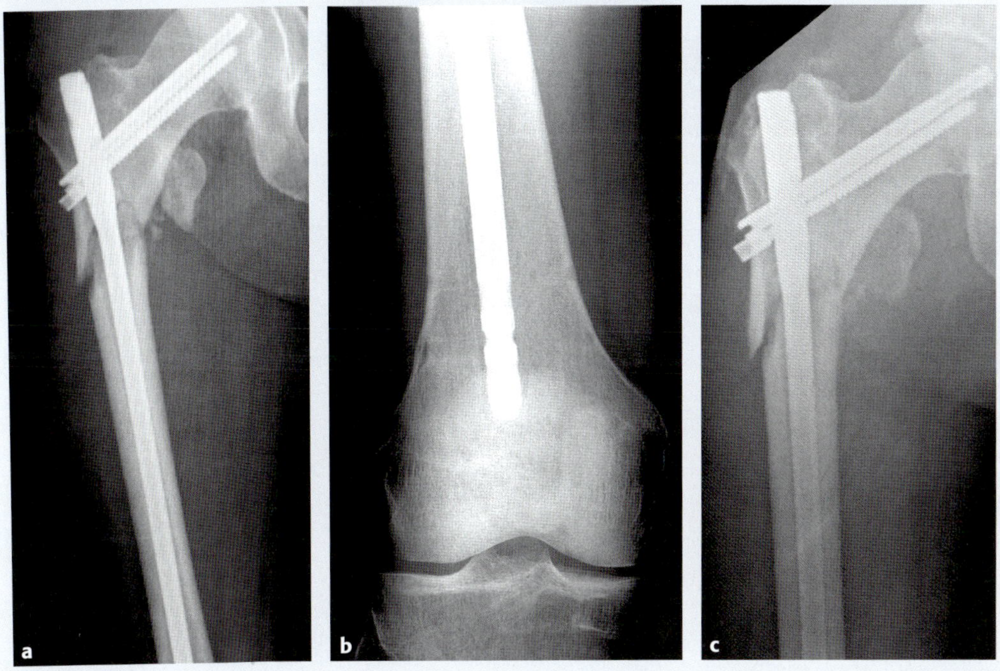

Fig 7.1-15a–c X-rays at 5 months following the intervention.
a Before dynamization, in the distal area of the femur.
b After the removal of the distal bolts.
c The effects of the dynamization can be seen in the proximal femur after weight bearing.

Analysis of failure and reflection

The unstable fracture in the proximal zone of the femur with clear surgical indication can be treated with an extramedullary or intramedullary implant. For biomechanical reasons the implant of choice here was the intramedullary nail, which is associated with femoral head and neck fixation. The intramedullary nail has biomechanical advantages since it is situated closer to the mechanical axis of the femur, reducing the purchase with respect to extramedullary plates, so the load transfer can be more efficient and the material fatigue can be reduced. The fracture is stabilized, and healing usually evolves with the formation of a hard callus.

A good alignment of the femur and, where possible, contact of the bone fragments at the fracture site must be achieved. Reduction of the fragments must be carried out before proceeding to the distal locking of the nail to allow interfragmentary axial compression. If dynamization does not achieve contact between the bone fragments and allow their axial compression, then the friction index on the fracture surface is not increased and the bone does not contribute to its own stability. In this case, the surgeon attempted with dynamization to convert the static stability achieved by the locked nail into dynamic stability, but the compact medullary region of the distal femur did not allow the nail to slide in and the fragments of the fracture to collapse, having also lost rotational stability.

A shorter nail or a less compact bone marrow might have facilitated the nail sinking into the distal zone and also allowed greater impact on the bone fragments and more stability of the fracture site, which could have resulted in fracture union.

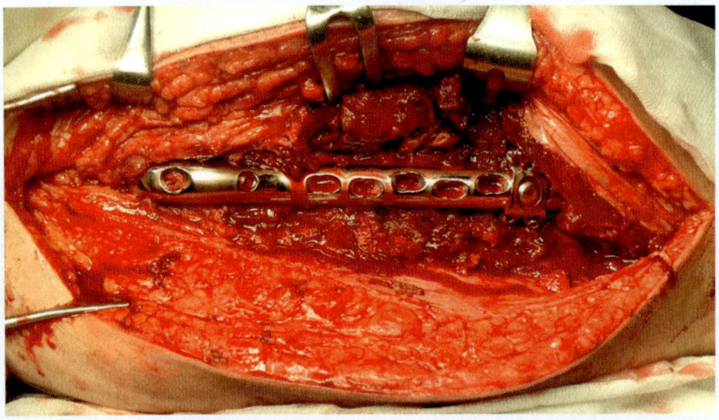

Fig 7.1-16 Intraoperative photograph with hook plate positioned to achieve axial compression and osteoperiosteal decortication at the level of the fracture site.

Final outcome

The clinical evolution improved with progressive reduction of the pain until pain disappeared completely and union with bone callus could be observed on the x-ray (**Fig 7.1-18**).

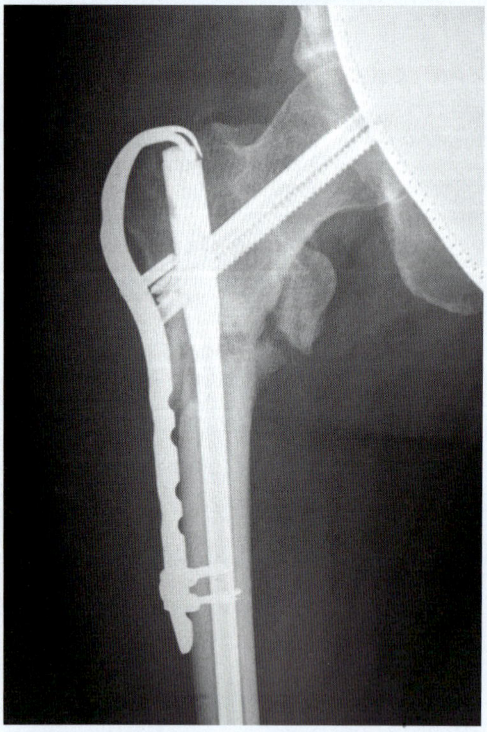

Fig 7.1-17 Postoperative AP control x-ray.

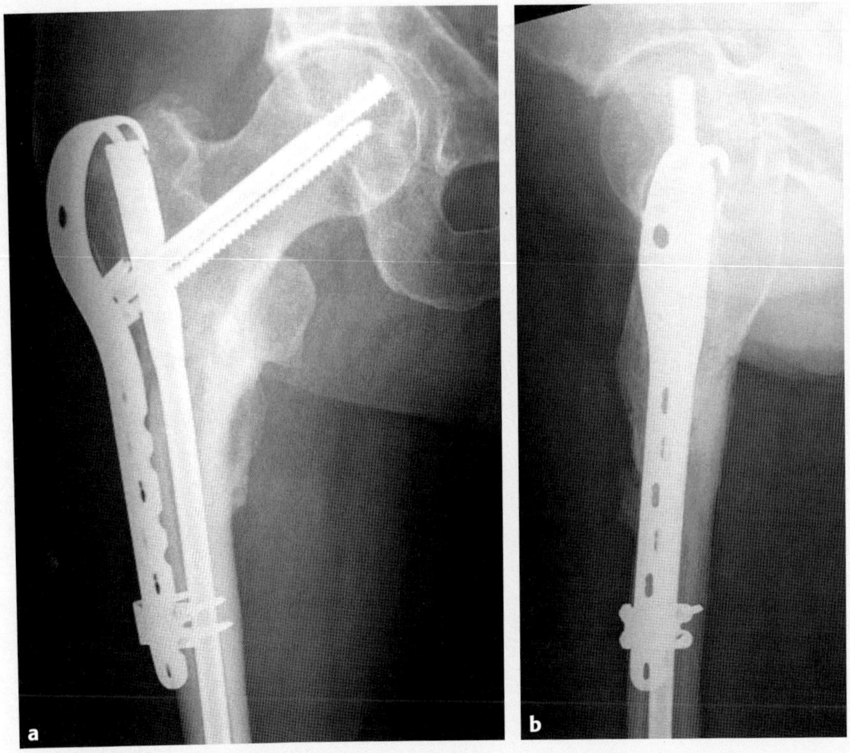

Fig 7.1-18a–b Final control x-rays showing good outcome with evolution of bone callus and fracture union.

Key points to remember

- Clinical assessment and correct preoperative planning are essential.
- Taking postoperative control x-rays and clinical images is very important to detect early failures.
- Signs of osteolysis around the implants indicate stability failures.
- Once the failure has been detected, it is essential to correct and resolve it early.
- The incorrect evolution of the callus consolidation in x-ray series shows the mechanical or biological failures.

References and suggested reading

Gautier E, Sommer C. Guidelines for the clinical application of the LCP. *Injury.* 2003 Nov;34 Suppl 2:B63–76.
Müller ME, Allgöwer M, Schneider R, et al. *Manual of Internal Fixation; techniques recommended by the AO-ASIF Group.* 3rd ed. Allgöwer M, ed. Berlin Heidelberg: Springer-Verlag; 1991.
Orozco Delclós R. *Errores en la Osteosíntesis.* Barcelona: Masson; 1993.
Perren SM. Evolution of the internal fixation of long bone fractures. The scientific basis of biological internal fixation: choosing a new balance between stability and biology. *J Bone Joint Surg Br.* 2002 Nov;84(8):1093–1110.
Rüedi TP, Murphy WM. *AO Principles of Fracture Management.* Stuttgart New York: Thieme; 2000.
Wagner M, Frigg R. *Internal Fixators—Conepts and Cases Using LCP and LISS.* New York: Thieme; 2006.

Section 8

The learning circle

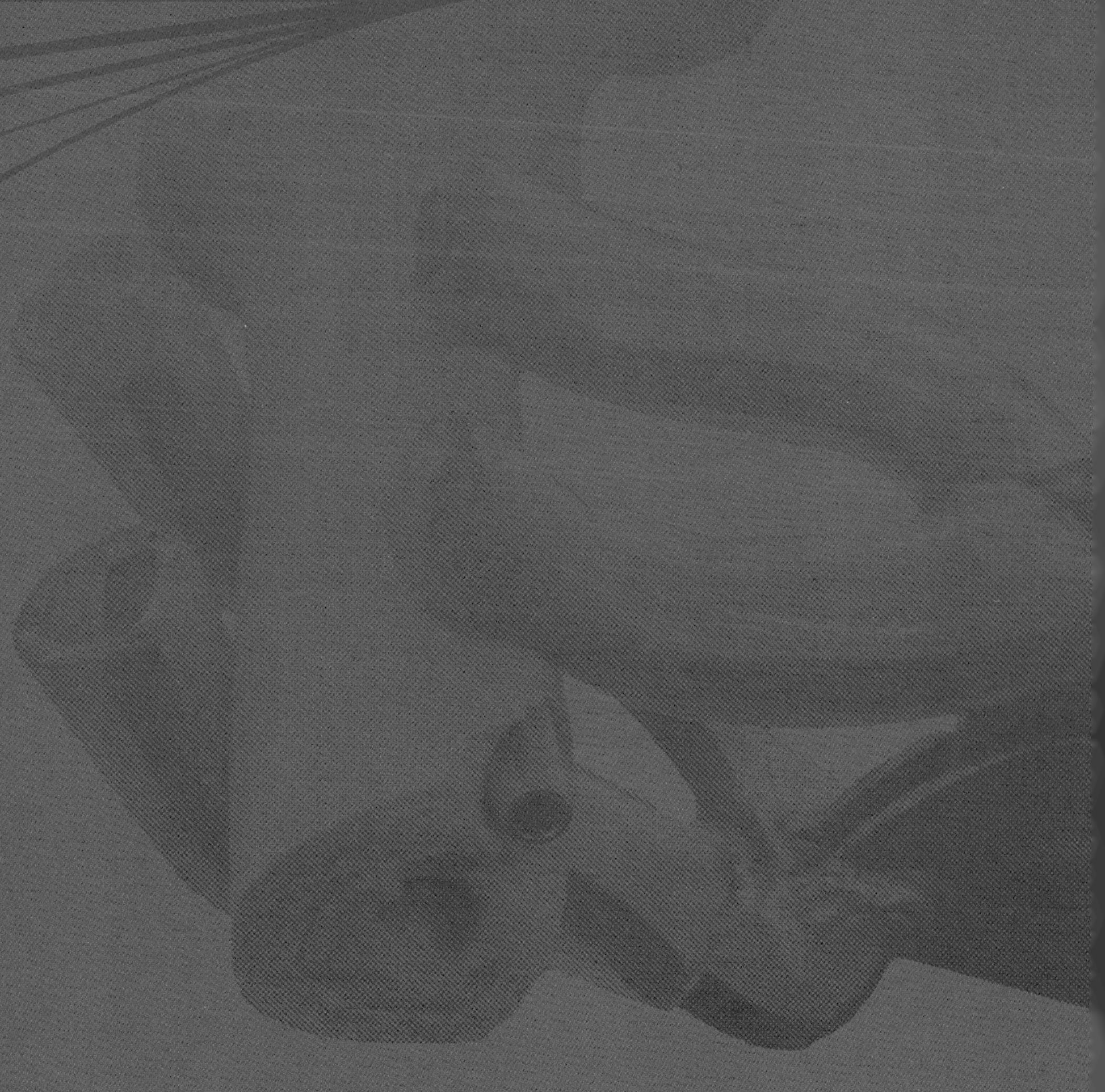

Section 8
The learning circle

8.1 The learning circle: tips and tricks to minimize failures

Jaime Quintero

To anticipate, recognize, and understand mistakes is the principle of wisdom.

Maurice E Müller [1993]

Preamble, context, and definitions

Over the past decades, errors and complications in medical practice have been a matter of extensive research covering all aspects of their causes, management, costs, and outcomes. Currently, society assumes that progress in medicine and the appearance of new technologies will decrease complications of illness and disease and that if complications occur, they probably arise from errors and misconduct from the medical side (ie, general, orthopedic, and trauma surgeons, as well as medical doctors). The abundance of information available publicly (eg, online) regarding specific cases and the media attention to specific cases have made these situations more relevant and usually have a negative impact on surgeons and healthcare providers.

In the fields of orthopedics and traumatology in particular, these aspects have received little attention in medical schools and in training program curricula. In many instances, product training activities by the medical industry have become more relevant than teaching the principles and basic science behind operative and nonoperative management of trauma and deformities (diseases) of the musculoskeletal system. When treating a case, surgeons tend to select an implant without considering the whole decision-making process which includes understanding the type of injury, the energy involved, the soft-tissue injuries, the patient, the associated injuries, and possible complications from the "first hit", ie, the injury itself.

Students, residents, and fellows must have a good understanding of patient safety programs while universities, healthcare providers, hospitals, and scientific societies have the obligation to support continuous medical education programs to provide learners with correct understanding and proper definitions of the different terms used in the current literature and hospital routine. Errors, complications, adverse events, and their consequences for patient safety must become part of the learning process. We must provide the highest possible rate of successful outcomes to achieve good safety.

As noted by Grober and Bohnen [2005], medicine is beginning to benefit from interdisciplinary and collaborative efforts between the healthcare sector and safety-critical industries such as the aviation industry and others with well-established record keeping and analysis of errors. Terms such as "incidents" and "accidents" express medicine's "near misses", "adverse events", and "failures" well. Whether human error or a disease-related complication caused an adverse event can be critical for administrative or legal consequences. A combined paper by medical and aviation experts [Münzberg et al, 2018] has shown that implementing a safety culture means more than just following important checklists. Interhuman behavior, ie, relationship between humans, might result in avoiding or facilitating hazardous situations. Human factors such as time pressure, deficient communication skills, staff shortages, stress, excessive demands, and poor teamwork need to be considered in the medical safety culture.

Walshe [2000] has summarized the definitions of adverse events by different health researchers and the three different key characteristics:

- Negativity: is an undesirable, untoward, or detrimental event to the healthcare process or to the patient.
- Patient involvement/impact: it must involve or have some negative impact on a patient with potential of harm. Some restricted definitions include events where the patient has suffered some definable and identifiable ill effect from the event.

- Causation: the event is a result of some part of the healthcare process (either through commission or omission).

Medical errors have had a broad spectrum of definitions over the years and the lack of a standardized nomenclature has led to multiple and overlapping definitions. The reader can find a thorough analysis of the different definitions and surrogate terms in the paper by Grober and Bohnen [2005].

According to the World Health Organization [2016], there are now more than 26 terms used for "medical error". However, they recommend using the definition by the United States National Coordinating Council for Medication Error Reporting and Prevention [2015]:

> Any preventable event that may cause or lead to inappropriate medication use or patient harm while the medication is in the control of the health care professional, patient, or consumer. Such events may be related to professional practice, health care products, procedures, and systems, including prescribing, order communication, product labelling, packaging, and nomenclature, compounding, dispensing, distribution, administration, education, monitoring of use.

We can easily extrapolate the different terms of this definition to our trauma and orthopedic practice, such as "healthcare products" = implants, "procedures" = operative techniques, "systems" = indication of different options and treatment modalities, "education" = acquisition and transfer of knowledge of the scientific basis of sound, proven and well-established principles and techniques. One could also classify errors based on the action plans (knowledge-based or rule-based errors) or errors in the execution. Additionally, and particularly in the field of trauma and orthopedics, errors can be classified according to violation of the well-established principles, namely errors in indication or in surgical technique, a wrong approach, the positioning of an implant in a nonreduced fracture, errors in dimension, type, and biomechanical function of the implant, and lack of stability with early loosening and failure with delayed or nonhealing of the fracture site.

A strong culture of safety will have a great impact in adverse events, failures, and complications. It will promote better communication, trust, and less risky behavior. Education in this context is paramount.

In the emergency department

One of the biggest problems in fracture care that may lead to disastrous consequences for patients and legal action for surgeons is the undiagnosed or "hidden" injury. Undiagnosed fractures, complex ligamentous injuries, or combined skeletal and severe soft-tissue injuries are often missed while first examining the patient in hospital, and often some of these injuries are diagnosed after the patient is discharged. The polytrauma patient with multiple skeletal injuries is an example. Often, emergency departments are crowded, residents and staff are overloaded with daily strenuous routine work, and a senior surgeon may be unavailable. Injuries that are frequently overlooked in the emergency department are, among others, posterior dislocation of the shoulder, scapular fractures, cervical fracture dislocations, sternoclavicular dislocations, femoral neck fractures associated with high-energy femoral shaft fractures, posterior dislocation of the knee, associated posterior malleolar fracture with tibial shaft fractures, syndesmotic injuries, and elbow dislocation associated with radial head fractures. In high-energy trauma, the neurovascular structures must be addressed, and repeated clinical examination of the injured limb is necessary during the resuscitation phase.

In our experience, one of the most frequent errors is inadequate reporting in the medical records of the general condition of the patient and/or of a complete and accurate medical examination with the description of the injuries, including the neurovascular status. In comatose patients it may be difficult to assess nerves and specific function of an extremity, but this must be recorded, and a thorough examination conducted later. Communicating with and informing the patient and relatives is essential to create an atmosphere of trust and confidence. Detailed explanation of the medical condition and further discussions must also be recorded.

The value of fellowships and mentorship during the learning process

Like other organizations, hospitals, and institutions, the AO group recognized the value of education and training by mentorship a long time ago and has a long tradition of offering short- and long-term fellowship programs to trainee surgeons where they can join a well-trained team of surgeons at renowned universities and/or institutions. This offers the trainee surgeon an opportunity to establish a unique personal relationship that, if it endures over time, evolves from one where the information flows mostly from mentor to trainee into a long-lasting friendship with a mutual exchange of information. The mentor imparts wisdom, shares knowledge, inspires and teaches the fellow, and most significantly shares her or his experience in prevention and early diagnosis of errors and complications and how to avoid them. This may of course also happen at the residency stage, but the fact that the fellow is adapting to a new environment while being away from her or his family and personal daily duties allows time for reflection, analysis, and improvement. Universities, scientific societies, and organizations like the AO need to continuously strive to offer their learners the best educational opportunities to improve their knowledge and skills in the process of identifying the factors that lead to complications, errors, and failures, and their adequate prevention and management. It is also of utmost importance to find emerging talent, like musical schools do, and to find those by the mentoring process who will become the leaders in disseminating this knowledge to the benefit of the patients. This aspect will certainly improve the performance of a trainee surgeon, will enhance her or his skills, knowledge, and understanding of how to deal with more complex cases while avoiding errors.

Preoperative planning, much more than a nice sketch

While literature in recent years has significantly emphasized the value of preoperative planning [Mast et al, 1989], one should bear in mind that planning does not just mean drawing a nice sketch showing the expected end result.

Trainee and even experienced surgeons often tend to look at an x-ray in the emergency department and then decide to apply the latest implant they saw in a booth at a congress or the one that was presented by an industrial representative in a product training. We have observed that this is common practice not just in the decision-making process in orthopedic trauma cases. When an x-ray of a hip or a knee case that has some degenerative findings is shown to a surgeon, the first question asked is: "Which prosthesis is best for this case?" The patient and their individual needs, such as expectations, level of activity, findings at the clinical examination, deformities, limitations, and pain, are usually not discussed. There is also rarely discussion about whether other treatment modalities may be preferable, such as a preservation procedure, arthroscopy, osteotomy, or just a wait-and-see approach with medication, physical therapy, and changing some habits.

Preoperative planning is an intellectual process which starts with the very first look at the patient. The type of patient, type of injury, quality of bone, conditions of the soft tissue and the neurovascular status are all factors that will determine the initial steps for an appropriate diagnosis and treatment. Appropriate x-ray imaging and computed tomographic scans lead to a proper classification that not only determine the mechanism of injury but also the prognosis based on the complexity of the morphology. The planning continues and will encourage the surgeon to take the first actions, temporary immobilization with an appropriate method while a final decision is being made between modality treatments. As Gawande [2011] points out, paying attention to small details and having clear goals produce excellent results as in all professions. However, the surgeon must also anticipate problems, prepare alternative plans, and be mentally prepared for unexpected events. It has repeatedly been said at medical educational events that failure to plan is planning to fail.

References and suggested reading

Gawande A. *Personal Best. Top athletes and singers have coaches. Should you?* The New Yorker. October 3, 2011.
Grober ED, Bohnen JM. Defining medical error. *Can J Surg.* 2005 Feb;48(1):39–44.
Mast J, Jakob RP, Ganz R. *Planning and reduction technique in fracture surgery.* Berlin: Springer-Verlag; 1989.
Müller ME. Foreword. In: Orozco Delclós R, ed. *Errores en la Osteosíntesis.* Barcelona: Masson; 1993:VIII.
Münzberg M, Russeler M, Egerth M, et al. [Safety Culture in Orthopaedic Surgery and Trauma Surgery—Where Are We Today?]. *Z Orthop Unfall.* 2018 Oct;156(5):579–585. German.
National Coordinating Council for Medication Error Reporting and Prevention. *What is a Medication Error?* New York; 2015. Available at: www.nccmerp.org/about-medication-errors. Accessed October 14, 2018.
Walshe K. Adverse events in health care: issues in measurement. *Qual Health Care.* 2000 Mar;9(1):47–52.
World Health Organization. *Medication Errors: Technical Series on Safer Primary Care.* Geneva: World Health Organization; 2016.

Section 9
Bizarre failures

Section 9
Bizarre failures

9.1 Difficult to classify

Miquel Videla Cés
Joan Girós Torres, Roberto Rivero Sosa, J Miquel Sales Pérez

These are my principles; if you do not like them, I have others.
Groucho Marx

When all aspects of a procedure are done correctly, the results are always similar. But we must bear in mind that conscious learning becomes subconscious knowledge, which does not make surgeons infallible but subject to performing occasional inadvertent errors. Most failures can be explained, as any surgeon throughout their professional career has made or almost made a mistake. In the process of evaluating the failure, the environmental conditions that may have caused the failure are assessed with a certain tolerance. However, there are failures that are difficult to classify and justify from a technical and/or medical point of view. These errors are used to discredit the principles of internal fixation by those who do not follow the principles on purpose. Fortunately, errors are not frequent, but when detected they can be used as an argument for discrediting and disavowing a technique.

From a technical point of view, an unjustifiable error is an error made by a surgeon who does not have proper training and embarks on the adventure of internal fixation without following advice or any recommendations. Unfortunately, this type of failure happens quite frequently. It is often due to surgeons' independent and stubborn personalities and the difficulty in convincing them of the best indication or best technical resource. Improvisation is usually their modus operandi; for example, it is not comparable to an improvisation by a professional jazz musician but rather by a street musician with little training [Orozco Delclós, 1993].

In a surgery, when you act without a sound technical basis and without following the technical principles, you may make serious mistakes. There is a saying about surgeons which is actually meant as a reproof: "Sometimes wrong; never in doubt". That is to say, information is inadequate; the science is ambiguous, one's knowledge and abilities are never perfect. Even in the simplest operation, it cannot be taken for granted that a patient will come through better off. Surgical skills can be taught; tenacity cannot [Gawande, 2002].

The more concerning problem with medical and surgical failures is when they are demonized. Doctors refrain from acknowledging and discussing them publicly. However, it is important to analyze and evaluate the failure. Jeffrey Cooper, the author of *Preventable anesthesia mishaps: a study of human factors. 1978* [Cooper et al, 2002], used a technique called "critical incident analysis" in an effort to learn about factors which contribute to errors. This technique had been used since the 1950s to analyze aviation disasters. Disasters do not occur for no reason. Instead they usually develop during a process. When things go wrong, it is usually because of an accumulation of failures.

The majority of errors that are of varying clinical significance are committed during the inevitable learning curve. This highlights the potential problems with implants, the inaccuracy of the measures, (ie, errors related to the implant dimensions with regard to length and thickness), and the lack of congruence and compatibility between materials, especially in the use of the new generation implants (ie, plates, nails, and screws).

In the weeks after a principles training course, the incidence of failures increases due to the lack of reflection on the basic concepts learned during the course and the implementation of the skills acquired during the practical activities using plastic models. Although very helpful, plastic models differ enormously from clinical practice where factors like surgical approach, the state of the soft tissues, and strict use of the principles play a decisive role.

There are occasional cases that fit not just in one particular category but in several categories of failures, eg, breaching the principles of osteosynthesis, choice of implant, or factors related to the surgical team or patient, which makes grouping them difficult.

Nowadays we can see on the internet samples of unbelievable x-ray results that could be fake surgeries or done by a very inexperienced surgeon as the ones shown in **Fig 9.1-1**, for instance.

Analyzing the critical incident, the author finds it hard to believe that in a hospital where intramedullary nailing is performed, a patient leaves the operating room with a femoral nail as an extramedullary fixator. The editors consider this example as "fake" surgery.

We present two complete cases of a humeral shaft fracture with one part of the intramedullary nail located outside the bone (AO/OTA 12B1) (**Fig 9.1-2**), and in Case 2, rescue surgery involved the extraction of the nail and a reintervention with an extramedullary plate (**Fig 9.1-3**).

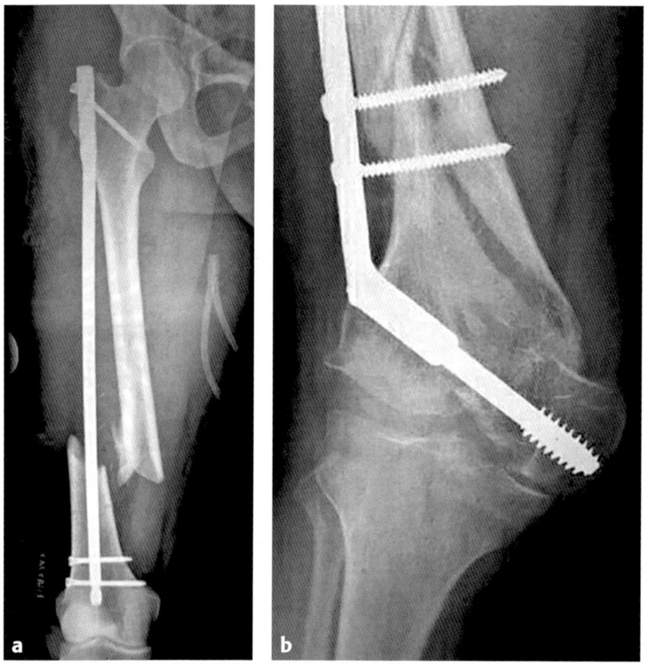

Fig 9.1-1a–b X-rays of distal femoral fractures: real or modified?

- **a** X-ray of an "intramedullary–extramedullary" femoral nail found online.
- **b** X-ray showing a distal femoral fracture treated with a dynamic hip screw (DHS) resulting in a valgus deformity of the axis of the knee. The medial condyle seems to be a proximal femoral allograft. Is this a 'fake' surgery or a surgery difficult to classify?

Miquel Videla Cés
Joan Girós Torres, Roberto Rivero Sosa, J Miquel Sales Pérez

Case description

Humeral shaft fracture treated with an intramedullary nail whose proximal half is outside the bone (**Fig 9.1-2**). Since the humerus is not a weight-bearing bone, 20–30° of misalignment is tolerated without a significant loss of function. Another technical mistake in this case was the excessive length of the proximal locking screw. These failures most likely arose due to the surgeon's inexperience.

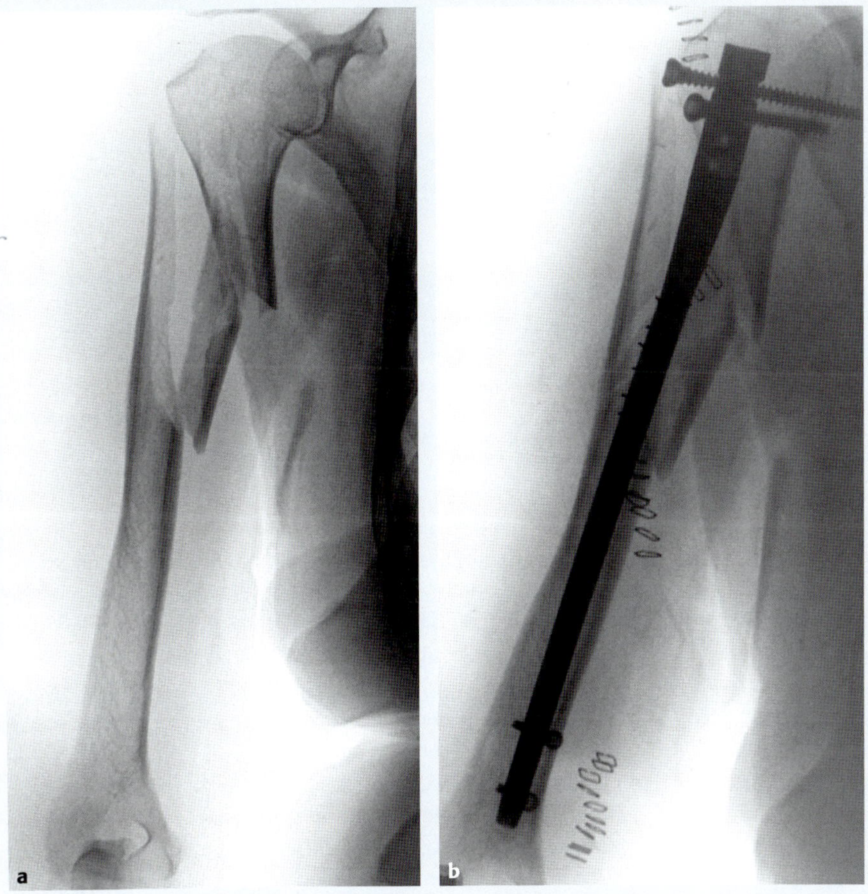

Fig 9.1-2a–b X-rays of a humeral shaft fracture.

CASE 2

Case description

An 80-year-old woman sustained a humeral shaft fracture that was treated with an intramedullary nail whose proximal half was completely outside the bone (AO/OTA 12B) (**Fig 9.1-3**). The locking screws were loose and the patient had pain and a disability. Rescue surgery was performed with a long PHILOS plate to achieve absolute stability and bone healing with a good axis. Bone healing was achieved 3 months after the second surgery. The patient was pain-free and had only a 30% loss of function of the affected limb.

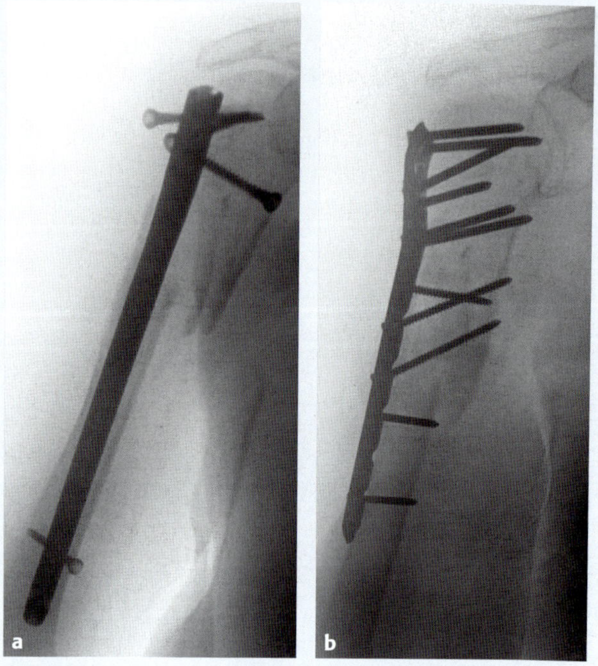

Fig 9.1-3a–b Humeral shaft fracture treated with an intramedullary nail whose proximal half is completely outside the bone (**a**). Rescue surgery was performed with a long PHILOS plate (**b**).

Analysis of failure and reflection

In an attempt to rationalize any error, we have not found any justification for Cases 1 and 2 in which errors or complications were the result of bad technical indication, without applying possible solutions.

Since most errors can probably be corrected by the surgeon who committed them or by another more experienced surgeon with more technical skills, it seems unjustifiable to allow chronic iatrogenesis either through ignorance of the prognosis, indecision, or waiting for nature and time to work wonders, thinking that patients heal despite the surgeon. It is not enough to ask what a surgeon could or should have done differently, but also present solutions so that she or he and also others may learn and succeed next time. The surgeon is often the final actor in a chain of events that has set her or him up to fail. Error experts therefore believe that the process and not the individuals involved in it require closer examination and correction [Gawande, 2002].

In some cases, the result of a surgery may seem, when first analyzed, the most irrational of the failures. We should always try to understand why surgery was done in a particular way, because sometimes the solution chosen, even though different from the norm, may have been the only viable solution given the particular circumstances.

On other occasions, we face multifactorial failures, among which inexperience of the surgeon and the surgical team play a role as well as technical defects and planning. On top of this, we must consider the patient's level of compliance as well as the state of the bone biology and porosity. When the failure is multifactorial, both analysis of the problem and the possible solution are often very limited (**Fig 9.1-4–Fig 9.1-10**).

Miquel Videla Cés
Joan Girós Torres, Roberto Rivero Sosa, J Miquel Sales Pérez

CASE 3

Case description

An 82-year-old man fell from standing height and sustained a simple pertrochanteric fracture with varus displacement (AO/OTA 31A1). In an initial attempt to treat the fracture, an angled blade plate was used, because internal fixation of the fracture was not possible. To solve this treatment failure, a dynamic hip screw (DHS) was chosen, which was a good decision in this case.

Analysis of failure and reflection

The rescue surgery of a simple pertrochanteric fracture with DHS is shown in **Fig 9.1-4**, but the surgeon was involved in a chain of failures: the fracture was not reduced, a wrong entry point was chosen for the barrel of the plate, and the surgeon seemed unaware that a sliding screw specific to the DHS existed. This accumulation of failures can only be attributed to a total ignorance of the technique.

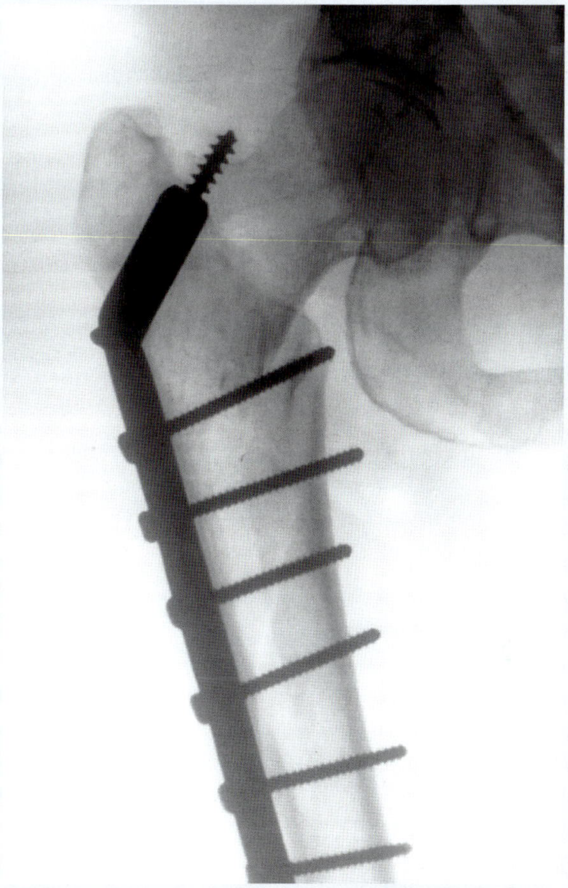

Fig 9.1-4 Attempt at a rescue surgery for a simple pertrochanteric fracture, showing a wrong entry point for a wrong sliding screw, a lack of reduction, and a remaining varus deformity of the fracture.

CASE 4

Case description

Fracture of the intertrochanteric region involving both the major and minor tuberosities.

Analysis of failure and reflection

Emergency surgery was performed by a poorly trained team and in an old-fashioned way using an old extramedullary implant, an angled blade plate, which is nowadays no longer used to treat acute proximal femoral fractures (**Fig 9.1-5**). A synthesis was chosen with an angled blade plate, which is technically very demanding. There was probably no preoperative planning nor were there any intraoperative control x-rays. The fact that the blade of the plate was placed away from the femoral neck, anchoring the implant far from the bony area for which it was designed, and finishing the operation while the bone had not been reduced show a total ignorance of the steps and technical difficulties involved in the correct treatment of this fracture.

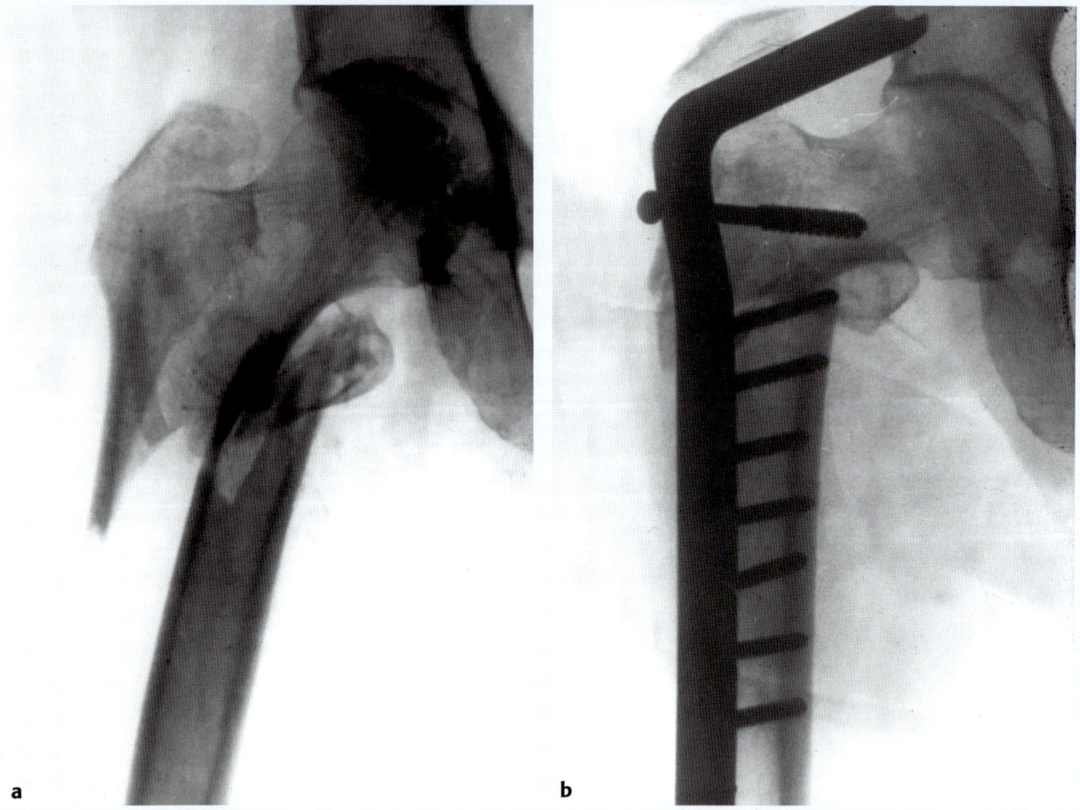

Fig 9.1-5a–b Attempt at internal fixation of an intertrochanteric fracture with an angled blade plate.

Miquel Videla Cés
Joan Girós Torres, Roberto Rivero Sosa, J Miquel Sales Pérez

Case description

The failed treatment of this radial diaphyseal fracture had serious consequences. The surgeon used screws whose heads were smaller than the holes in the plate, and the plate was not molded to fit the anatomical curvature of the radius. Minimal movement of the forearm in the immediate postoperative period resulted in the fracture becoming unstable, the heads of the screws going through the holes in the plate like buttons through buttonholes, and the whole assembly becoming dismantled (**Fig 9.1-6**).

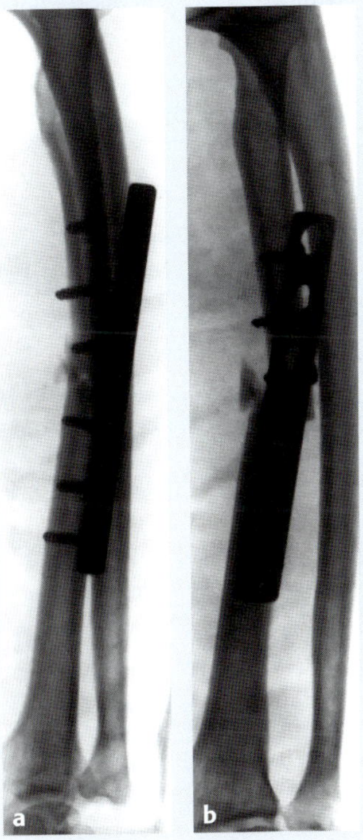

Fig 9.1-6a–b Fracture of the radial diaphysis, treated with a dynamic compression plate 4.5 and 3.5 mm screws.

Analysis of failure and reflection

The responsibility of the failure rests with the surgical team, as it can only be attributed to the surgeons', assistants', and operating room personnel's total ignorance of the implant and how it should be used.

CASE 6

Case description

Comminuted fracture of the patella with bursting of the articular surface. Tension band wiring has become the preferred method of internal fixation for patellar fractures (**Fig 9.1-7**).

Analysis of failure and reflection

The failure in this case was due to the fact that the surgeons did not follow the principle of anatomical reduction of joint surfaces, but instead focused only on the tension band. The tension band is particularly suitable for simple transverse fractures of the patella but not for comminuted patellar fractures, as it is very difficult to maintain the congruence of several small fragments only with K-wires and cerclage wires. The cannulated screws that the surgeon decided to use were also not helpful in maintaining joint reduction of the patellar fracture.

The problem is not the bone healing process, but the appearance of femoropatellar arthritis that is likely to occur in the medium term.

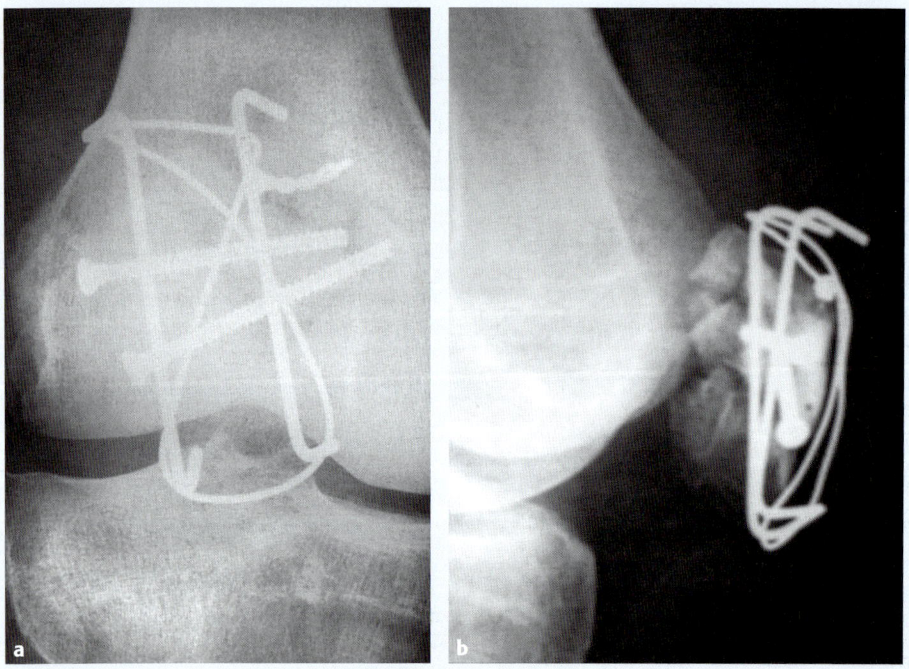

Fig 9.1-7a–b Tension band wiring of the unreduced patella.

Miquel Videla Cés
Joan Girós Torres, Roberto Rivero Sosa, J Miquel Sales Pérez

Case description

A male patient fell from a height of about 2 m onto his feet, sustaining a simple intraarticular metaphyseal fracture of the tibial pilon (**Fig 9.1-8a–b**).

The fracture was treated with open reduction and minimal internal fixation. The aim was to restore the ankle joint, which was achieved satisfactorily (**Fig 9.1-8c–d**).

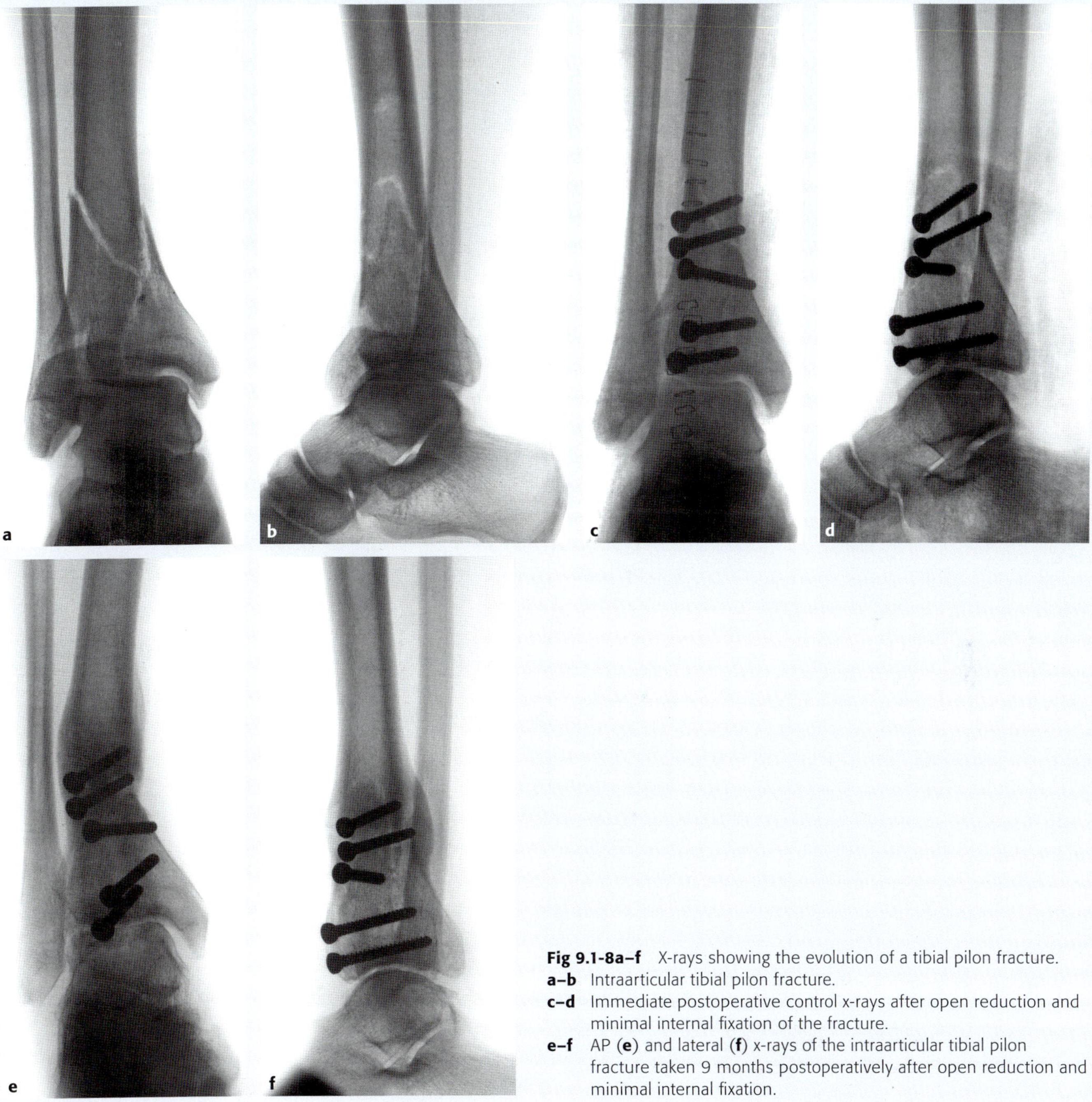

Fig 9.1-8a–f X-rays showing the evolution of a tibial pilon fracture.
a–b Intraarticular tibial pilon fracture.
c–d Immediate postoperative control x-rays after open reduction and minimal internal fixation of the fracture.
e–f AP (**e**) and lateral (**f**) x-rays of the intraarticular tibial pilon fracture taken 9 months postoperatively after open reduction and minimal internal fixation.

Analysis of failure and reflection

The analysis of the case shows that the surgeon did not use cancellous bone screws for the osteosynthesis of the joint segment, which may have been due to a lack of knowledge about the existence of screws with thread pitch for cancellous bone. Nor did she or he use any other implant to fix the joint segment to the diaphyseal segment. The immediate postoperative x-ray showed a good congruence of the articular surface with a good axis of the tibia, but the weight pressing down on the soft and unstable, ie, immature or fibrous, callus as a result of lack of fixation caused a consolidation of the tibial axis in varus malalignment as seen in the 9-month postoperative control x-rays (**Fig 9.1-8e–f**). The presence of an irritating hypertrophic callus in the diaphyseal and metaphyseal areas is a reflection of the instability of the fracture despite having direct reduction performed using a long surgical incision.

Minimum stability required in a fracture should be achieved with the minimum amount of essential material, which is not synonymous with a minimum number of implants if they do not offer the required stability for the correct consolidation of the fracture site.

The surgeon acted more like a carpenter than a qualified technician who should have known the material and understood the principles of internal fixation very well.

Miquel Videla Cés
Joan Girós Torres, Roberto Rivero Sosa, J Miquel Sales Pérez

Case description

The x-rays without clinical background information were provided by AOTrauma Latin America. Inexplicably, the proximal half of the ulna was fixed to the distal half of the radius, leaving the distal ulnar fragments and the proximal radial fragments unconnected and on each side of the newly formed bone (**Fig 9.1-9**).

The authors consider this to be a severe open injury and they must assume that the surgeon had particular reasons to perform this shocking surgery. The result shows that the patient was unable to make a pronation/supination movement and the elbow could be flexed only at the expense of the ulnar insertion of the anterior brachialis muscle.

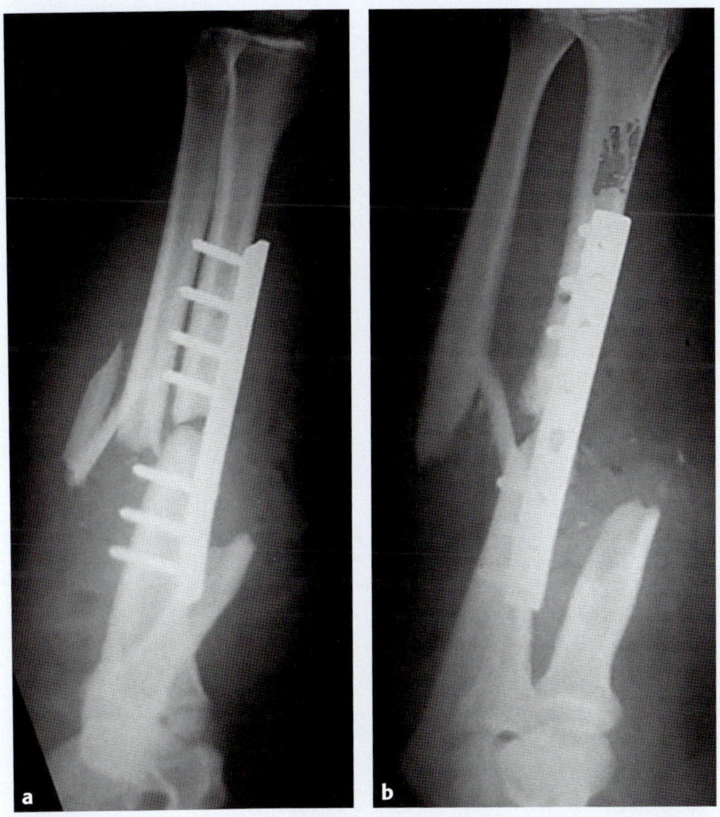

Fig 9.1-9a–b Internal fixation of the proximal half of the ulna to the distal half of the radius. This could be the perfect forearm arthrodesis or an unclassifiable and crazy internal fixation.

Analysis of failure and reflection

The authors do not know if any serious soft-tissue problems forced the surgeon to make this surgical decision. If not, and although they cannot classify the type of failure, they can only assume that a lack of knowledge of the topographical anatomy and of the functional and physiological basis of the upper extremity is likely to have been the reason.

CASE 9

Case description

An 84-year-old woman with high comorbidity and cognitive impairment sustained a pertrochanteric fracture. She was treated with a dynamic hip screw (DHS) and transferred to a nursing home. She was readmitted to the emergency department after suffering a casual fall with a serious deformity, pain in the right leg, and an inability to walk.

The x-rays (**Fig 9.1-10**) showed a catastrophic situation with a loss of fracture reduction and complete loosening of the implant. The severe failure presented by the patient implied a multifactorial etiology.

We must be very clear that elderly patients with high comorbidity and cognitive impairment cannot make any kind of functional commitment, so the patient ambulated without assistance or supporting aids, and without any protection.

The complete disassembly of the DHS and the removal of the plate and all screws from the cortex showed not only that the patient had severe osteoporosis, but also the technique of drilling and screwing was deficient, probably because drills with a diameter larger than needed for the 4.5 mm cortex screws were used.

We must also take into account that the nursing home staff could have contributed more to preventing new falls in this frail patient.

"Disasters do not simply occur, they evolve."

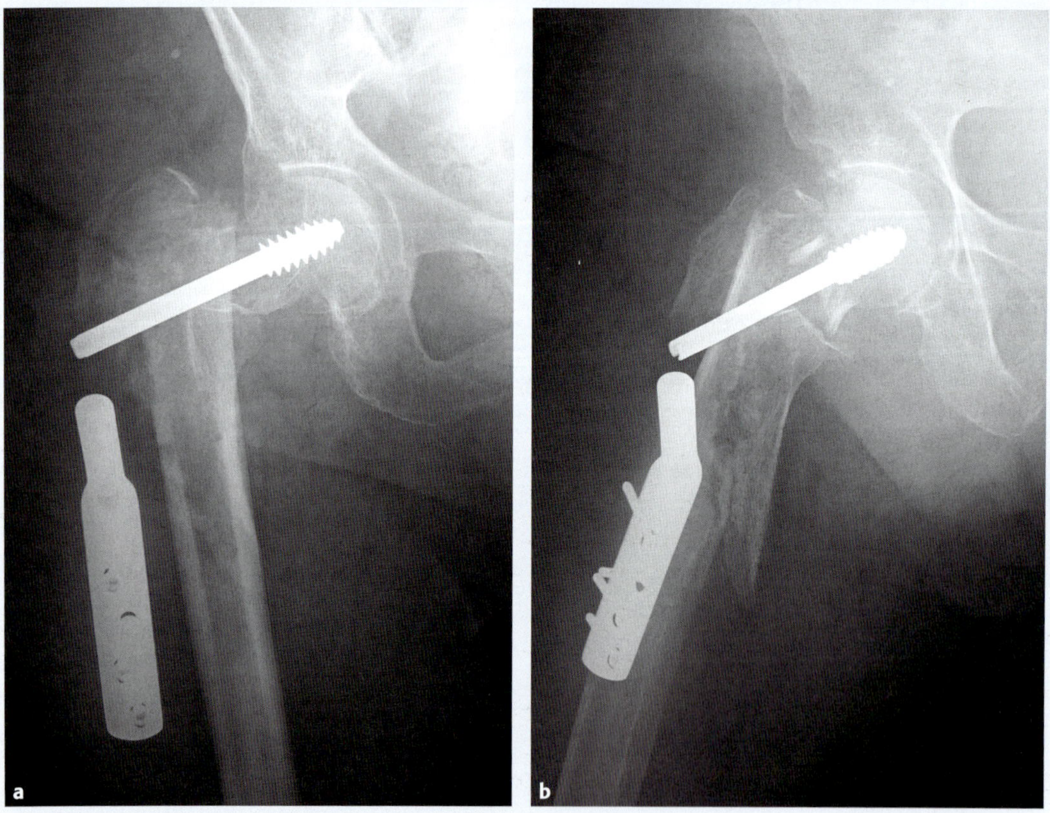

Fig 9.1-10a–b Dynamic hip screw failure.

Analysis of failure and reflection

This unfortunate case summarizes the multifactorial etiology of failure. The biomechanical factors of the implant and the choice of implant itself in relation to the anatomical and biomechanical characteristics of the fracture played an important role, as well as the psychological deterioration and biology of the patient. Also, the surgical and technical defects as well as the lack of control and prevention of new falls may have been decisive.

As all these cases have shown, failures usually have detrimental consequences for the patient and should therefore be prevented. However, failures also teach surgeons a lesson, which helps them improve (**Fig 9.1-11**).

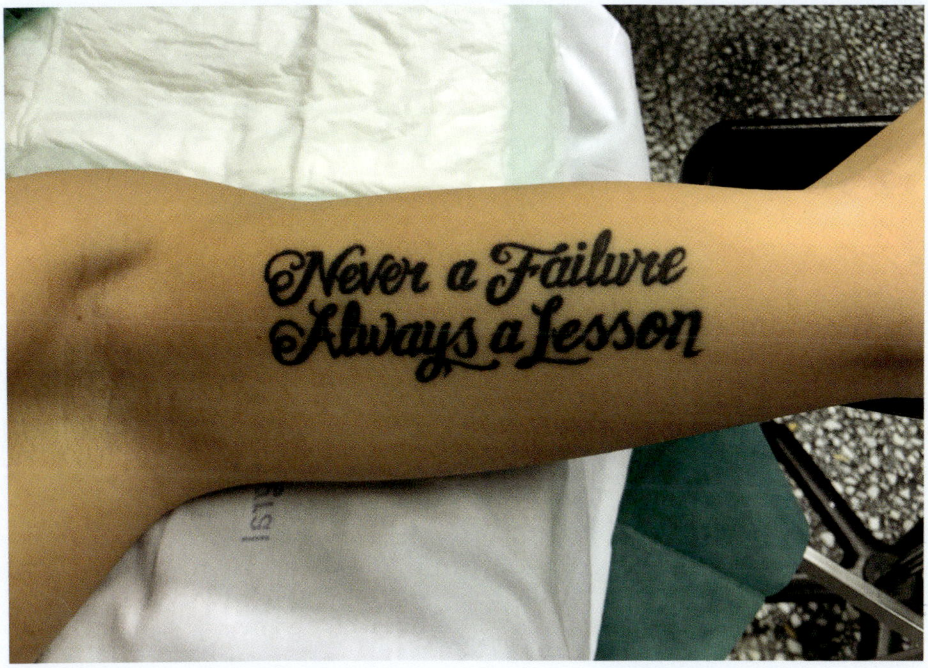

Fig 9.1-11 Lesson learned.

References and suggested reading

Cooper JB, Newbower RS, Long CD, et al. Preventable anesthesia mishaps: a study of human factors. 1978. *Qual Saf Health Care.* 2002 Sep;11(3):277–282.

Gawande A. Education of a Knife. In: Gawande A, ed. *Complications: a surgeon's notes on an imperfect science.* New York: Metropolitan Books; 2002:11–34.

Gawande A. When Doctors Make Mistakes. In: Gawande A, ed. *Complications: a surgeon's notes on an imperfect science.* New York: Metropolitan Books; 2002:47–74.

Orozco Delclós R. Errores injustificables. In: Orozco Delclós R, ed. *Errores en la Osteosíntesis.* Barcelona: Masson; 1993:190–191. Spanish.

Appendix

Glossary

AO/OTA Fracture and Dislocation Classification

Gustilo-Anderson Classification of Open Fractures

Glossary

Glossary

The glossary provides the working definitions for terms that have been used by authors within the book. We hope that the glossary will help readers to understand the text and also be useful for surgeons taking postgraduate examinations.

abduction	Movement of a part, in the coronal plane, away from the midline.
absolute stability	See stability, absolute.
aiming device	A device to guide a wire, or a drill bit, into the correct direction.
allograft	Bone, or tissue, transplanted from one individual to another individual of the same species.
anatomical position	The reference position of the body: standing facing the observer, with the palms of the hands facing forwards.
anatomical reduction	Reinstatement of the exact prefracture shape of the bone.
antibiotic	Any biologically derived drug, or naturally occurring substance, that can inhibit the growth of, or destroy, microorganisms.
arthrodesis	Fusion of a joint by bone as a planned outcome of a surgical procedure.
articular fracture	The entire articular block is separated from the diaphysis.
articular fracture, multifragmentary	A fracture in which part of the joint is depressed and there are more than one articular fracture fragments.
articular fracture, partial	Only part of the joint is involved in the fracture, while the remainder remains attached to the diaphysis. There are several varieties.
augmentation	Surgical procedure for the controlled reinforcement with Traumacen V + cement (55% ceramics components, 45% PMMA) introduced through the implant in severe osteoporotic fractures of the proximal femur and humerus.
augmentation plate	See wave plate.
autograft	A graft of tissue from one site to another within the same individual.
bicortical screw	A screw that gains purchase in both the near cortex and the far cortex.
biological internal fixation	A technique of biologically respectful surgical exposure, fracture reduction, and fixation, which favors the preservation of the blood supply at the fracture site and, thereby, optimizes the healing potential of the bone and soft tissues.
bone graft	Bone removed from one skeletal site and placed into another. Bone grafts are used to stimulate bone union (osteoinduction) and also to restore skeletal continuity where there has been bone loss—see allograft, autograft.
bone healing	See healing.
bone resorption	Removal of bone by osteoclasts. This is an integral element of bone remodeling, either during normal bone turnover, growth, or after fracture. Pathological removal of bone by activated osteoclasts and giant cells occurs if bone is dead, when bone is infected, and around implants where there is excessive movement.
bone substitute	Nonosseous biological, or inorganic, material that can be used in place of, or to augment, bone graft, in order to fill a defect.

bridging plate — A plate that spans the fracture site and is attached to each main fragment of a multifragmentary fracture, maintaining axial and rotational alignment and length. It is not fixed to, nor does it disturb, the blood supply of intervening fragments.

buttress — A construction that resists axial load by applying force at 90° to the axis of potential deformity.

calcar — Meaning "spur" in Latin, the medial cortex of the femoral neck, proximal to the lesser trochanter, which transmits the majority of the compressive forces generated in the femoral neck during loadbearing (calcar femorale).

callus — A tissue of immature bone and cartilage that is formed at the site of bony repair and which bridges a fracture—see healing, indirect.

cancellous bone — Spongy trabecular bone found mostly at the proximal and distal ends of diaphyseal bones, and the interiors of small bones, such as the carpal and tarsal bones.

combination hole — The plate hole of the locking compression plate (LCP) that consists of two parts: the nonthreaded dynamic compression unit (DCU; shaped like the holes of a dynamic compression plate) and the threaded part which has a reciprocal thread for the engagement of the head of a locking head screw (LHS).

compartment syndrome — Raised pressure in a closed osteofascial compartment that results in local tissue ischemia. It is a true surgical emergency.

complex regional pain syndrome (CRPS) — Neuropathic pain with associated sudomotor and vasomotor disturbances, which develops after trauma, another inciting event, or a period of immobilization of the part. The diagnostic criteria are broad and there are no specific tests for the diagnosis of this condition. There are two types (CRPS I and CRPS II) that have the same signs and symptoms, the difference being that an identifiable peripheral nerve lesion is associated with CRPS II. CRPS is also known as fracture disease, algodystrophy, reflex sympathetic dystrophy, and Sudeck's atrophy.

compression — The act, or effect, of pressing together, usually in order to achieve, or increase, stability.

compression, interfragmentary — Bone fragments are pressed together, either with a lag screw, or a plate, in order to produce absolute stability.

compression screw — See lag screw.

conventional plate — Any plate with smooth holes that can accommodate any unthreaded screw head of matching dimensions.

conventional screw — Any screw with a smooth outer surface of the head (ie, without threads) that is used for fracture, or plate, fixation.

coronal plane — The vertical plane of the body passing from side to side, so that a coronal bisection of the body would cut it into a front half and a back half. Also called the frontal plane.

corrosion — This is an electrochemical process that results in the destruction of metal by the liberation of ionic metal.

cortical bone — The dense bone forming the tubular element of the shaft, or diaphysis (middle part), of a long bone. The term is also applied to the dense, thin shell covering the cancellous bone of the metaphysis.

corticotomy — A special osteotomy where the cortex is surgically divided, but the medullary contents and the periosteum are not injured.

critical strain level — The strain level at which a tissue disrupts or ceases to perform its normal physiological function.

debridement — The surgical excision from a wound injury zone, or area of other pathology, of foreign material and all avascular, contaminated, or infected tissue.

deep infection — Bacterial, or fungal, infection involving fascia and/or muscles and/or bone and/or implants with an associated inflammatory response.

deformation, elastic — A temporary change in length, or shape, of a material that will return to its former state when the deforming force is released.

deformation, plastic — A change in length or shape of a material of such magnitude that it is permanent and will not recover when the deforming force is released.

deformity — Any abnormality of the form of a body part.

delayed union — Fracture healing is not taking place by the expected time that is expected for healing of a particular fracture in a particular patient—see nonunion.

diaphysis — The cylindrical, or tubular, part of a long bone between the metaphyseal ends, often referred to as the shaft.

diastasis screw — A positioning screw that is inserted into the fibula and tibia in order to maintain their normal anatomical relationship at the distal tibiofibular syndesmosis. The screw thread must gain purchase in both bones as compression must not be applied—see position screw.

dislocation — A displacement of a joint such that no part of one articular surface remains in contact with the other articular surface. Sometimes used incorrectly to denote fracture displacement.

displacement — The condition of being out of place. A fracture is displaced if the fragments are not perfectly anatomically aligned.

distal — Away from the center of the body, more peripheral.

dorsal — Pertaining to the back—or dorsum—of the body in the anatomical position. An exception is the foot; the top of the foot, even though it faces forwards in the anatomical position, is called the dorsum.

ductility — The degree of permanent (plastic) deformation that a material tolerates before it breaks. The ductility of a material determines the degree to which an implant, such as a plate, can be contoured without breaking.

dynamic compression plate (DCP) — A plate with chamfered oval holes through which eccentrically placed screws can be inserted to create compression across a fracture site.

dynamic compression unit (DCU) — The nonthreaded part of an LCP combination hole that is shaped like the hole of a dynamic compression plate (DCP).

dynamic locking — When an interlocking screw is inserted into the oval locking hole of an intramedullary nail, it controls rotation and alignment but allows some (controlled) impaction of the fracture during weight bearing—see dynamization.

dynamization — Diverting some or all of the mechanical load away from a fixation device in order to load the fracture site, with a view to enhancing bone formation.

early total care (ETC) — Definitive treatment, in polytrauma patients, of all injuries, including major long-bone fractures, within 24 hours of injury.

epiphysis — The end of a long bone that bears the articular component. The epiphysis develops from the cartilaginous element between the joint surface and the growth plate (physis)—see metaphysis.

external fixation — Skeletal stabilization using pins, wires, or screws that protrude through the skin and are linked externally by bars, or other devices.

extraarticular fracture — The fracture does not involve the articular surface but is within the end segment of a long bone and may be within the joint capsule.

far cortex — The cortex more distant from the operator—see near cortex. Sometimes referred to as the transcortex.

fasciocutaneous flaps — Soft-tissue flaps, based on a perforating artery, which include the skin, the subcutaneous tissues, and the deep fascia.

fasciotomy — The surgical division of the fascial wall of an osteofascial muscle compartment, usually to release high intracompartmental pressure—see compartment syndrome.

fatigue failure If any material is subjected to multiple loading cycles, it may develop microscopic cracks and eventually fail at a stress well below its tensile strength, and often below the yield strength of the pristine material.

fibrocartilage Tissue consisting of elements of cartilage and of fibrous tissue. It is the normal constituent of the menisci of the knee and the triangular fibrocartilage at the wrist. It also forms as a repair tissue after injury to articular cartilage.

fixed-angle device An implant with two or more parts that are solidly connected at a given angle so that it will resist forces tending to angulate one part with respect to the other. Such devices are used to prevent angular displacement of fractures. Fixed angle devices may be manufactured as a single, solid device (eg, 95° angled blade plate), or produced by mechanically coupling two implants (eg, a locking compression plate with a locking head screw).

fracture disease A condition characterized by disproportionate pain, soft-tissue swelling, patchy bone loss, and joint stiffness—see complex regional pain syndrome.

fracture fixation Application of a mechanical device to a broken bone to allow healing in a controlled position and (usually) to facilitate early functional rehabilitation. The surgeon determines the degree of reduction required and the mechanical environment at the fracture locus, which in turn influence the mode of bone healing.

fracture treatment, goal According to Müller et al, the goal of fracture treatment is to restore optimal function of the limb in respect to mobility and load-bearing capacity, while avoiding complications.

fragility fracture A fracture that occurs through bone weakened by osteopenia or osteoporosis during normal daily activities or following a fall from standing height or less.

guide wire A wire inserted into bone to allow precise positioning of a drill, reamer, or implant. The wire can act as a visual aid for the direction of insertion of an instrument, or implant, or can physically direct it, eg, cannulated drill.

Haversian system Cortical bone is composed of a system of small channels (osteons) about 0.1 mm in diameter. Each osteon consists of concentric layers, or lamellae, of compact bone tissue that surround a central canal, the Haversian canal. These channels contain the blood vessels and are remodeled after a disturbance of the blood supply to bone. There is a natural turnover of the Haversian system by continuous osteonal remodeling; this process is part of the dynamic and metabolic nature of bone. It is also involved in the adaptation of bone to an altered mechanical environment.

healing The biological process that returns an injured part to its preinjury condition. Bone healing is regarded as complete when bone has regained normal stiffness and strength.

healing, contact One form of direct bone healing that occurs between two fragments of bone maintained in motionless contact (absolute stability). The fracture is repaired by direct osteonal remodeling.

healing, direct It is observed following internal fixation with absolute stability. It is characterized by the absence of callus; there is no resorption of bone at the fracture site. Bone forms by osteonal remodeling without intermediate repair tissue, the osteons proceeding directly across the fracture contact areas. Direct fracture healing was formerly called primary healing.

healing, gap One form of direct bone healing in which there is absolute stability, but a very small gap remains between the fracture fragments. Lamellar bone forms in the gap and is then remodeled by penetrating osteons.

healing, indirect Bone healing by callus formation in fractures treated either with relative stability or left untreated.

hook plate A plate that is bent so that it captures a fracture fragment, which can then be reduced by applying tension to the plate. The hook can be part of a specially designed plate for a specific anatomical site or improvised by cutting and bending the end of a conventional plate.

impacted fracture A fracture in which the opposing bony surfaces are driven into each other, with the effect that they behave as a single unit. This is a combined clinical and radiological diagnosis.

Injury Severity Score (ISS)
An anatomical scale that was developed to ascribe a numerical value to the extent and severity of trauma in patients with injuries to multiple systems. The highest abbreviated injury scale, or AIS, (range 0 to 5) is calculated for a maximum of three systems (eg, head trauma, musculoskeletal trauma, abdominal injuries). Each AIS is then squared and the three squared scores added together to calculate the ISS (maximum = 3 x 5^2 = 75)—see polytrauma.

interlocking screw
Also called (inter)locking bolt. It couples an intramedullary nail to the bone to maintain length and alignment, and to control rotation.

internal fixator/infix
Mechanical device that remains deep to the skin and bridges a fracture zone—similar to external fixation—providing an angularly locked, extramedullary splint resulting in relative stability. This can be achieved with an LCP or LISS.

intertrochanteric fracture
A fracture of the proximal femur that passes between the greater and lesser trochanters.

ischemia
Reduction in blood flow resulting in tissue hypoxia.

lag screw
A screw that passes across a fracture plane through a glide hole in the near fragment, to grip the opposite fragment in a threaded hole, thereby producing interfragmentary compression when it is tightened.

LC-DCP
See limited-contact plate.

LCP
See locking plate and internal fixator.

less invasive stabilization system (LISS)
See locking plate and internal fixator.

limited-contact plate
A plate designed to limit contact with the underlying bone, which preserves the maximum possible periosteal blood supply. The most common variety is the limited-contact dynamic compression plate (LC-DCP).

locking attachment plate (LAP)
Block plate that overlaps the LCP system for large fragments. Indicated in periprosthetic and intramedullary peri-implant fractures. The screws placed through the lateral arms of the plate offer the possibility of avoiding the intramedullary implant obtaining a solid fixation in cortical bone being an alternative to the cables.

locking compression plate (LCP)
See locking plate and internal fixator.

locking head screw (LHS)
A screw with a thread cut into its head, providing a mechanical coupling, or linkage, to a compatibly threaded screw hole in a plate, thereby creating a fixed-angle combination device.

locking plate
A plate with threaded screw holes that allow mechanical coupling to a locking head screw (LHS). The less invasive stabilization system (LISS) and locking compression plates (LCPs) have combination holes that will accept either conventional screw heads or threaded screw heads.

malunion
Fracture healing in a position of deformity.

Masquelet technique
A method for managing acute bone defects by stabilizing a fracture and then filling the bone defect with acrylic cement. After 6–8 weeks a vascular biomembrane forms between the cement and the related tissues. Second-stage surgery then removes the cement but preserves the biomembrane. Autogenous bone graft is used to replace the cement and growth factors produced by the biomembrane promote incorporation of the graft and fracture healing.

metaphysis
In the adult, this is the segment of a long bone located between the articular surface and the shaft. It consists mostly of cancellous bone within a thin cortical shell.

minimally invasive osteosynthesis (MIO)
Any fracture fixation undertaken using small skin incisions and designed to limit surgical trauma to the deeper soft tissues. Examples include percutaneous K-wiring, external fixator and "closed" intramedullary nailing, as well as minimally invasive plate osteosynthesis (MIPO).

minimally invasive plate osteosynthesis (MIPO)	Reduction and fixation with a plate of any design, without direct surgical exposure of the fracture site, using small skin incisions and subcutaneous or submuscular insertion of the plate.
minimally invasive surgery (MIS)	Any surgical procedure undertaken using small skin incisions. Examples include laparoscopic abdominal surgery, arthroscopy, MIPO, and "closed" intramedullary nailing.
monocortical screw	A screw that purchases only in the near cortex.
multifragmentary fracture	A fracture with more than one fracture plane so that there are three, or more, pieces. The proximal and distal fragments will not have direct contact following anatomical reduction. The term is used in the AO/OTA Fracture and Dislocation Classification as a fracture type.
negative-pressure wound therapy (NPWT)	See vacuum-assisted wound closure.
near cortex	The cortex nearer the operator and on the side of insertion of an implant: sometimes called the cis-cortex.
nonunion	The fracture remains mobile and healing has stopped. The fracture will not unite without surgical intervention. A nonunion is usually due to inadequate mechanical, or biological, conditions—see union, pseudarthrosis, and delayed union.
osteoarthritis	A degenerative condition of synovial joints which is characterized by loss of articular cartilage, subchondral bone sclerosis, bone cysts, and the formation of osteophytes. It is now more commonly referred to as degenerative joint disease (DJD).
osteomyelitis	An acute, or chronic, inflammatory condition affecting bone and the contents of its medullary cavity, usually the result of infection.
osteopenia	A reduction in bone mass of between 1 and 2.5 standard deviations below the mean for a young adult (ie, a T score of -1 to -2.5)—see osteoporosis.
osteoporosis	A reduction in bone mass of more than 2.5 standard deviations below the mean for a young adult (ie, a T score of less than -2.5)—see osteopenia, fragility fracture, and pathological fracture.
osteosynthesis	A term coined by Albin Lambotte to describe the "synthesis" (derived from the Greek for making together or fusing) of a fractured bone by a surgical intervention using implants. It includes external fixation.
osteotaxis	See external fixation.
osteotomy	Controlled surgical division of a bone.
pathological fracture	A fracture through abnormal bone, which occurs at normal physiological load or stress.
perioperative	The period of time around the operation, including the immediate preoperative assessment, anesthesia, and the first 24 hours following surgery.
periosteal	about periosteum.
periosteum	The fibrovascular membrane covering the exterior surface of a bone. The deep cell layer (cambium) has osteogenic potential.
periprosthetic fracture	A fracture that occurs in close relationship to a component of a joint prosthesis, most commonly the intramedullary stem of a joint replacement.
pertrochanteric fracture	A fracture of the proximal femur that involves the greater trochanter.
"personality" of the fracture	A term coined by EA Nichol (1965) to express the combination of attributes of a fracture that determine its outcome after treatment. There are three key factors: the patient, the soft tissues, and the fracture itself.
plate screw	A screw inserted through a plate to compress the plate to the bone. The preload created and friction hold the plate in place.

Poller screw	A blocking screw across the intramedullary canal inserted to redirect an intramedullary nail during its insertion.
polytrauma	A syndrome of multiple injuries to one or more body systems, or cavities, with sequential systemic reactions that may lead to dysfunction, or failure, of remote uninjured organs and vital systems. It can also be defined as an injury severity score (ISS) of ≥ 15.
position screw	A position screw is placed between two adjacent bones, or fracture fragments, to maintain their normal, relative anatomical relationship without applying compression. After restoration of the normal relationship of the bones, a pilot hole is drilled and tapped through both the near and far cortices of each bone. A fully threaded screw is then inserted and the absence of a glide hole means that no compression is generated between the head of the screw and the far cortex. The syndesmotic diastasis screw used in type C ankle fractures is an example of a position screw—see diastasis screw.
prebending (precontouring-premolding) of a plate	Preoperative, or intraoperative, contouring of a plate to the shape of the bone.
preload	The application of interfragmentary compression keeps the fragments together until a tensile force is applied which exceeds the compressive force (preload).
preshaped plate	A plate that is designed and shaped during manufacture to fit a specific anatomical site, so that intraoperative contouring of the plate is usually not needed.
protection (plate)	A plate, or other implant, that reduces the load exerted on a lag screw fixation, thereby protecting it from overload. This was formerly referred to as a neutralization device (plate).
pseudarthrosis	It literally means false joint. When a nonunion is mobile and allowed to persist for a long period, the bone ends become sclerotic and the intervening soft tissues differentiate to form a type of synovial articulation—see delayed union, union.
reconstruction plate	A notched plate that can be bent on the flat as well as in the conventional manner, producing complex 3D shapes for fixation of fractures in irregularly shaped bones, such as the pelvis, or the distal humerus.
reduction	The realignment of a displaced fracture.
reduction, direct	Hands, or instruments, directly manipulate fracture fragments under vision.
reduction, indirect	Fragments are manipulated by applying corrective forces at a distance from the fracture zone, by distraction, or by other means, without exposing the fracture site.
refracture	A reoccurrence of a fracture after it has been solidly bridged by bone, at a level of load otherwise tolerated by normal bone. The resulting fracture line may coincide with the original fracture line or be within the area of bone that has undergone changes as a result of the fracture and its treatment.
relative stability	See stability, relative.
remodeling (of bone)	The process of transformation of external bone shape (external remodeling) or of internal bone structure (internal remodeling, or remodeling of the Haversian system).
rigidity	See stiffness.
sagittal plane	This is a vertical plane of the body passing from front to back, so that a sagittal bisection of the body would cut it into a right half and a left half.
sarcopenia	The loss of skeletal muscle mass and strength, as a result of aging.
scintigraphy	Three-dimensional image that reflects biological processes at the cellular level after the injection of substances that contain radioactive isotopes.
screw	Any device exploiting helical geometry for converting rotational movement into rectilinear longitudinal motion.

second look Surgical inspection of a wound, or injury zone, 24–72 hours after the initial management of the injury.

segmental If the shaft of a bone is broken at two levels, leaving a separate shaft segment between the two fracture sites, it is called a "segmental" fracture complex.

self-drilling screw A screw with a sharp, pointed drill tip bearing cutting flutes, which drills its own pilot hole and cuts its own thread.

shear A shearing force is one which tends to cause one segment of a body to slide upon another, as opposed to tensile forces, which tend to elongate a body.

simple fracture There is a single fracture plane producing two fracture fragments.

single-photon emission computed tomography (SPE-CT) A nuclear medicine imaging technique using gamma rays and a detector to produce tomograms and 3D information.

splinting A splint is made of stiff material that is applied to a fractured body region to reduce motion at the fracture site. It can be applied externally (plaster cast, functional brace, external fixator) or internally (plate, intramedullary nail, internal fixator).

stability, absolute Fixation of fracture fragments so that there is effectively no interfragmentary displacement of the fracture surfaces under physiological load. This allows direct bone healing.

stability, relative A fixation, or support construction, that allows small amounts of interfragmentary motion in proportion to the load applied. This results in indirect healing by external callus formation.

stable fixation Fixation of a fracture that allows early motion of the adjacent joints and provides a mechanical environment that allows fracture healing before failure of the implant.

stiffness The ability of a material to resist deformation. It is defined as the relationship between load applied and the resulting elastic deformation. The inherent stiffness of a material is expressed by its modulus of elasticity (Young's modulus).

strain Change in length of a material when a given force is applied. Normal strain is the ratio of deformation (lengthening or shortening) to original length. It has no dimensions but is often expressed as a percentage.

strain theory by Perren With a small fracture gap, any interfragmentary motion will result in a relatively large change in length (ie, high strain). If this exceeds the strain tolerance of the intervening tissue, healing will not take place. If a larger fracture gap is subjected to the same amplitude of movement, the relative change in length of each intervening tissue component will be smaller (ie, less strain). If the critical strain level is not exceeded, there will be normal tissue function and indirect healing by callus.

strain tolerance The ability of tissue to undergo deformation due to an applied force and continue to perform its normal physiological function. The maximum strain tolerance is the maximum amount of deformation at which a tissue can still perform its normal physiological function. No tissue can function normally when a deforming force causes the tissue to disrupt. This is the critical strain level.

strength The ability of a material to resist the application of force without deformation. The strength of a material can be expressed as ultimate tensile strength, ultimate bending strength, or ultimate torsional strength. Strength determines the level of load that an implant can resist.

stress concentration The build-up of stresses in an implant, or bone, where there is a defect, a change in cross section, a hole, or a scratch—see stress distribution.

stress distribution If bending stresses are distributed over a long, unsupported segment of a plate, the stress per unit area is correspondingly low, which reduces the risk of fatigue failure.

stress protection — Using a plate to reduce peak loads applied to a screw fixation—see protection (plate). In older texts, this term may be applied to the concept that a rigid implant, such as a plate, applied firmly to bone, protects the underlying bone from stress and, thereby, induces bone resorption. This observed phenomenon is now understood to be due to the vascular impact of the tightly applied plate on the underlying cortex—see stress shielding.

stress riser — A defect (eg, empty screw hole in a plate or an empty drill hole in a bone) that brings about a concentration of stress—see stress concentration.

stress shielding — Bone deprived of functional stimulation by having its physiological stresses reduced by a load-sharing implant may react by becoming less dense, according to Wolff's law (1872).

Sudeck's atrophy — See complex regional pain syndrome.

syndesmosis screw — See diastasis screw and position screw.

tap — The process by which a thread is cut in a predrilled hole. It also refers to the instrument used to cut the thread.

tension band — The principle by which an implant, attached to the tension side of a bending fracture, converts the tensile force into a compressive force at the cortex beneath the implant. While wires, cables, and sutures are often used for tension band fixation, plates and external fixators, when appropriately placed, can also function as tension bands.

thread(ed) hole — A pilot hole is drilled and a tap is used to cut the helical groove that receives the thread of the screw. The result is a threaded hole.

toggling — Slight movement at the couple between a screw and a plate, or an intramedullary nail. Implants may be designed to allow toggle (eg, intramedullary nails) where the tolerances of the assembly do not permit an exact fit. Toggle between plates and screws may occur during plate failure with loosening of the implant.

torque — The moment produced by a rotational force. As an example, torque is applied to drive home and tighten a screw. The moment is equal to the product of lever arm (unit meter) and force (unit Newton) producing torsion and rotation about an axis (the unit of torque is a Newton-meter).

traction table — An operating table with attachments that allow safe and precise positioning of the patient and the application of tension, or compression, through a limb to reduce a fracture, whilst allowing access for surgery and radiological imaging. Also known as a fracture table.

translation — Displacement of one bone fragment in relation to another, usually at right angles to the long axis of the bone, or in the plane of the fracture.

union — Union strictly means "as one". The bone has healed and regained its normal stiffness and strength. In clinical terms, this means there is no movement or tenderness at the fracture site and no pain on stressing the fracture site. Radiologically, there should be evidence of bone trabeculae bridging the fracture site.

vacuum-assisted wound closure — An open wound is sealed with an impervious, adherent dressing and low pressure suction is applied beneath the dressing to remove any exudates and to encourage the formation of granulation tissue.

valgus — Angulation of the distal part away from the midline in the anatomical position.

varus — Angulation of the distal part towards the midline in the anatomical position.

wave plate — The central section of a wave plate is contoured to stand off the near cortex over a distance of several holes. This leaves a gap between the plate and the bone, which preserves the biology of the underlying bone, provides a space for the insertion of bone graft, and increases the stability because of the distance of the waved portion of the implant from the neutral axis of the shaft. Such plating is useful in nonunion treatment.

working length — The distance across a fracture site between the two nearest points where the implant (usually an intramedullary nail, or bridging plate) and the bone are coupled.

AO/OTA Fracture and Dislocation Classification

For further educational material about the classification and access to the complete Fracture and Dislocation Classification Compendium, please use the QR code.

Humerus

Bone: Humerus 1

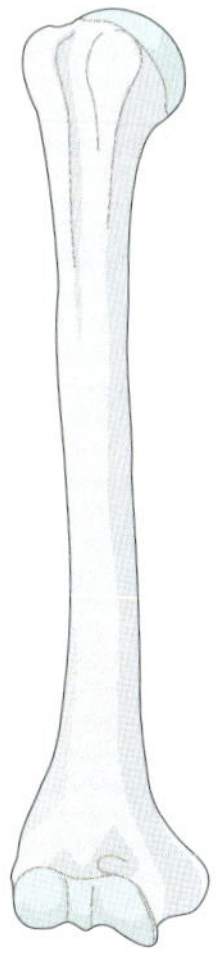

11

Location: Humerus, **proximal end segment** 11

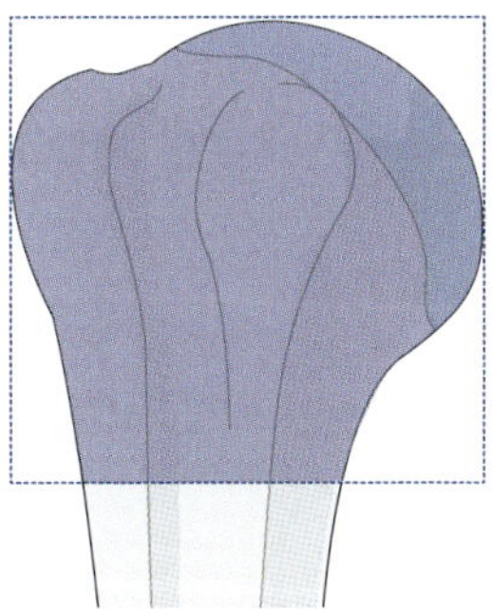

Types:

Humerus, proximal end segment,
extraarticular, unifocal, 2-part fracture
11A

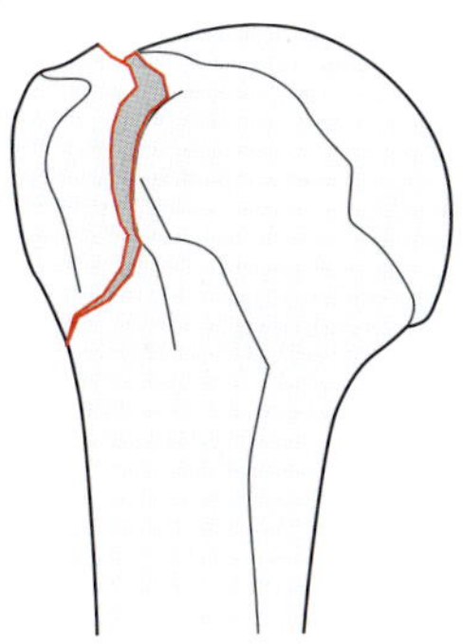

Humerus, proximal end segment,
extraarticular, bifocal, 3-part fracture
11B

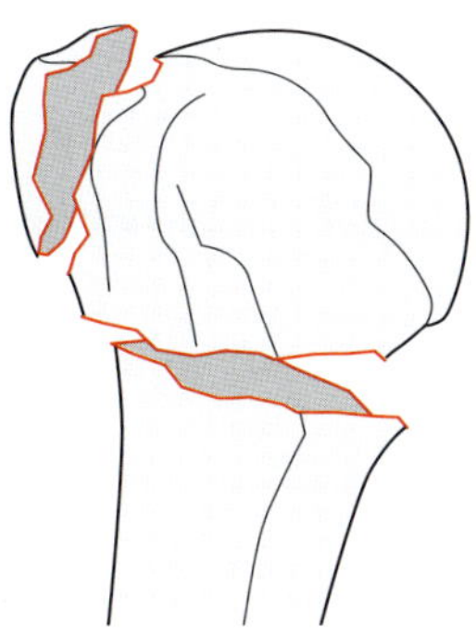

Humerus, proximal end segment,
articular or 4-part fracture
11C

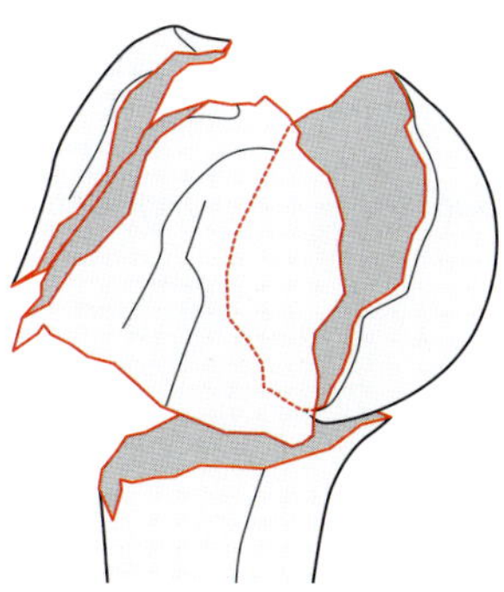

Qualifications *are optional and applied to the fracture code where the asterisk is located as a lower-case letter within rounded brackets. More than one qualification can be applied for a given fracture classification, separated by a comma. For a more detailed explanation, see the compendium introduction.*

11A

Type: Humerus, proximal end segment, **extraarticular, unifocal, 2-part fracture** 11A

Group: Humerus, proximal end segment, extraarticular, unifocal, 2-part, **tuberosity fracture** 11A1

Subgroups:

Greater tuberosity fracture
11A1.1

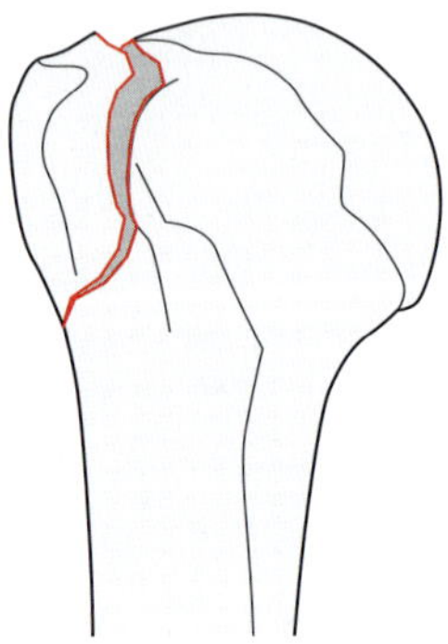

Lesser tuberosity fracture
11A1.2

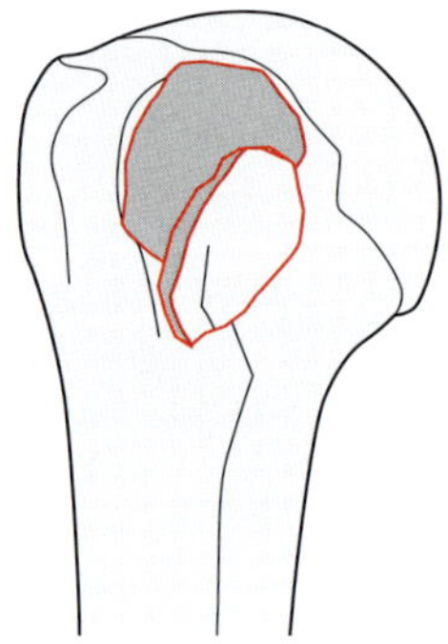

Group: Humerus, proximal end segment, extraarticular, unifocal, 2-part, **surgical neck fracture** 11A2

Subgroups:

Simple fracture
11A2.1

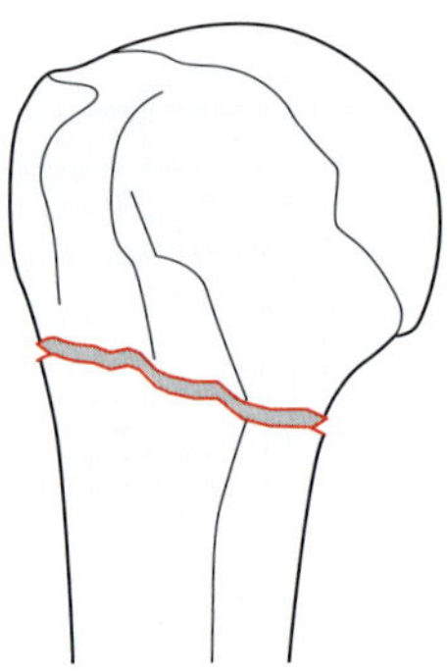

Wedge fracture
11A2.2

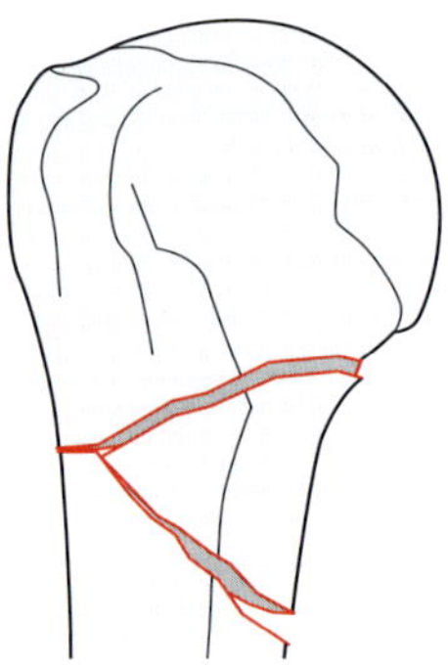

Multifragmentary fracture
11A2.3

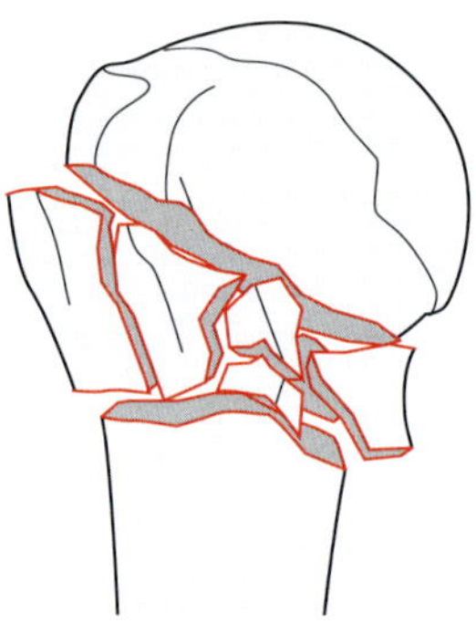

Group: Humerus, proximal end segment, unifocal, 2-part, extraarticular **vertical fracture** 11A3

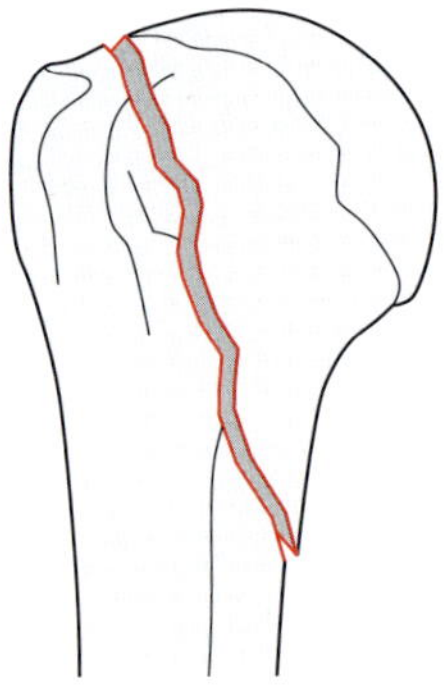

11B

Type: Humerus, proximal end segment, **extraarticular, bifocal, 3-part fracture** 11B

Group: Humerus, proximal end segment, extraarticular, bifocal, 3-part, **surgical neck fracture** 11B1

Subgroups:
With greater tuberosity fracture
11B1.1*

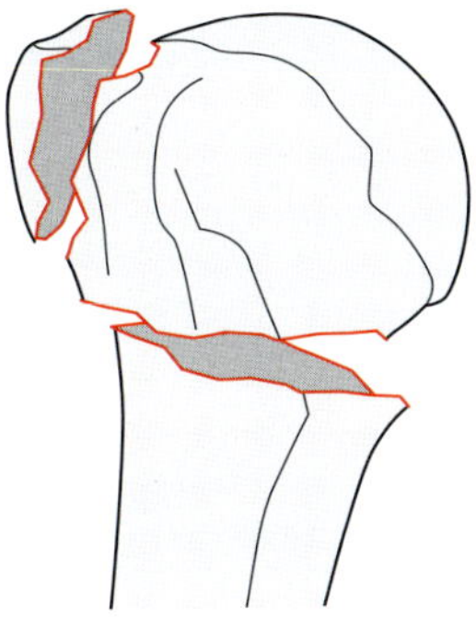

With lesser tuberosity fracture
11B1.2*

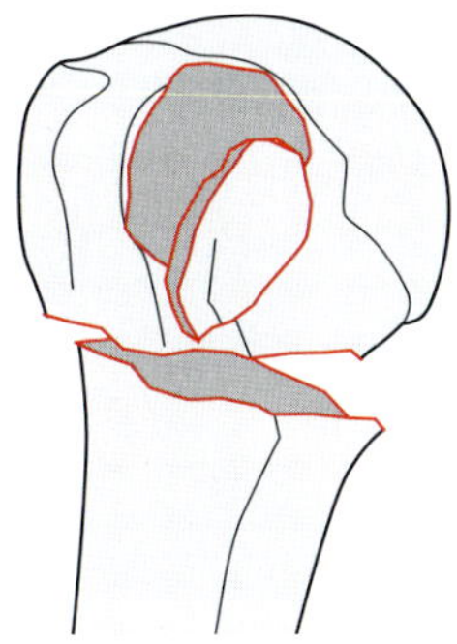

*Qualifications:
u Intact wedge
v Fragmentary wedge

11C

Type: Humerus, proximal end segment, **articular or 4-part fracture** 11C

Group: Humerus, proximal end segment, articular or 4-part, **anatomical neck fracture** 11C1

Subgroups:
Valgus impacted fracture
11C1.1*

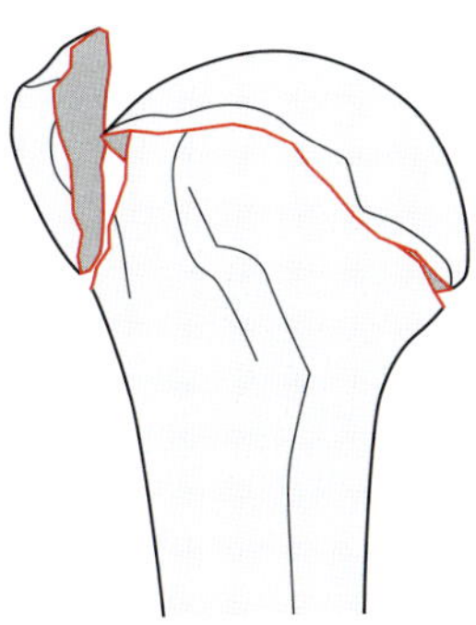

*Qualifications:
n **Greater tuberosity**
o Lesser tuberosity
p Both tuberosities

Isolated anatomical neck fracture
11C1.3

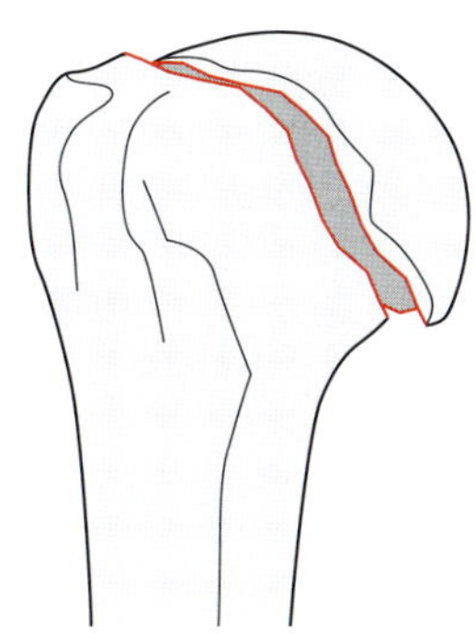

Group: Humerus, proximal end segment, articular or 4-part, **anatomical neck fracture associated with metaphyseal fracture** 11C3

Subgroups:

With a multifragmentary metaphyseal segment with intact articular surface
11C3.1

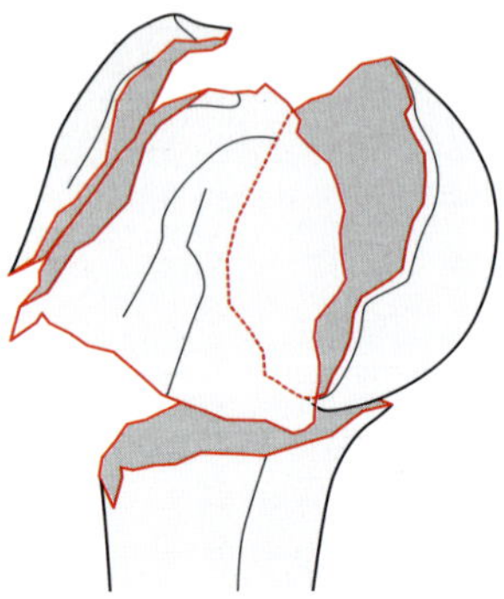

With a multifragmentary metaphyseal segment with articular fracture
11C3.2*

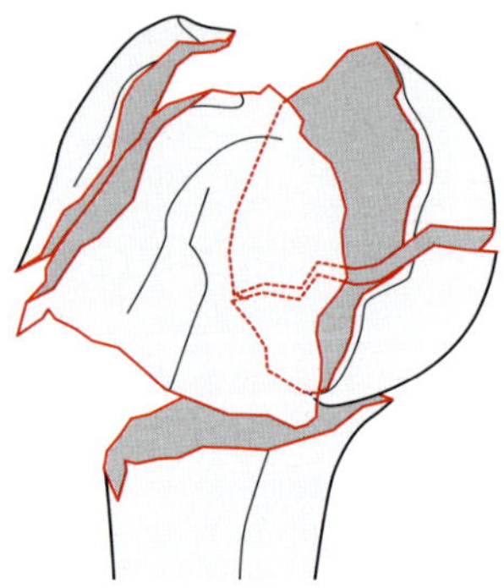

With a multifragmentary metaphyseal fracture, with diaphyseal extension and articular fracture
11C3.3*

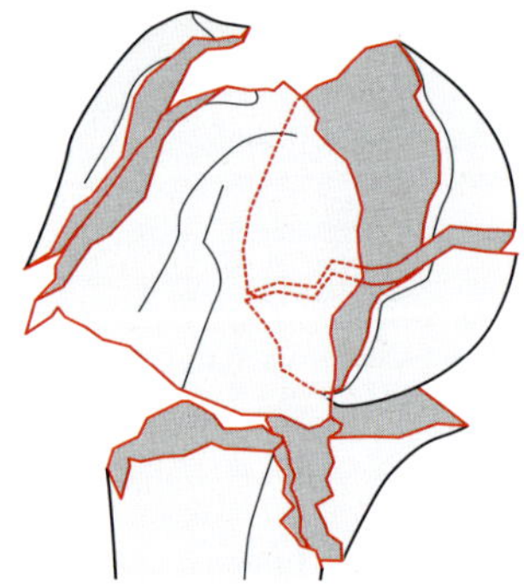

*Qualifications:
x **Simple articular**
y Multifragmentary articular

12

Location: Humerus, **diaphyseal segment** 12

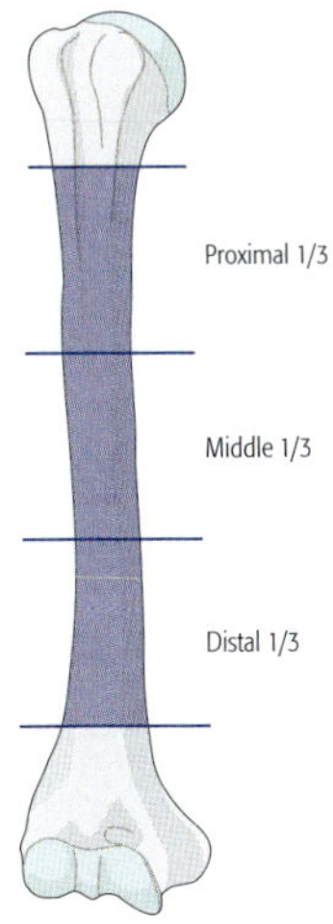

Types:

Humerus, diaphyseal segment,
simple fracture
12A

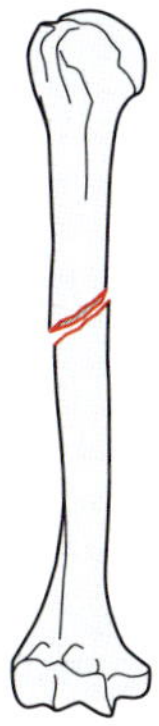

Humerus, diaphyseal segment,
wedge fracture
12B

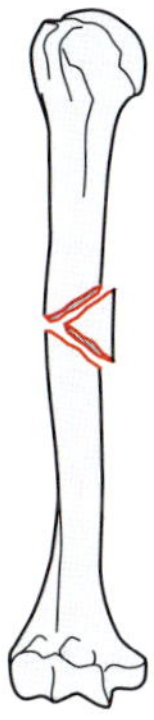

Humerus, diaphyseal segment,
multifragmentary fracture
12C

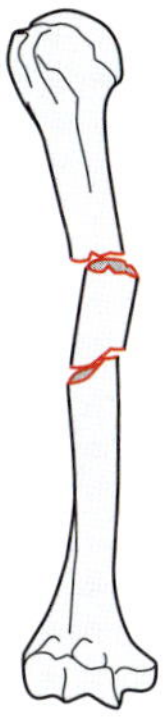

12A

Type: Humerus, diaphyseal segment, **simple fracture** 12A

Groups:

Humerus, diaphyseal segment, simple,
spiral fracture
12A1*

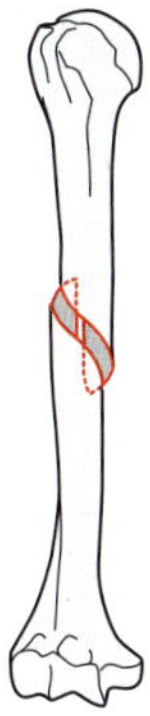

Humerus, diaphyseal segment, simple,
oblique fracture (≥30°)
12A2*

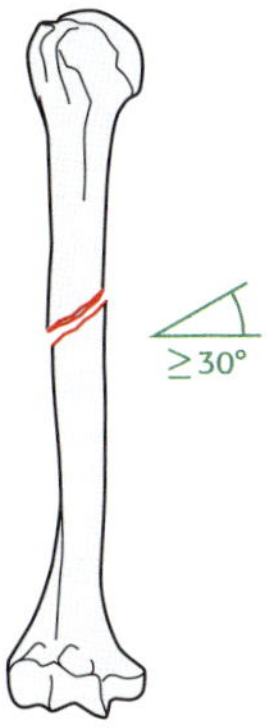

Humerus, diaphyseal segment, simple,
transverse fracture (<30°)
12A3*

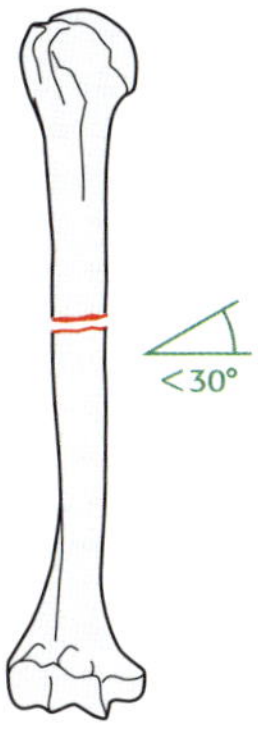

*Qualifications:
- a Proximal 1/3
- b **Middle 1/3**
- c Distal 1/3

12B

Type: Humerus, diaphyseal segment, **wedge fracture** 12B

Groups:

Humerus, diaphyseal segment,
intact wedge fracture
12B2*

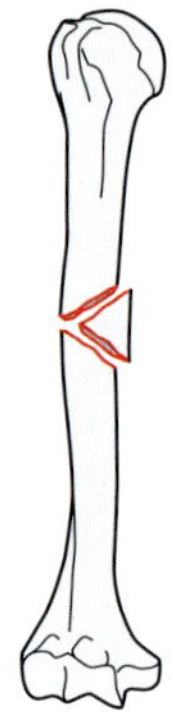

Humerus, diaphyseal segment,
fragmentary wedge fracture
12B3*

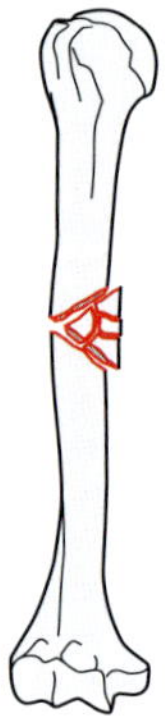

*Qualifications:
a Proximal 1/3
b **Middle 1/3**
c Distal 1/3

12C

Type: Humerus, diaphyseal segment, **multifragmentary fracture** 12C

Groups:

Humerus, diaphyseal segment, multifragmentary,
intact segmental fracture
12C2*

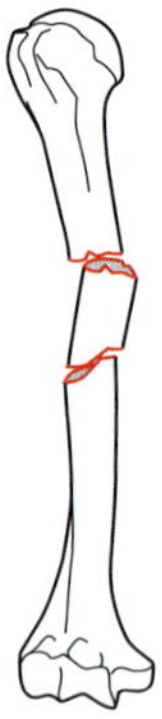

Humerus, diaphyseal segment, multifragmentary,
fragmentary segmental fracture
12C3*

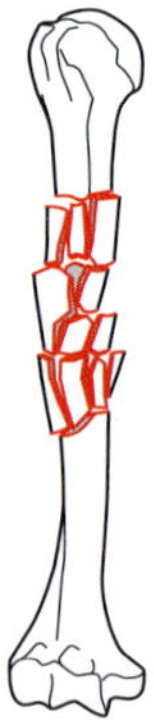

*Qualifications:
i Proximal diaphyseal-metaphyseal
j **Pure diaphyseal**
k Distal diaphyseal-metaphyseal

13

Location: Humerus, **distal end segment** 13

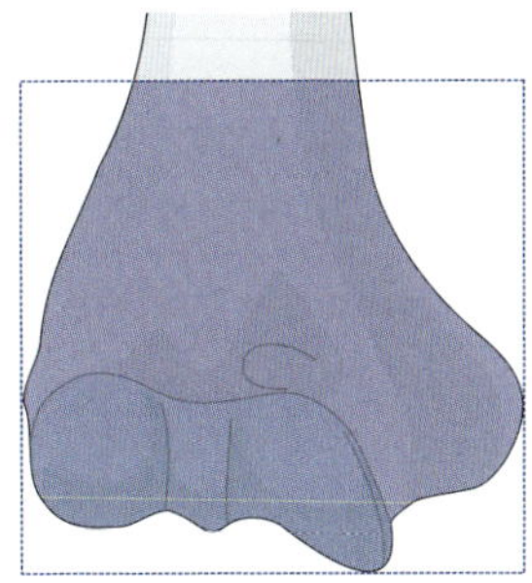

Types:

Humerus, distal end segment,
extraarticular fracture
13A

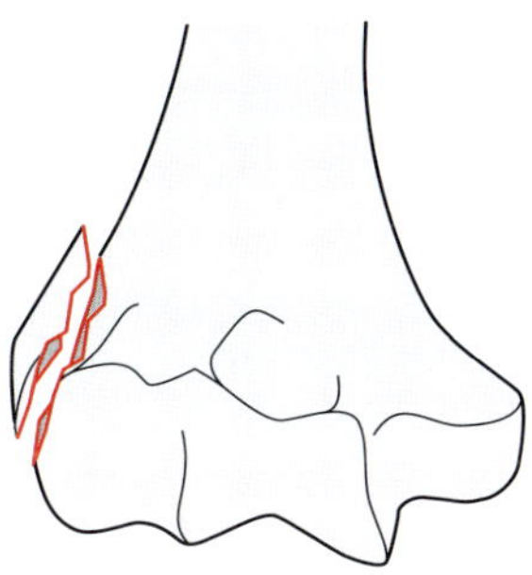

Humerus, distal end segment,
partial articular fracture
13B

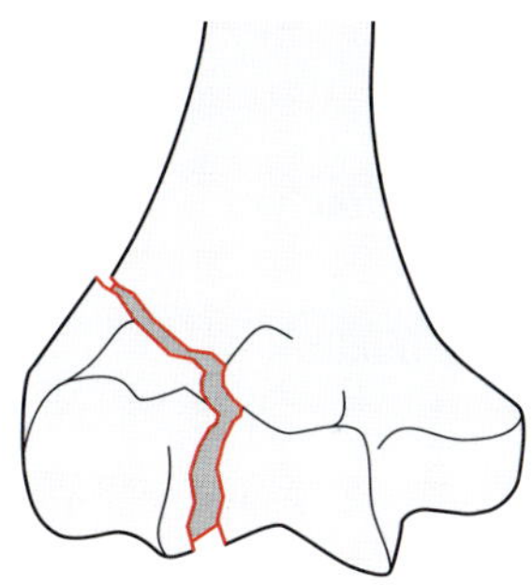

Humerus, distal end segment,
complete articular fracture
13C

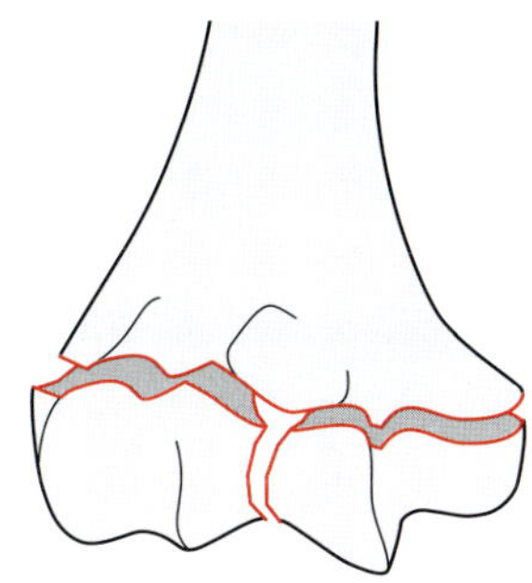

13A

Type: Humerus, distal end segment, **extraarticular fracture** 13A

Group: Humerus, distal end segment, extraarticular, **avulsion fracture** 13A1

Subgroups:

Lateral epicondyle fracture
13A1.1

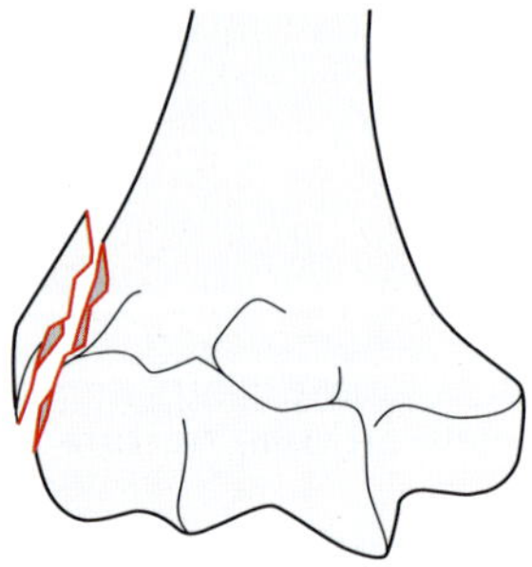

Medial epicondyle fracture
13A1.2

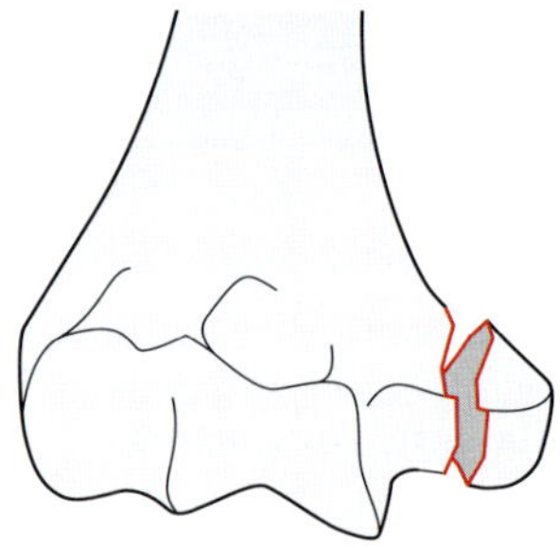

Group: Humerus, distal end segment, extraarticular, **simple fracture** 13A2

Subgroups:

Spiral fracture
13A2.1

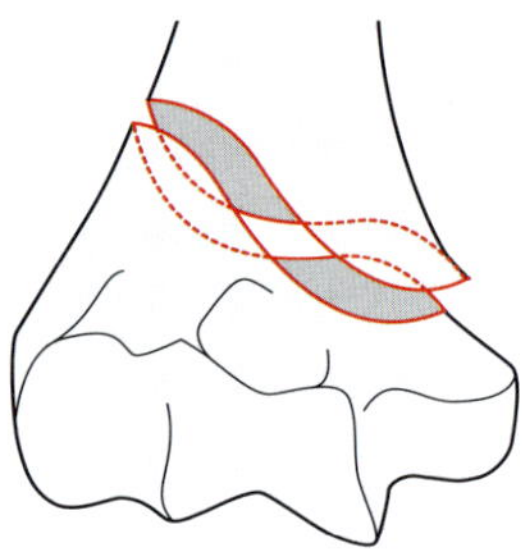

Oblique fracture
13A2.2

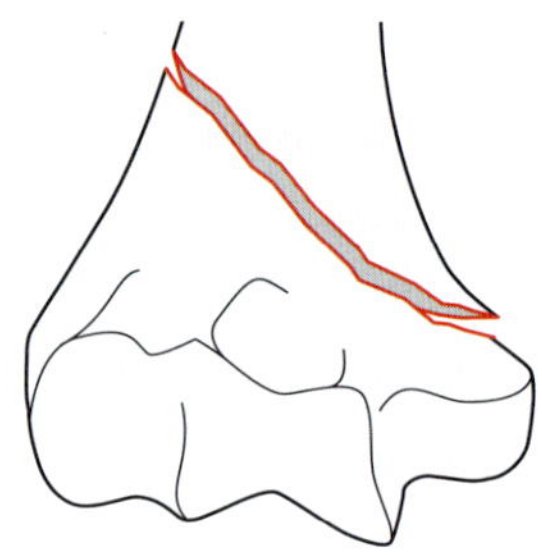

Transverse fracture
13A2.3

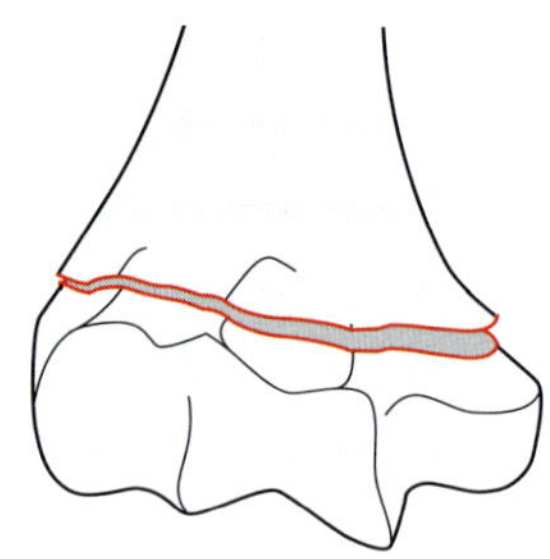

Group: Humerus, distal end segment, extraarticular, **wedge or multifragmentary fracture** 13A3

Subgroups:

Intact wedge fracture
13A3.1*

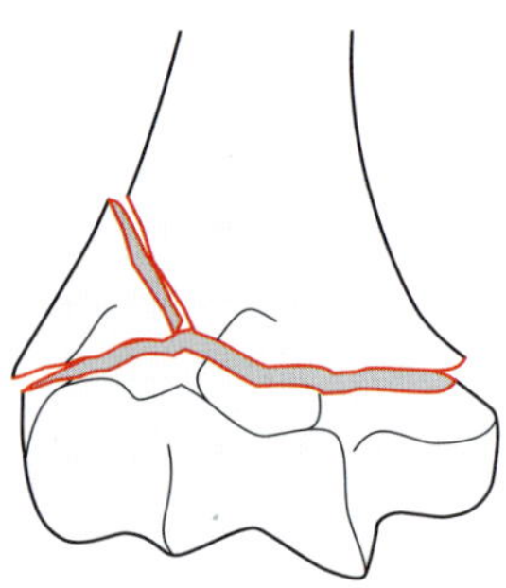

Fragmentary wedge fracture
13A3.2*

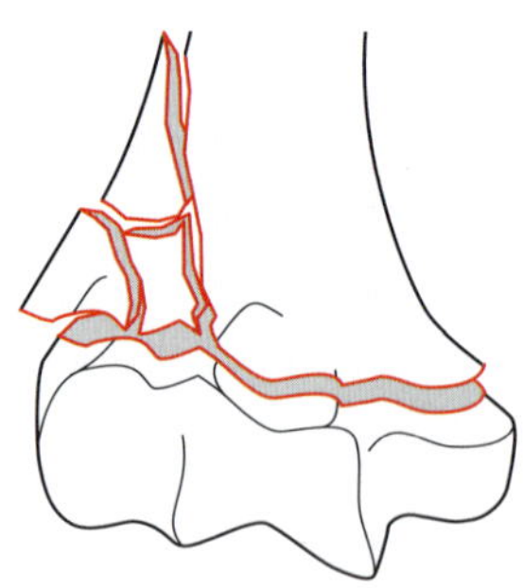

Multifragmentary fracture
13A3.3

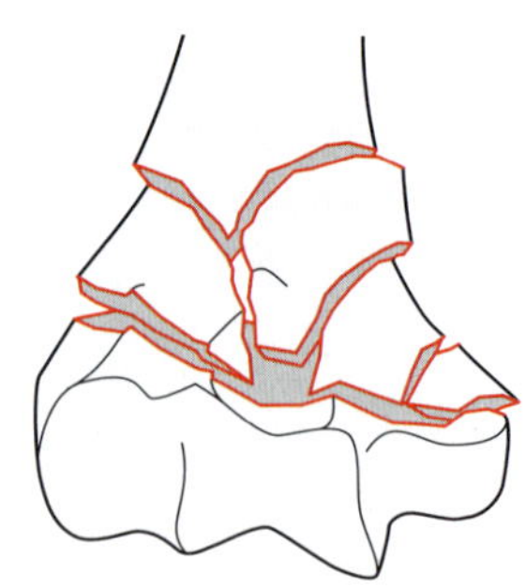

*Qualifications:
f **Lateral**
h Medial

13B

Type: Humerus, distal end segment, **partial articular fracture** 13B

Group: Humerus, distal end segment, partial articular, **lateral sagittal fracture** 13B1

Subgroups:

Simple transtrochlear fracture
13B1.1

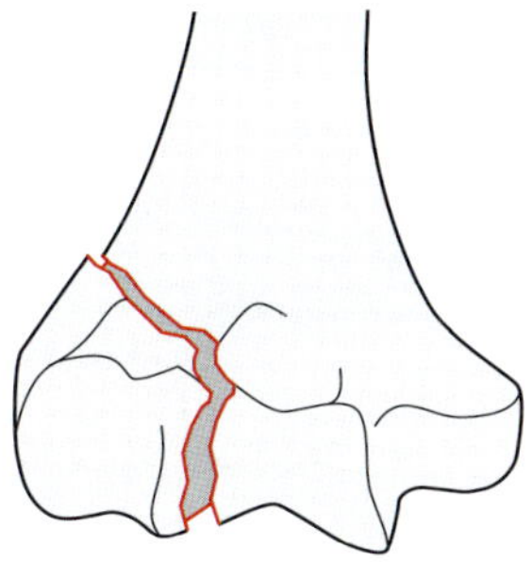

Capitellum fracture
13B1.2*

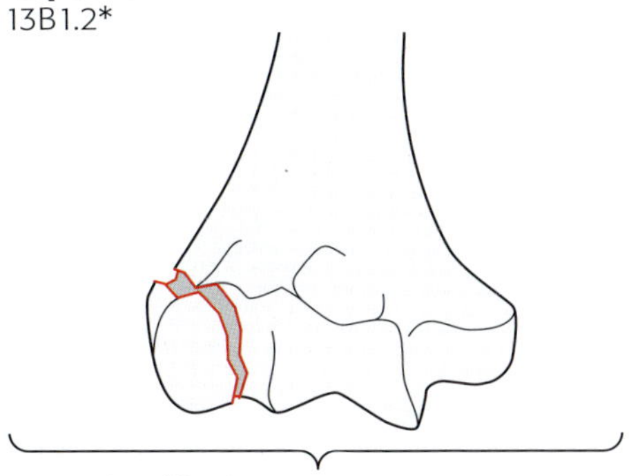

*Qualifications:
q **Transcapitellar**
r Between capitellum and trochlea

Fragmentary transtrochlear fracture
13B1.3

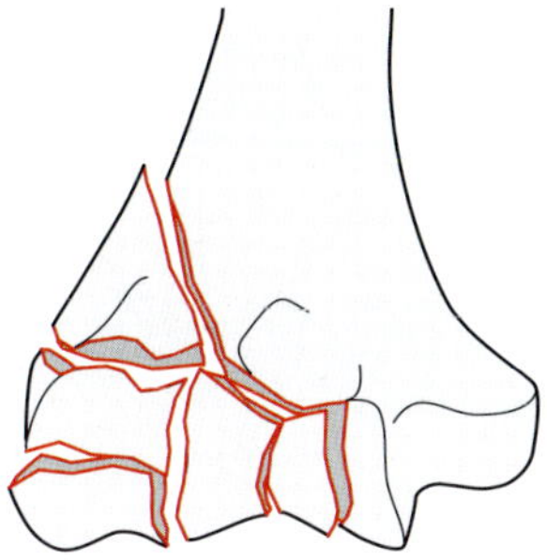

Group: Humerus, distal end segment, partial articular, **medial sagittal fracture** 13B2

Subgroups:

Simple transtrochlear fracture through the trochlear groove
13B2.1

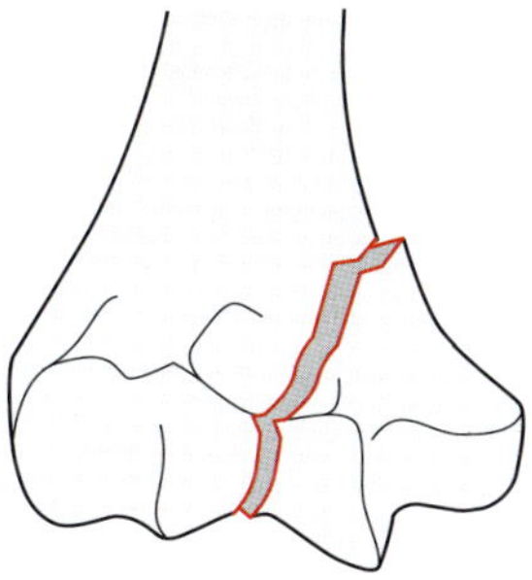

Simple transtrochlear fracture through the medial articular surface
13B2.2

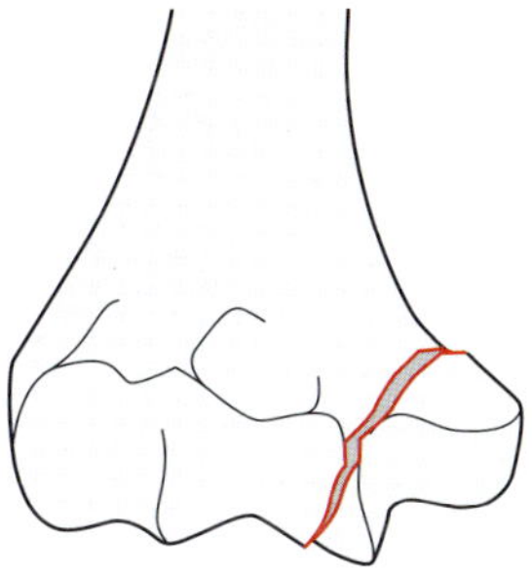

Fragmentary transtrochlear fracture
13B2.3

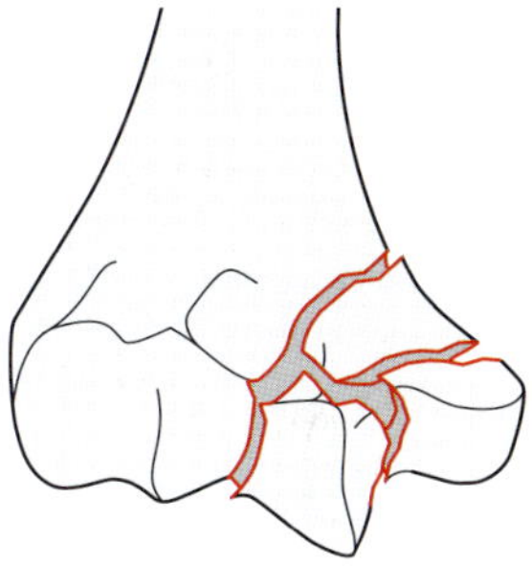

Group: Humerus, distal end segment, partial articular, **frontal/coronal plane fracture** 13B3

Subgroups:

Capitellum fracture
13B3.1

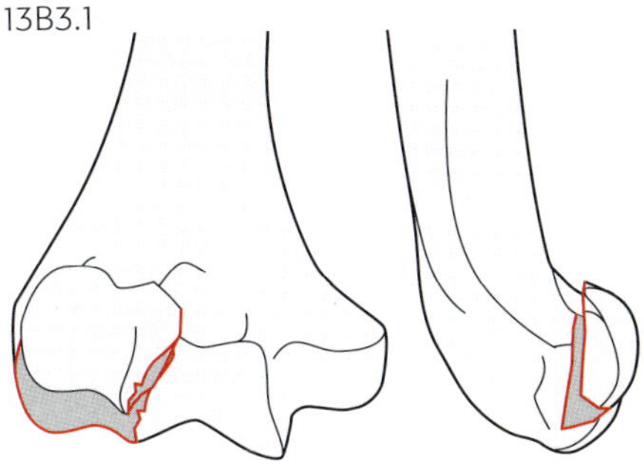

Trochlea fracture
13B3.2

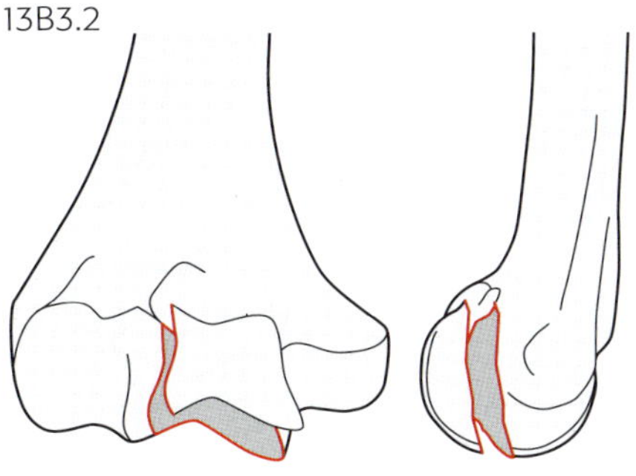

Capitellum and trochlea fracture
13B3.3

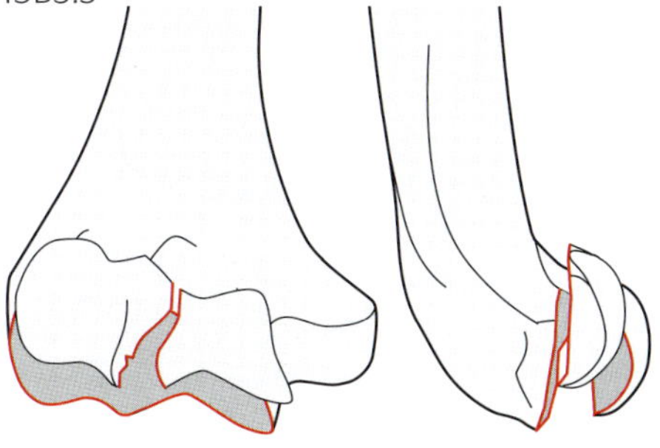

13C

Type: Humerus, distal end segment, **complete articular fracture** 13C

Group: Humerus, distal end segment, complete, **simple articular, simple metaphyseal fracture** 13C1

Subgroups:

Above the transcondylar axis
13C1.1

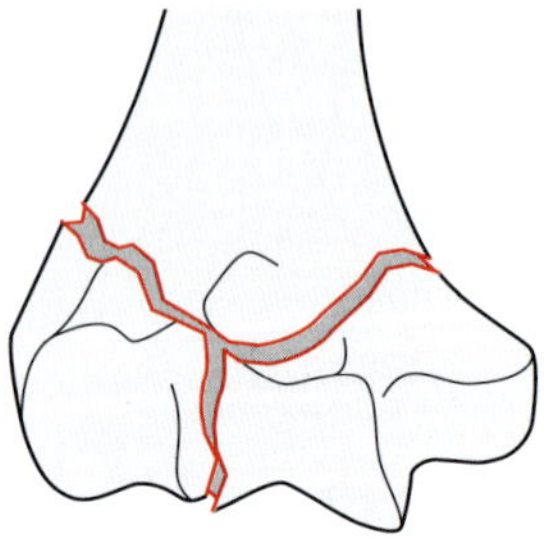

Through or below the transcondylar axis
13C1.3

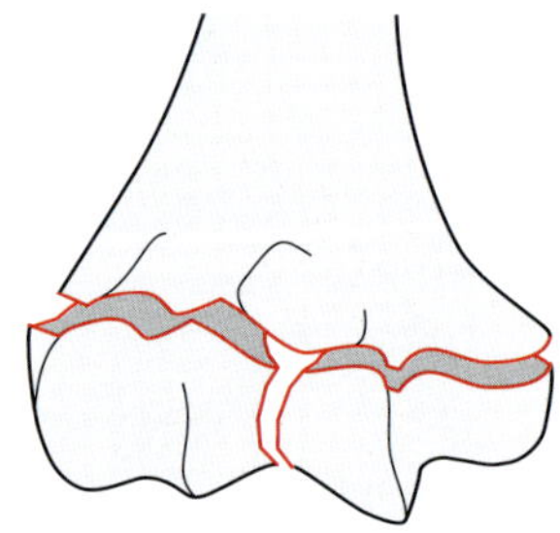

Group: Humerus, distal end segment, complete, **simple articular, wedge or multifragmentary metaphyseal fracture** 13C2

Subgroups:

Intact wedge fracture
13C2.1*

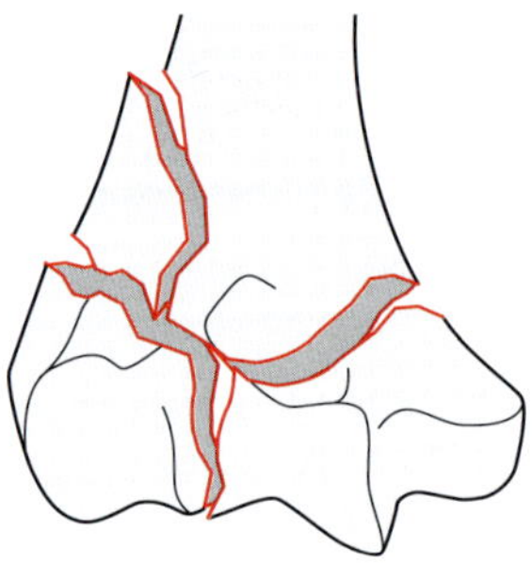

Fragmentary wedge fracture
13C2.2*

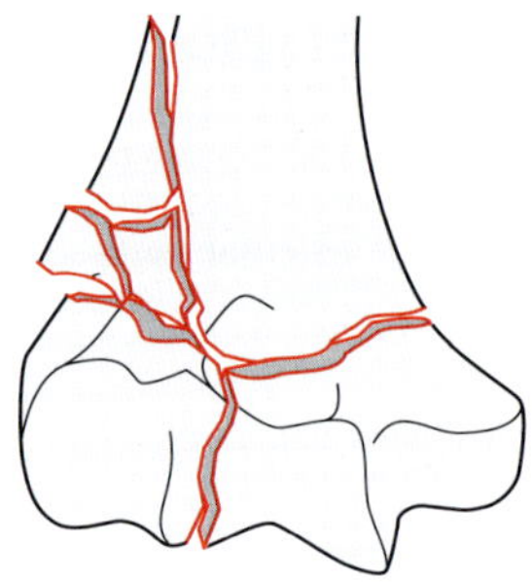

Multifragmentary fracture
13C2.3

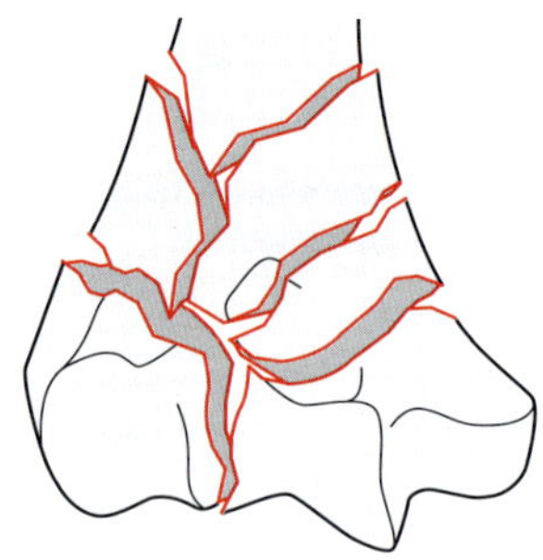

*Qualifications:
f **Lateral**
h Medial
u **Intact wedge**

Group: Humerus, distal end segment, complete, **multifragmentary articular fracture, wedge or multifragmentary metaphyseal fracture** 13C3

Subgroups:

Simple metaphyseal fracture
13C3.1*

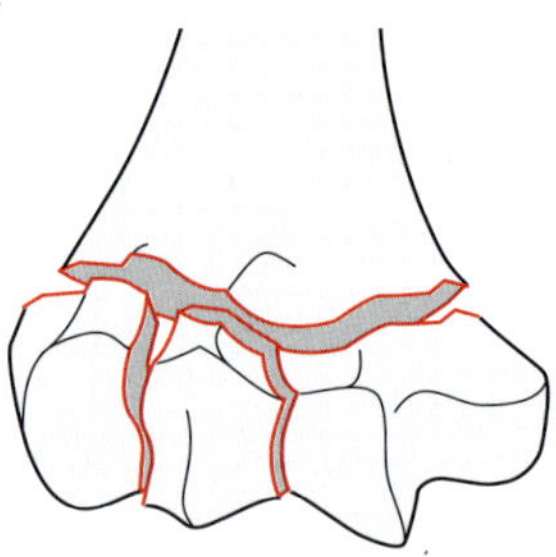

Wedge metaphyseal fracture
13C3.2*

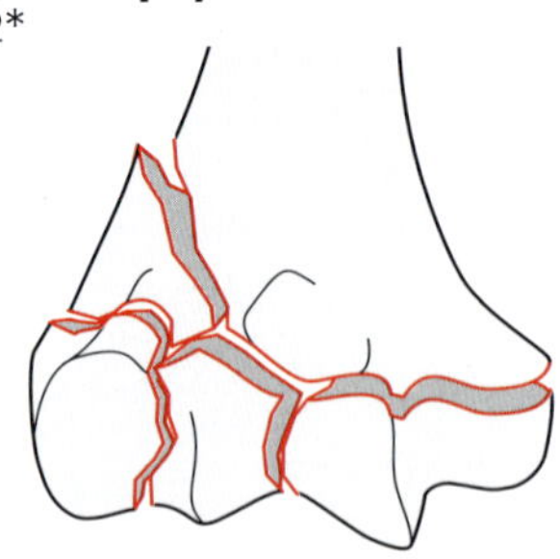

Multifragmentary metaphyseal fracture
13C3.3

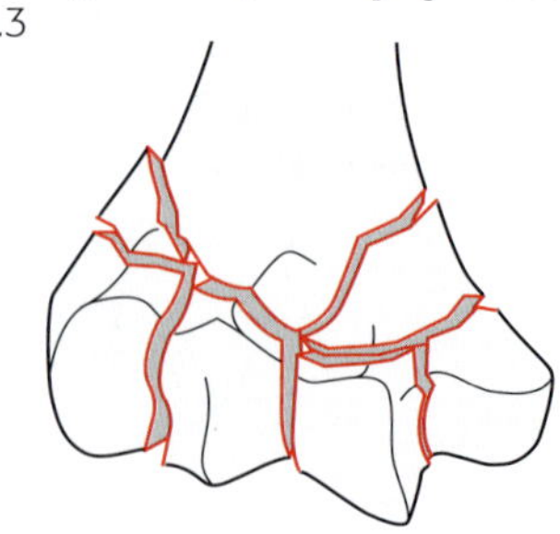

*Qualifications:
s **Proximal to transcondylar axis**
t Distal to transcondylar axis

*Qualifications:
f **Lateral**
h Medial
l Fragmentary
u **Intact wedge**

Qualifications *are optional and applied to the fracture code where the asterisk is located as a lower-case letter within rounded brackets. More than one qualification can be applied for a given fracture classification, separated by a comma. For a more detailed explanation, see the compendium introduction.*

Radius and Ulna

Bone: Radius 2R/**Ulna** 2U

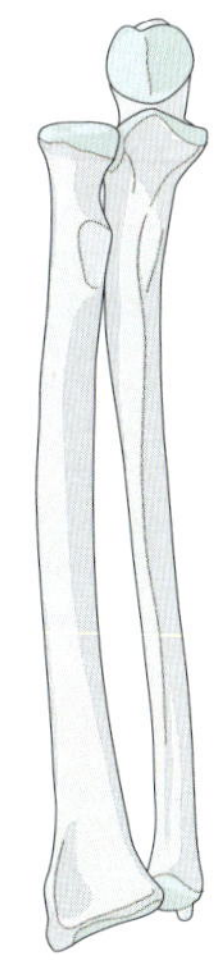

2R1/2U1

Location: Radius or Ulna, **proximal end segment** 2R1/2U1

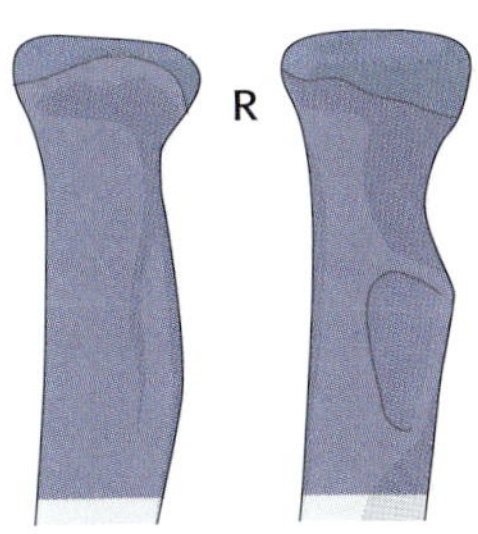

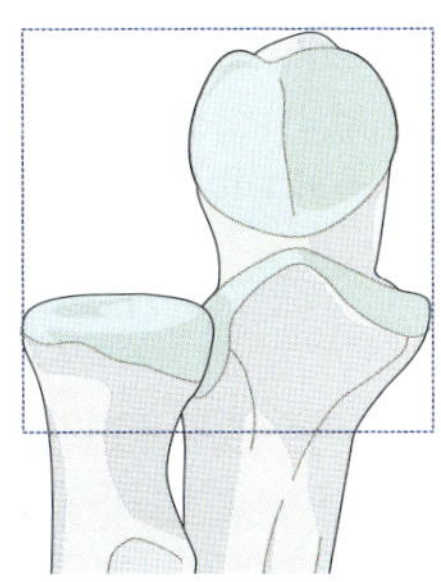

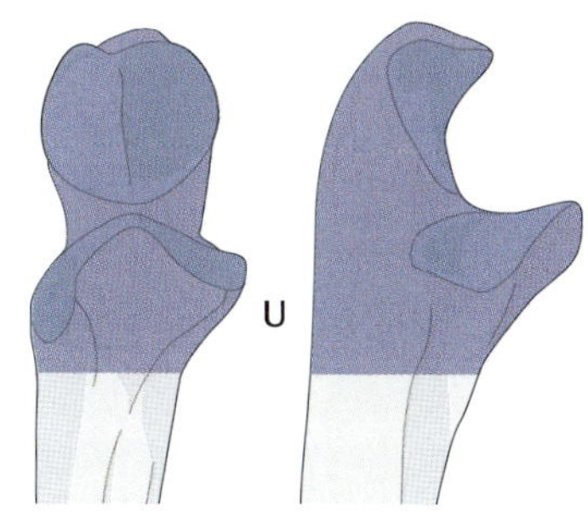

→ To facilitate the coding of radius and ulna fractures, they are now coded independently.
→ The end segment location of either bone is determined by using the two bones as a unit.

Types:

Radius, proximal end segment,
extraarticular fracture
2R1A

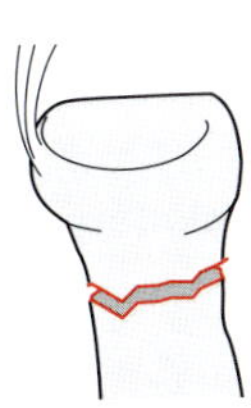

Radius, proximal end segment,
partial articular fracture
2R1B

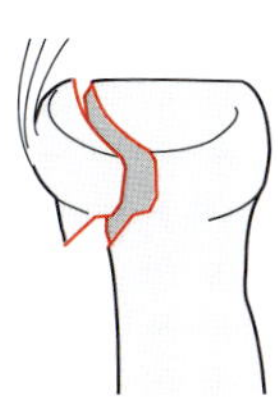

Radius, proximal end segment,
complete articular fracture
2R1C

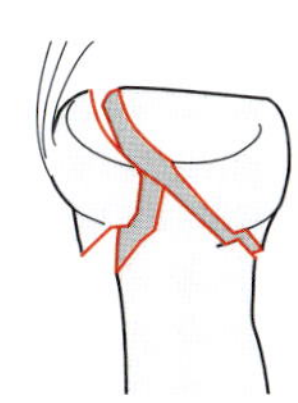

Ulna, proximal end segment,
extraarticular fracture
2U1A

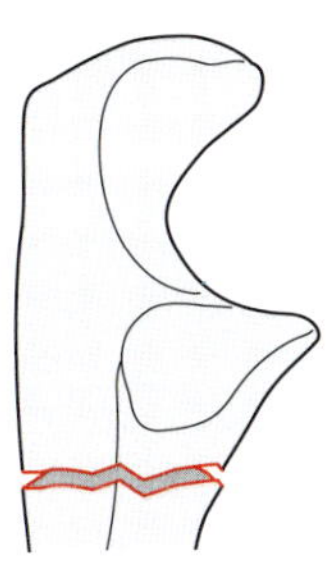

Ulna, proximal end segment,
partial articular fracture
2U1B

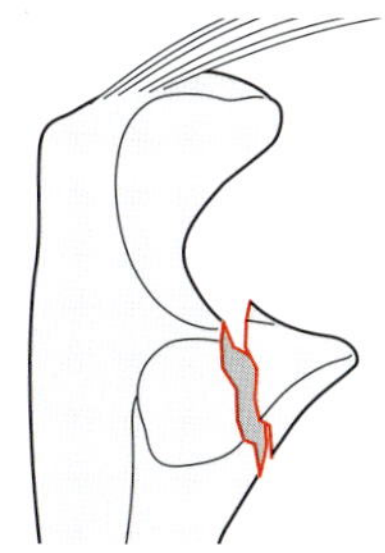

Ulna, proximal end segment,
complete articular fracture
2U1C

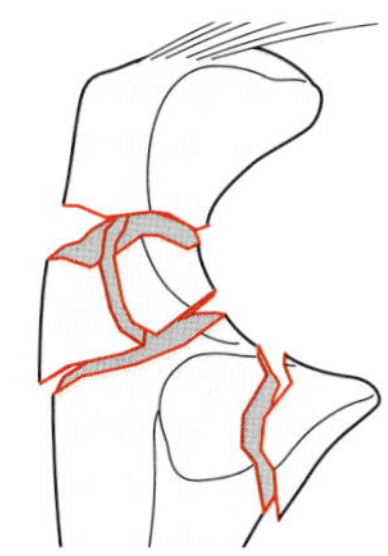

Qualifications *are optional and applied to the fracture code where the asterisk is located as a lower-case letter within rounded brackets. More than one qualification can be applied for a given fracture classification, separated by a comma. For a more detailed explanation, see the compendium introduction.*

2R1A/2U1A

Type: Radius, proximal end segment, **extraarticular fracture** 2R1A

Groups:

Radius, proximal end segment, extraarticular, **avulsion of bicipital tuberosity**
2R1A1

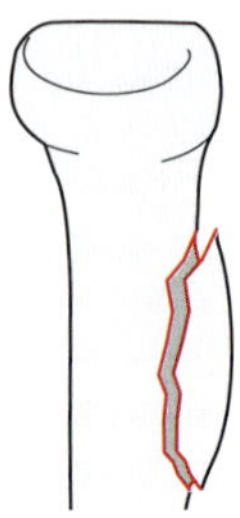

Radius, proximal end segment, extraarticular, **neck, simple**
2R1A2

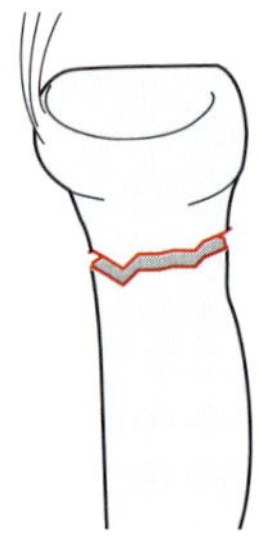

Radius, proximal end segment, extraarticular, **neck, multifragmentary**
2R1A3

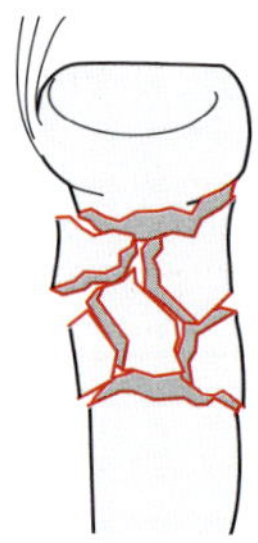

Type: Ulna, proximal end segment, **extraarticular fracture** 2U1A

Groups:

Ulna, proximal end segment, extraarticular, **avulsion of triceps insertion**
2U1A1

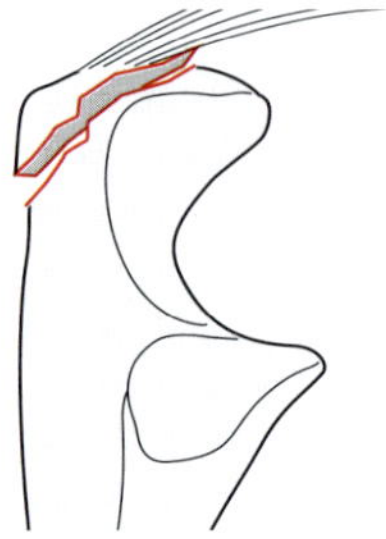

Ulna, proximal end segment, extraarticular, **metaphyseal simple fracture**
2U1A2

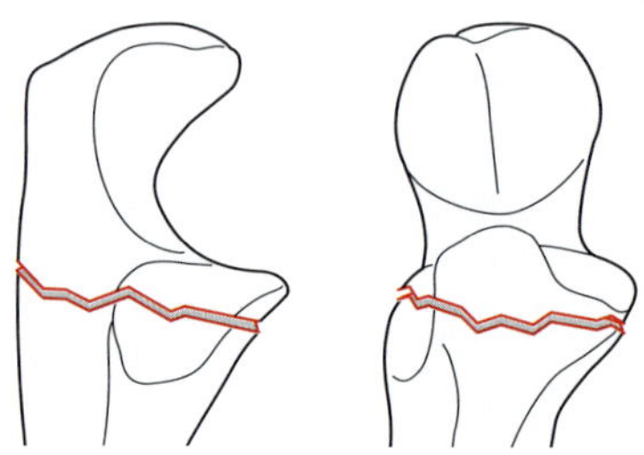

Ulna, proximal end segment, extraarticular, **metaphyseal multifragmentary fracture**
2U1A3

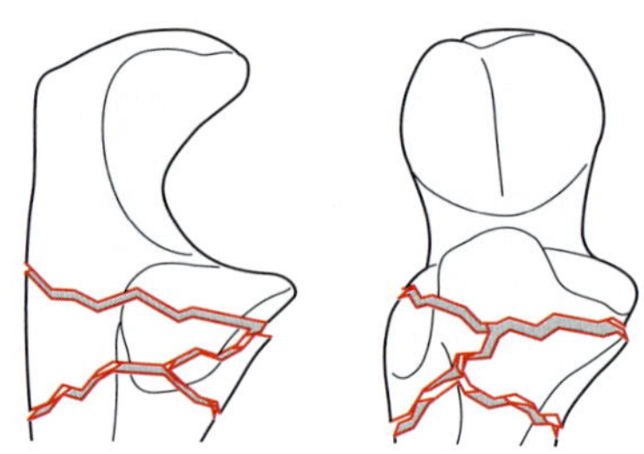

2R1B/2U1B

Type: Radius, proximal end segment articular, **partial articular fracture** 2R1B

Groups:

Radius, proximal end segment articular, partial articular, **simple fracture**
2R1B1

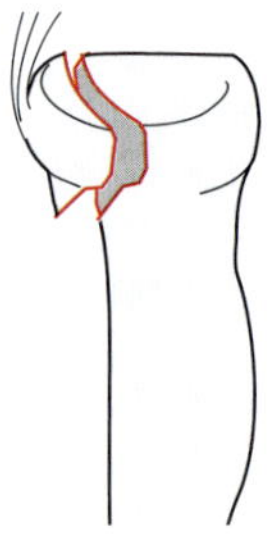

Radius, proximal end segment articular, partial articular, **fragmentary fracture**
2R1B3

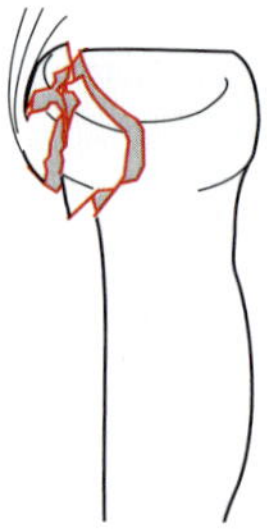

Type: Ulna, proximal end segment, **partial articular fracture** 2U1B

Groups:

Ulna, proximal end segment, partial articular,
olecranon fracture
2U1B1*

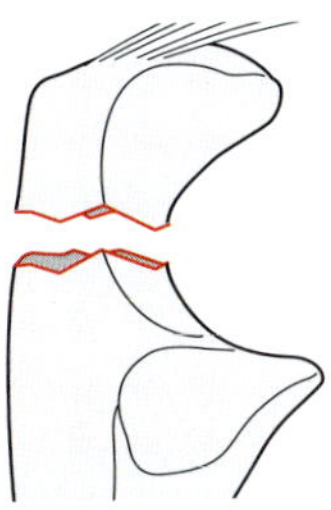

*Qualifications:
d **Simple**
e Multifragmentary

Ulna, proximal end segment, partial articular,
coronoid fracture
2U1B2*

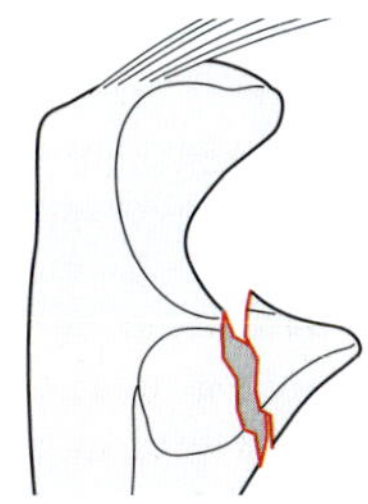

*Qualifications:
n Involving sublime facet
o Tip (avulsion)
p **<50%**
q ≥50%

2R1C/2U1C

Type: Radius, proximal end segment articular, **complete articular fracture** 2R1C*

Groups:

Radius, proximal end segment articular,
complete articular, **simple fracture**
2R1C1

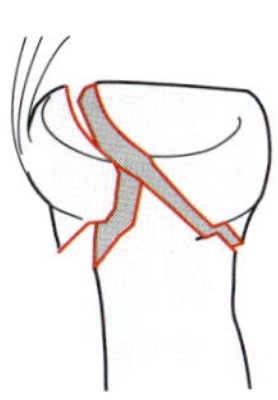

Radius, proximal end segment articular,
complete articular, **multifragmentary fracture**
2R1C3

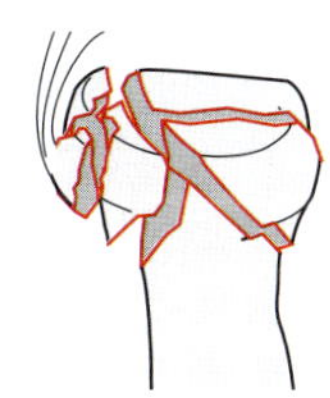

Type: Ulna, proximal end segment, **complete articular fracture** 2U1C

Groups:

Ulna, proximal end segment, complete articular,
olecranon and coronoid fracture
2U1C3*

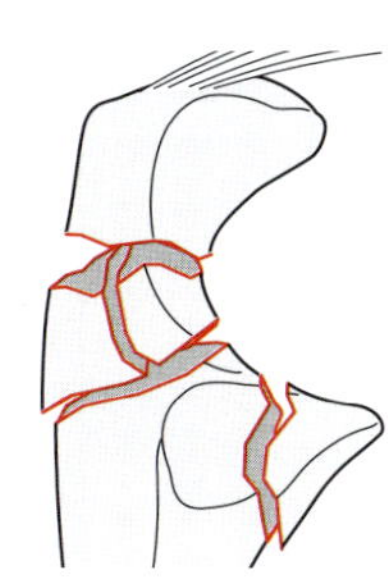

*Qualifications:
d Simple
r Multifragmentary olecranon
s **Multifragmentary involving coronoid process**

2R2/2U2

Location: Radius or ulna,
diaphyseal segment 2R2/2U2

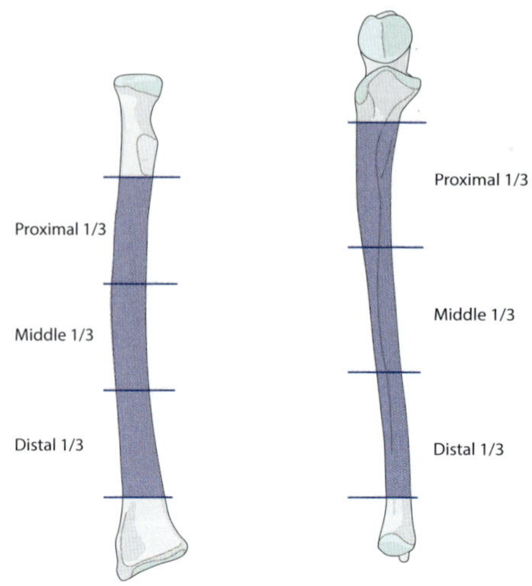

Types:

Radius, diaphyseal segment,
simple fracture
2R2A

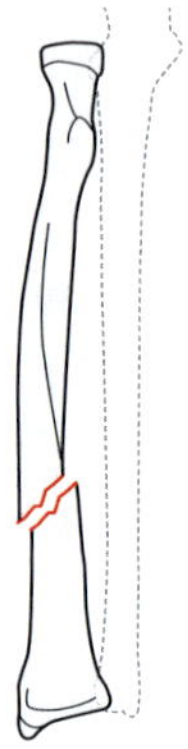

Radius, diaphyseal segment,
wedge fracture
2R2B

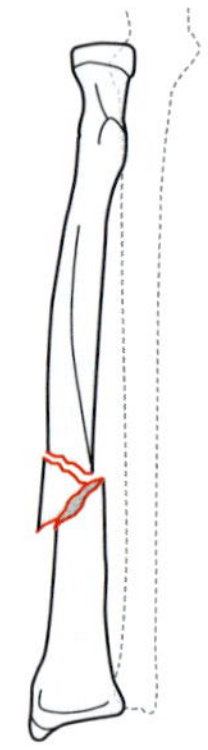

Radius, diaphyseal segment,
multifragmentary fracture
2R2C

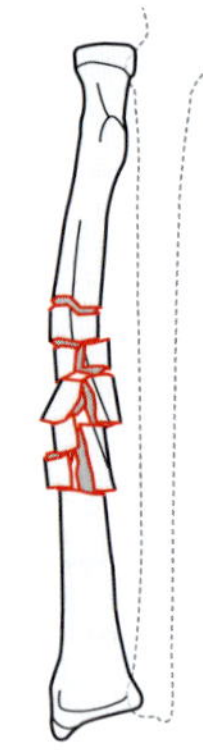

Ulna, diaphyseal segment,
simple fracture
2U2A

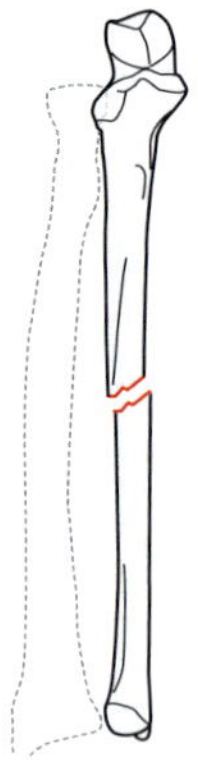

Ulna, diaphyseal segment,
wedge fracture
2U2B

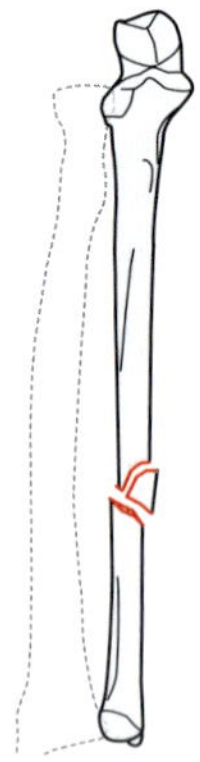

Ulna, diaphyseal segment,
multifragmentary fracture
2U2C

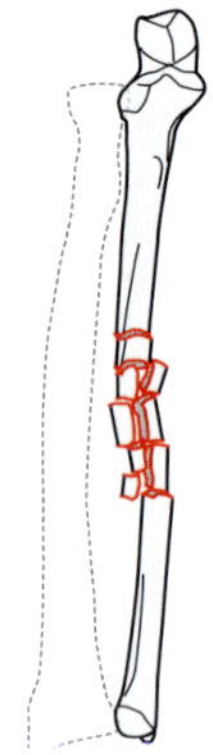

2R2A/2U2A

Type: Radius or ulna, diaphyseal segment, **simple fracture** 2R2A/2U2A

Groups:

Radius, diaphyseal segment, simple,
spiral fracture
2R2A1*

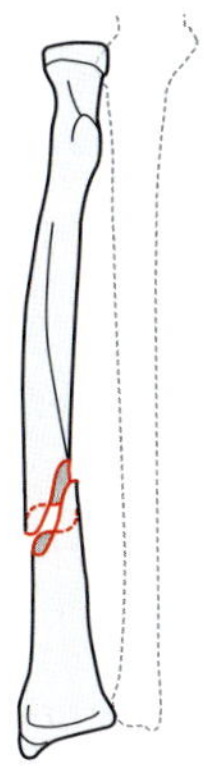

Radius, diaphyseal segment, simple,
oblique fracture (≥30°)
2R2A2*

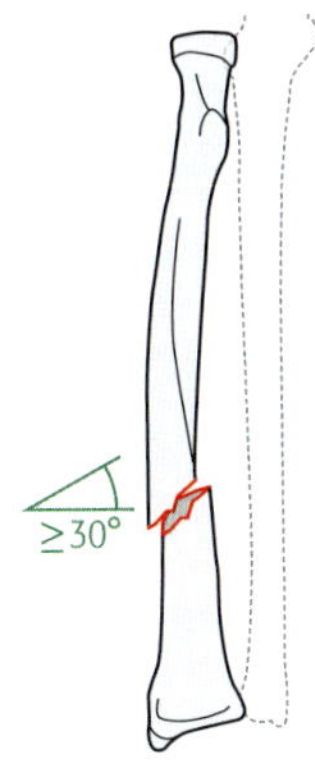

Radius, diaphyseal segment, simple,
transverse fracture (<30°)
2R2A3*

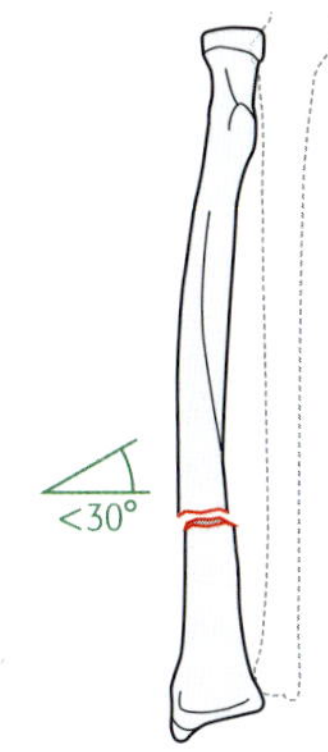

Ulna, diaphyseal segment, simple,
spiral fracture
2U2A1*

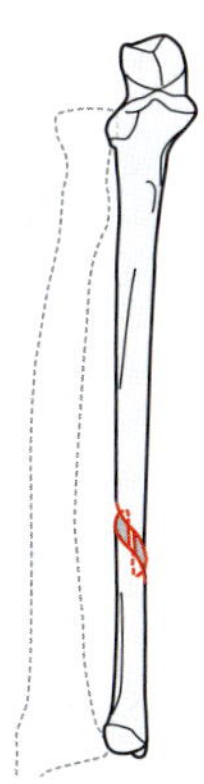

Ulna, diaphyseal segment, simple,
oblique fracture (≥30°)
2U2A2*

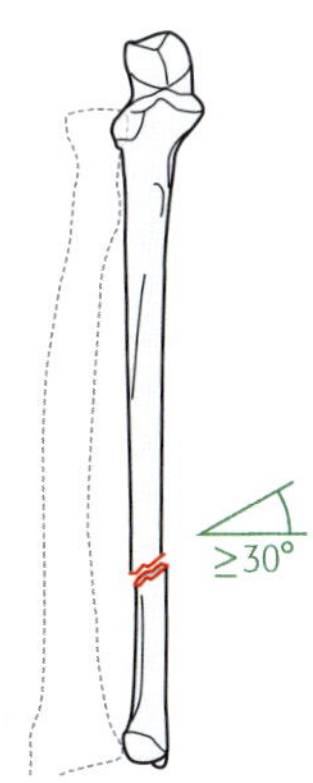

Ulna, diaphyseal segment, simple,
transverse fracture (<30°)
2U2A3*

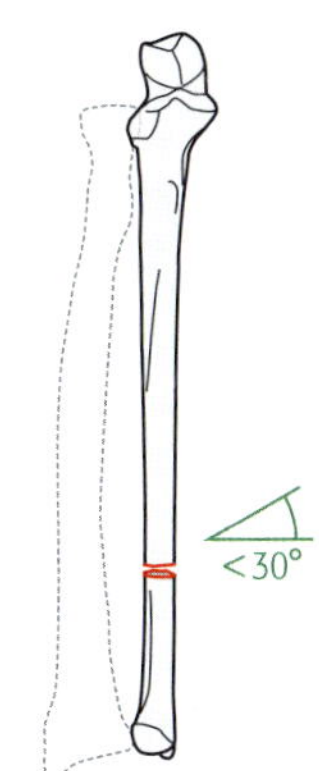

*Qualifications for radius and ulna:

a Proximal 1/3
b Middle 1/3
c **Distal 1/3**

2R2B/ 2U2B

Type: Radius or ulna, diaphyseal segment, **wedge fracture** 2R2B/2U2B

Groups:

Radius, diaphyseal segment,
intact wedge fracture
2R2B2*

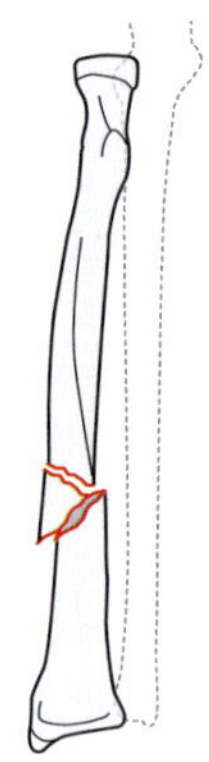

Radius, diaphyseal segment,
fragmentary wedge fracture
2R2B3*

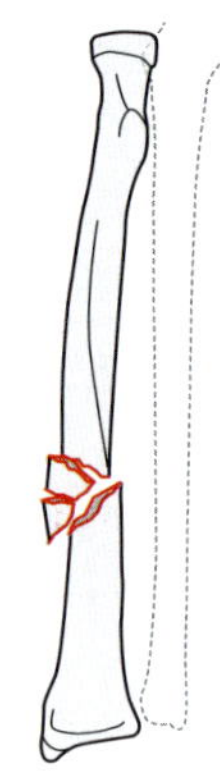

Ulna, diaphyseal segment,
intact wedge fracture
2U2B2*

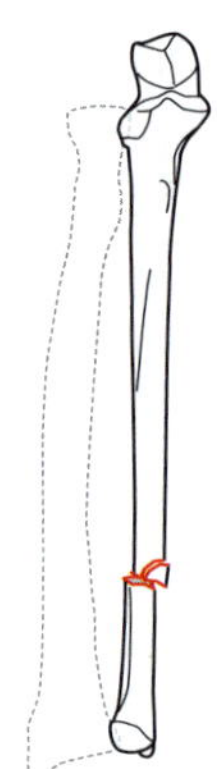

Ulna, diaphyseal segment,
fragmentary wedge fracture
2U2B3*

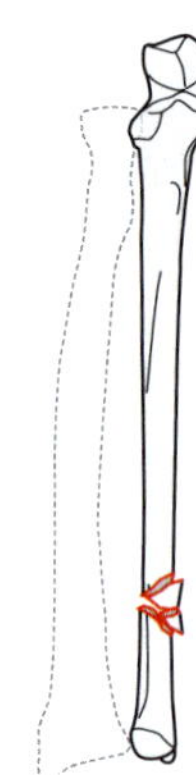

*Qualifications for radius and ulna:
- a Proximal 1/3
- b Middle 1/3
- c **Distal 1/3**

2R2C/2U2C

Type: Radius or ulna, diaphyseal segment, **multifragmentary fracture** 2R2C/2U2C

Groups:

Radius, diaphyseal segment, multifragmentary,
intact segmental fracture
2R2C2*

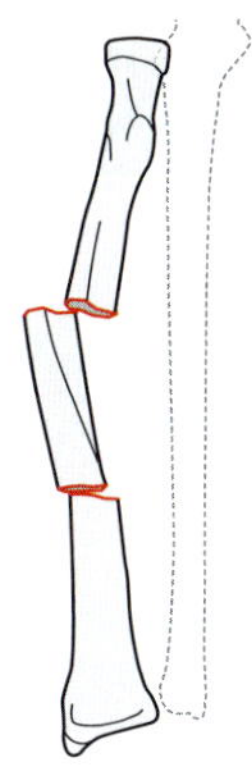

Radius, diaphyseal segment, multifragmentary,
fragmentary segmental fracture
2R2C3*

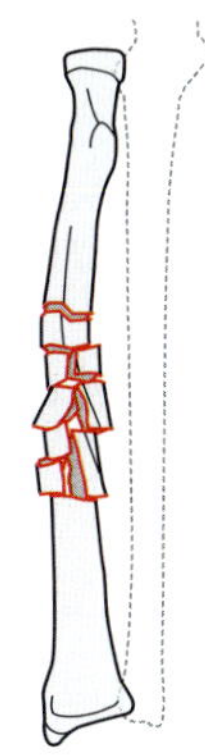

Ulna, diaphyseal segment, multifragmentary,
intact segmental fracture
2U2C2*

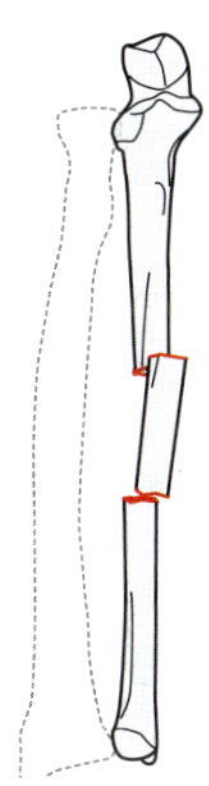

Ulna, diaphyseal segment, multifragmentary,
fragmentary segmental fracture
2U2C3*

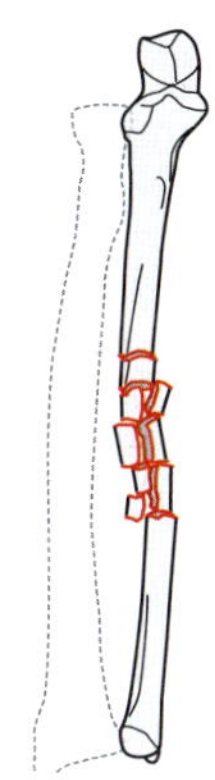

*Qualifications for radius and ulna:
- i Proximal diaphyseal-metaphyseal
- j **Pure diaphyseal**
- k Distal diaphyseal-metaphyseal

→ **Galeazzi** and **Monteggia** fracture patterns can be coded as follows:
The code for the fracture pattern is the radius or ulna fracture code with qualifier of (g) for Galeazzi or (m) for Monteggia representing disruption of the radio-ulnar joint. For more information about Galeazzi and Monteggia fractures, please refer to the Appendix.

2R3/2U3

Location: Radius/Ulna, **distal end segment** 2R3/2U3

U

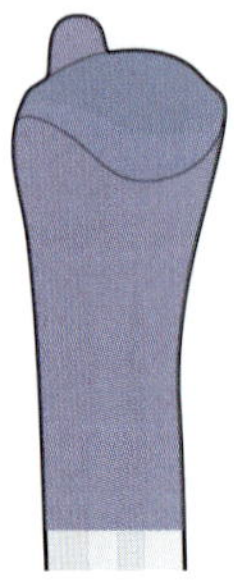

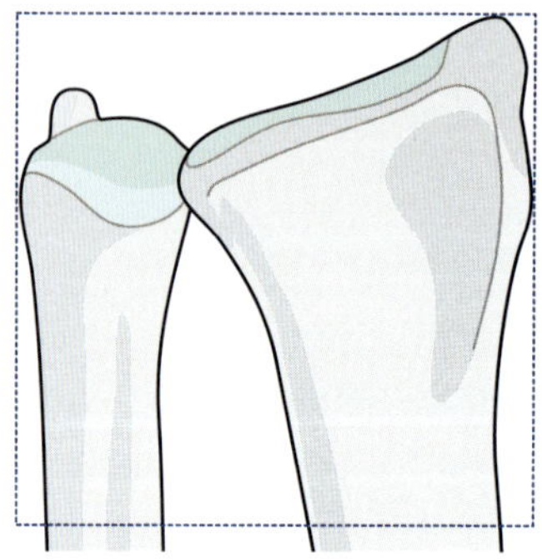

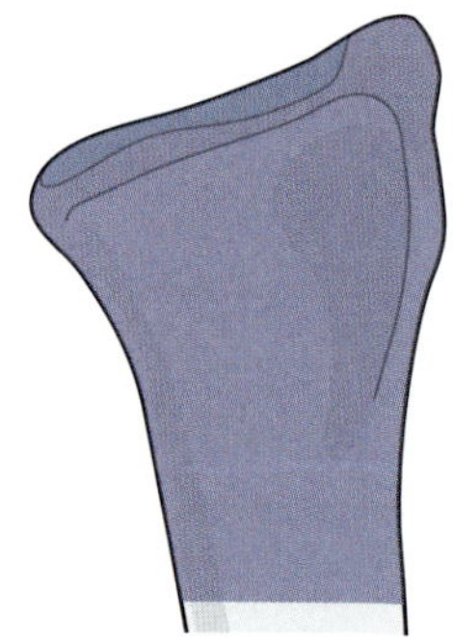

R

Types:

Radius, distal end segment,
extraarticular fracture
2R3A

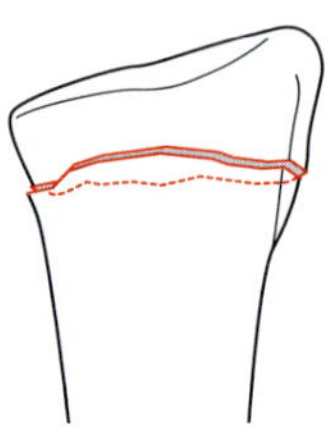

Radius, distal end segment,
partial articular fracture
2R3B

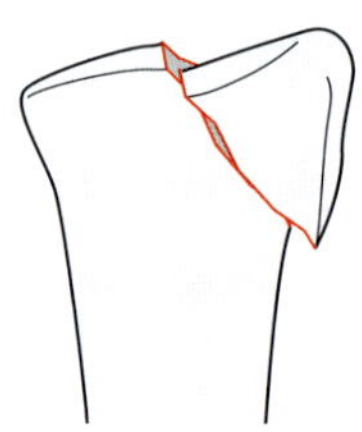

Radius, distal end segment,
complete articular fracture
2R3C

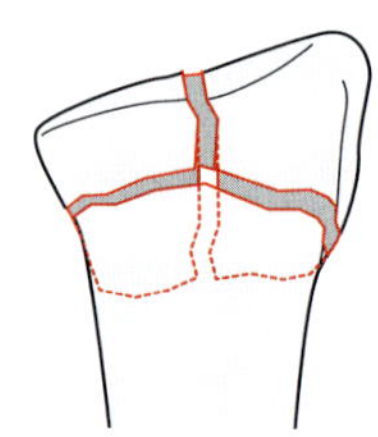

Ulna, distal end segment,
extraarticular fracture
2U3A

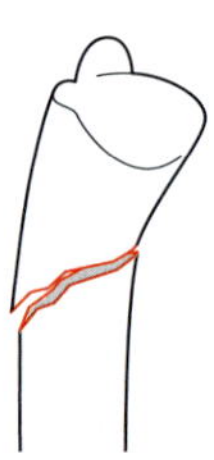

Ulna, distal end segment,
partial articular fracture
2U3B

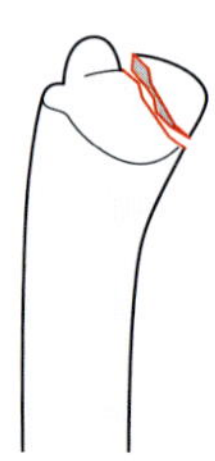

Ulna, distal end segment,
complete articular fracture
2U3C

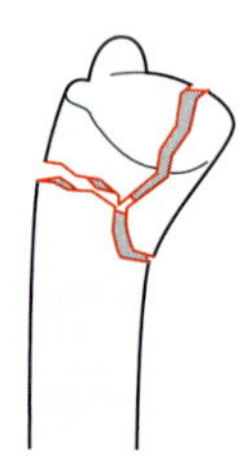

2R3A

Type: Radius, distal end segment, **extraarticular fracture** 2R3A

Group:
Radius, distal end segment, extraarticular,
radial styloid avulsion fracture
2R3A1

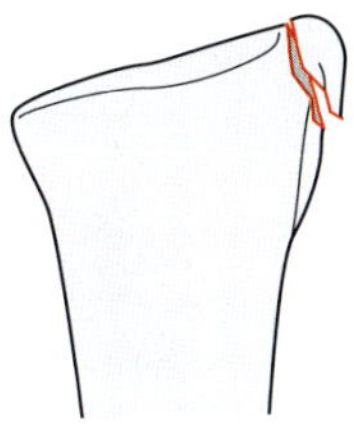

Group: Radius, distal end segment, extraarticular, **simple fracture** 2R3A2

Subgroups:

Transverse, no displacement/tilt (may be shortened)
2R3A2.1

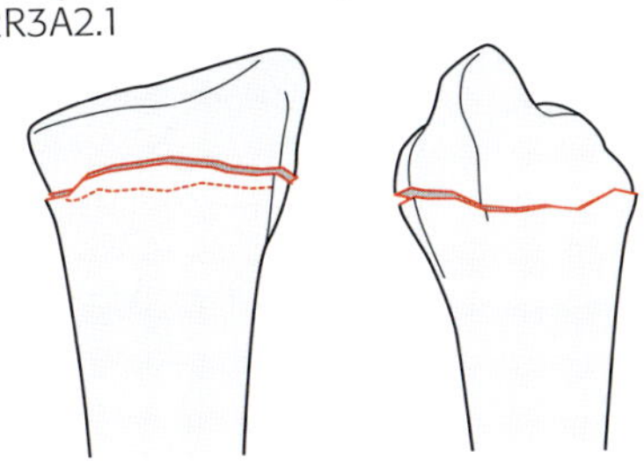

Dorsal displacement/tilt (Colles)
2R3A2.2

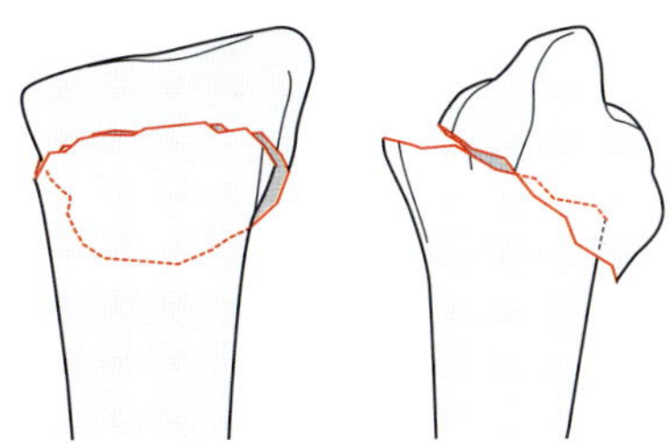

Volar displacement/tilt (Smith's)
2R3A2.3

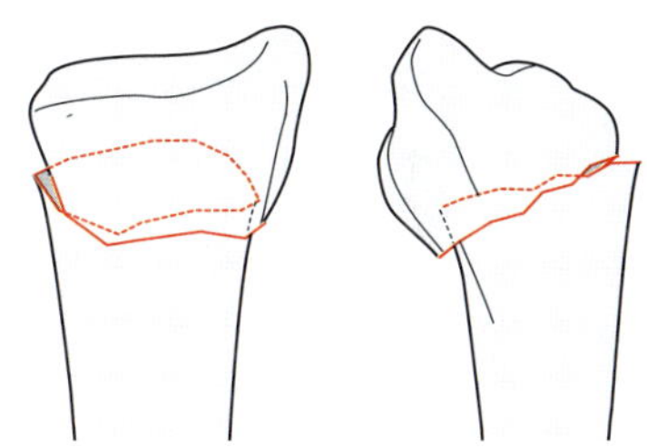

Group: Radius, distal end segment, extraarticular, **wedge or multifragmentary fracture** 2R3A3

Subgroups:

Intact wedge fracture
2R3A3.1

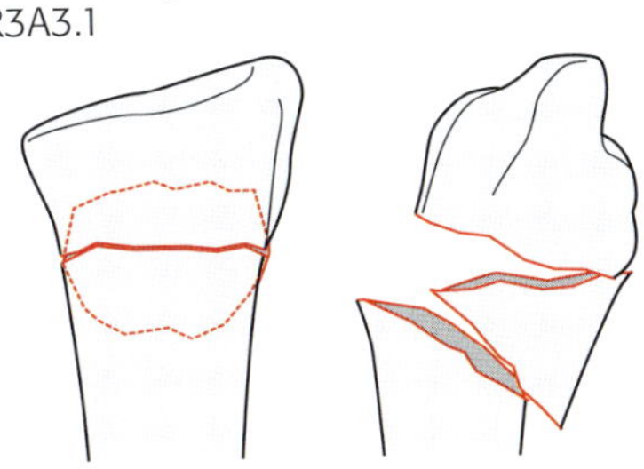

Fragmentary wedge fracture
2R3A3.2

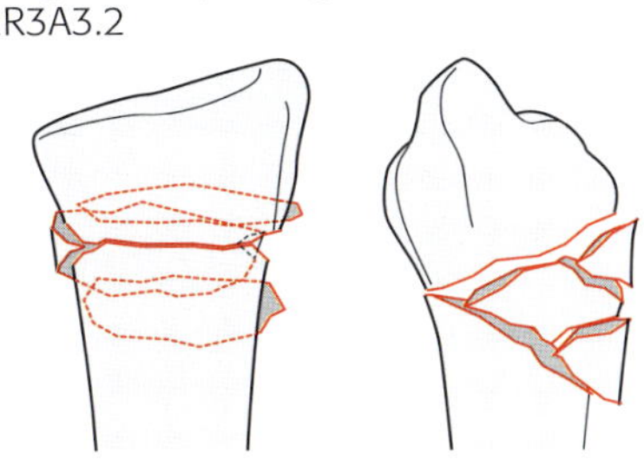

Multifragmentary fracture
2R3A3.3

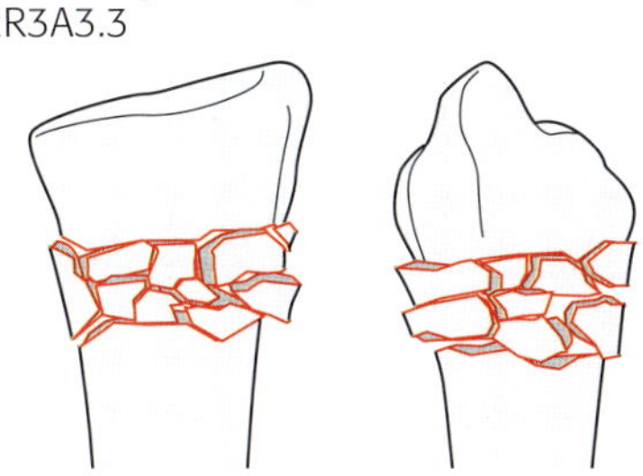

2U3A

Type: Ulna, distal end segment, **extraarticular fracture** 2U3A

Group: Ulna, distal end segment, extraarticular, **styloid process fracture** 2U3A1

Subgroups:

Tip of styloid fracture
2U3A1.1

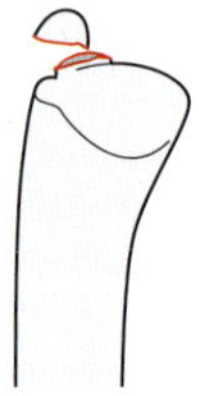

Base of styloid fracture
2U3A1.2

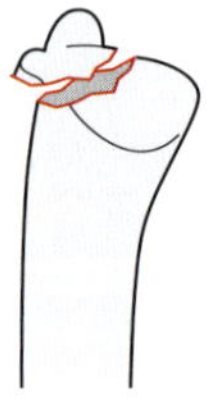

Group: Ulna, distal end segment, extraarticular, **simple fracture** 2U3A2

Subgroups:

Spiral fracture
2U3A2.1

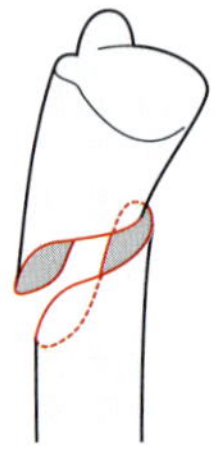

Oblique fracture (≥30°)
2U3A2.2

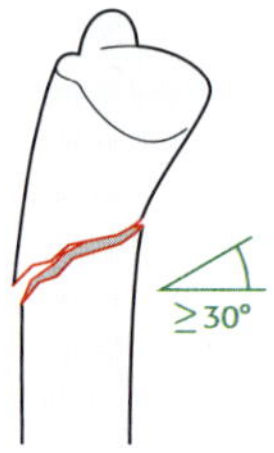

Transverse fracture (<30°)
2U3A2.3

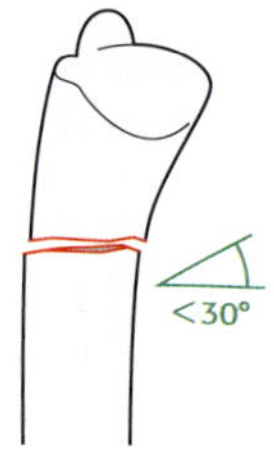

Group: Ulna, distal end segment, extraarticular, **multifragmentary fracture** 2U3A3

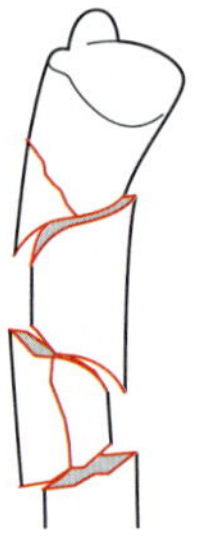

2R3B

Type: Radius, distal end segment, **partial articular fracture** 2R3B

Group: Radius, distal end segment, partial articular, **sagittal fracture** 2R3B1

Subgroups:
Involving scaphoid fossa
2R3B1.1

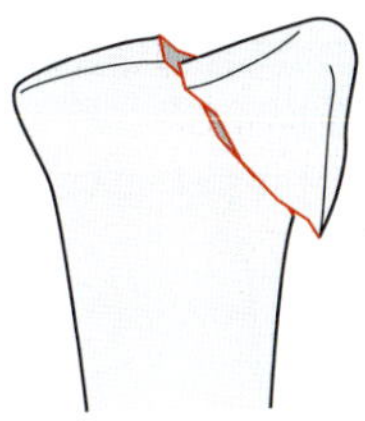

Involving lunate fossa
2R3B1.3

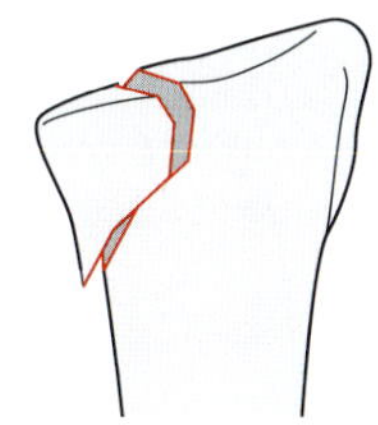

Group: Radius, distal end segment, partial articular, **dorsal rim (Barton's) fracture** 2R3B2

Subgroups:
Simple fracture
2R3B2.1

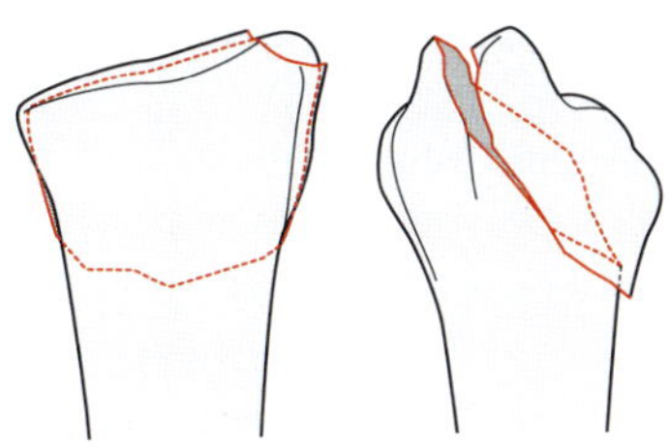

Fragmentary fracture
2R3B2.2

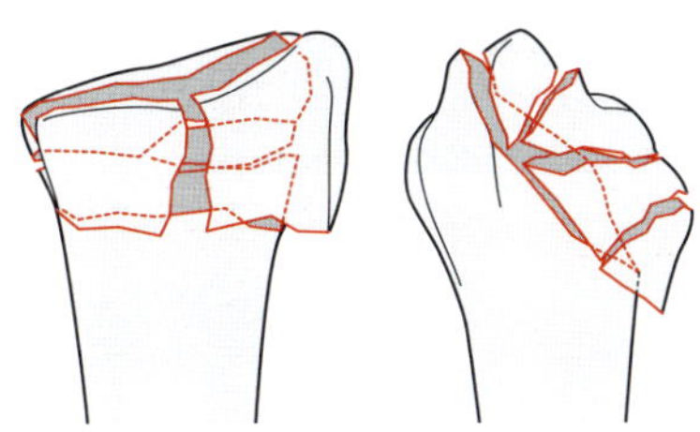

With dorsal dislocation
2R3B2.3

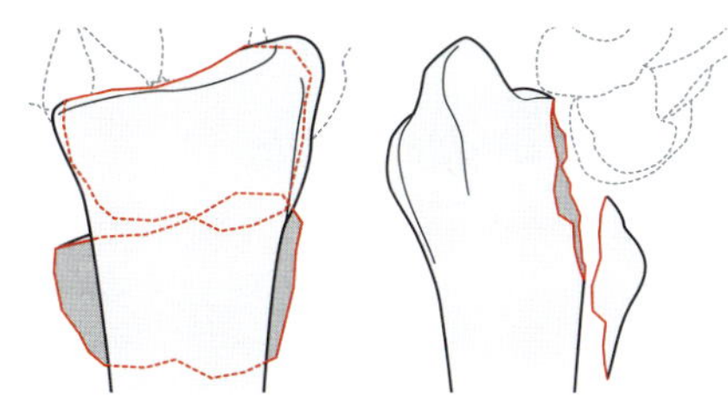

Group: Radius, distal end segment, partial articular, **volar rim (reverse Barton's, Goyrand-Smith's II) fracture** 2R3B3

Subgroups:
Simple fracture
2R3B3.1

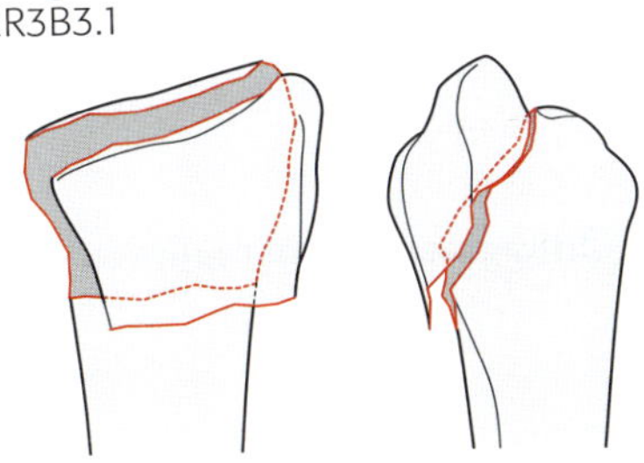

Fragmentary fracture
2R3B3.3

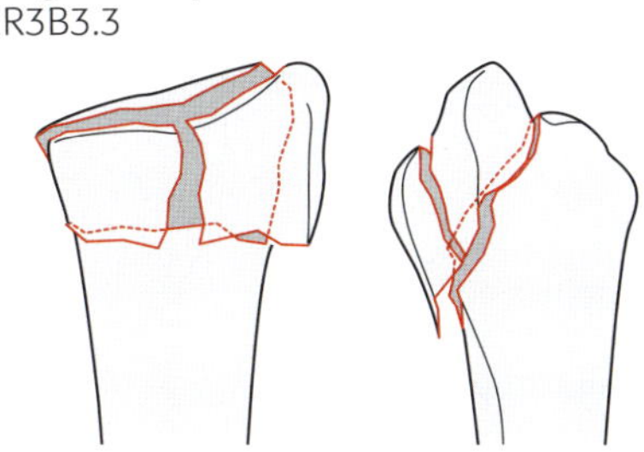

2R3C

Type: Radius, distal end segment, **complete articular fracture** 2R3C

Group: Radius, distal end segment, complete, **simple articular and metaphyseal fracture** 2R3C1

Subgroups:

Dorsomedial articular fracture
2R3C1.1*

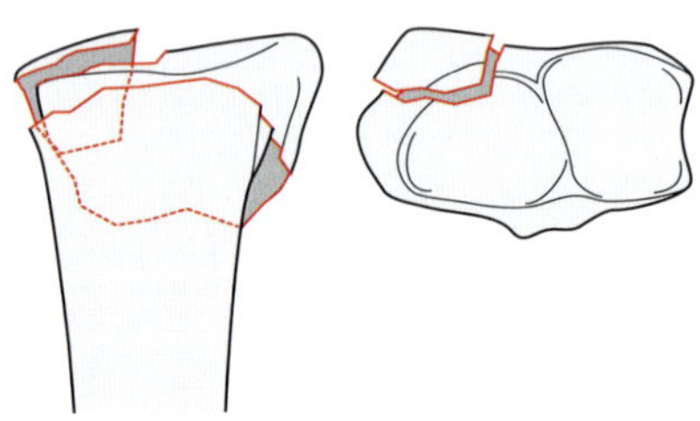

Sagittal articular fracture
2R3C1.2*

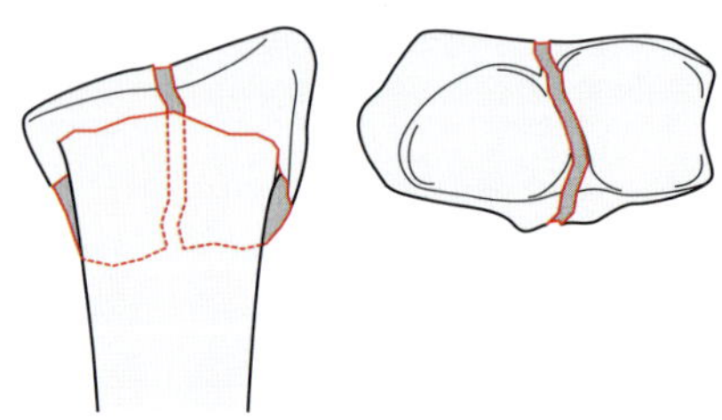

Frontal/coronal articular fracture
2R3C1.3*

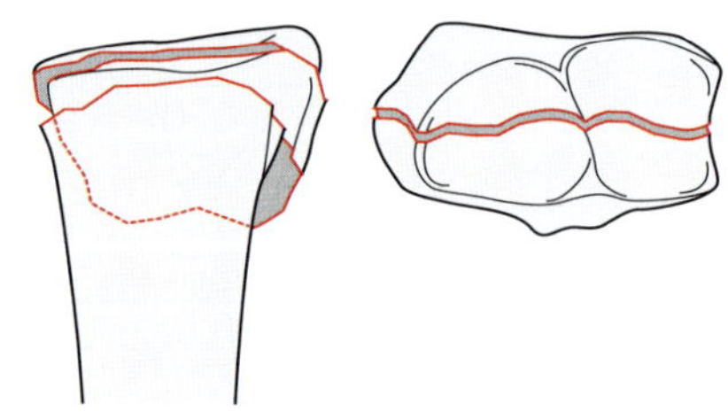

*Qualifications:
t DRUJ stable
u DRUJ unstable

Group: Radius, distal end segment, complete, simple articular, **metaphyseal multifragmentary fracture** 2R3C2

Subgroups:

Sagittal articular fracture
2R3C2.1*

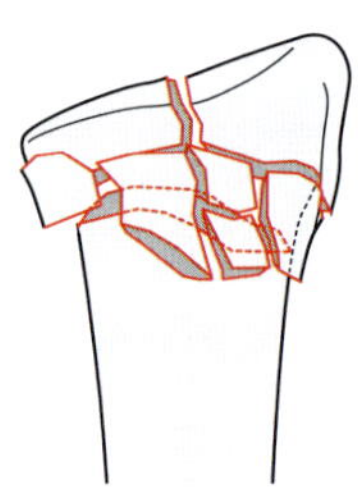

Frontal/coronal fracture
2R3C2.2*

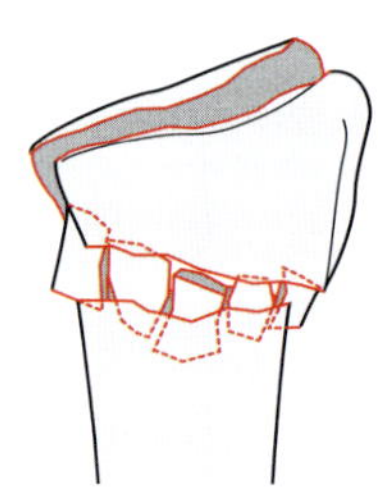

Extending into the diaphysis
2R3C2.3*

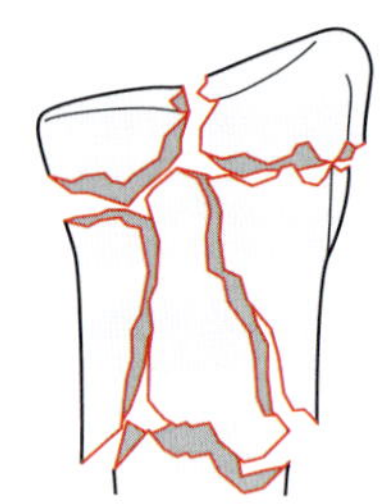

*Qualifications:
t DRUJ stable
u DRUJ unstable

Group: Radius, distal end segment, complete, **articular multifragmentary fracture, simple or multifragmentary metaphyseal fracture** 2R3C3

Subgroups:

Simple metaphyseal fracture
2R3C3.1*

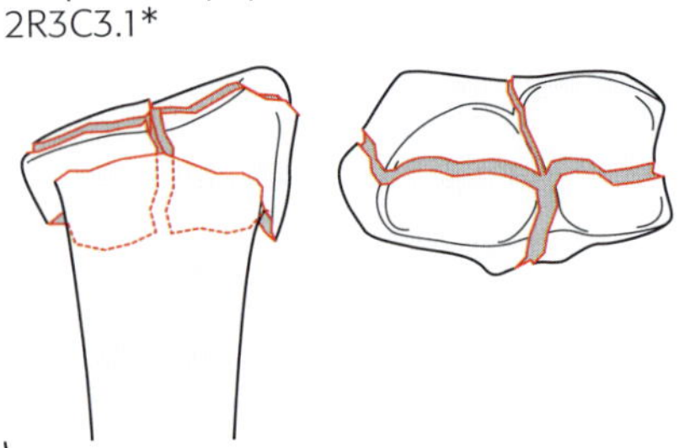

Metaphyseal multifragmentary fracture
2R3C3.2*

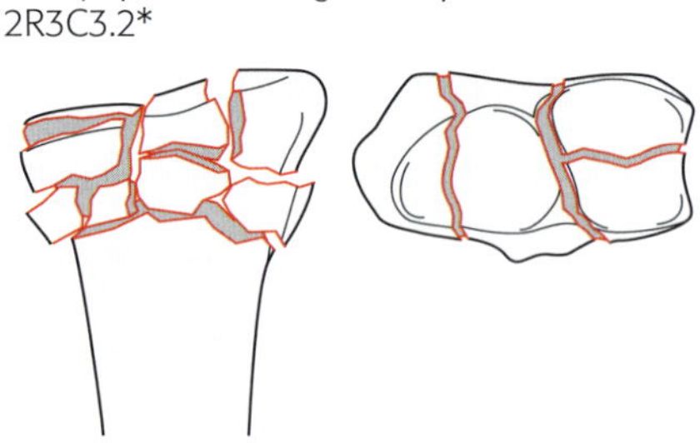

Extending into the diaphysis
2R3C3.3*

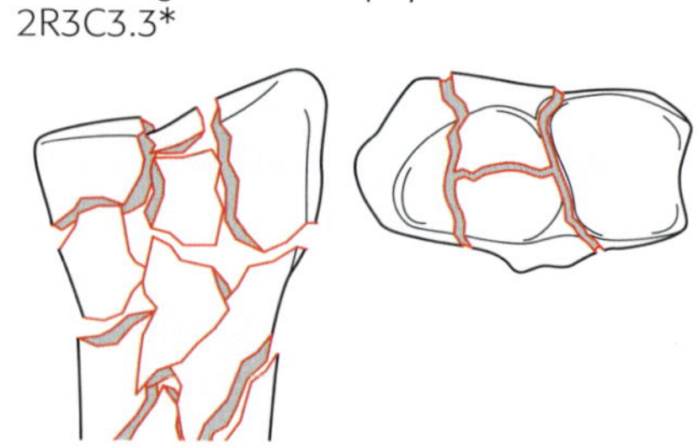

*Qualifications:
t DRUJ stable
u DRUJ unstable

Qualifications *are optional and applied to the fracture code where the asterisk is located as a lower-case letter within rounded brackets. More than one qualification can be applied for a given fracture classification, separated by a comma. For a more detailed explanation, see the compendium introduction.*

Femur

Bone: Femur 3

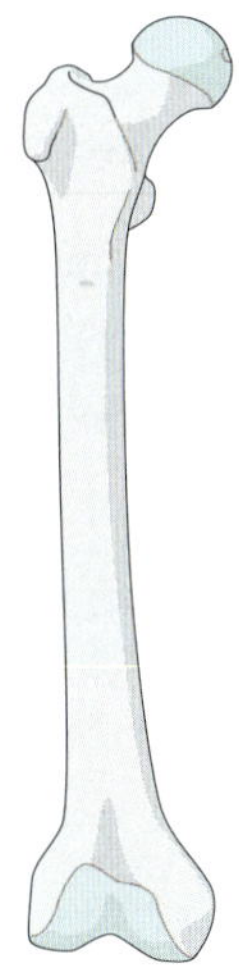

31

Location: Femur, **proximal end segment** 31

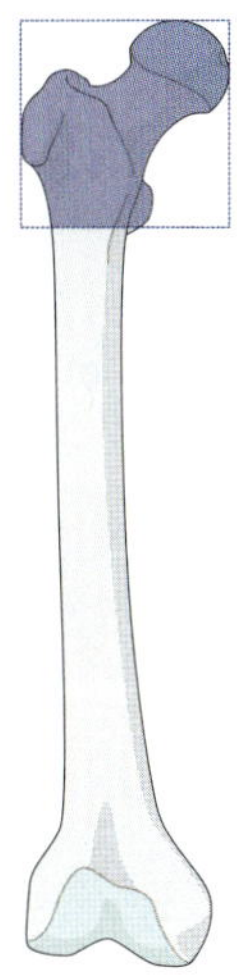

Types:

Femur, **trochanteric region fracture**
31A

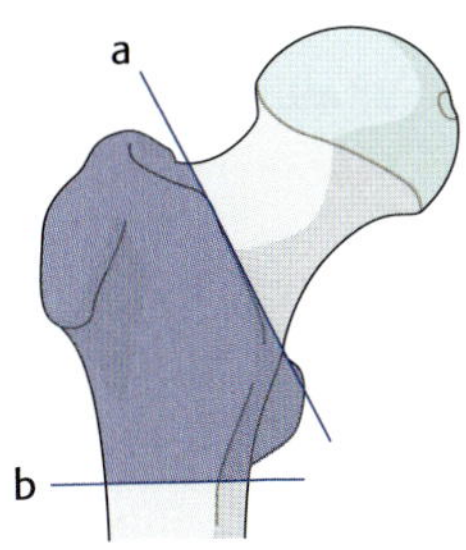

Any fracture centered below the intertrochanteric line (a) and above a horizontal transverse line at the inferior border of the lesser trochanter(b).

Femur, **neck fracture**
31B

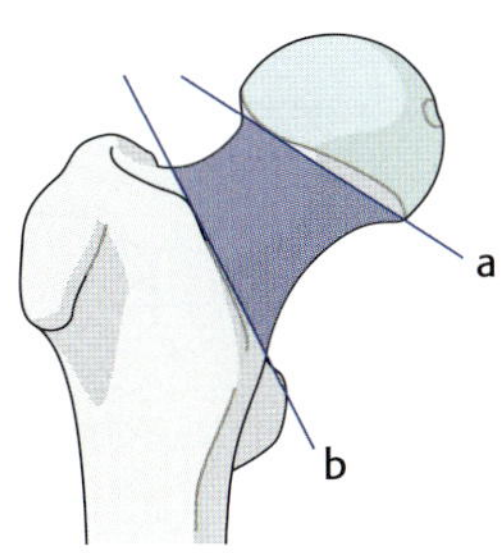

Any fracture centered between a line drawn at the distal extent of femoral head articular cartilage (a) and the intertrochanteric line distally (b) are subcapital or femoral neck fractures.

Femur, **head fracture**
31C

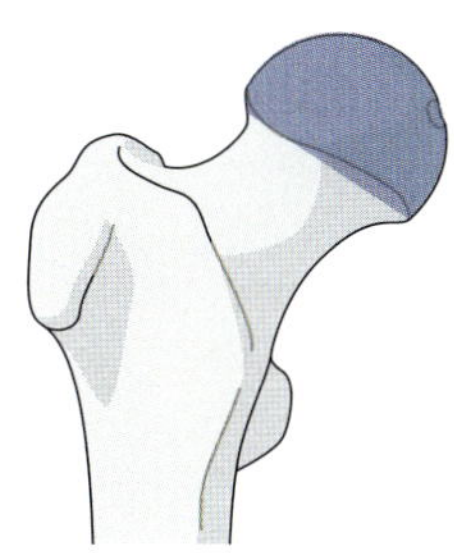

Fractures through the portion of the proximal segment covered with articular cartilage.

Qualifications *are optional and applied to the fracture code where the asterisk is located as a lower-case letter within rounded brackets. More than one qualification can be applied for a given fracture classification, separated by a comma. For a more detailed explanation, see the compendium introduction.*

31A

Type: Femur, proximal end segment, **trochanteric region fracture** 31A

Group: Femur, proximal end segment, trochanteric region, **simple pertrochanteric fracture** 31A1

Subgroups:

Isolated single trochanter fracture
31A1.1*

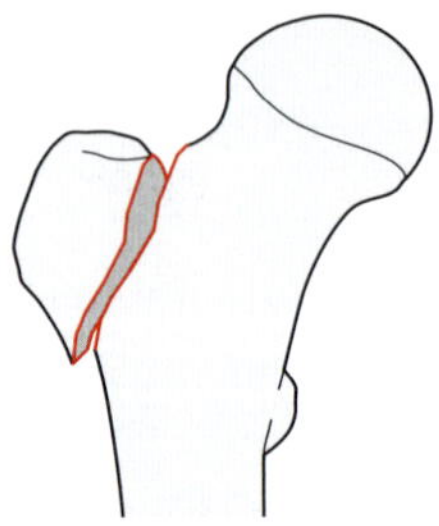

*Qualifications:
n **Greater trochanter**
o Lesser trochanter

Two-part fracture
31A1.2

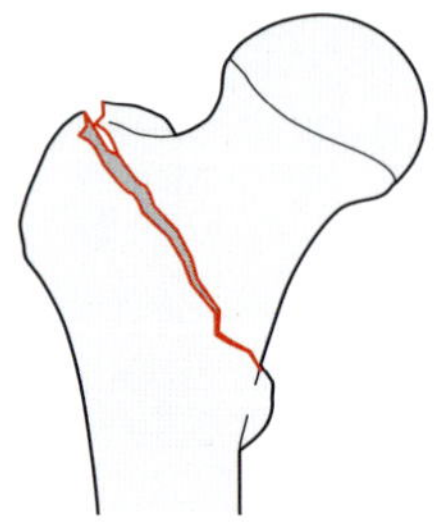

Lateral wall intact (>20.5 mm) fracture
31A1.3

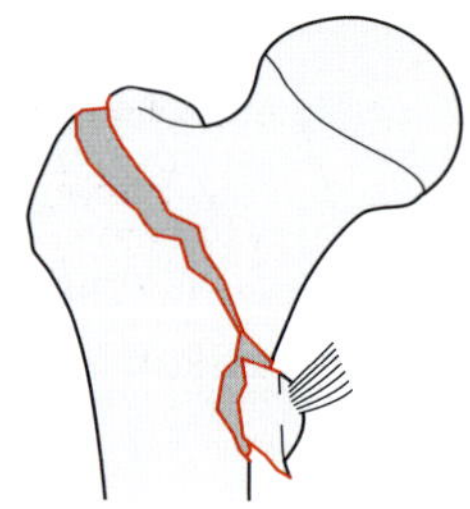

Group: Femur, proximal end segment, trochanteric region, **multifragmentary pertrochanteric, lateral wall incompetent (≤ 20.5 mm) fracture** 31A2

Subgroups:

With 1 intermediate fragment
31A2.2

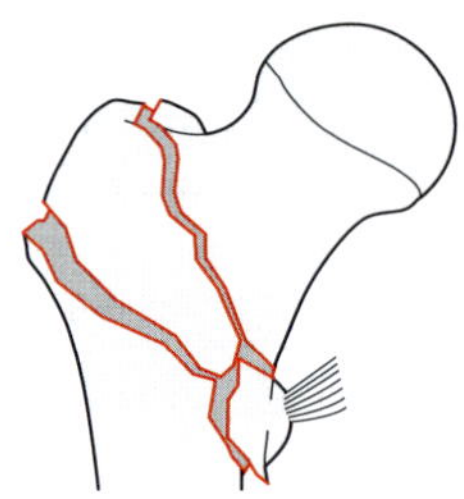

With 2 or more intermediate fragments
31A2.3

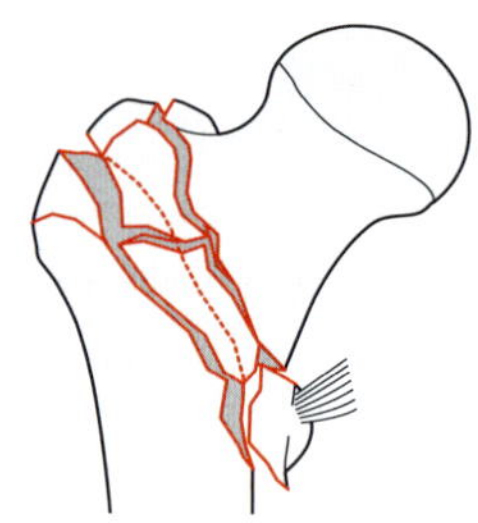

→ For more information about calculating the lateral wall thickness, please refer to the Appendix.

Group: Femur, proximal end segment, trochanteric region, **intertrochanteric (reverse obliquity) fracture** 31A3

Subgroups:

Simple oblique fracture
31A3.1

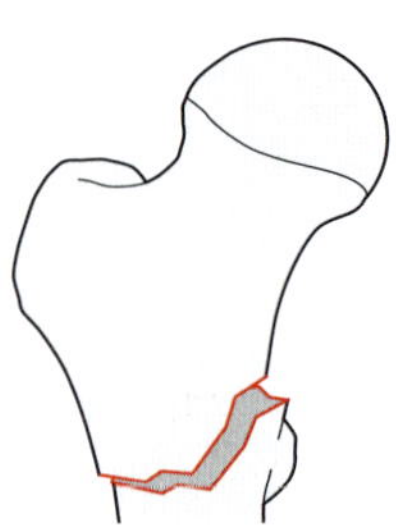

Simple transverse fracture
31A3.2

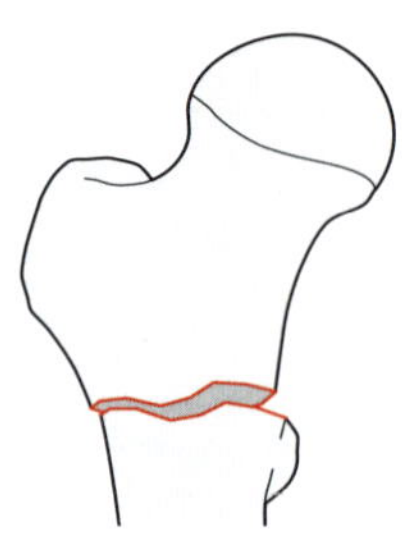

Wedge or multifragmentary fracture
31A3.3

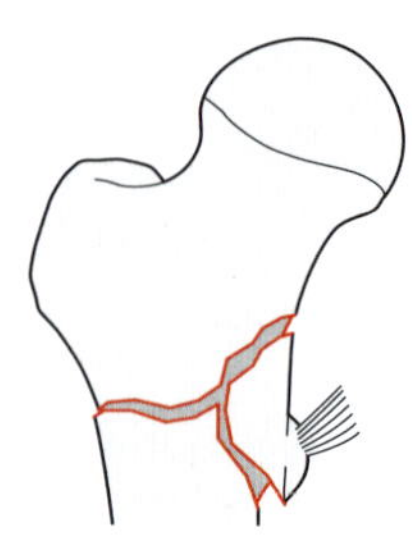

31B

Type: Femur, proximal end segment, **femoral neck fracture** 31B

Group: Femur, proximal end segment, femoral neck, **subcapital fracture** 31B1

Subgroups:

Valgus impacted fracture
31B1.1

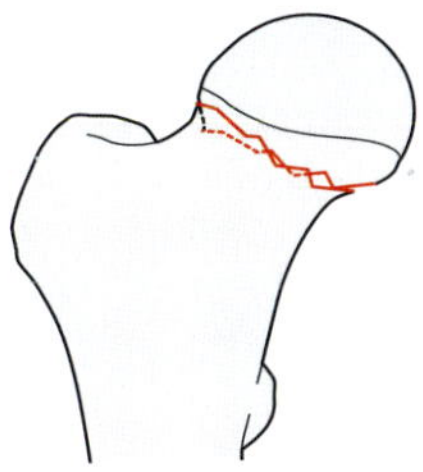

Nondisplaced fracture
31B1.2

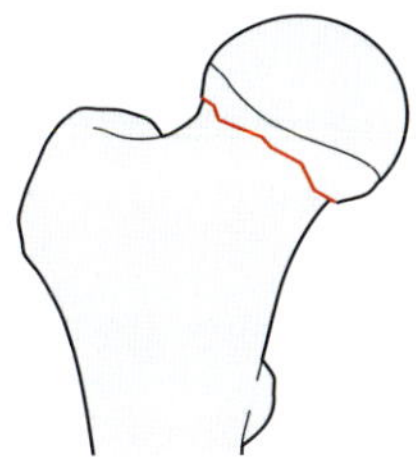

Displaced fracture
31B1.3

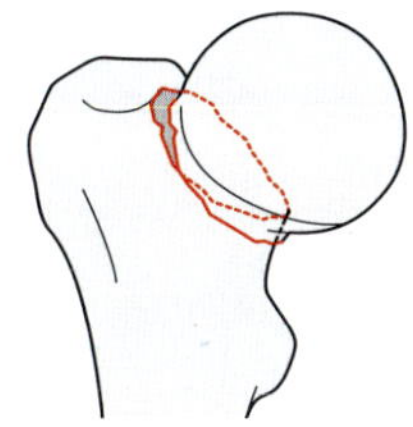

Group: Femur, proximal end segment, femoral neck, **transcervical fracture** 31B2

Subgroups:

Simple fracture
31B2.1*

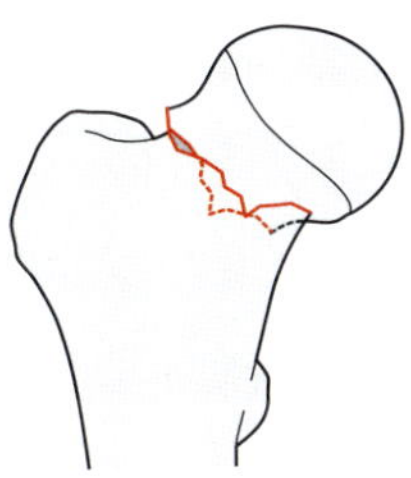

Multifragmentary fracture
31B2.2*

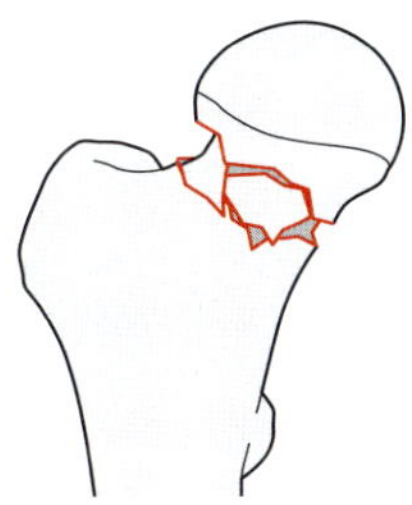

Shear fracture
31B2.3*

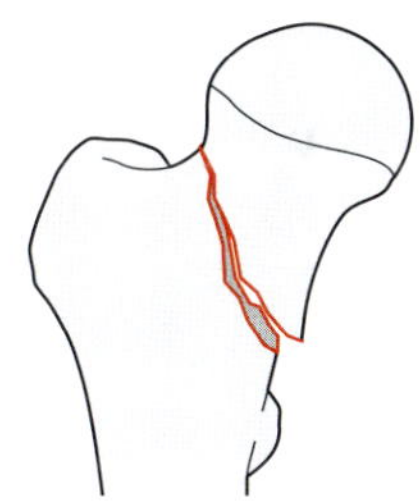

*Qualifications:
p Pauwels 1 (<30°)
q Pauwels 2 (30–70°)
r Pauwels 3 (>70°)

Group: Femur, proximal end segment, femoral neck, **basicervical fracture** 31B3

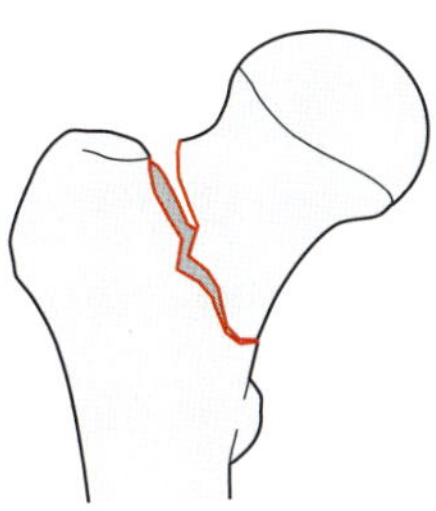

31C

Type: Femur, proximal end segment, **femoral head fracture** 31C

Group: Femur, proximal end segment, femoral head, **split fracture** 31C1

Subgroups:

Avulsion of ligamentum teres fracture
31C1.1

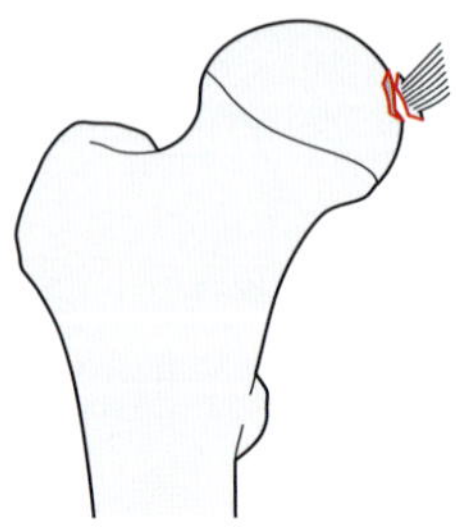

Split, infrafoveal fracture
31C1.2

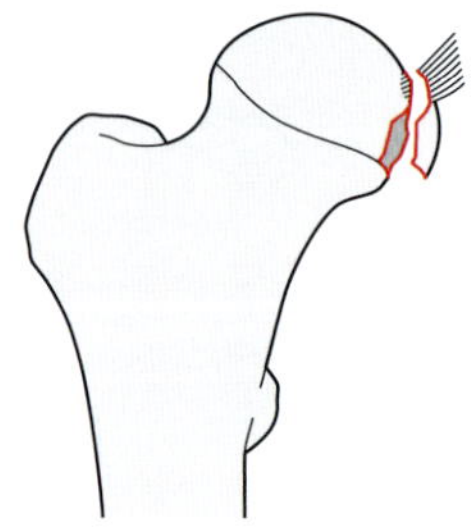

Split, suprafoveal fracture
31C1.3

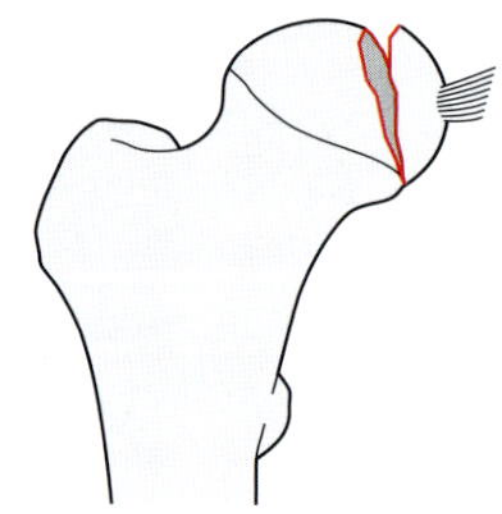

Group: Femur, proximal end segment, femoral head, **depression fracture** 31C2

Subgroups:

Chondral lesion
31C2.1

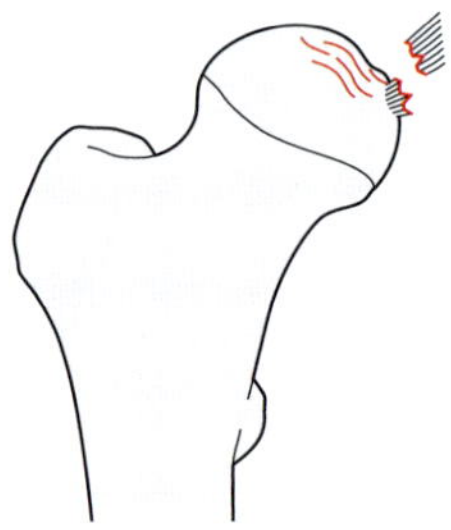

Depression impaction fracture
31C2.2

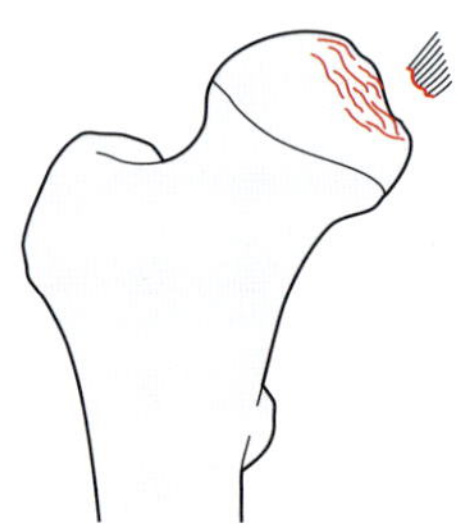

Split depression fracture
31C2.3

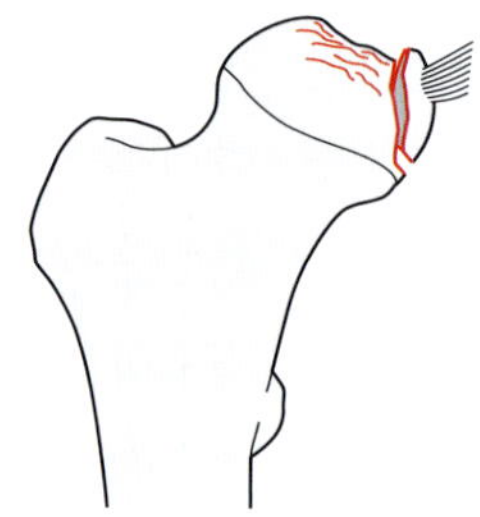

→ Associated dislocations are coded using the dislocation direction universal modifier in square brackets [5_].

32

Location: Femur, **diaphyseal segment** 32

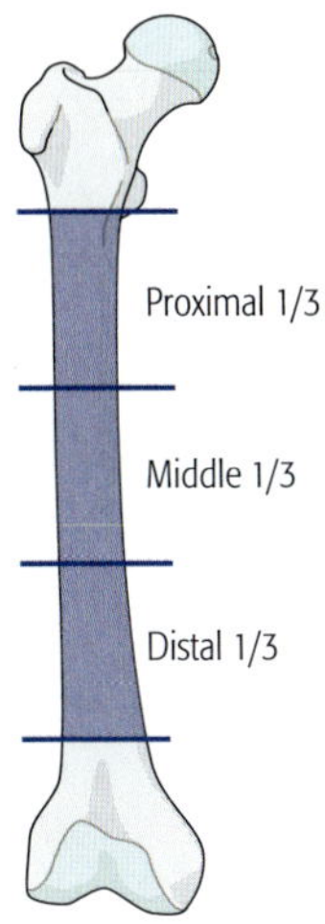

Types:

Femur, diaphyseal segment,
simple fracture
32A

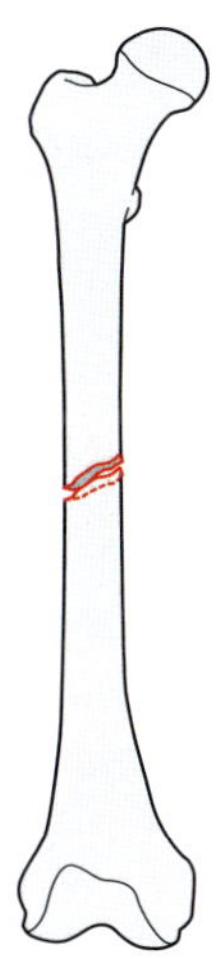

Femur, diaphyseal segment,
wedge fracture
32B

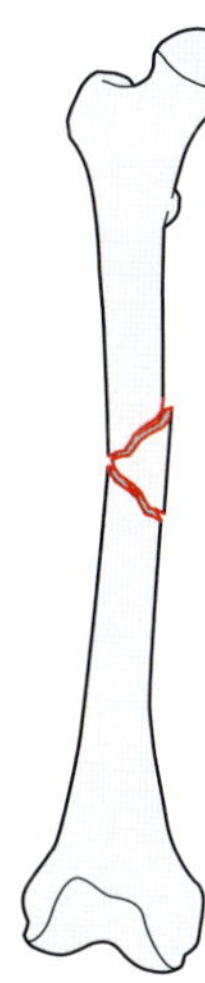

Femur, diaphyseal segment,
multifragmentary fracture
32C

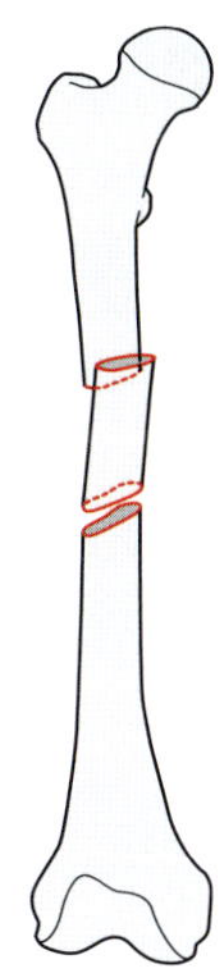

32A

Type: Femur, diaphyseal segment **simple fracture** 32A

Groups:

Femur, diaphyseal segment, simple, **spiral fracture**
32A1*

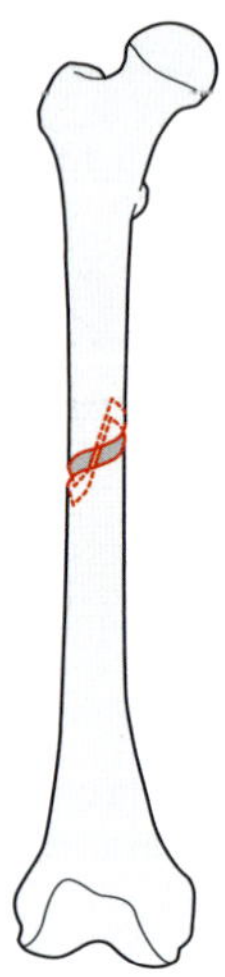

Femur, diaphyseal segment, simple, **oblique fracture (≥30°)**
32A2*

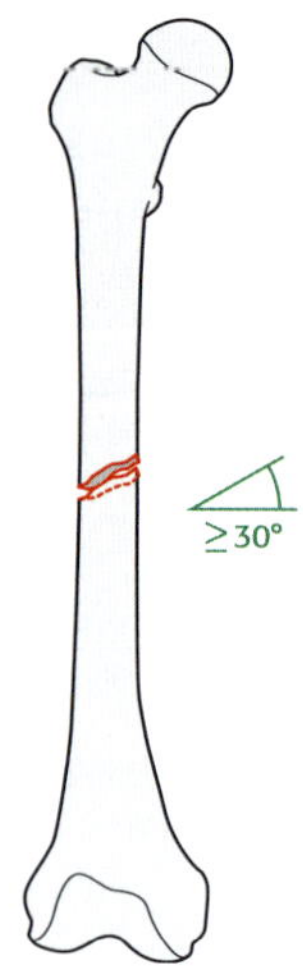

Femur, diaphyseal segment, simple, **transverse fracture (<30°)**
32A3*

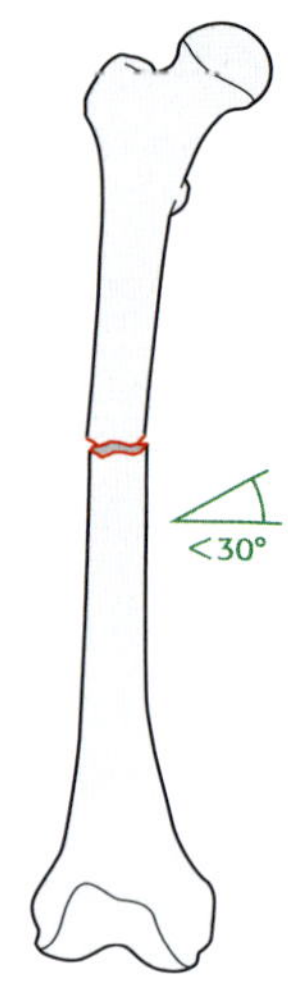

*Qualifications:
a Proximal 1/3
b **Middle 1/3**
c Distal 1/3

32B

Type: Femur, diaphyseal segment, **wedge fracture** 32B

Groups:

Femur, diaphyseal segment, **intact wedge fracture**
32B2*

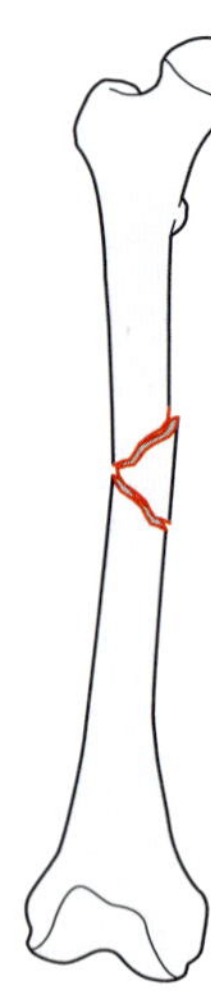

Femur, diaphyseal segment, **fragmentary wedge fracture**
32B3*

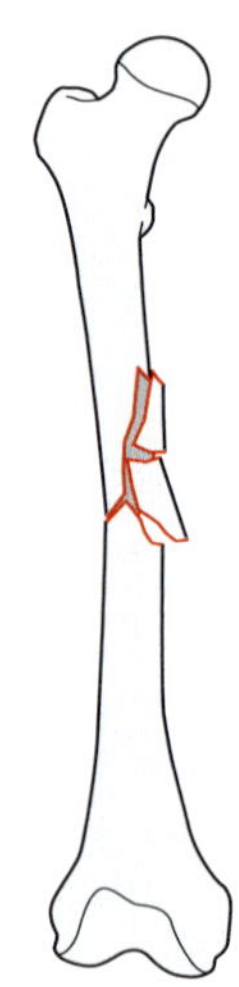

*Qualifications:
a Proximal 1/3
b **Middle 1/3**
c Distal 1/3

32C

Type: Femur, diaphyseal segment, **multifragmentary fracture** 32C

Groups:

Femur, diaphyseal segment, multifragmentary, **intact segmental fracture** 32C2*

Femur, diaphyseal segment, multifragmentary, **fragmentary segmental fracture** 32C3*

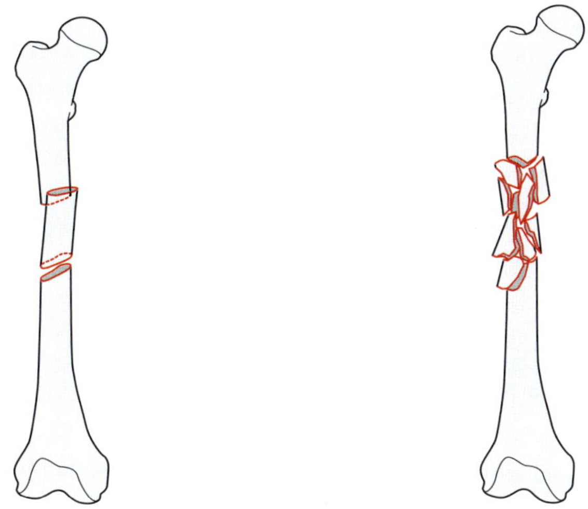

*Qualifications:
- i Proximal diaphyseal-metaphyseal
- j **Pure diaphyseal**
- k Distal diaphyseal-metaphyseal

33

Location: Femur, **distal end segment** 33

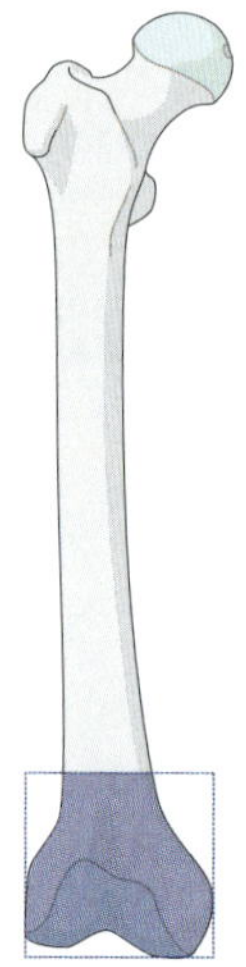

Types:

Femur, distal end segment, **extraarticular fracture** 33A

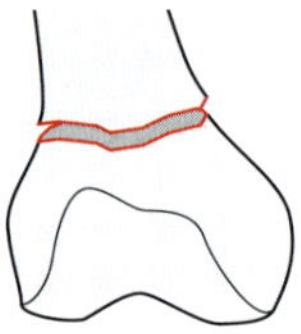

Femur, distal end segment, **partial articular fracture** 33B

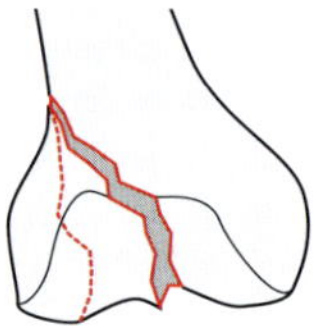

Femur, distal end segment, **complete articular fracture** 33C

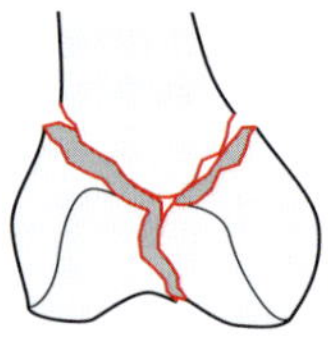

33A

Type: Femur, distal end segment, **extraarticular fracture** 33A

Group: Femur, distal end segment, extraarticular, **avulsion fracture** 33A1

Subgroups:

Lateral epicondyle fracture 33A1.1

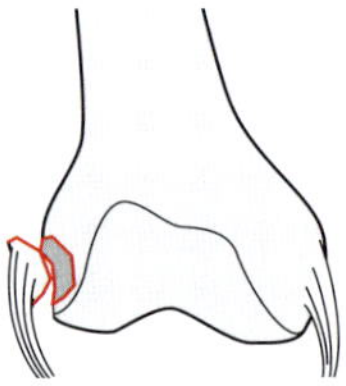

Medial epicondyle fracture 33A1.2

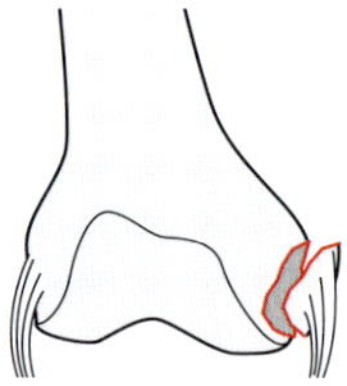

Group: Femur, distal end segment, extraarticular, **simple fracture** 33A2

Subgroups:

Spiral fracture 33A2.1

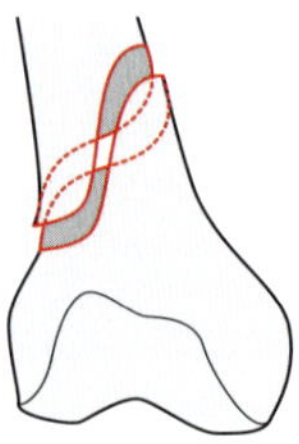

Oblique fracture 33A2.2

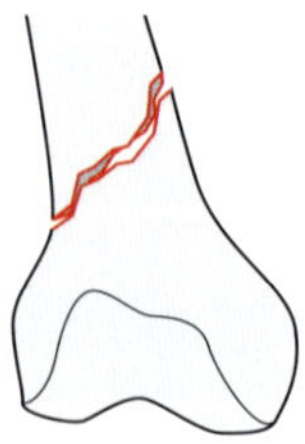

Transverse fracture 33A2.3

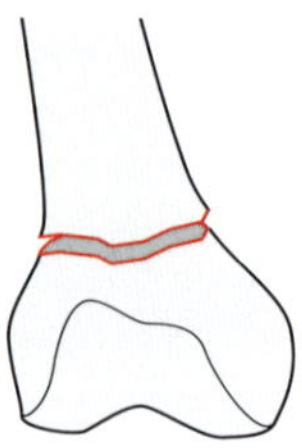

Group: Femur, distal end segment, extraarticular, **wedge or multifragmentary fracture** 33A3

Subgroups:

Intact wedge fracture
33A3.1*

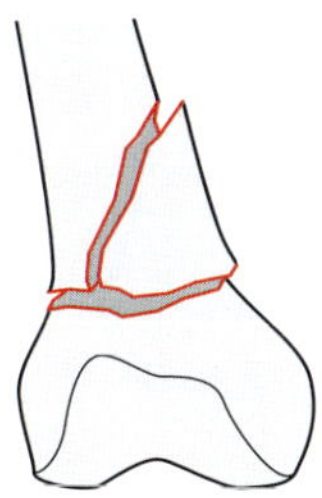

Fragmentary wedge fracture
33A3.2*

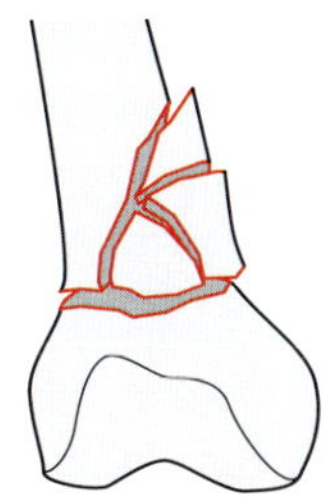

Multifragmentary fracture
33A3.3

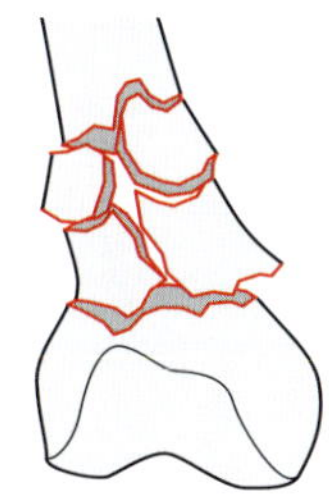

*Qualifications:
f Lateral
h **Medial**

33B

Type: Femur, distal end segment, **partial articular fracture** 33B

Group: Femur, distal end segment, partial articular, **lateral condyle, sagittal fracture** 33B1

Subgroups:

Simple through the notch
33B1.1

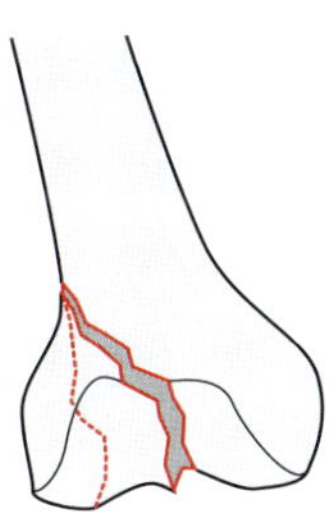

Simple through the load bearing surface
33B1.2

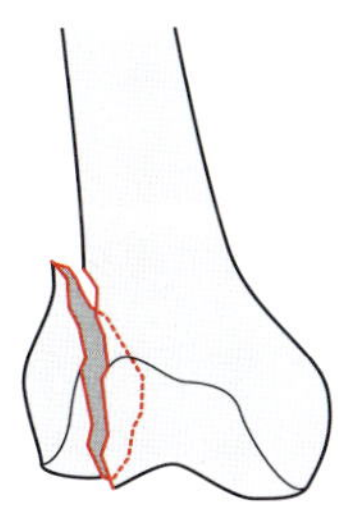

Fragmentary fracture
33B1.3

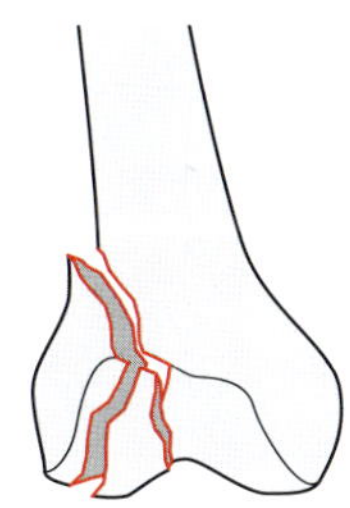

Group: Femur, distal end segment, partial articular, **medial condyle, sagittal fracture** 33B2

Subgroups:

Simple through the notch
33B2.1

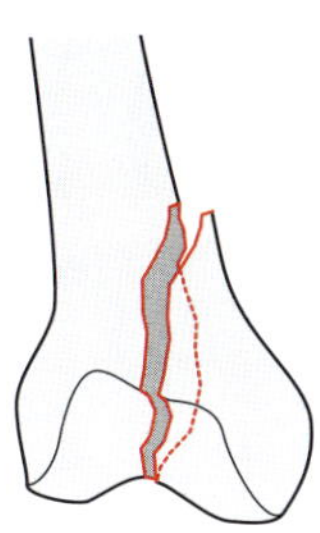

Simple through the load bearing surface
33B2.2

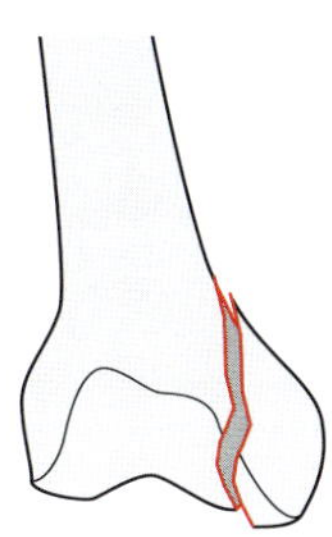

Fragmentary fracture
33B2.3

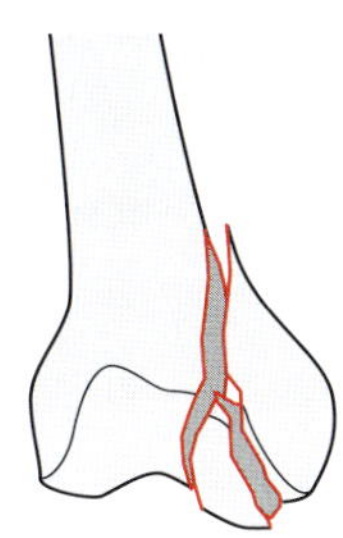

Group: Femur, distal end segment, partial articular, **frontal/coronal fracture** 33B3

Subgroups:

Anterior and lateral flake fracture
33B3.1

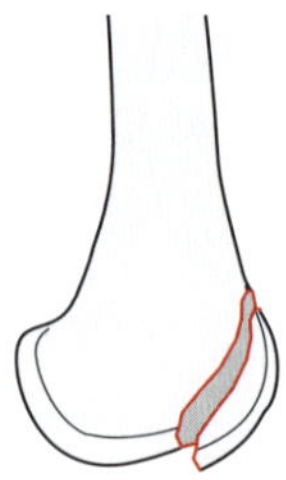

Posterior unicondylar fracture (Hoffa)
33B3.2*

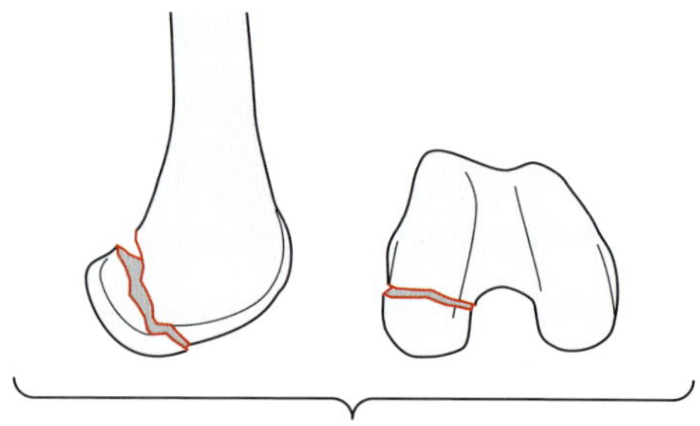

Posterior bicondylar fracture (bilateral Hoffa)
33B3.3

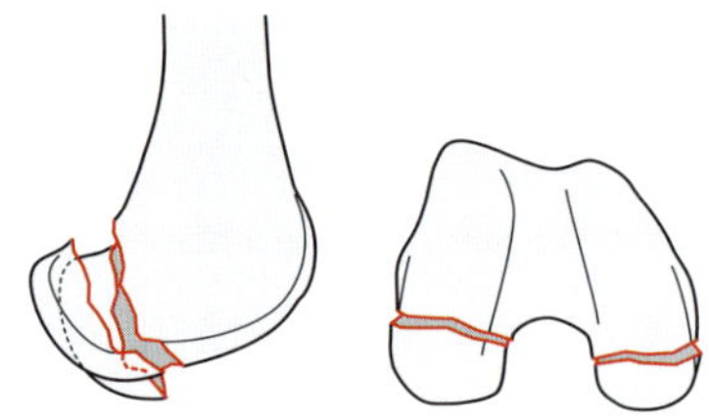

*Qualifications:
f **Lateral**
h Medial

33C

Type: Femur, distal end segment, **complete articular fracture** 33C

Group: Femur, distal end segment, complete, **simple articular, simple metaphyseal fracture** 33C1

Subgroups:

Above transcondylar axis
33C1.1

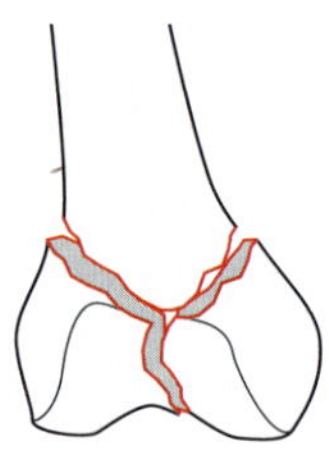

Through or below transcondylar axis
33C1.3

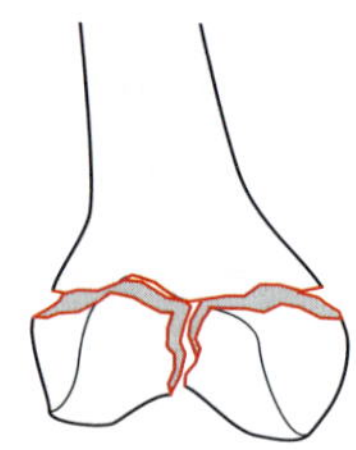

Group: Femur, distal end segment, complete, **simple articular, wedge or multifragmentary metaphyseal fracture** 33C2

Subgroups:

Intact wedge metaphyseal fracture
33C2.1*

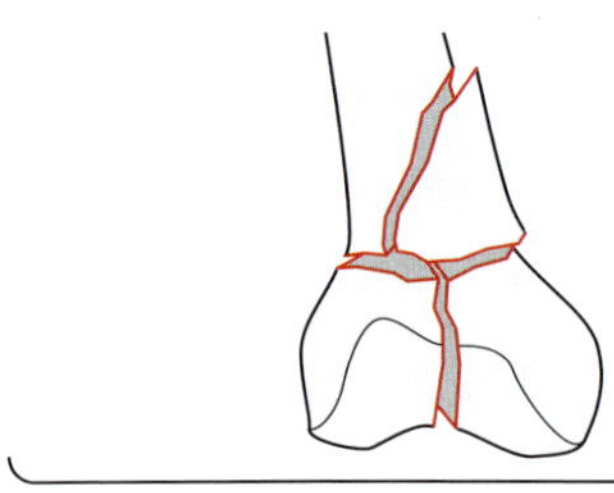

Fragmentary wedge metaphyseal fracture
33C2.2*

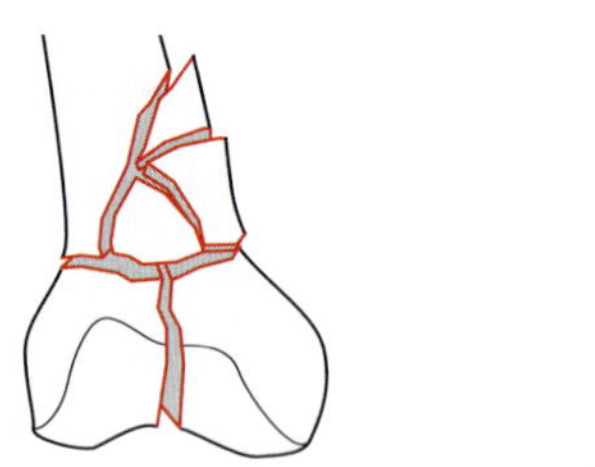

Multifragmentary metaphyseal fracture
33C2.3

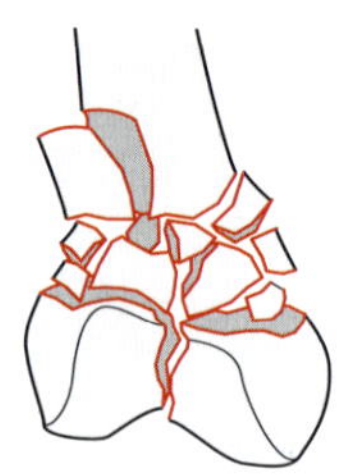

*Qualifications:
f Lateral
h **Medial**

Group: Femur, distal end segment, complete, **multifragmentary articular fracture, simple, wedge or multifragmentary metaphyseal fracture** 33C3

Subgroups:

Simple metaphyseal fracture
33C3.1

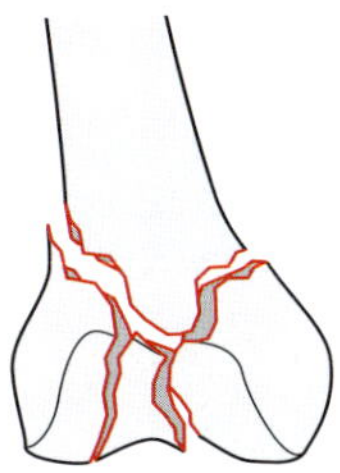

Wedge metaphyseal fracture
33C3.2*

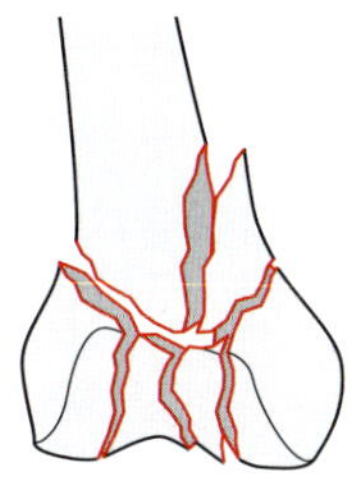

*Qualifications:
f Lateral
h **Medial**
s **Intact**
l Fragmentary

Multifragmentary metaphyseal fracture
33C3.3

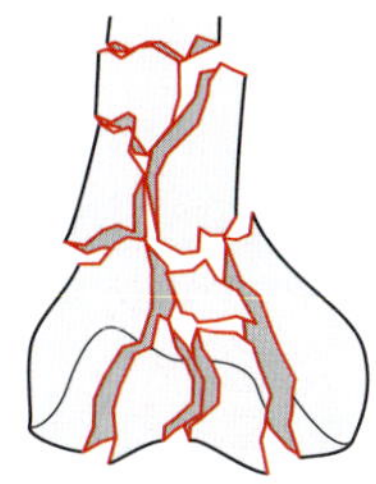

Qualifications *are optional and applied to the fracture code where the asterisk is located as a lower-case letter within rounded brackets. More than one qualification can be applied for a given fracture classification, separated by a comma. For a more detailed explanation, see the compendium introduction.*

Tibia

Bone: Tibia 4

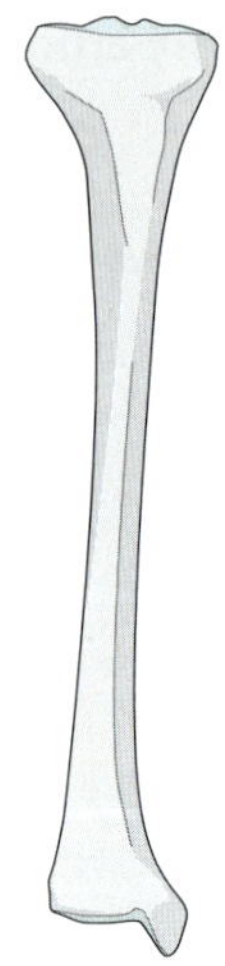

41

Location: Proximal end segment 41

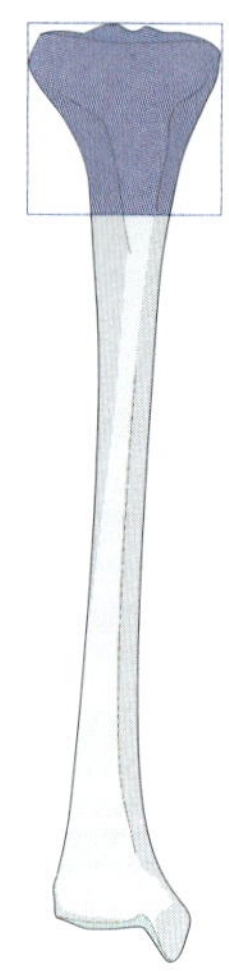

Types:

Tibia, proximal end segment,
extraarticular fracture
41A

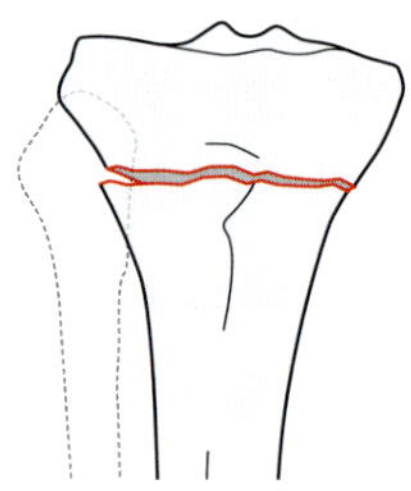

Tibia, proximal end segment,
partial articular fracture
41B

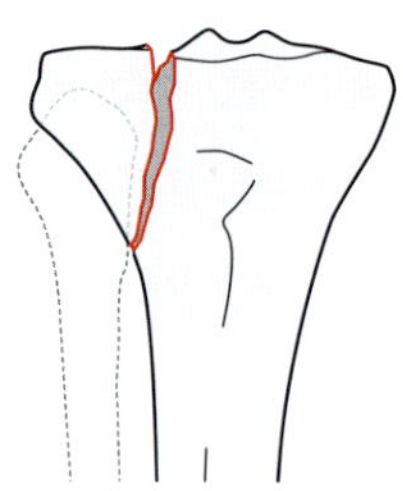

Tibia, proximal end segment
complete articular fracture
41C

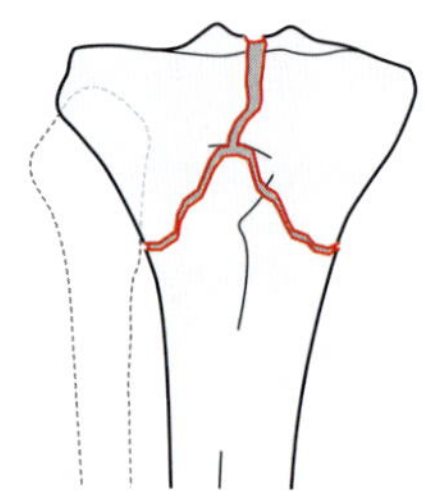

→ To facilitate the coding of tibia and fibula fractures, they are now coded independently. The use of an "F" is required to designate the fibula.

Qualifications *are optional and applied to the fracture code where the asterisk is located as a lower-case letter within rounded brackets. More than one qualification can be applied for a given fracture classification, separated by a comma. For a more detailed explanation, see the compendium introduction.*

41A

Type: Tibia, proximal end segment, **extraarticular fracture** 41A

Group: Tibia, proximal end segment, extraarticular, **avulsion fracture** 41A1

Subgroups:

Of the capsular attachments
41A1.1*

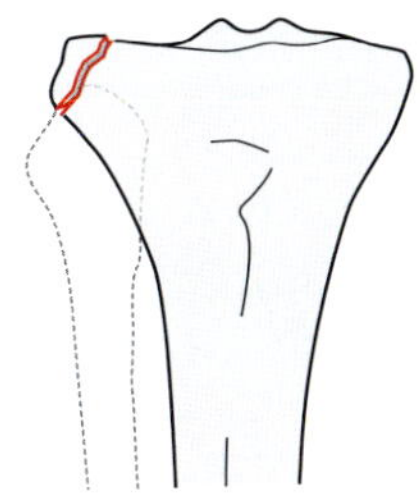

Of the tibial tubercle
41A1.2

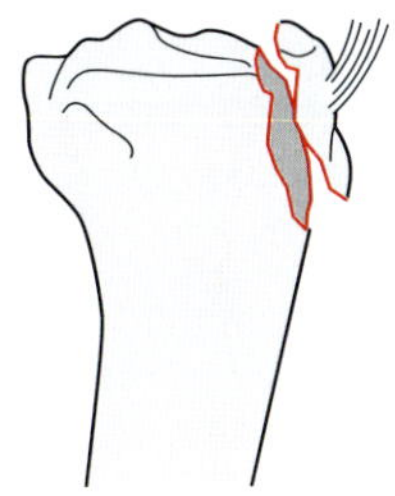

Of tibial spine (cruciate attachment)
41A1.3*

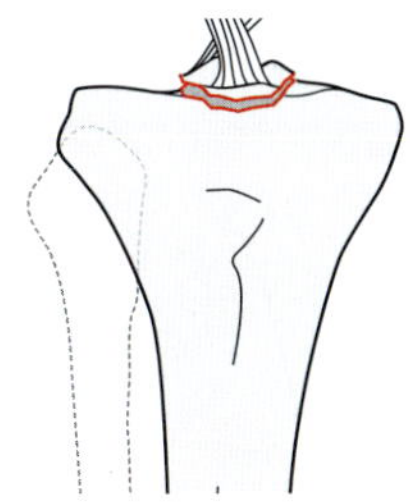

*Qualifications (41A1.1):
n **Lateral (Segond)**
h Medial

*Qualifications (41A1.3):
o **Anterior**
p Posterior

Group: Tibia, proximal end segment, extraarticular, **simple fracture** 41A2

Subgroups:

Spiral fracture
41A2.1

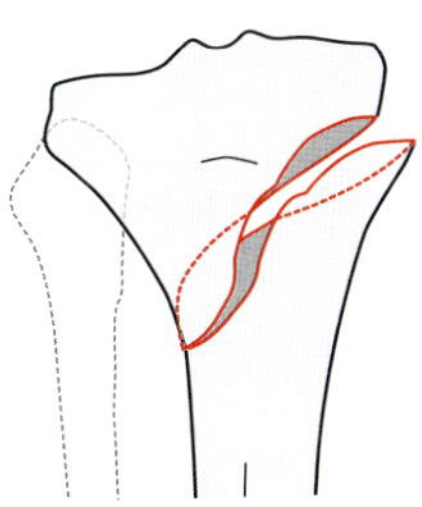

Oblique fracture
41A2.2

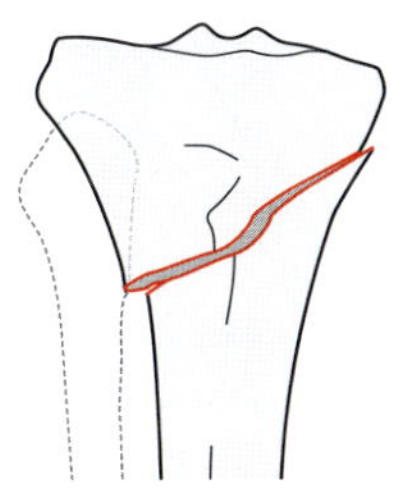

Transverse fracture
41A2.3

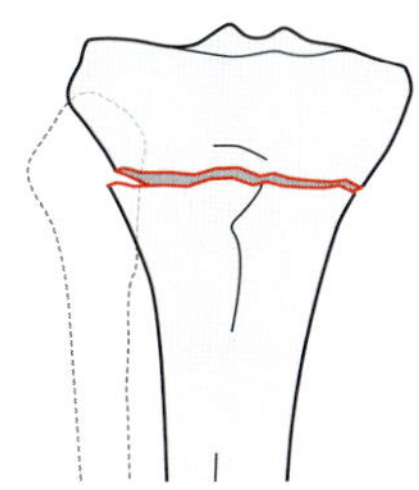

Group: Tibia, proximal end segment, extraarticular, **wedge or multifragmentary fracture** 41A3

Subgroups:

Intact wedge fracture
41A3.1*

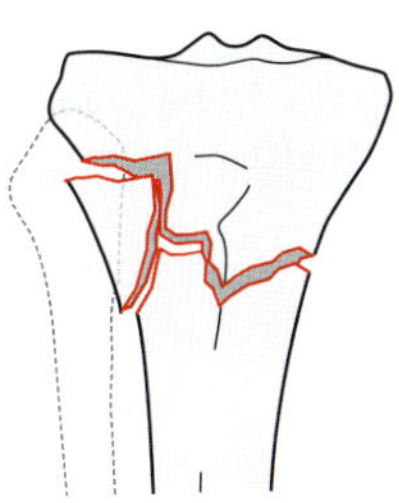

Fragmentary wedge fracture
41A3.2*

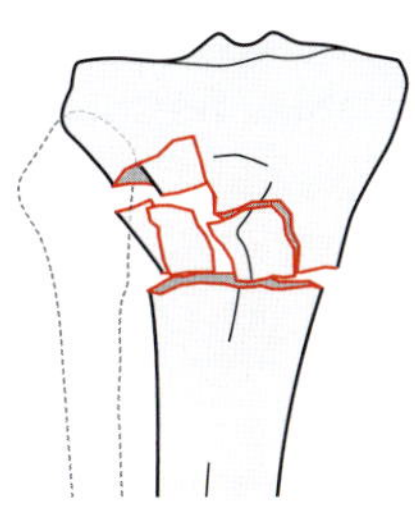

Multifragmentary fracture
41A3.3

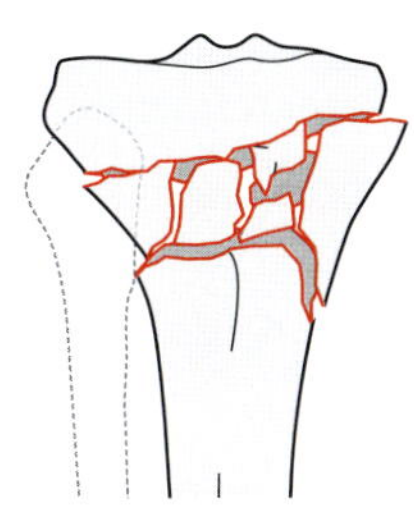

*Qualifications:
f **Lateral**
h Medial

41B

Type: Tibia, proximal end segment, **partial articular fracture** 41B

Group: Tibia, proximal end segment, partial articular, **split fracture** 41B1

Subgroups:

Lateral plateau fracture
41B1.1

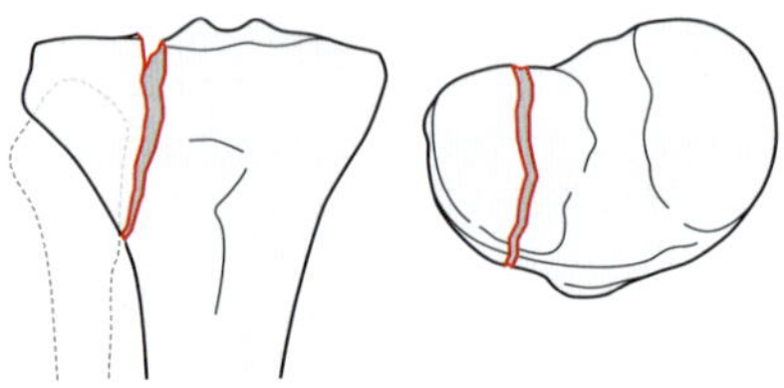

Medial plateau fracture
41B1.2

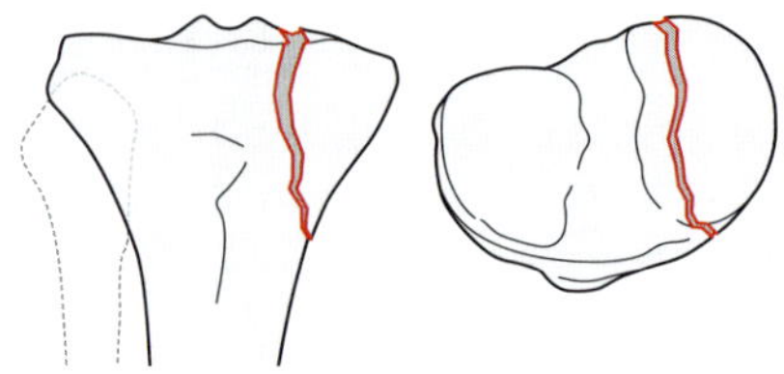

Oblique, involving the tibial spines and 1 of the tibial plateaus
41B1.3*

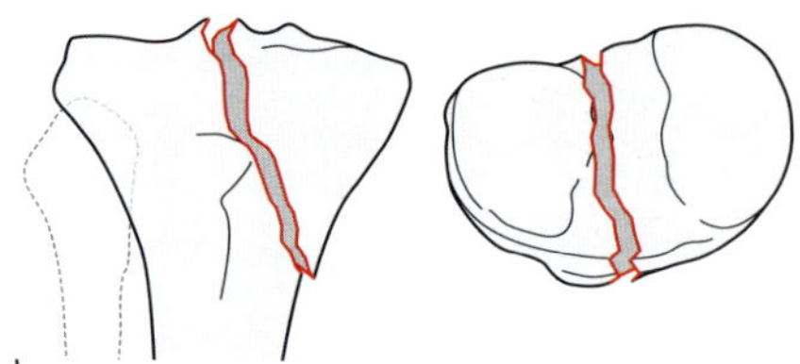

*Qualifications:
f Lateral
h **Medial**

Group: Tibia, proximal end segment, partial articular, **depression fracture** 41B2

Subgroups:

Lateral plateau fracture
41B2.1*

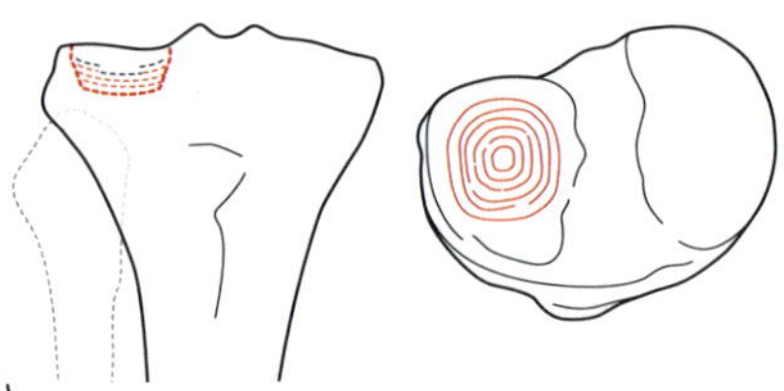

*Qualifications:
t Anterolateral (AL)
u **Posterolateral (PL)**
x Central

Medial plateau fracture
41B2.2

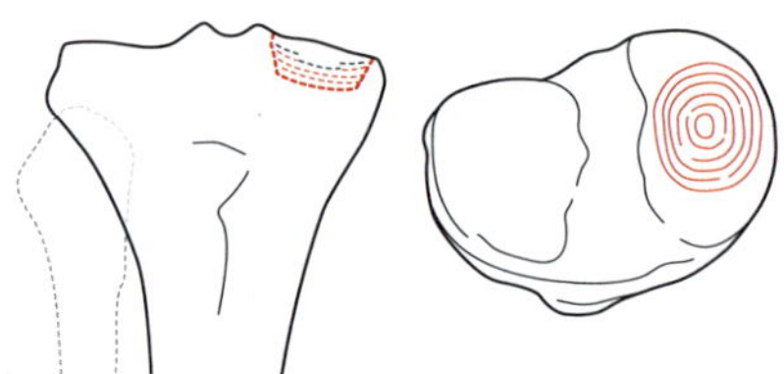

*Qualifications:
v Anteromedial (AM)
w Posteromedial (PM)
x **Central**

→ For more information about the division of the proximal tibia into quadrants, please refer to the Appendix.

Group: Tibia, proximal end segment, partial articular, **split-depression fracture** 41B3

Subgroups:

Lateral plateau fracture
41B3.1*

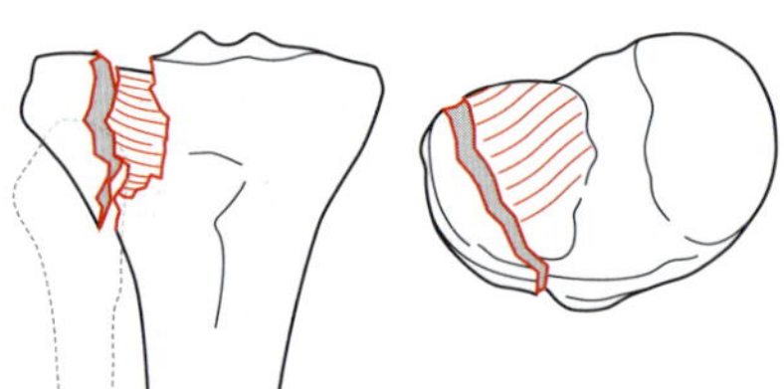

*Qualifications:
t Anterolateral (AL)
u **Posterolateral (PL)**
x Central

Medial plateau fracture
41B3.2*

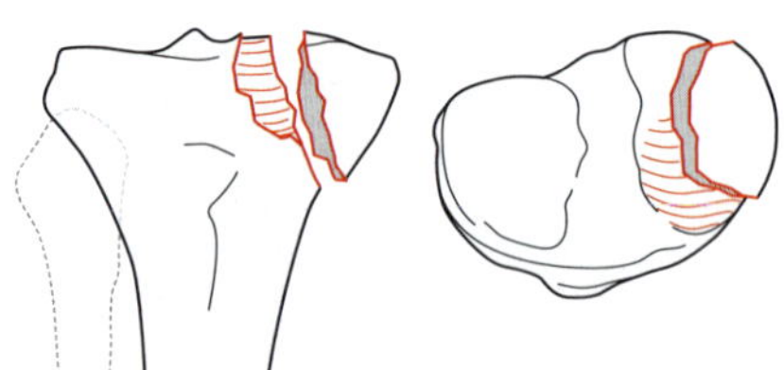

*Qualifications:
v **Anteromedial (AM)**
w Posteromedial (PM)
x Central

Involving the tibial spines and 1 of the tibial plateaus
41B3.3*

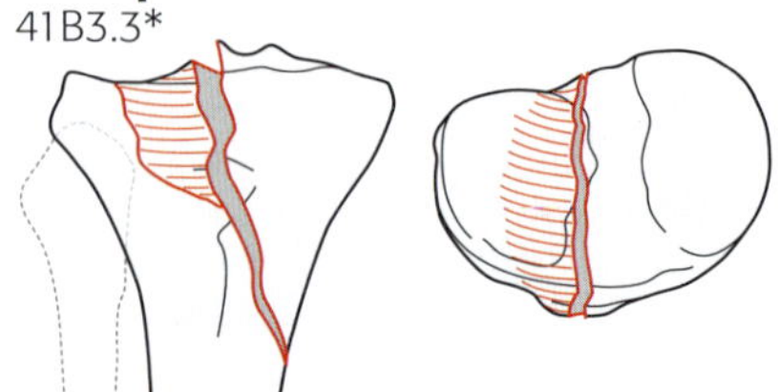

*Qualifications:
f **Lateral**
h Medial

→ For more information about the division of the proximal tibia into quadrants, please refer to the Appendix.

41C

Type: Tibia, proximal end segment, **complete articular fracture** 41C

Group: Tibia, proximal end segment, complete, **simple articular, simple metaphyseal fracture** 41C1

Subgroups:

Without intercondylar eminence fracture
41C1.1

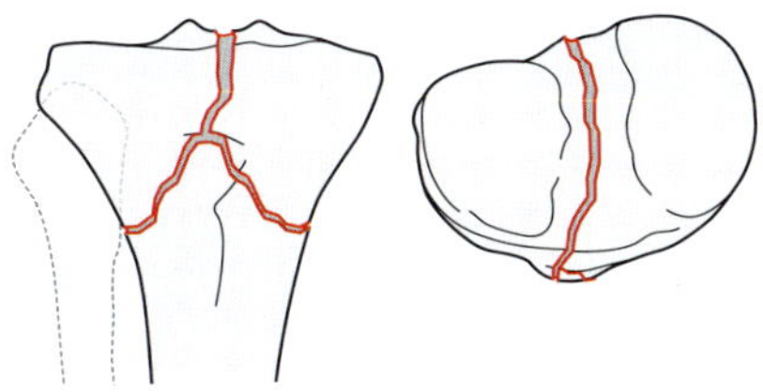

With intercondylar eminence fracture
41C1.2

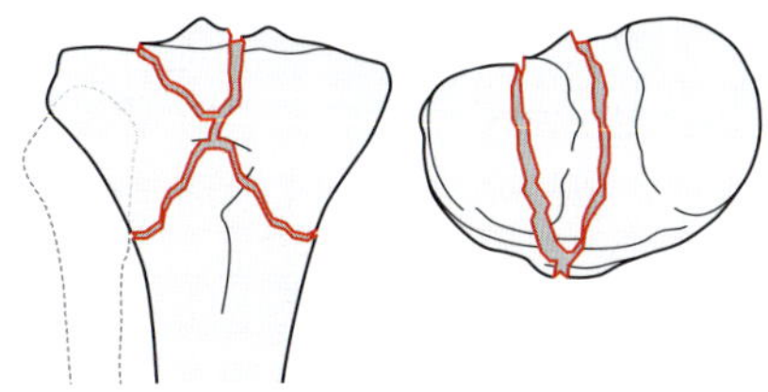

Group: Tibia, proximal end segment, complete, **simple articular, wedge or multifragmentary metaphyseal fracture** 41C2

Subgroups:

Intact wedge fracture
41C2.1*

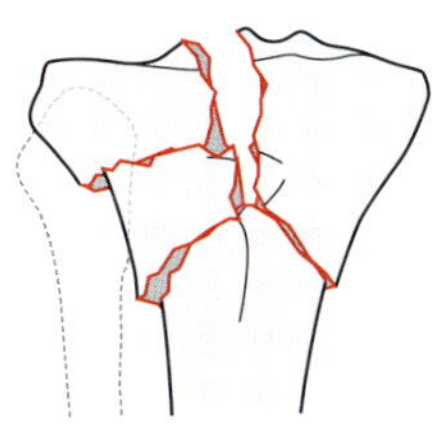

Fragmentary wedge fracture
41C2.2*

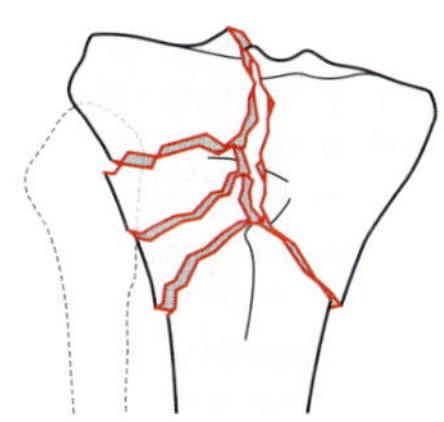

Multifragmentary metaphyseal fracture
41C2.3

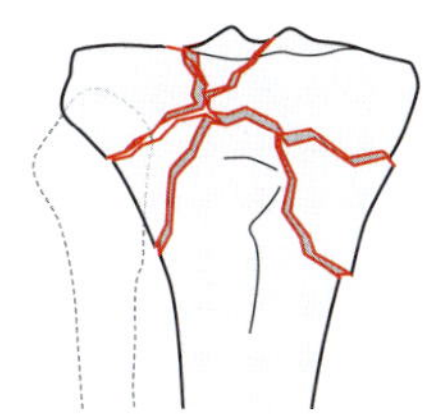

*Qualifications
- f **Lateral**
- h Medial

Group: Tibia, proximal end segment, complete, **fragmentary or multifragmentary metaphyseal fracture** 41C3

Subgroups:

Fragmentary lateral plateau fracture
41C3.1*

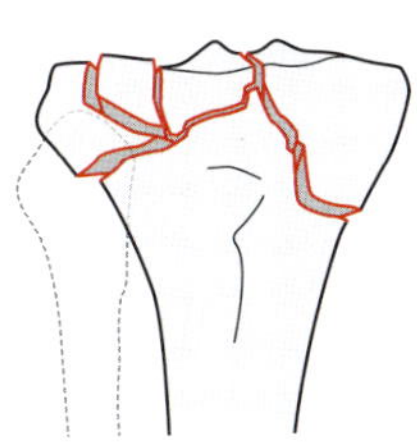

Fragmentary medial plateau fracture
41C3.2*

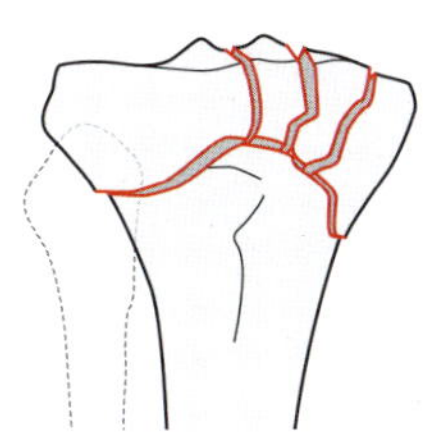

Multifragmentary medial and lateral plateau fracture
41C3.3*

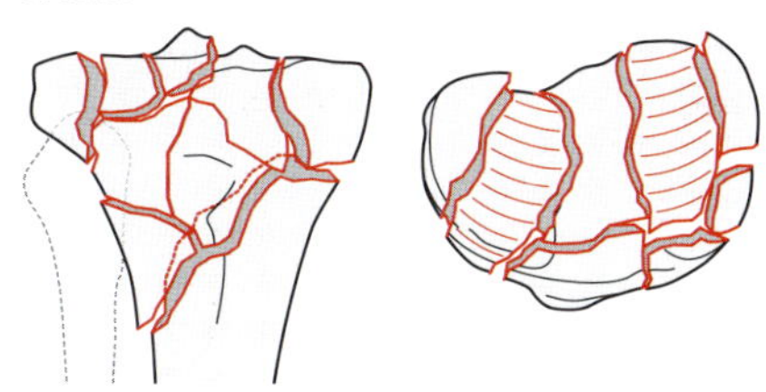

*Qualifications:
- d Simple metaphysis
- e Multifragmentary metaphysis
- s Metadiaphyseal extension
- t Anterolateral (AL)
- u Posterolateral (PL)
- v Anteromedial (AM)
- w Posteromedial (PM)
- x Central

42

Location: Tibia, **diaphyseal segment** 42

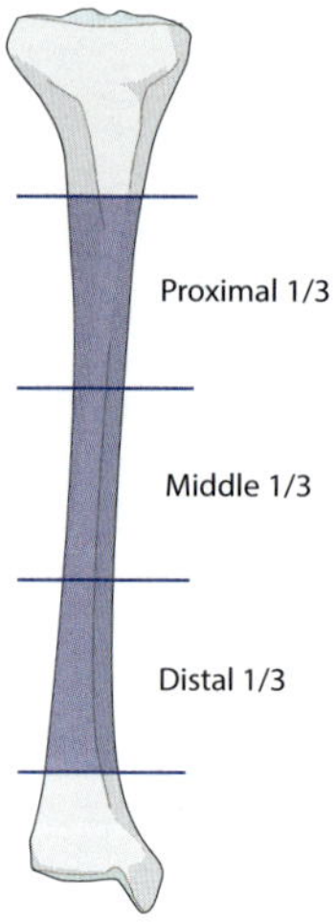

Types:

Tibia, diaphyseal segment
simple fracture
42A

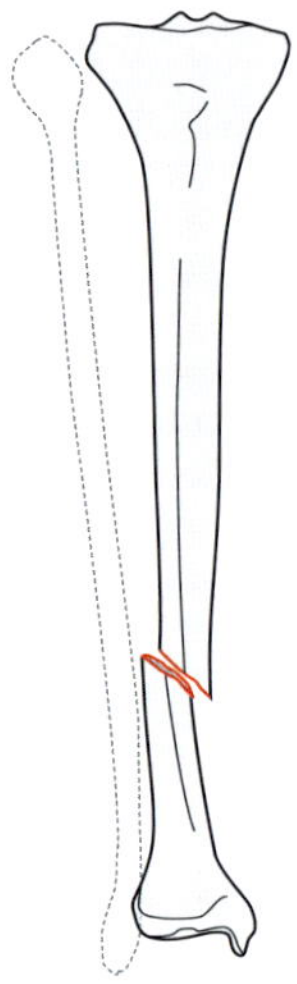

Tibia, diaphyseal segment,
wedge fracture
42B

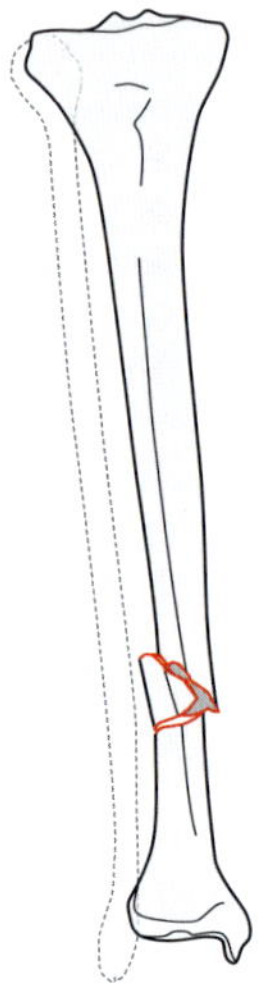

Tibia, diaphyseal segment,
multifragmentary fracture
42C

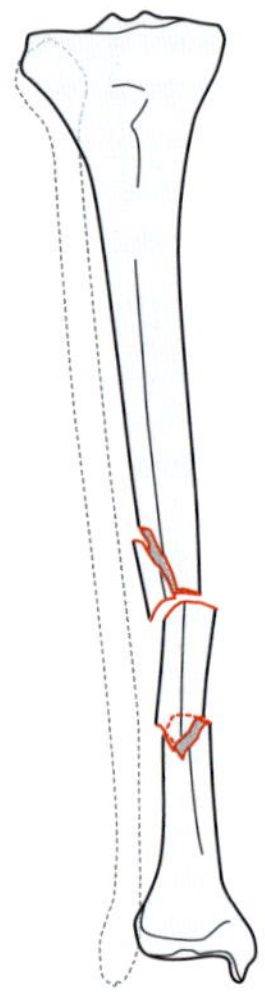

42A

Type: Tibia, diaphyseal segment, **simple fracture** 42A

Groups:

Tibia, diaphyseal segment, simple, **spiral fracture** 42A1*

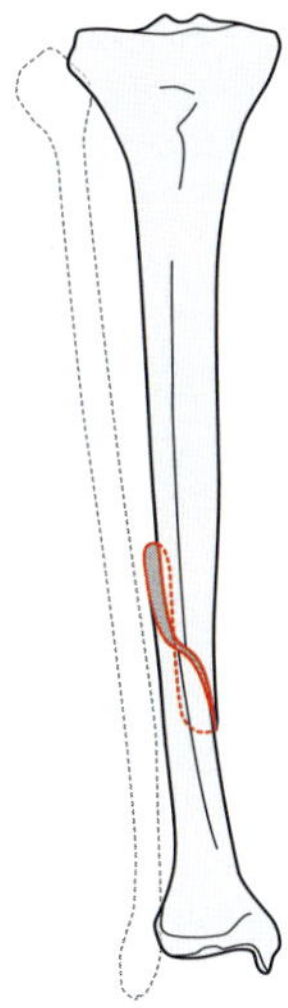

Tibia, diaphyseal segment, simple, **oblique fracture (≥ 30°)** 42A2*

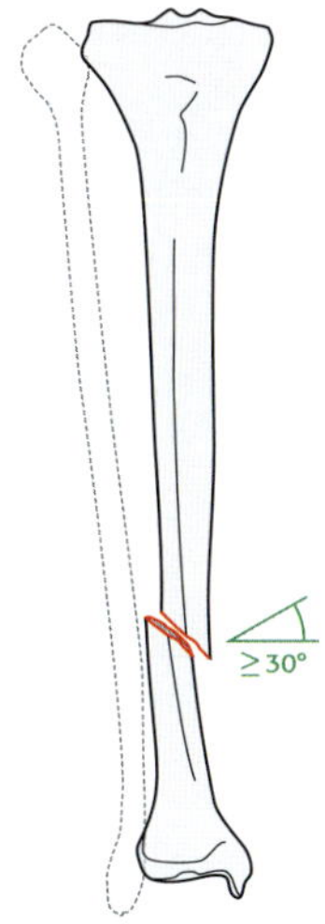

Tibia, diaphyseal segment, simple, **transverse fracture (<30°)** 42A3*

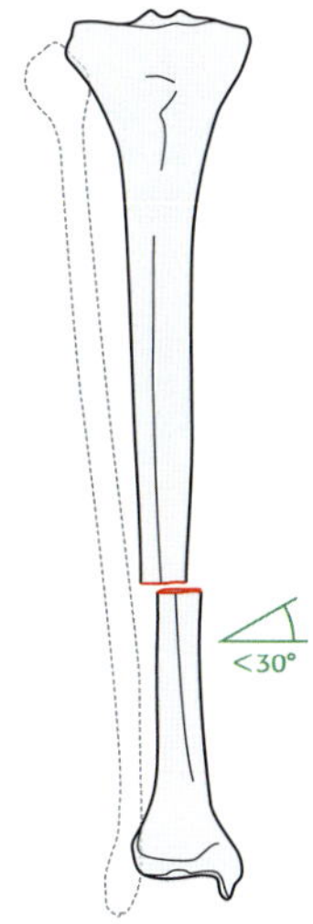

*Qualifications:
- a Proximal 1/3
- b Middle 1/3
- c **Distal 1/3**

42B

Type: Tibia, diaphyseal segment, **wedge fracture** 42B

Groups:

Tibia, diaphyseal segment, **intact wedge fracture** 42B2*

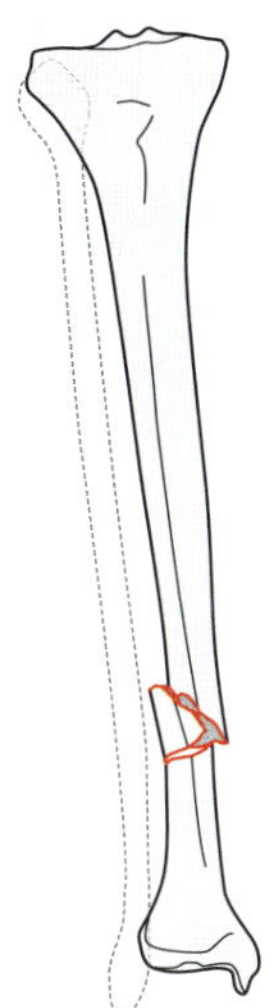

Tibia, diaphyseal segment, **fragmentary wedge fracture** 42B3*

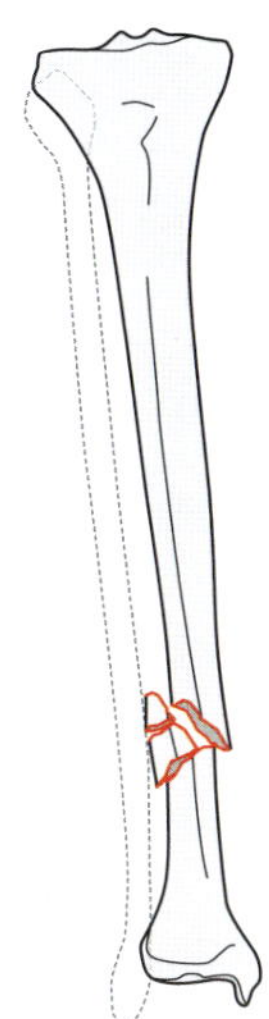

*Qualifications:
- a Proximal 1/3
- b Middle 1/3
- c **Distal 1/3**

42C

Type: Tibia, diaphyseal segment, **multifragmentary fracture** 42C

Groups:

Tibia, diaphyseal segment, multifragmentary, **intact segmental fracture** 42C2

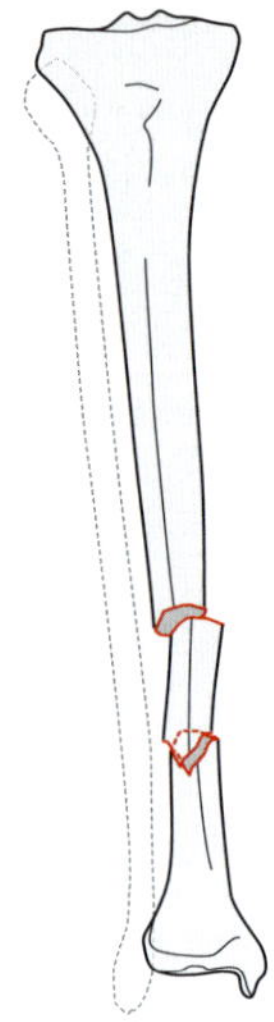

Tibia, diaphyseal segment, multifragmentary, **fragmentary segmental fracture** 42C3*

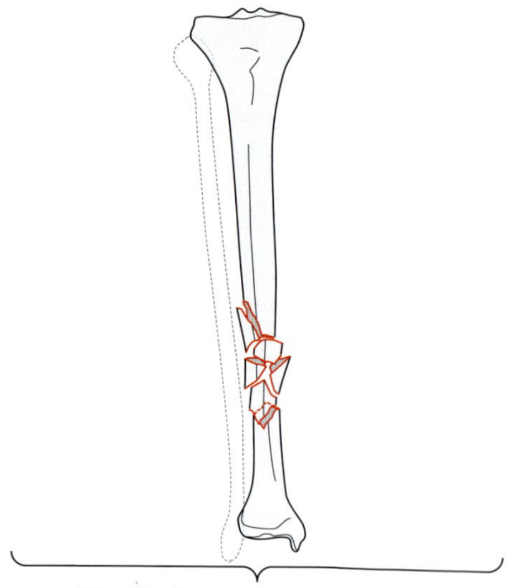

*Qualifications:
- i Proximal diaphyseal-metaphyseal
- j **Pure diaphyseal**
- k Distal diaphyseal-metaphyseal

43

Location: Tibia, **distal end segment** 43

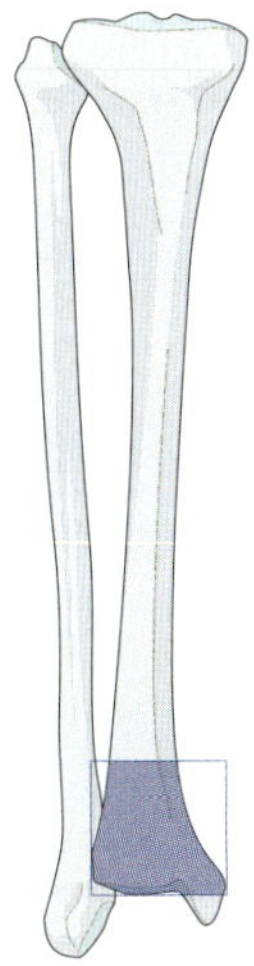

Types:

Tibia, distal end segment, **extraarticular fracture** 43A

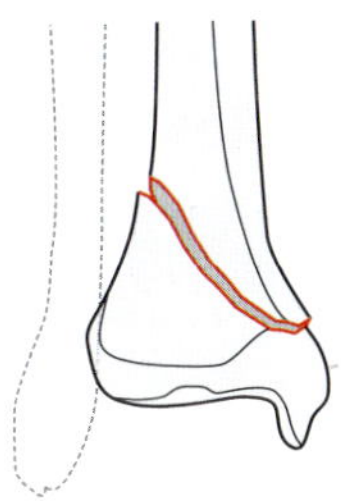

Tibia, distal end segment, **partial articular fracture** 43B

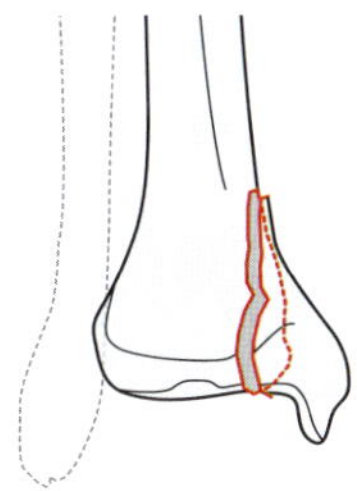

Tibia, distal end segment, **complete articular fracture** 43C

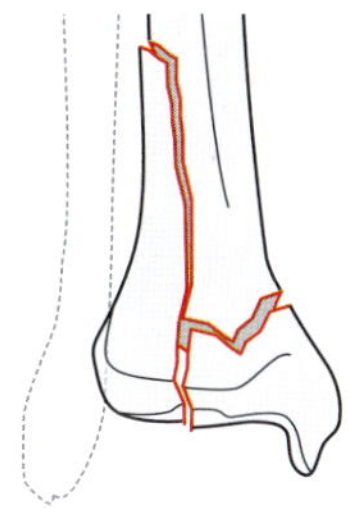

43A

Type: Tibia, distal end segment, **extraarticular fracture** 43A

Group: Tibia, distal end segment, extraarticular, **simple fracture** 43A1

Subgroups:

Spiral fracture 43A1.1

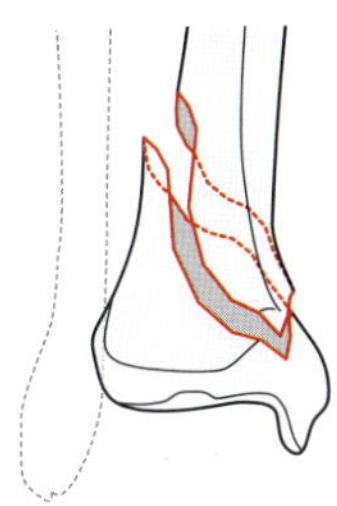

Oblique fracture 43A1.2

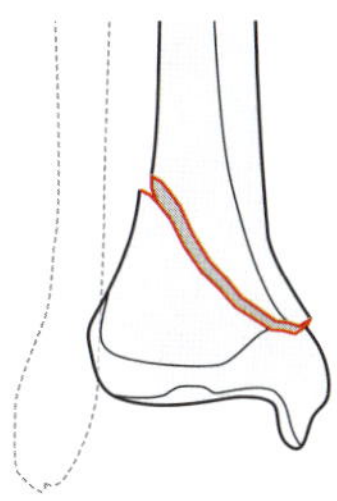

Transverse fracture 43A1.3

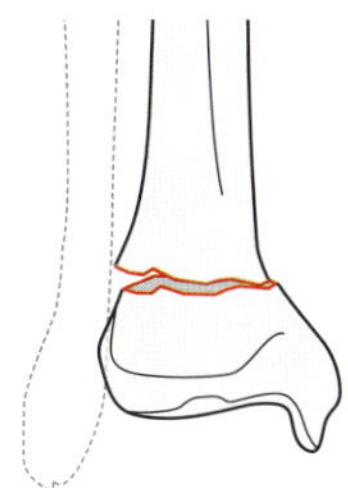

Group: Tibia, distal end segment, extraarticular, **wedge fracture** 43A2

Subgroups:

Posterolateral impaction fracture
43A2.1

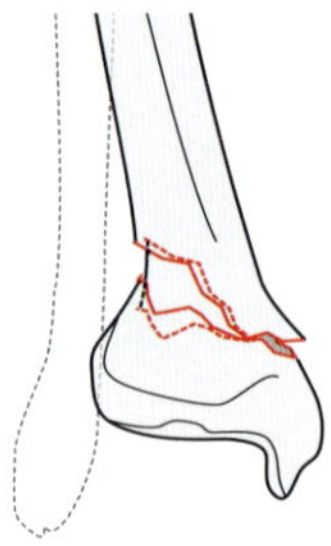

Anteromedial wedge fracture
43A2.2

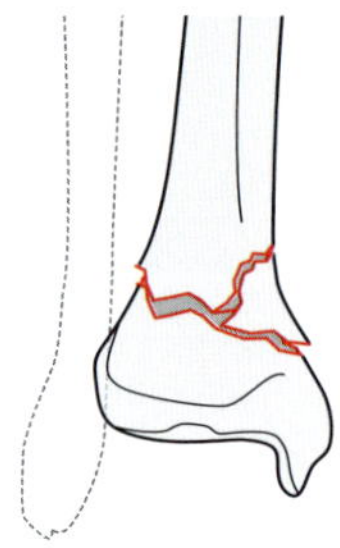

Fracture extending into diaphysis
43A2.3

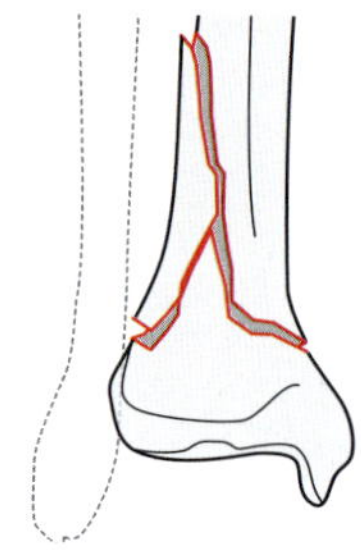

Group: Tibia, distal end segment, extraarticular, **multifragmentary fracture** 43A3

Subgroups:

With 3 intermediate fragments
43A3.1

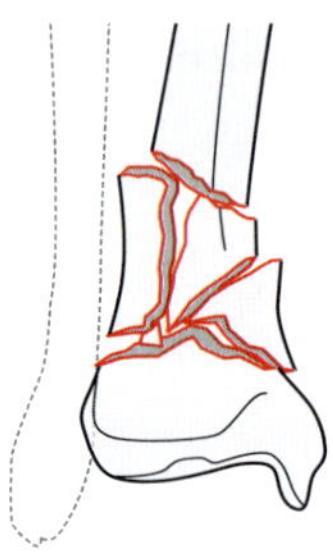

With more than 3 intermediate fragments
43A3.2

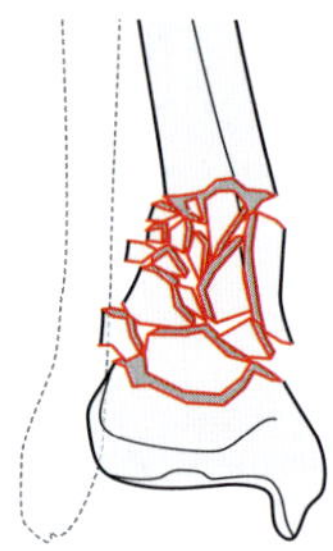

Extending into diaphysis
43A3.3

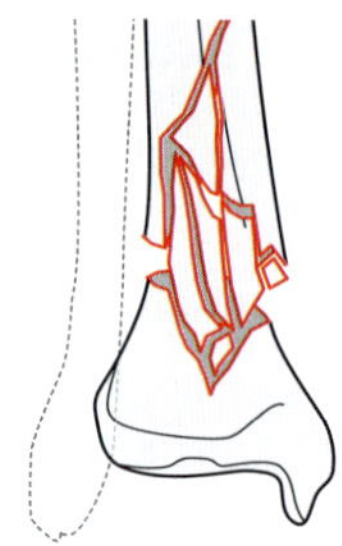

43B

Type: Tibia, distal end segment, **partial articular fracture** 43B

Group: Tibia, distal end segment, partial articular, **split fracture** 43B1

Subgroups:

Frontal/coronal fracture
43B1.1*

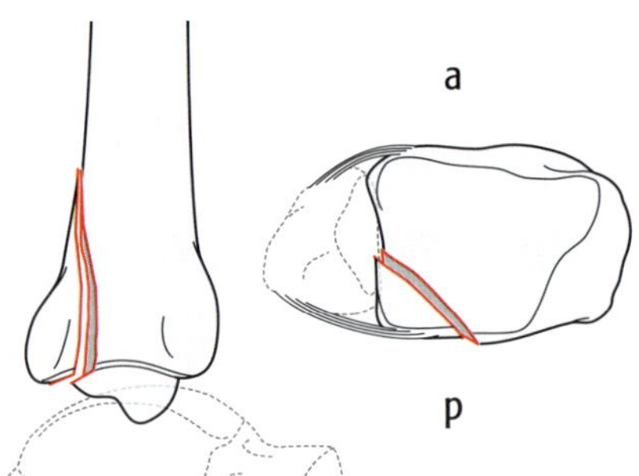

*Qualifications:
- o Anterior
- y **Posterior Volkmann**

Sagittal fracture
43B1.2*

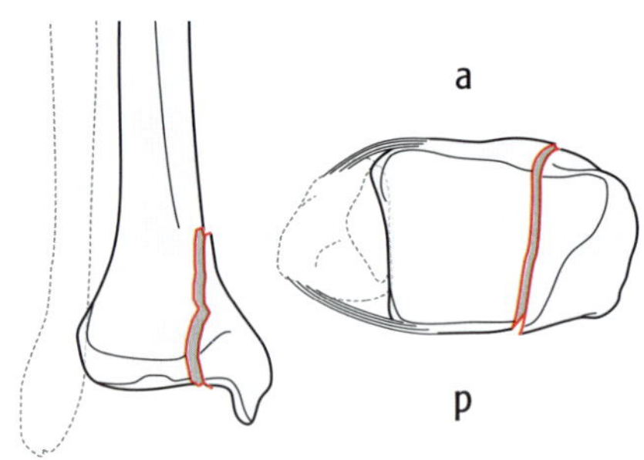

*Qualifications:
- f Lateral
- z **Medial articular surface including medial malleolus**

Fragmentary metaphyseal fracture
43B1.3

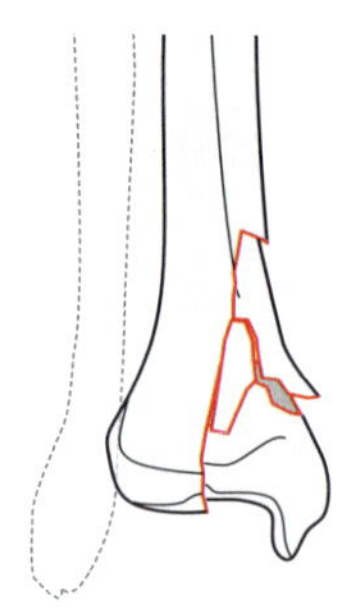

Group: Tibia, distal end segment partial articular, **split depression fracture** 43B2

Subgroups:
Frontal/coronal fracture
43B2.1*

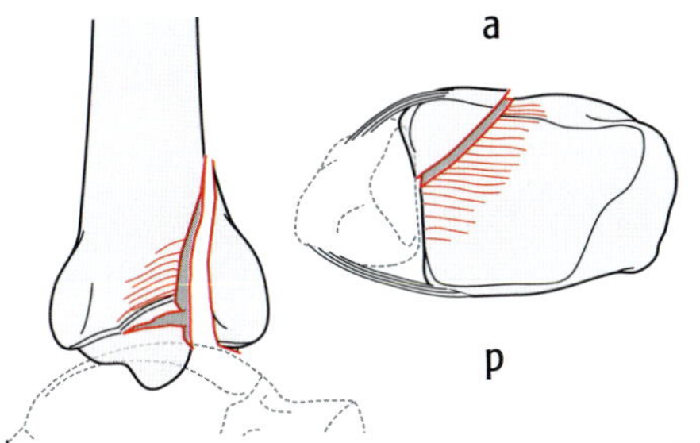

Sagittal fracture
43B2.2*

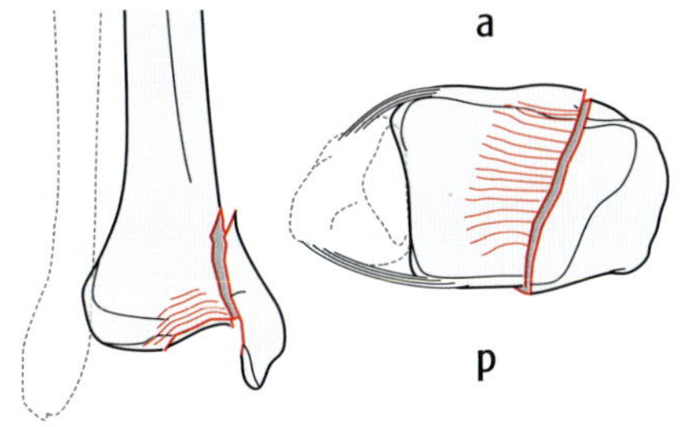

Central fragment fracture
43B2.3

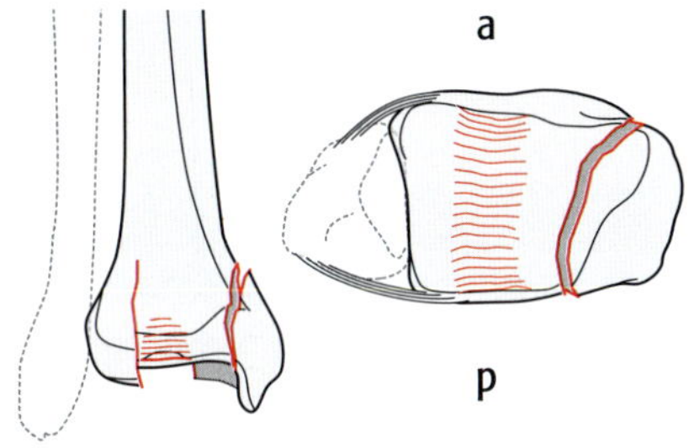

*Qualifications (43B2.1):
- o **Anterior**
- y Posterior Volkmann

*Qualifications (43B2.2):
- f Lateral
- h **Medial**

Group: Tibia, distal end segment, partial articular, **depression fracture** 43B3

Subgroups:
Frontal/coronal fracture
43B3.1*

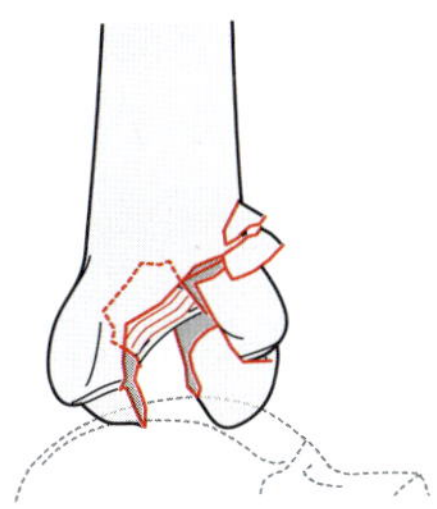

Sagittal fracture
43B3.2*

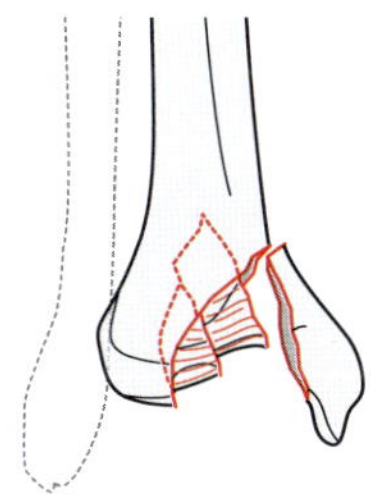

Fragmentary metaphyseal fracture
43B3.3

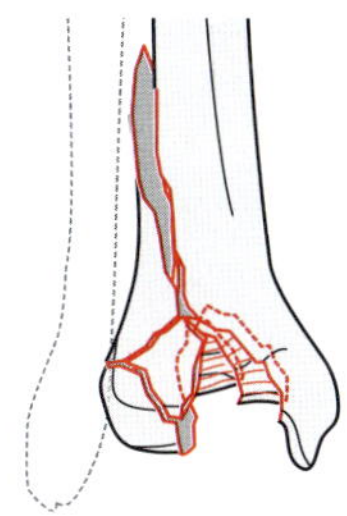

*Qualifications (43B3.1):
- o **Anterior**
- y Posterior Volkmann

*Qualifications (43B3.2):
- f Lateral
- h **Medial**

43C

Type: Tibia, distal end segment, **complete articular fracture** 43C

Group: Tibia, distal end segment, complete, **simple articular, simple metaphyseal fracture** 43C1

Subgroups:
Without impaction
43C1.1*

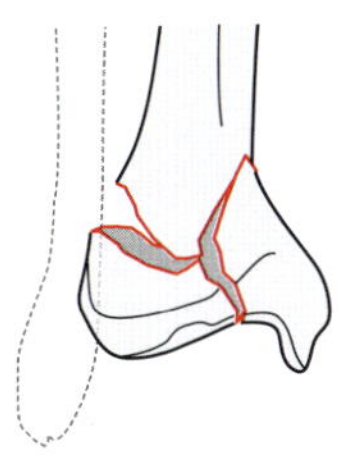

With epiphyseal depression
43C1.2

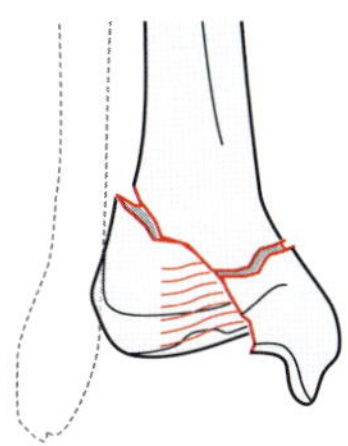

Extending into diaphysis
43C1.3

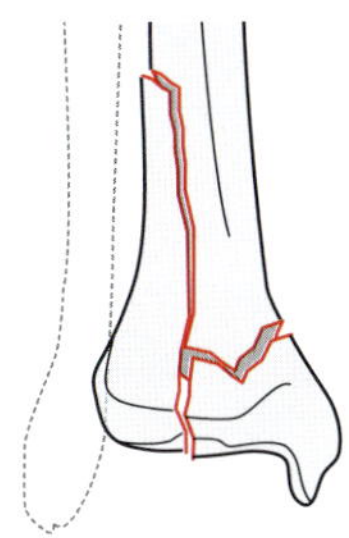

*Qualifications (43C1.1):
- q Frontal/coronal plane
- r **Sagittal plane**

Group: Tibia, distal end segment, complete, **simple articular, multifragmentary metaphyseal fracture** 43C2

Subgroups:

With asymmetric impaction
43C2.1*

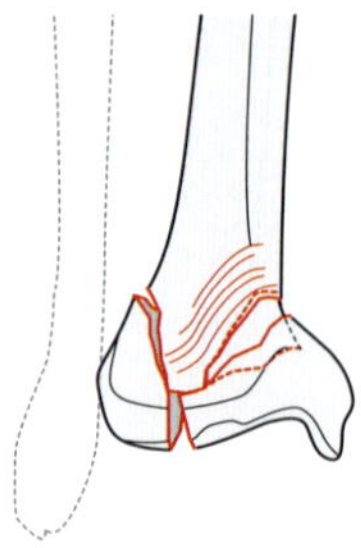

*Qualifications:
q Frontal/coronal plane
r **Sagittal plane**

Without asymmetric impaction
43C2.2

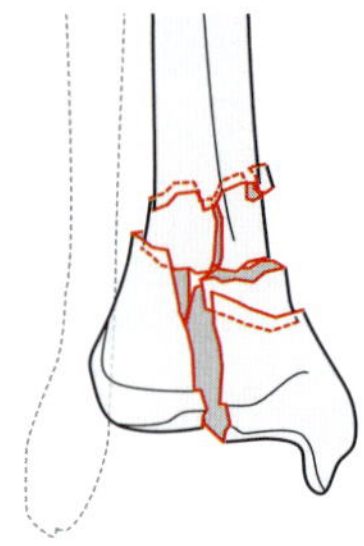

Extending into diaphysis
43C2.3

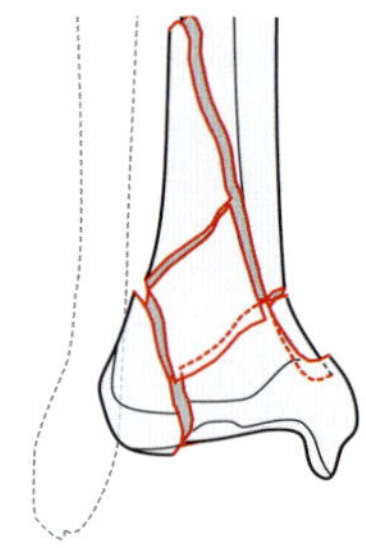

Group: Tibia, distal end segment, complete, **multifragmentary articular and metaphyseal fracture** 43C3

Subgroups:

Epiphyseal fracture
43C3.1

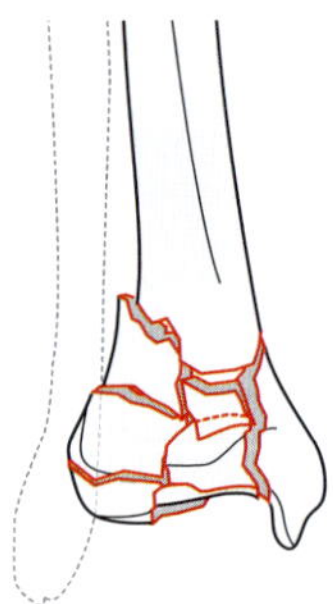

Epiphyseal-metaphyseal fracture
43C3.2

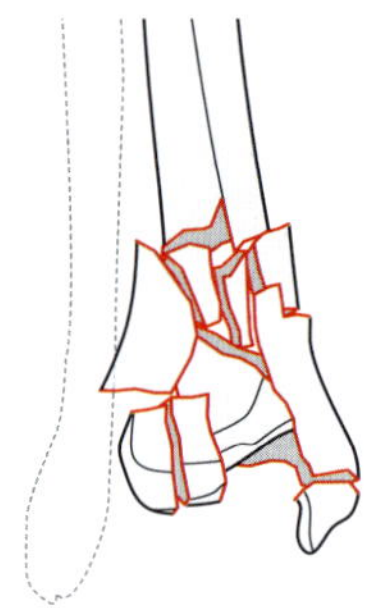

Epiphyseal-metaphyseal-diaphyseal fracture
43C3.3

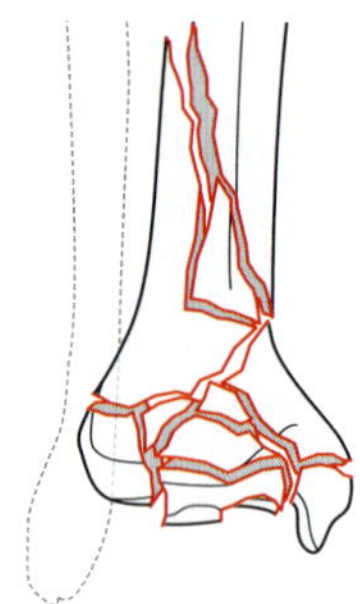

Qualifications *are optional and applied to the fracture code where the asterisk is located as a lower-case letter within rounded brackets. More than one qualification can be applied for a given fracture classification, separated by a comma. For a more detailed explanation, see the compendium introduction.*

Fibula

Bone: Fibula 4F

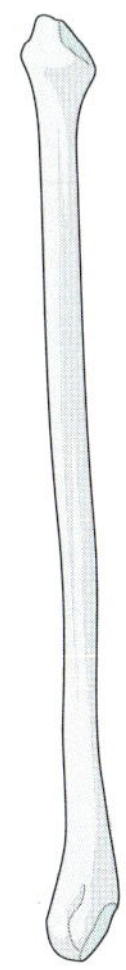

4F1

Location: Fibula, **proximal end segment** 4F1

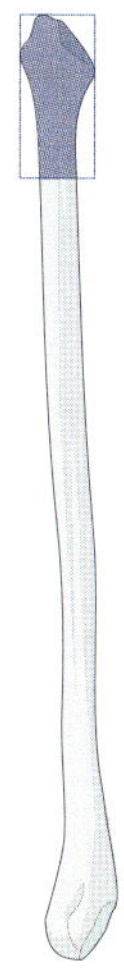

Types:

Fibula, proximal end segment,
simple fracture
4F1A*

Fibula, proximal end segment,
multifragmentary fracture
4F1B*

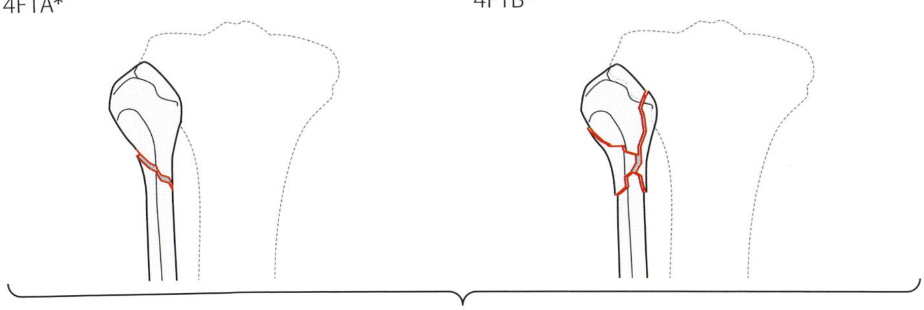

*Qualifications:
n Extraarticular
o Intraarticular

→ To facilitate the coding of tibia/fibula fractures, they are now coded independently. The use of an "F" is required to designate the fibula.

Qualifications *are optional and applied to the fracture code where the asterisk is located as a lower-case letter within rounded brackets. More than one qualification can be applied for a given fracture classification, separated by a comma. For a more detailed explanation, see the compendium introduction.*

4F2

Location: Fibula, **diaphyseal segment** 4F2

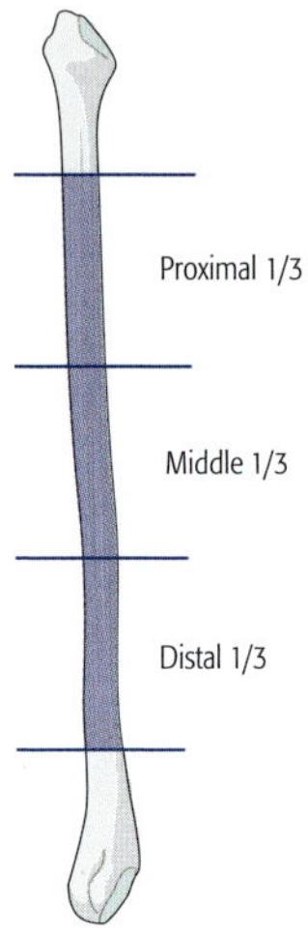

Types:

Fibula, diaphyseal segment,
simple fracture
4F2A*

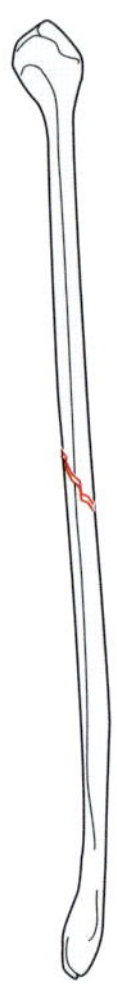

Fibula, diaphyseal segment,
wedge or multifragmentary fracture
4F2B*

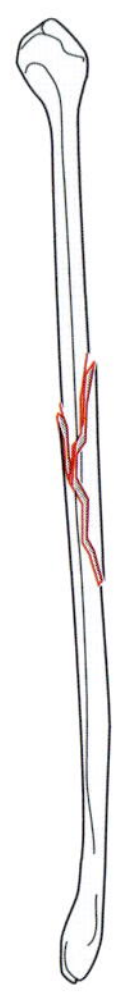

*Qualifications:
a Proximal 1/3
b **Middle 1/3**
c Distal 1/3

4F3

Location: Fibula, **distal end segment**
(excluding lateral malleolar fractures 44) 4F3

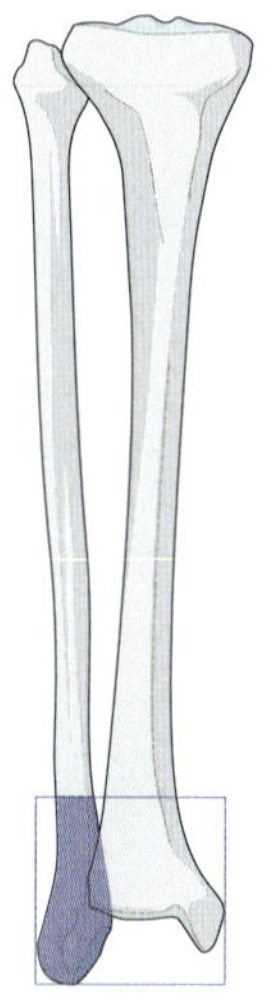

Types:

Distal end segment,
simple fracture
4F3A

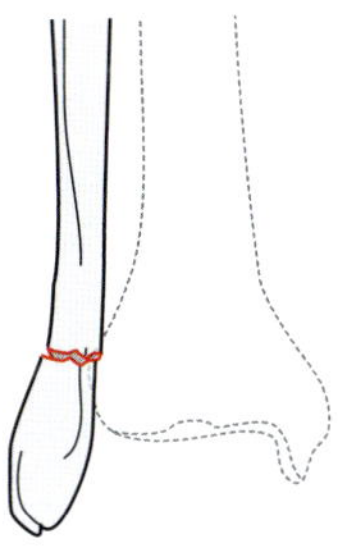

Distal end segment
wedge or multifragmentary fracture
4F3B

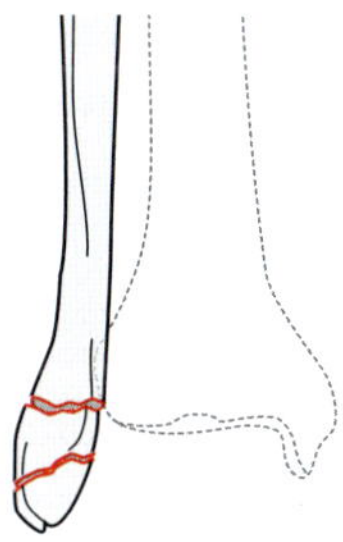

→ The fibular fracture code is used only if the distal fibula fracture is NOT part of a malleolar fracture (44). For further information, please refer to the Appendix.

Qualifications *are optional and applied to the fracture code where the asterisk is located as a lower-case letter within rounded brackets. More than one qualification can be applied for a given fracture classification, separated by a comma. For a more detailed explanation, see the compendium introduction.*

Universal modifiers

The universal modifiers are descriptive terms of fracture morphology, displacement, associated injury, or location that are generalizable to most fractures. They provide detail that are optional for users.

Universal modifiers may be added to the end of the fracture code within square brackets, eg, [1].

Multiple universal modifiers may be contained within the same set of squared brackets and separated by a comma.

Example: A proximal humerus fracture-dislocation with **displacement, anterior dislocation, cartilage injury, and osteopenia** = 11A1.2**[2,5a,8e,9]**

Example: Humerus, proximal end segment, articular or 4-part fracture, with multifragmentary metaphyseal fracture and articular fracture with an **anterior dislocation** = 11C3.2**[5a]**

List of universal modifiers

1		**Nondisplaced**	
2		**Displaced**	
3		**Impaction**	
	3a	Articular	
	3b	Metaphyseal	
4		**No impaction**	
5		**Dislocation**	
	5a	Anterior (volar, palmar, plantar)	
	5b	Posterior (dorsal)	
	5c	Medial (ulnar)	
	5d	Lateral (radial)	
	5e	Inferior (with hip is also obturator)	
	5f	Multidirectional	
6		**Subluxation/ligamentous instability**	
	6a	Anterior (volar, palmar, plantar)	
	6b	Posterior (dorsal)	
	6c	Medial (ulnar)	
	6d	Lateral (radial)	
	6e	Inferior (with hip is also obturator)	
	6f	Multidirectional	
7		**Diaphyseal extension**	
8		**Articular cartilage injury#**	
	8a	ICRS Grade 0	Normal
	8b	ICRS Grade 1	Superficial indentation (A) and /or superficial fissures and cracks (B)
	8c	ICRS Grade 2	Abnormal lesions extending down to 50% of cartilage depth
	8d	ICRS Grade 3	Severely abnormal with defects extending down >50% of cartilage depth (A); down to calcified layer (B); down to subchondral bone but not through (C); blisters included (D)
	8e	ICRS Grade 4	Severely Abnormal Cartilage loss through subchondral bone
9		**Poor bone quality**	
10		**Replantation**	
11		**Amputation associated with a fracture**	
12		**Associated with a nonarthroplasty implant**	
13		**Spiral type fracture**	
14		**Bending type fracture**	

#This grading system is used with the permission of the International Cartilage Repair Society.[38]

Gustilo-Anderson Classification of Open Fractures

Gustilo-Anderson Classification of Open Fractures

Grade	Wound size	Contamination	Soft-tissue damage	Soft-tissue damage
I	< 1 cm	Clean	Minimal	Simple with minimal comminution
II	1–10 cm	Moderate	Moderate with some muscular damage	Moderate comminution
IIIA	> 10 cm	High	Severe with associated crush injury	Moderate–soft-tissue cover possible
IIIB	> 10 cm	High	Severe loss of cover	Requires reconstructive procedures
IIIC	> 10 cm	High	Severe vascular injury requiring repair	Requires reconstructive procedures

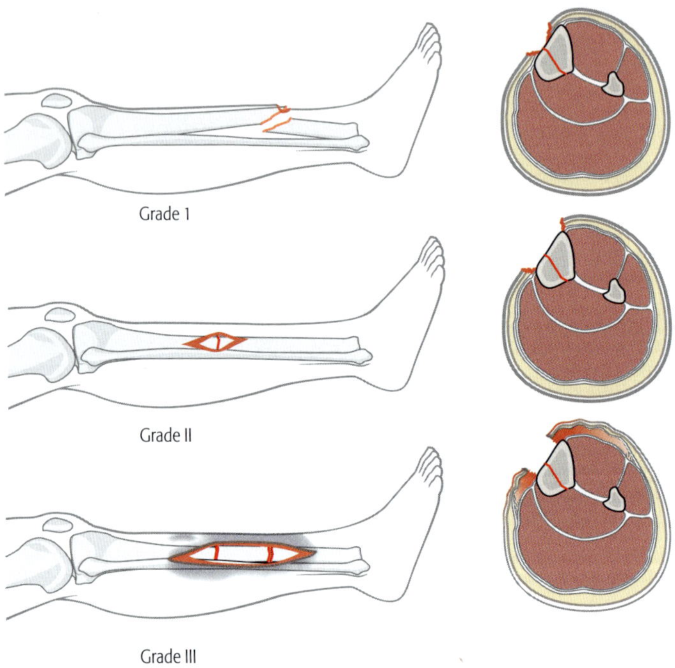

Gustilo RB, Anderson JT. Prevention of infection in the treatment of one thousand and twenty-five open fractures of long bones: retrospective and prospective analyses. *J Bone Joint Surg Am.* 1976 Jun;58(4):453–458.